D0938609

Community Health Nursing
Concepts and Practice

Community Health Nursing
Concepts and Practice
Second Edition

Barbara Walton Spradley, R.N., M.N.

Public Health Nursing, School of Public Health,
University of Minnesota, Minneapolis

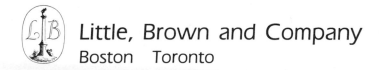
Little, Brown and Company
Boston   Toronto

To the memory of my husband, James P. Spradley

Library of Congress Cataloging in Publication Data
Spradley, Barbara Walton.
    Community health nursing.

    Includes bibliographies and index.
    1. Community health nursing.   2. Public health
nursing.   I. Title.   [DNLM: 1. Community Health Nursing.
WY 106 S766c]
RT98.S68   1985   610.73'43   84-28876
ISBN 0-316-80744-3

Copyright © 1985 by Barbara Walton Spradley

All rights reserved. No part of this book may be reproduced in any form or by any electronic or mechanical means including information storage and retrieval systems without permission in writing from the publisher except by a reviewer who may quote brief passages in a review.

Library of Congress Catalog Card No. 84-28876

ISBN 0-316-80744-3

9 8 7 6 5 4 3 2 1

HAL

Published simultaneously in Canada by Little, Brown & Company (Canada) Limited

Printed in the United States of America

The author and publisher would like to thank the following sources for granting permission to use their material:
    Figure 1–2: From *Health Is a Community Affair*, Harvard University Press, 1967. Reprinted by permission of the publisher.
    Table 2–1: From A.P.H.A. Position Paper, *American Journal of Public Health, 65*, 189–93, 1975. Reprinted by permission of the American Public Health Association.
    Figures 2–4 and 2–5: From J. J. Hanlon and G. E. Pickett, *Public Health: Administration and Practice*, 8th edition, St. Louis, 1984, Times Mirror/Mosby College Publishing. Reprinted by permission of the publisher.
    List on page 117: From Sr. Theresa Stanley, "Ethics as a Component of the Curriculum," in *Nursing and Health Care* 1:2 (September 1980). © Technomic Publishing Company, Inc., 1980. Reprinted by permission of the publisher.
    List on page 118: From J. B. Thompson and H. O. Thompson, *Ethics in Nursing*, 1981. Reprinted by permission of the publisher, Macmillan Publishing Company.
    Figure 5–7: From Leah Curtin, "A Proposed Model for Critical Ethical Analysis," in *Nursing Forum 17* (1978). Reprinted by permission.
    Figure 7–9: Adapted from P. Hersey and K. Blanchard, *Management of Organizational Behavior: Utilizing Human Resources*, 3rd Edition (1977). Reprinted by permission of Prentice-Hall Publishing Company.
    Figure 8–3: From G. D. Friedman, *Primer of Epidemiology*. Reprinted by permission of the publisher, McGraw-Hill Publishing Company.
    Table 8–5: Adapted from H. R. Leavell and E. G. Clark, *Preventive Medicine for the Doctor in His Community*, 1965. Reprinted by permission of McGraw-Hill Publishing Company.
    Figure 8–6: From P. Moore and J. Flynn, "Users of coin-operated computerized sphygmomanometry and reasons for utilization: A descriptive study," *American Journal of Public Health 74*, 4, 368–370. Reprinted by permission of the American Public Health Association.
    Figure 12–4: Adapted from R. G. Hirschowitz, "Crisis/Transition Sequence," in *Levinson Letter*. Reprinted by permission of the Levinson Institute, Cambridge, Mass.

(continued on p. 614)

Contents

Contents

two   Tools for Practice   155

7   The Nursing Process in Community Health   157

8   Epidemiology   181

9   Working with Populations and Groups   224

10   The Helping Relationship and Contracting   266

Contents

Contents

Contributing Authors

Beverly Dorsey, R.N., B.S.
Director, Ambulatory Care Services
University Hospitals
University of Minnesota
Minneapolis, Minnesota

Sara T. Fry, R.N., M.S., M.A.
Assistant Professor
School of Nursing
University of Virginia
Charlottesville, Virginia

Terry W. Miller, R.N., M.S.N., P.H.N.
Curriculum Coordinator and Instructor
Department of Nursing
School of the Applied Arts and Sciences
San Jose State University
San Jose, California

Elaine Richard, R.N., M.S.
Director of Occupational Health
HealthLine
St. Joseph's Hospital
Tampa, Florida

Shirley J. Thompson, Ph.D.
Associate Professor
Department of Epidemiology and Biostatistics
School of Public Health
University of South Carolina
Columbia, South Carolina

Sarah L. Turner, R.N., M.P.H., Ph.D.
Associate Professor
College of Nursing
University of South Carolina
Columbia, South Carolina

Preface

The first edition of *Community Health Nursing: Concepts and Practice* was
written to capture the essence of community health nursing, to clarify its
meaning for the practitioner, and to share enthusiasm for a field whose
complex nature demands and fosters creativity, leadership, and innovation.
As a basic text, the second edition, like the first, is designed to give un-
dergraduate nursing students a comprehensive introduction to the field of
community health nursing.

Several topics have assumed greater significance for community health
nursing since the publication of the first edition of this book. Consequently
their inclusion makes this second edition more comprehensive, while at the
same time they provide a sharp focus on issues of current and future concern
to community health nurses. Seven new chapters cover these issues. They
include health care organization and financing, values and ethics, an expanded
discussion of children's health, occupational health, and the health of older
adults, home health care, and the political arena. Finally, the importance of
environmental health has been given greater emphasis. Rather than presented
separately, however, it has been woven as a major thread throughout the
text through discussion of environmental health concepts and numerous
environmental health illustrations.

In response to feedback from colleagues, the basic organization and content
of the first edition has been retained with changes made primarily for refinement
and updating. An exception is the chapter on epidemiology which has been

essentially rewritten by two nurse epidemiologists. The host-agent-environment model has been eliminated in this edition since epidemiologic thinking has advanced to include a broader, multiple-causation view rendering the earlier model less effective for understanding the conditions influencing health and disease states.

Another change in the second edition is the introduction in chapter 3 of a conceptual model for community health nursing. The model serves to clarify the definition of this field and provides a conceptual framework for understanding community health nursing practice in the remainder of the book.

Community health nursing, now more than ever, is a challenging, evolving field of nursing practice — one that is on the cutting edge of many innovations in health care delivery. It is, at the same time, a field of nursing surrounded by some confusion. *Community Health Nursing: Concepts and Practice* was originally written to clarify the nature and practice of community health nursing. This second edition seeks to further clarify the conceptual and philosophical foundations influencing its definition. Recent years have seen considerable discussion and debate about what community health nursing is versus what public health nursing is. The two terms have been used synonymously in this and other texts as well as in the field. The rationale continues to be that nurses who incorporate public health theory and principles into their practices, emphasizing communities of people or a population-oriented view, are true public health practitioners. Confusion enters when community health nursing is defined by where, instead of how, it is practiced. Dramatic increases in ambulatory and home care are creating an escalating demand for nurses to practice in the community; many of these nurses, however, practice basic nursing or other nursing specialties — not community health nursing as it is defined here. The challenge for the nurse who wishes to practice community health nursing lies in incorporating public health knowledge with basic nursing knowledge to offer preventive, health promoting, protective services that benefit population groups. At the beginning practitioner level the nurse may have limited impact on populations but a public health orientation must be germaine to his or her practice. At advanced levels of practice with advanced preparation in public health the nurse can become a public or community health nurse specialist.

In this edition we continue to use the terms community health nurse and public health nurse interchangeably based on the belief that either label is appropriate so long as it describes a practitioner whose work incorporates public health theory and skills.

This book is organized into four major parts, each providing the reader with a different perspective on community health nursing. Part one introduces the conceptual foundations with expanded discussion of community health in chapter 1 and a new chapter 2 on the history of public health and the organization and financing of health care services. These set the stage for expanded coverage of the nature and scope of community health nursing practice in chapter 3. Roles and settings for practice are covered in chapter 4, followed by a new chapter on values and health emphasizing the importance of awareness of values in health care. This prepares the reader for a better understanding of the cultural dimension covered in chapter 6.

Part two examines several important tools for community health nursing practice. These include application of the nursing process, epidemiology, working with populations and groups, the helping relationship and contracting, health teaching, and crisis prevention and intervention.

Part three, Care of Communities, first describes how to assess a community's health in chapter 13. The remaining chapters focus on specific target communities or populations, including children, families, working adults, the elderly, and the home care population.

Part four explores the expanding influence of community health nurses through leadership, management of planned change, and involvement in the political arena.

Acknowledgments

I am indebted to many people for support, encouragement, and ideas in the preparation of this second edition. Six individuals lent their expertise and made substantial contributions: Sara Fry wrote the chapter on values, Shirley Thompson and Sarah Turner rewrote the chapter on epidemiology, Elaine Richard coauthored the chapter on occupational health, Beverly Dorsey contributed to the chapter on home health, and Terry Miller wrote the chapter on politics.

I wish to thank Marla Salmon and my faculty colleagues in the Program in Public Health Nursing, School of Public Health, University of Minnesota for their ideas and encouragement. My thanks also go to the many community colleagues who supported and contributed to my efforts: in particular, Esther Tatley of Chicago County Public Health Nursing Service, Barbara O'Grady of Ramsey County Nursing Service, Linda Stein of Ramsey County Community Health Services, and Elaine Saline of the Ramsey County Mental Health Consortium.

I would like to thank the many people who provided their suggestions and assistance as reviewers throughout the revision process. These include Linda Daniel of the University of Michigan, Peggy Drapo and Charlotte Patrick of Texas Women's University, Debby Hogan and Barbara Morgan of the University of Rhode Island, Kathy Jordan of Tennessee State University, Nashville, Sheila Warren of Mt. St. Mary's College, Newburgh, NY, and Von Best Whitaker at the University of Missouri, Columbia.

I could not and probably would not have completed this project without the patient encouragement of my editor, Ann West. To her I owe a great debt of gratitude. I am also grateful to Lauren Green and the other helpful people at Little, Brown.

Finally, I am thankful to the many friends and family members who provided essential encouragement. In particular I wish to thank Bob and Karen Veninga for their unfailing love and support; Janet Hagberg, Bill Svrluga, Ruth Warland, and David and Carolyn McCurdy for their friendship; my daughters, Sheryl, Deborah and Laura for their encouragement; and my mother, Lois Walton, and sister, Lindie Bacon, for their love and prayers.

one

Conceptual Foundations

1

Community Health

Community Influence

Human beings are social creatures. All of us, with rare exceptions, live out our lives in the company of other people. An Eskimo lives in a small, tightly knit community of close relatives; a rural Mexican lives in a small village with hardly more than two hundred members. In complex societies most people find their lives influenced by many overlapping communities such as their professional society, political party, neighborhood, and city. Even those who try to escape community membership always begin their lives in some type of group and usually continue to depend on groups for material and emotional support. Communities are an essential and permanent feature of human experience.

The communities in which people live have a profound influence on their collective health and well-being. It is well known, for example, that the rate of alcoholism is very low among members of the Orthodox Jewish community. In this religious and cultural community firm rules and procedures for drinking control its use. Drunkenness is negatively evaluated and sobriety is viewed as a virtue. Consequently, alcoholism among Orthodox Jews is practically unknown (U.S. Department of Health, Education and Welfare [USDHEW], 1967, p. 26). A few years ago an illness, Legionnaires' disease, was named after its emergence to public attention at a national convention of the American Legion. This community, a voluntary organization with members in many parts of the country, was, for a brief period, peculiarly affected by a disease. Although many people tend to think of health and illness as individual matters, it has been established that they are also community matters. Recent experiences in many parts of the nation with acquired immune deficiency syndrome (AIDS) demonstrate the point (Valdiserri, Brandon, & Lyter, 1984). Communities can influence the spread of disease, provide barriers to protect members from health hazards, organize in ways to combat outbreaks of infectious disease, and promote practices that contribute to individual and community health.

Roles and Functions in Community Health

These facts are the basis for a challenging field of practice — community health. Many different professionals work in community health to form a complex team. The city planner designing an urban renewal project necessarily becomes involved in community health. The social worker counseling on child abuse or the use of chemical substances among adolescents is involved in community health. A physician treating patients affected by a sudden outbreak of hepatitis and seeking to find the source is engaged in community health practice. Prenatal clinics, meals for the elderly, genetic counseling centers, legislation to restrict smoking in public places, educational programs for the early detection of cancer, and hundreds of other activities are all part of the community health effort.

Professional nurses are an integral part of community health practice. Their roles and activities are so varied that it is impossible to describe the "typical" community health nurse. They work in every conceivable kind of community health agency from state public health departments to community-based advocacy groups. Their duties range from examining infants in a well-baby clinic or teaching elderly stroke victims in their homes to carrying out epidemiologic research or engaging in health policy analysis and decision making. Community health nursing is a specialty area. It combines all the basic elements of professional, clinical nursing with community health practice. This book examines the unique contribution that community health nursing makes to our health care system. Our discussion of the concepts and theories that make community health nursing an important specialty within nursing begins with the broader field of community health, which provides the context as well as essential content for community health nursing practice.

Community health, also known as public health, is sometimes misunderstood. Even many health professionals tend to think of community health in limiting terms such as sanitation, poverty area clinics, and massive efforts to prevent health problems. Although these are a part of its ever-broadening practice, community health is much more. In order to understand the nature and

4

significance of this field, it is necessary to look more closely at the concepts of community and health.

Community

Broadly defined, a community is a collection of people who share some important feature of their lives. Some communities, such as a tiny village in Appalachia, are composed of people who share almost everything. They live in the same location, work at a limited number of jobs, attend the same churches, and make use of the single health clinic and visiting physician or nurse. Other communities, such as the American Legion, are large, scattered, and composed of people who may share only their interest and involvement in that particular group. Although most communities share many aspects of their experience, three primary criteria are useful for identifying communities that relate to community health practice: geography, common interest, and health problem.

Geography

A community is often defined by its geographic boundaries. A city, town, or village is a geographic community. Consider the community of Hayward, Wisconsin. Located in northwestern Wisconsin, it is set in the north woods environment, far removed from any urban center, and in a climatic zone characterized by extremely harsh winters. With a population of less than twenty-five hundred, it is considered a rural community. The population has certain identifiable characteristics such as age and sex ratios, and its size fluctuates with the seasons; summers bring hundreds of tourists and seasonal residents. Hayward is a social system as well as a geographic location. The families, schools, hospital, churches, stores, and government institutions are linked in a complex network. This community, like others, has an informal power structure. It has a communication system that includes gossip, the newspaper, the co-op store bulletin board, and the radio station. In one sense, then, a community consists of a collection of people located in a specific place and is made up of institutions organized into a social system.

Local communities such as Hayward vary in size. A few miles south of Hayward lie several other communities, including Northwoods Beach and Round Lake, but these three, along with other towns and isolated farms, form a larger community called Sawyer County. If you worked for a health agency serving only Hayward, that community would be of primary concern; however, if you worked for the Sawyer County Health Department, you would focus on this larger community. A community health nurse employed by the State Health Department in Madison, Wisconsin, would have an interest in Sawyer County and Hayward, but only as one small part of the larger community of Wisconsin.

Frequently, a single part of a city can be treated as a community. In Seattle, for example, the skid row district near the waterfront is a community of many transients. For certain purposes in community health, it is useful to identify a geographic area as a community.

Common Interest

A community can also be identified by a common interest. A collection of people, widely scattered geographically, can have an interest that binds the members together. The members of a church in a large metropolitan area, a group of migrant workers, or the members of a national professional organization can all be treated as communities. Sometimes within a fairly small geographic area, a group of people become a community by promoting their common interest. The younger families in the northern part of Sawyer County, Wisconsin, may emerge as a community through a common interest in the needs of their children for better schools. The residents in an industrial community may develop a common interest in air or water pollution issues, while others who work but do not live there may not share that interest. The kinds of shared interests that lead to the formation of communities are almost infinitely varied.

Health Problem Solving

Frequently in community health practice a community is an area with fluid boundaries within which a problem can be identified and solved. The shape of this community varies with the size of the geographic area affected and the number of resources needed to address a problem. Such a community is called "a community of solution" (National Commission on Community Health Services, 1967). A water pollution problem may involve several counties whose agencies and personnel must work together to control upstream water supply, industrial waste disposal, and city water treatment. This group of counties forms a community of solution around a health problem. In another instance, several schools may collaborate with law enforcement and health agencies to study patterns of students' drug use and possible preventive approaches. The boundaries of this community of solution form around the schools and agencies involved. Figure 1-1 depicts some communities of solution related to one city.

Community health workers, including the community health nurse, need to understand the complex nature of communities. What are the characteristics of the people in terms of age, sex, race, and socioeconomic level? How does the community interact with other communities? What is its past history? Is the community undergoing rapid change? Many of these questions as

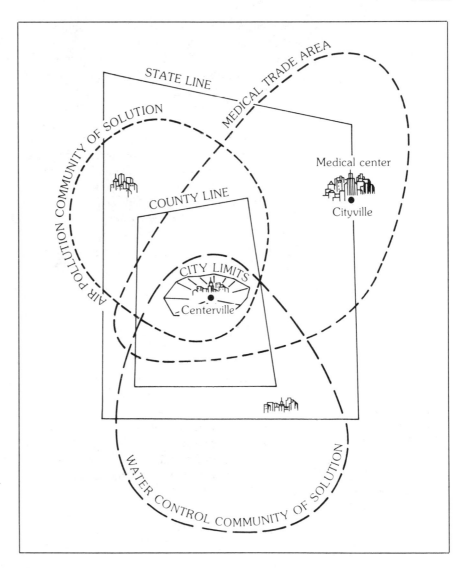

Figure 1-1
A city's communities of solution. State, county, and
city boundaries (shown in
solid lines) may have little
or no bearing on health
solution boundaries.

well as the tools needed to assess a community for health purposes are discussed in chapter 13.

Health

In 1946, the World Health Organization defined health as a state of complete physical, mental, and social well-being and not merely as the absence of disease or infirmity. Our understanding of the concept of health builds on this classic definition. We recognize that health is not just the absence of illness but the presence of a positive capacity to lead an energetic, satisfying, and productive life. We value a strong emphasis on well-being or ''wellness'' as we have come to know it. We are growing to understand health broadly through holistic perspectives.

Yet health is an elusive concept. For each person it has acquired dozens of meanings in the course of ordinary conversations. As children, we were encouraged to eat proper foods in order to grow strong and healthy. We later heard of people who "lost" their health. Under the treatment of physicians these people may have "regained" their health. Like barnacles slowly accumulating on the hull of an ocean barge, multiple meanings became attached to the concept of health. Although health is widely accepted as desirable, the exact nature of health is often unclear and ambiguous. In order to clarify the concept for our use in considering community health practice, the distinguishing features of health shall be briefly characterized; then the implications of this concept for the activities of professionals in the field can be examined more fully.

A Relative Concept

Health is a relative, not an absolute, concept. Our language tends to impose on us a black-and-white way of thinking about health. Most people contrast health with illness or disease. A person has one condition or the other — that is, a person can move from one category to the other, from sick to well again — in an absolute sense. This kind of thinking must be set aside if we are to grasp the nature and significance of community health practice.

Health, according to the concept used in this text, always involves many levels. We are all familiar with degrees of illness. We classify a person with terminal cancer or end-stage renal disease as very ill. Someone else recovering

Figure 1-2
The wellness–illness continuum. The level (degree) of illness increases as one moves toward total disability or death; the level of wellness increases as one moves toward optimal health. This continuum shows the relative nature of health. At any given time a person can be placed at some point along the continuum.

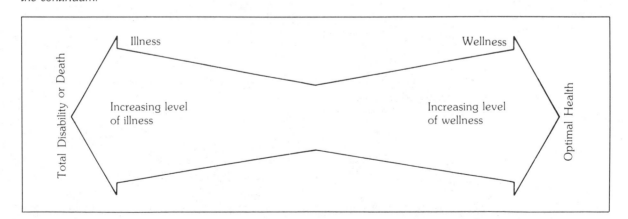

8

from a cholecystectomy is less ill, yet another person with infectious mono-nucleosis may be mildly ill. These are degrees or levels of illness. In the same manner we can identify degrees of wellness. From a mildly well person who functions minimally with a disease such as chronic arthritis to a robust 70-year-old person who is functioning at an optimal level of wellness, we see variations in degrees of health. Health always involves a continuum — a range of degrees — from optimal health at one end to death or total disability at the other (see Figs. 1-2, 1-3). The health of an individual, family, group, or community moves back and forth along this continuum throughout life.

By thinking of health relatively, as a matter of degree, we can avoid the strong tendency to polarize its meaning and thus limit our practice. Traditionally, the majority of health care was focused on treatment of acute and chronic conditions at the illness end of the continuum. Gradually the emphasis shifted to include attention to the wellness end of the continuum. Community health practice ranges over the entire continuum; it always works to improve the degree of health in individuals, families, groups, and communities. However, community health practice particularly emphasizes the promotion and preservation of positive health and the prevention of illness or injury.

A State of Being

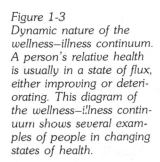

Figure 1-3
Dynamic nature of the wellness–illness continuum. A person's relative health is usually in a state of flux, either improving or deteriorating. This diagram of the wellness–illness continuum shows several examples of people in changing states of health.

Health refers to a state of being. Individuals and communities have many different qualities and characteristics. We might describe a person in such terms as *energetic, outgoing, enthusiastic, beautiful, caring, loving,* and *intense.* Together, these qualities become the essence of a person's existence; they describe a state of being. Similarly, a specific geographic community might be characterized by the terms *congested, deteriorating, unattractive, dirty,* and *disorganized.* These characteristics suggest diminishing degrees of vitality. Again, they describe a state of being.

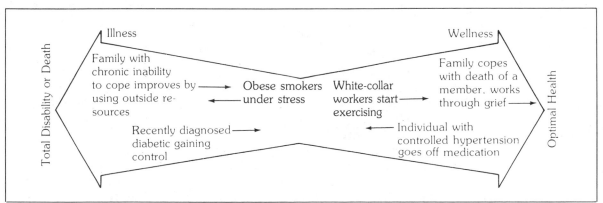

Health, as a set of qualities or a state of being, involves the total person or the total community. That is, all the dimensions of life affecting everyday functioning determine an individual's or a community's health. Physical, psychological, spiritual, and sociocultural experiences influence one's present condition. Thus, an individual's placement on the wellness–illness continuum can only be known if we consider that person from a holistic perspective (Fig. 1-4). Wellness is a relative state of well-being; illness is a relative state of ill-being.

As we consider an aggregate of people in terms of health, it sometimes becomes useful to speak of the "health of a community." With aggregates as well as individuals, health as a state of being does not merely involve the physical condition but includes psychological, spiritual, and sociocultural factors as well.

Subjective and Objective Dimensions

Health involves subjective and objective dimensions. Subjectively, a healthy person is one who feels well, who experiences the sensation of a vital, positive state. Healthy people are full of life and vigor, capable of physical and mental productivity. They feel minimal discomfort and displeasure with the world around them. Again, people experience varying degrees of vitality and well-being. The state of feeling well fluctuates. Some mornings we wake up feeling more energetic and enthusiastic than other mornings. How a person feels varies day by day, even hour by hour; nonetheless, it can be a strong indicator of that person's health state.

Health also involves the objective dimension of ability to function. A healthy individual or community is one that can carry out necessary activities and achieve enriching goals. Unhealthy people not only feel ill but are limited, to some degree, in their ability to carry out daily activities. Indeed, levels of illness or wellness are largely measured in terms of ability to function (Terris, 1975). A person confined to bed is labeled sicker than an ill person managing self-care. A family that meets its members' needs is healthier than one that has poor communication patterns and is unable to provide adequate physical and emotional resources. Degree of functioning is directly related to state of health.

The ability to function can be observed. A man dresses and feeds himself and goes to work. Despite financial exigencies, a family nourishes its members through a supportive emotional climate. A community fails to provide adequate resources and services for its members. These performances, to some degree, can be regarded as indicators of health status.

Underlying performance are the values an individual, family, or community places on actions. Some activities such as walking and taking care of personal needs are functions almost everyone values. Other actions (for example, sports such as running) have more limited appeal. In assessing the health

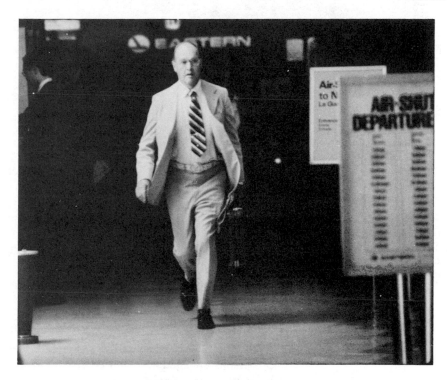

Figure 1-4
Rushing to catch his air shuttle, this businessman is experiencing work stress and an unhealthy life-style that is likely to move his health state to the illness end of the continuum.

of individuals and communities, the community health nurse can observe their ability to function but must also know their values, which may contrast sharply with those of the professional.

Subjective (feeling well or ill) and objective (function) dimensions together provide us with a clearer picture of people's health. When they feel well and demonstrate functional ability, they are close to the wellness end of the wellness-illness continuum. Even those with a disease such as arthritis or diabetes may feel well and perform well within their capacity. These people can be considered healthy. Figure 1-5 depicts the relationships between the subjective and objective views of health.

Health as a Resource

Health can be viewed as an important resource, both of individuals and communities. The relationship between health and community has been summarized by Henkel (1970, p. 2):

1. The health and well-being of an individual physically, emotionally, and socially is one of his most important assets.

11

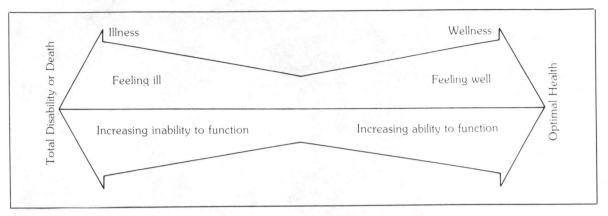

Total Disability or Death

Illness

Feeling ill

Increasing inability to function

Wellness

Feeling well

Increasing ability to function

Optimal Health

Figure 1-5
Subjective and objective
views of the wellness–
illness continuum.

2. Through judicious use of this asset he will be able to achieve more effectively his goals in life.
3. To develop this asset to the greatest possible level requires the concerted and cooperative efforts of many people.
4. Society as a whole will ultimately benefit from healthy citizens.

The implications of this view of health have far-reaching consequences for persons engaged in health care. No longer can we justify concentrating the majority of our efforts exclusively on healing the sick or even on the prevention of disease. For centuries health work has focused on the illness end of the wellness–illness continuum. We now live in an age when it is not only possible to promote health but our mandate and responsibility to do so (USDHEW, 1979).

As important as health promotion is the need for health assessment. When one considers health status from the perspective just discussed, its measurement becomes more feasible as well as necessary. Health promotion and health assessment are essential aspects of community health nursing and are discussed in detail in later chapters.

Elements of Community Health Practice

We have examined the definitions of community and of health. Together, these concepts provide the foundation for understanding community health. In acute care the health of an individual is the primary focus. Community health broadens that focus to concentrate on families, groups, and the community at large. The community becomes the recipient of service, and health becomes the product. Viewed from another perspective, community health is concerned with the interchange between population groups and their total environment and the impact of that interchange on collective health.

Just as a whole is greater than the sum of its parts, the health of a community is more than the sum of the health of its individual citizens. A community that achieves high-level wellness is composed of healthy citizens, functioning in an environment that protects and promotes health. Community health, as a field of practice, seeks to provide the organizational structure, resources, and activities needed to accomplish the goal of an optimally healthy community.

What is the difference between community health and public health? Theoretically there is none. Both are organized community efforts aimed at the promotion, protection, and preservation of the public's health. Historically, however, as a field of practice, public health has been associated with official or government efforts. This is in contrast to private health efforts directed toward solving selected health problems. The latter augments the former. Community health practice encompasses both because its focus includes all health agencies and efforts, public or private, concerned with community health. In this text, the term *community health* refers to this broader perspective while recognizing the fundamental concepts and principles of public health to be its birthright and foundation for practice.

Winslow's 1920 definition of public health is still timely and forms the basis for our definition of community health in this text: "Public health is the science and art of preventing disease, prolonging life, and promoting health and efficiency through organized community efforts for the sanitation of the environment, the control of communicable infections, the education of the individual in personal hygiene, the organization of medical and nursing services for the early diagnosis and preventive treatment of disease, and the development of the social machinery to insure everyone a standard of living adequate for the maintenance of health, so organizing these benefits as to enable every citizen to realize his birthright of health and longevity" (cited in Hanlon & Pickett, 1984, p. 4).

One of the challenges community health practice faces is to remain responsive to community health needs. As a result, its structure is complex; numerous health services and programs are currently available or will be developed in the future. Examples include health education, family planning, accident prevention, environmental protection, immunization, nutrition, early periodic screening and developmental testing, school programs, mental health, and industry and occupational health.

Community health practice can best be understood by examining six basic elements, which when combined encompass its services and programs: (1) promotion of healthful living, (2) prevention of health problems, (3) treatment of disorders, (4) rehabilitation, (5) evaluation, and (6) research.

Promotion of Healthful Living

Promotion of healthful living is now recognized as one of the most important elements of community health practice. Health promotion programs and activities include many forms of health education, demonstration of healthful practices, and efforts to provide a greater number of health-promoting options. Wellness programs in business and industry are an example. Health education, although a useful tool, has limited significance alone unless accompanied by desire, opportunity, and resources that encourage more healthful practices (Milio, 1976). In Maryland an intensive health education effort to teach families about safety and to reduce childhood injuries at home made no significant difference (Dershewitz & Williamson, 1977). This was due, in part, to expecting too broad a range of behavior changes. A similar effort in New York City to reduce childhood injuries from window falls combined home visits, health education, follow-up, and provision of free window guards (supplied by the health department) with highly successful results (Spiegel & Lindaman, 1977).

Demonstration of such healthful practices as eating more nutritious foods and exercising more regularly is often performed by individual health workers. In addition, groups and health agencies that support the rights of nonsmokers, encourage physical fitness programs for all ages, or demand that food products be properly labeled demonstrate the importance of these practices and create public awareness.

The goal of health promotion is to raise individuals', families', groups', and communities' levels of wellness. Community health accomplishes this goal through a three-pronged effort: (1) to increase understanding of health, (2) to raise community standards for health, and (3) to assist in developing more positive health practices. More specifically, the U.S. Public Health Service has outlined 15 target areas with specific objectives and plans for their implementation (Public Health Service, 1983). They are:

Preventive health services
    Family planning
    Pregnancy and infant care
    Immunizations
    Sexually transmissible diseases
    High blood pressure control
Health protection
    Toxic agent control
    Occupational safety and health
    Accidental injury control
    Fluoridation of community water supplies
    Infectious agent control
Health promotion
    Smoking cessation
    Reduction of alcohol and drug abuse
    Improved nutrition
    Exercise and fitness
    Stress control

It is difficult to provide health-promoting options, that is, opportunities to make more healthful choices, without reexamining and, in many instances, restructuring organizational patterns and policies as well as increasing personal and societal resources. At the local level, many health agencies are offering services at hours more convenient to their clientele and, in some cases, are providing transportation or other means of easier access to service. Furthermore, community residents are forming stronger bonds of partnership with health workers in order to understand and solve their own health problems as well as to assume greater responsibility for achieving positive health for themselves and their communities.

Prevention of Health Problems

Prevention of health problems constitutes a major part of community health practice. Prevention means anticipating and obviating problems or discovering them as early as possible in order to avert or minimize possible disability and impairment. It is practiced on three levels in community health: (1) primary prevention, (2) secondary prevention, and (3) tertiary prevention (Leavell & Clark, 1965, p. 20).

Primary prevention obviates the occurrence of a health problem. It keeps it from happening at all: "It precedes disease or dysfunction and is applied to a generally healthy population" (Shamansky & Clausen, 1980, p. 106). For example, a community health nurse who encourages an elderly couple to install safety devices, such as a grab bar by the bathtub or a hand rail on the front steps, is preventing injuries from falls. Local health departments help control and prevent communicable diseases such as rubeola or polio-myelitis by providing regular immunization programs. Primary prevention involves anticipatory planning and action on the part of community health professionals who must project themselves into the future, envision potential needs and problems, and then design programs to counteract them so that they never occur. A nutritionist who instructs a group of overweight women to follow a well-balanced diet during weight loss is preventing the possibility of nutritional deficiency. The concepts of primary prevention and planning for the future are foreign to many social groups who may resist on the basis of conflicting values. The "Parable of the Dangerous Cliff" (Fig. 1-6) illustrates such a value conflict.

Secondary prevention seeks to detect and treat existing health problems at the earliest possible stage. Pathology is now involved. Hypertension screening centers, which have been formed in many communities, help identify a high-risk group and encourage early treatment. Another example is breast and testicular self-examination programs. Secondary prevention attempts to discover a health problem at a point when intervention may lead to its control or eradication. This is the reasoning behind water and soil testing for contaminants and hazardous chemicals in community environmental health. It also prompts community health nurses to watch for early signs of child abuse in a family,

15

Parable of the Dangerous Cliff

'Twas a dangerous cliff, as they freely confessed,
  Though to walk near its crest was so pleasant;
But over its terrible edge there has slipped
  A duke, and full many a peasant.
The people said something would have to be done
  But their projects did not at all tally.
Some said, "Put a fence around the edge of the cliff";
  Some, "An ambulance down in the valley."
The lament of the crowd was profound and was loud,
  As their hearts overflowed with their pity;
But the cry of the ambulance carried the day
  As it spread through the neighboring city.
A collection was made, to accumulate aid,
  And the dwellers in highway and alley,
Gave dollars or cents.
Not to furnish a fence
But "An ambulance down in the valley."
"For the cliff is all right if you're careful," they said;

"And if folks ever slip and are dropping,
  It isn't the slipping that hurts them so much
As the shock down below when they're stopping."
So for years (we have heard), as these mishaps occurred,
  Quick forth would the rescuers sally,
To pick up the victims who fell from the cliff,
  With the ambulance down in the valley.
Said one, in his plea, "It's a marvel to me
  That you'd give so much greater attention
To repairing results than to curing the cause;
  You had much better aim at prevention.
    For the mischief, of course, should be stopped at its source,
Come neighbors and friends, let us rally.
  It is far better sense to rely on a fence
Than an ambulance down in the valley."
"He is wrong in his head," the majority said;
  "He would end all our earnest endeavor.
He's a man who would shirk this responsible work,
  But we will support it forever.

Aren't we picking up all, just as fast as they fall,
  and giving them care liberally?
A superfluous fence is of no consequence,
If the ambulance works in the valley."
The story looks queer as we've written it here,
  But things oft occur that are stranger,
More humane, we assert, than to take care of the hurt,
  Is the plan of removing the danger.
The very best plan is to safeguard the man,
  And attend to the thing rationally;
To build up the fence and try to dispense
  With the ambulance down in the valley.
Better still! Cut down the hill!

—Author Unknown

Figure 1-6
"Parable of the Dangerous Cliff."

16

emotional disturbances in a group of widows, or excessive drinking among adolescents.

Tertiary prevention attempts to reduce the extent and severity of a health problem to its lowest possible level. Rehabilitation of persons following a stroke, postmastectomy exercise programs, and Alcoholics Anonymous support groups are examples. The clients involved have an existing illness or disability whose impact on their lives is lessened through tertiary prevention. In broader community health practice we use tertiary prevention to minimize the effects of an existing unhealthy community condition. An example of such prevention is warning urban residents about rats in the sewer system.

Health assessment of individuals, families, and communities is an important part of preventive practice. One must determine health status in order to anticipate problems and select appropriate preventive measures. A community health nurse who discovers that a young mother has herself been a victim of child abuse institutes early treatment for the mother to prevent abuse and foster adequate parenting of her children. If assessment of a community reveals inadequate facilities and activities to meet the future needs of its increasing population of senior citizens, agencies and groups collaborate to plan and develop the needed resources.

Health problems are most effectively prevented by maintaining healthy life-styles and healthy environments. To these ends, community health practice directs many of its efforts to provide safe and satisfying living and working conditions, nutritious food, and clean air and water. This area of practice is sometimes referred to as preventive medicine.

Treatment of Disorders

Treatment of disorders, which focuses on illnesses and health problems, is the remedial aspect of community health practice. The first of its three major functions is to provide *direct service* to people with health problems. A family, unable to afford the purchase of a wheelchair for a son with multiple sclerosis, is provided one through a community agency. If the wife in an older couple is newly diagnosed as diabetic, home visits from a community health nurse, for assistance with diet planning, administration of insulin, and personal care, are arranged. A neighborhood health center forms an educational and support group for people needing to lose weight. Many kinds of community agencies provide direct health or health-related services.

Second, the remedial aspect of community health practice includes *indirect service* by assisting people with health problems to obtain treatment. In many instances a community agency may not be able to provide needed care and will refer the individuals or groups concerned to a more appropriate resource. A young woman with postpartum bleeding, assisted by the community health nurse, gets an immediate appointment with a physician at the local clinic. A social worker helps a family that is plagued by personal and economic problems to enter a family therapy and counseling program. A number of community agencies provide information and referral services.

Third, treatment of disorders also includes the development of *programs to correct unhealthy conditions.* One community with a high incidence of alcoholism and drug abuse initiated a chemical dependency counseling and treatment center. In another community, the health department developed new regulations for industrial waste disposal as a result of increased pollution of the water supply. Individual community members and health workers also take corrective action to remedy situations such as a case of apparent child abuse, poor nutrition in a school's lunch program, or inhumane conditions and treatment in a nursing home.

Rehabilitation

Rehabilitation, the fourth element of community health practice, focuses on reducing disability and, as much as possible, restoring function. People whose handicaps are congenital or acquired through illness or accident such as stroke, heart condition, amputation, or mental illness can be helped to regain some measure of lost function or to develop new compensating skills. For example, a factory worker who lost his leg in an industrial accident received good medical and nursing care, prosthetic fittings, and physical and occupational therapy; he thus retrained to assume successfully an office job.

In community health, the need to reduce disability and restore function applies equally to families, groups, and communities as well as to individuals. Many groups form for rehabilitative purposes, such as Alcoholics Anonymous, halfway houses for discharged psychiatric patients, or ostomy clubs. Rehabilitation services are often needed and sought by whole communities such as a ghetto area that desires to provide decent, safe playgrounds for its children (Fig. 1-7).

As an element of community health practice, rehabilitation becomes increasingly significant when disease trends and changes in life expectancy are considered. Chronic conditions have replaced acute as the major causes of morbidity; these include such cripplers as cardiovascular disease and cancer, the increased incidence of accidents, and environmentally caused conditions. As a result, the need for long-term care and rehabilitation has increased, stimulated further by a greater proportion of elderly persons in the population.

Evaluation

Evaluation is the means by which community health practice is analyzed and improved. Evaluation of health and health care should be an integral part of every kind of health service from individual practice to national and international programs. Whether done on the single case or program level, evaluation helps solve problems and provides direction for future health care

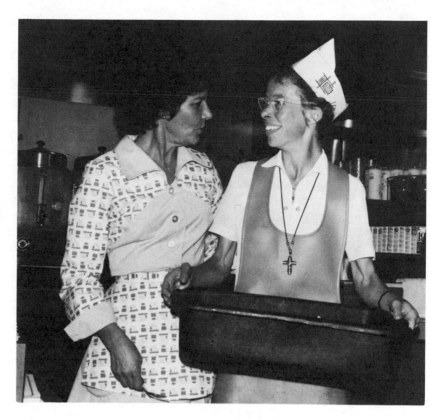

Figure 1-7
This retarded young adult,
functioning well within her
capacity, demonstrates that
community health efforts
can enable people to
achieve a high level of
health despite disability.

efforts. Its goals are to determine needs and the success of present activities as well as to develop improved services. In one community, evaluation of mental health services revealed a need for more comprehensive psychiatric emergency care on a 24-hour basis. If a psychiatric crisis occurred during the night, police were the only persons available to help and jail the only place where the mentally ill could be taken. The deficiency was corrected by providing 24-hour psychiatric emergency service in the community mental health center. A community health nurse, in another instance, developed a contract with a family to whom she was making home visits. The parents wanted to learn how to cope with their adolescent boys. Specific, written objectives and a plan for measuring the outcomes enabled the couple and the nurse to evaluate the successful completion of this helping relationship.

Research

Research, a critical element of community health practice, provides a means for solving problems and exploring improved methods of health service. Community health conducts and utilizes scientific investigations at all levels from federal agencies such as the U.S. Public Health Service to state and local groups conducting research. Biostatistics and epidemiology are the primary public health measurement and analytic sciences underlying community health practice. Chapter 8 addresses these sciences in more detail.

Researchers in community health investigate the characteristics and patterns of illness and health. Conditions such as food poisoning, trauma, alcoholism, lung cancer, child abuse, drug dependency, or suicide are studied for possible causes and means of prevention. Health and healthful behavior are analyzed, for example, in nutrition projects and studies of normal human growth and behavior, for better understanding of ways to promote healthful living.

Community health researchers explore ways to improve health care. After a survey in Berkeley, California, revealed many deficiencies in day care centers, specific recommendations for improvement of health services for children enrolled in day care centers were made (Chang, Zukerman, & Wallace, 1978). A team of community health nurses in North Carolina studied nursing intervention with high-risk school children for the purpose of improving school nurse practice (Long et al., 1975). Other research projects might focus on the effectiveness of drug treatment programs, long-term stroke rehabilitation, or improved treatment approaches to obesity.

Community health researchers also examine the impact of social and environmental changes on health and health services provision. For example, one study focused on the possible causes of wife-battering (Parker & Schumacher, 1977), while another concentrated on the epidemiology and prevention of drowning (Dietz & Baker, 1974). A growing number of studies center around needs and care of the elderly. Others investigate ways to improve health services planning and policy development through such efforts as studies of community needs and program utilization.

Community Health Characteristics

Several characteristics of community health practice deserve special emphasis. First, community health practice, unlike the individualized focus of acute health care, has a group orientation. It is concerned with the health status of people in the aggregate, people who are parts of groups. These groups or communities, in turn, are multiple and overlapping. Thus community health must deal with a complex set of interacting physical, psychological, sociocultural, and biologic variables that influence human behavior and impinge on aggregate health (Williams, 1977).

Second, in community health practice the promotion of health and prevention of illness are of first-order priority. There is minimal emphasis on curative care. Some corrective actions are always needed, such as clean up of a toxic waste dump site, stricter enforcement of day care standards, or home care of the ill; however, community health best serves its constituents through preventive and health promoting actions (Hilbert, 1977). These include services to mothers and infants, prevention of environmental pollution, school health programs, senior citizen fitness classes, "workers'-right-to-know" legislation that warns against hazards in the workplace, and numerous others.

Third, community health practice uses measurement and analysis. The need to collect and examine data before decision making is fundamental to community health practice. Analysis of health states, environmental factors, health-related services, economic patterns, and social policy are among the many foci of community health evaluation and research, described further in chapter 8.

Finally, community health practice utilizes principles from management and organization theory to provide effective organization and management of health care services. Chapter 2 elaborates on this subject.

Summary

Community health is much more than environmental programs and massive efforts to control communicable disease. To comprehend the nature and significance of community health we must understand the concepts of community and of health.

A community, broadly defined, is a collection of people who share some important feature of their lives. More specifically, it is helpful in community health practice to identify communities in terms of three criteria: geography, common interest, and health problem. Sometimes a community, such as a city, county, or neighborhood, is formed by geographic boundaries. At other times a community may be identified by its common interest; examples are a religious community, a group of migrant workers, or a gathering of residents concerned about air pollution. A community may also be defined as a community of solution, that is, a pooling of efforts by people and agencies toward solving some health-related problem.

Health is an abstract concept that can be understood more clearly when we recognize its distinguishing features. First, health is a relative, not an absolute, concept. People are not either sick or well in an absolute sense but have levels of illness or wellness. These levels may be plotted along a continuum ranging from optimal health to total disability or death. This is known as the wellness–illness continuum. Thus, a person's state of health is dynamic, varying from day to day and even hour to hour.

Second, health is a state of being. That is, the characteristics of a person, family, or community can be said to describe the essence of their existence. These characteristics portray people and therefore suggest the presence or absence of vitality. As a state of being, health also involves the total person. All the dimensions of life — physical, psychological, social, and spiritual — affect health.

Third, health has both subjective and objective dimensions. The subjective aspect involves feeling well; the objective aspect refers to the ability to function. How one feels can indicate one's state of health. At the wellness end of the wellness–illness continuum, people feel well; at the illness end, they feel ill. The ability to function, which is observable and often used to measure health status, may be present anywhere along the continuum. Most often, performance diminishes dramatically toward the illness end.

Community health practice is concerned with preserving and promoting the health of the community. It incorporates six basic elements: (1) promotion of healthful living, (2) prevention of health problems, (3) treatment of disorders, (4) rehabilitation, (5) evaluation, and (6) research.

Important characteristics of community health practice include its emphasis on aggregates, promotion of health and prevention of illness, use of measurement and analysis, and effective management and organization of health services.

Study Questions

1. Identify a community of people for whom you have some concern. What makes it a community? What characteristics does this population group share?
2. Place the community you selected on the wellness–illness continuum. What factors influenced your decision?
3. Describe three preventive actions (one primary, one secondary, and one tertiary) that might be taken to move the community you selected closer to optimal wellness.
4. Place yourself on the wellness–illness continuum. What factors influenced your decision?

References

Chang, A., Zukerman, S., & Wallace, H. (1978). Health services needs of children in day care centers. *American Journal of Public Health, 68,* 373–377.

Dershewitz, R., & Williamson, J. (1977). Prevention of childhood injuries: A controlled clinical trial. *American Journal of Public Health, 67,* 1148–1153.

Dietz, P., & Baker, S. (1974). Drowning: Epidemiology and prevention. *American Journal of Public Health, 64,* 303–312.

Hanlon, J. J., & Pickett, G. E. (1984). *Public health: Administration and practice.* 8th edition. St. Louis: Times Mirror/Mosby.

Henkel, B. (1970). *Community health* (2nd ed.). Boston: Allyn and Bacon.

Hilbert, M. S. (1977). Prevention. *American Journal of Public Health, 67,* 353–356.

Leavell, H. R., & Clark, E. G. (1965). *Preventive medicine for the doctor in his community: An epidemiological approach* (3rd ed.). New York: McGraw-Hill.

Long, G., Whitman, C., Johansson, M., Williams, C., & Tuthill, R. (1975). Evaluation of a school health program directed to children with history of high absence. *American Journal of Public Health, 65,* 383–393.

Milio, N. (1976). A framework for prevention: Changing health-damaging to health-generating life patterns. *American Journal of Public Health, 66,* 435–439.

National Commission on Community Health Services. (1967). *Health is a community affair.* Cambridge: Harvard University Press.

Parker, B., & Schumacher, D. (1977). The battered wife syndrome and violence in the nuclear family of origin: A controlled pilot study. *American Journal of Public Health, 67,* 760–761.

Public Health Service. (1983). Public Health Service implementation plans for attaining the objectives for the nation. *Public Health Reports,* September-October 1983 Supplement, 1-177.

Shamansky, S., & Clausen, C. (1980). Levels of prevention: Examination of the concept. *Nursing Outlook, 28,* 104–108.

Spiegel, C., & Lindaman, F. (1977). Children can't fly: A program to prevent childhood morbidity and mortality from window falls. *American Journal of Public Health, 67,* 1143–1147.

Terris, M. (1975). Approaches to an epidemiology of health. *American Journal of Public Health, 65,* 1037–1045.

U.S. Department of Health, Education and Welfare, National Institute of Mental Health. (1967). *Alcohol and alcoholism.* Washington, DC: U.S. Government Printing Office.

Valdiserri, R. O., Brandon, W. R., & Lyter, D. W. (1984). AIDS surveillance and health education: Use of previously described risk factors to identify high-risk homosexuals. *American Journal of Public Health, 74,* 259–260.

Williams, C. A. (1977). Community health nursing — What is it? *Nursing Outlook, 25,* 250–254.

Selected Readings

Anderson, O. (1972). Health-services systems in the United States and other countries: Critical comparisons. In E. Jaco (Ed.), *Patients, physicians and illness: A sourcebook in behavioral science and health* (2nd ed.) (pp. 295–295). New York: Free Press.

Blum, H. (1981). *Planning for health: Generics for the eighties* (2nd ed.). New York: Human Sciences Press.

Braden, C. (1976). *Community health: A systems approach.* New York: Appleton-Century-Crofts.

Brown, J. (1978). *The health care dilemma.* New York: Human Sciences Press.

Dunn, H. (1961). *High-level wellness.* Arlington, VA: Beatty.

Hanlon, J. J., & Pickett, G. E. (1984). *Public health: Administration and practice.* 8th edition. St. Louis: Times Mirror/Mosby.

Hilbert, M. S. (1977). Prevention. *American Journal of Public Health, 67,* 353–356.

Lauzon, R. (1977). An epidemiological approach to health promotion. *Canadian Journal of Public Health, 68,* 311–317.

Leavell, H. R., & Clark, E. G. (1965). *Preventive medicine for the doctor in his community: An epidemiological approach* (3rd ed.). New York: McGraw-Hill.

Leininger, M., & Buck, G. (Eds.). (1974). *Health care issues.* Philadelphia: Davis.

Lerner, M. (1973). Conceptualization of health and social well-being. *Health Service Research, 8,* 6–12.

Milio, N. (1975). *The care of health in communities.* New York: Macmillan.

Milio, N. (1976). A framework for prevention: Changing health-damaging to health-generating life patterns. *American Journal of Public Health, 66,* 435–439.

National Commission on Community Health Services. (1967). *Health is a community affair.* Cambridge: Harvard University Press.

National League for Nursing. (1973). *Community health — Strategies for change.* New York: National League for Nursing.

Parsons, T. (1972). Definitions of health and illness in the light of American values and social structure. In E. Jaco (Ed.), *Patients, physicians and illness: A sourcebook in behavioral science and health* (2nd ed.) (pp. 107–127). New York: Free Press.

Public Health Service. (1979). *Healthy people: The surgeon general's report on health promotion and disease prevention* (DHEW Publication No. PHS 79–55071). Washington, DC: U.S. Government Printing Office.

Rosen, G. (1958). *A history of public health.* New York: MD Publications.

Shamansky, S., & Clausen, C. (1980). Levels of prevention: Examination of the concept. *Nursing Outlook, 28,* 104–108.

Shamansky, S., & Pesznecker, B. (1981). A community is . . . . *Nursing Outlook, 29,* 182–185.

Terris, M. (1975). Approaches to an epidemiology of health. *American Journal of Public Health, 65,* 1037–1045.

Terris, M. (1975). Evolution of public health and preventive medicine in the United States. *American Journal of Public Health, 65,* 161–169.

Torrens, P. (1978). *The American health care system: Issues and problems.* St. Louis: C. V. Mosby.

2

Organization and Financing of Community Health Services

Service delivery systems directed at restoring or promoting the public's health have evolved over centuries. That evolution is marked by many successes as well as failures in our efforts to accomplish the goal of a healthier world society. The structure, function, and financing of health care systems have changed dramatically over time in response to changing societal needs and demands, scientific advancements, more effective methods of service delivery, new technology, and development of varying approaches to resource acquisition and allocation (Hanlon & Pickett, 1984, p. 143). We have made considerable progress. At the same time we are faced with many problems, particularly those of escalating health care costs and system emphasis on illness rather than wellness.

This chapter describes the current organization of community health services in the United States and gives an overview of historical and legislative events that have influenced health planning and system structure and function. It also discusses the changing picture of health care financing and its incentives and disincentives for enhancing the public's health. More extensive treatment of these important subjects can be found in the selected readings at the close of the chapter.

Historical Perspectives

Health care as we know it today has changed dramatically from previous centuries. Yet from the beginning of time there is reason to believe that personal and community hygiene and health care were practiced. Many primitive tribes appeared to engage in sanitary practices such as burial of excreta, removal of the dead, and isolation of members with certain illnesses along with treatment of the sick using a variety of therapeutic agents administered by a "healer." Whether these activities were purely superstitions or derived from survival needs is unknown. Nonetheless, records show that their descendants in Eqypt and the Middle East, as early as 3000 B.C., were building drainage systems and practicing personal cleanliness (Hanlon & Pickett, 1984, p. 22). The biblical record in Leviticus describes the Hebrew hygienic code, circa 1500 B.C., as a prototype for personal and community sanitation. Even more advanced were the Athenians, circa 1000–400 B.C., who emphasized personal hygiene, diet, and exercise in addition to a sanitary environment albeit for the benefit of the wealthy. Their successors, the Romans, added many more community health measures such as laws regulating environmental sanitation and nuisances, and construction of paved streets, aqueducts, and a subsurface drainage system.

The Middle Ages (from about A.D. 500 to 1500) marked a distinct change in health beliefs and practices based on the philosophy that to pamper the body was evil. Neglected personal hygiene, improper diets, and accumulation of refuse and body wastes soon led to widespread epidemics and pandemics of disease including cholera and leprosy. Increased trade between Europe and Asia, military conquests, and Christian crusaders to the Middle East only furthered the spread of disease. Bubonic plague, known as the Black Death, in the mid 1300s was the most devastating of pandemics, reportedly killing about 43 million people, half the population of the known world (Hanlon & Pickett, 1984, p. 25). In response to this, the first known quarantine measure was instituted in 1377 at the port of Ragusa (now Dubrovnik) where travelers from plague areas were required to wait two months and be free of disease before entry was allowed. Marseilles, in 1383, passed the first quarantine law (Hanlon & Pickett, 1984, p. 25). During this regressed period in history, health care, what little existed, was private and reserved for the wealthy few, and public health problems were minimally and ineffectively addressed.

By the end of the Middle Ages more enlightened European thinkers began to challenge the prevailing beliefs and conditions. They no longer believed that disease was a punishment for sin, although traces of stigma regarding leprosy, tuberculosis, and cancer can be found yet today, and venereal disease is still regarded by some as punishment for immoral conduct. Concepts of human dignity and rights and an emphasis on the search for scientific truth influenced new efforts at reform during the late eighteenth century that continued through the nineteenth century.

Despite these signs of improvement, many serious problems persisted. Hundreds of pauper children died in England's abusive but legally approved workhouses and apprentice slavery system. Most of Europe continued in deplorable conditions of misery and filth. Many householders dumped their refuse out windows or doors into the streets. Stinking rivers and water supplies were seriously contaminated. Numerous diseases including cholera, typhus, typhoid, smallpox, and tuberculosis took a tremendous toll on human life.

Around the turn of the nineteenth century, England became increasingly concerned about social and sanitary reform. The first sanitary legislation, passed in 1837, established vaccination stations in London. One of the most notable reformers, Edwin Chadwick, published his "Report on an Inquiry into the Sanitary Conditions of the Laboring Population of Great Britain" (Hanlon & Pickett, 1984, p. 28) in 1842. Chadwick, the father of modern public health, believed that disease and poverty were related and could be changed. His efforts resulted in passage of the English Public Health Act and establishment of a General Board of Health for England in 1848 (Lewis, 1952). Conditions improved and scientific study advanced in England and concurrently in France, Germany, Scandinavia, and other European countries. England, however, set the pace for application of research, particularly with reference to public health measures, through steadily improved legislation. These laws subsequently became the pattern for American sanitary ordinances.

U.S. Health Care Development

Early health care in the American colonies consisted of private practice with infrequent governmental action for the public good. Action was usually in the form of isolated local responses to specific dangers or nuisances such as the 1647 regulation to prevent pollution of Boston Harbor or the 1701 Massachusetts law requiring ship quarantine and isolation of smallpox patients. New York City in the late 1700s formed a public health committee to monitor, among other public concerns, water quality, sewer construction, marsh drainage, and burial of the dead.

The U.S. Constitution, adopted in 1789, made no direct reference to public health nor was the federal government active in health matters. It was the responsibility of each sovereign state to manage its own health affairs. The first federal intervention for health problems was the Marine Hospital Service Act of 1798. It subsidized medical and hospital care for disabled seamen. During the early years a scourge of epidemics, especially yellow fever, smallpox, cholera, typhoid, and typhus, caused many deaths throughout the colonies. Quarantine efforts under local control proved ineffective. Congress, in 1873, finally instituted the national port quarantine system, which was regulated and enforced by the Marine Hospital Service. Epidemics were quickly brought under control, causing society to recognize the benefits of uniform central government policy. Improvements in public health and sanitation generally throughout the states, however, were held back by delayed progress in coping with other competing needs such as police and fire protection.

The Shattuck report, a landmark document, made a tremendous impact on sanitary progress. Lemuel Shattuck, a layman and legislator, chaired a legislative committee that studied health and sanitary problems in the commonwealth of Massachusetts. In 1850, he produced the "Report of the Sanitary Commission of Massachusetts." It described public health concepts and methods upon which much of today's public health practice is based. Among his many recommendations, Shattuck advocated the establishment of state and local boards of health, environmental sanitation, collection and use of vital statistics, systematic study of diseases, control of food and drugs, urban planning, establishment of nurses' training schools (there were none before this time), and preventive medicine. Unfortunately, it was almost 25 years before the recommendations were appreciated and truly implemented. A similar report by John C. Griscom conducted about the same time concluded that illness, premature death, and poverty were directly related. He also recommended sanitary reform (Fig. 2-1).

Precursors to an organized health care "system" in the United States came in the form of offical health agencies. Initially development occurred at the local level. Many cities established local boards of health in the late 1700s and early to mid-1800s. Among the earliest were Baltimore, Maryland (1798), Charleston, South Carolina (1815), and Philadelphia (1818). As their efforts expanded from handling public "nuisances" to dealing with epidemics and complex public health problems, they recognized that employment of full-time staff was needed and formed health departments. The first full-time county health departments were established in 1911 in North Carolina and Washington state. Massachusetts formed the nation's first state board of health in 1869 and a few years later the first state department of health. At the national level, the Marine Hospital Service, now broadened in function, became the Public Health and Marine Hospital Service in 1902. Congress gave it a more clearly defined organizational structure and specific functions for its director, the surgeon general. In 1912 it was renamed the U.S. Public Health Service.

Rapidly expanding through the years of World War I and the Great Depression, the U.S. Public Health Service strengthened its research activity based in the National Institutes of Health (founded 1912), added demonstration projects, and initiated greater cooperation with the states. Responding to increasingly complex needs, it added such programs significant to public

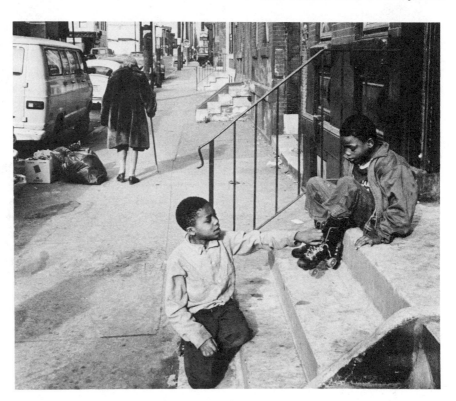

Figure 2-1
Poverty and environmental conditions have a direct influence on people's health.

health as the Children's Bureau (1912), the National Leprosarium at Carville, Louisiana (1917), examination of arriving aliens (1917), the Division of Venereal Diseases (1918), the Food and Drug Administration (1927), and the Narcotics Division (1929), which later became the Division of Mental Hygiene. Title VI of the 1935 Social Security Act promoted stronger federal support of state and local public health services including health manpower training.

As the number of health, welfare, and educational services proliferated, the need for consolidation prompted the creation of the Federal Security Agency in 1939. In 1953 it became the Department of Health, Education and Welfare, now the Department of Health and Human Services. Other significant events included the establishment, during World War II, of the Communicable Disease Center in Atlanta, currently the National Centers for Disease Control, and the development, after World War II, of the National Office of Vital Statistics, now called the National Center for Health Statistics.

The private sector actually responded first to America's health problems and to this day continues to complement and supplement the government's role in provision of health services. Voluntary health agencies began to emerge by the late 1800s. The first of these was the Anti-Tuberculosis Society of Philadelphia formed in 1892 to educate the public and the government about tuberculosis, then causing 10 percent of all deaths. Other agencies followed. The National Society to Prevent Blindness was formed in 1908, the Mental Health Association in 1909, the American Cancer Society in 1913, and several, including the National Easter Seal Society for Crippled Children and Adults and the Planned Parenthood Federation of America, in 1921. Also in the late 1800s, organized charities like the Red Cross, previously denounced for promoting dependent poverty, began to be recognized for their contributions to health and welfare. Philanthropy, too, became respected with the establishment of the Rockefeller Foundation (1913) followed by others like the Carnegie-Mellon and Kellogg foundations.

Many health-related professional associations over the years have influenced the quality and type of community health services delivery. Among these, the National Organization for Public Health Nursing, formed in 1912, significantly influenced early organization and quality of public health nursing services. It later became the National League for Nursing (1950) and continues to promote quality efforts in community health. The American Public Health Association, founded in 1872, to this day maintains a prominent role in the dissemination of public health information and advocacy for the nation's health.

Health Care Organization

The historical record demonstrates that for many centuries people have attempted to address community health needs. Responsibility for these shifted between individuals and governing institutions. Each arm, public and private, offered a unique perspective, different skills, and different resources. Lack of coordination between them, however, and no method for comprehensive planning and delivery of health services left huge gaps in some areas, duplication in others. It has only been within the past 100 years that the two arms have gradually begun to work together to create an emerging system of health care (Roemer, 1984). How does that system work today? What are its strengths and weaknesses? To answer these questions, we will first examine its structure. Why look at structure? Because it becomes the operational base for assessment, diagnosis, planning, implementation, and evaluation of services, and because it provides a framework for intersystem and intrasystem communication and coordination.

Health services occur at four levels: local, state, national, and international. Each, like ever-widening concentric circles, concerns itself with the health needs of the populations that its boundaries encompass. The organization of these services can be classified under one of two types, government or private.

Government Health Organization

Government health agencies, the tax-supported arm of the community health effort, perform an important function in community health practice. They are the official public health and welfare agencies whose areas of jurisdiction and types of service are dictated by law. They coordinate activities that often can be carried out only by group or community-wide action, for example, proper sewage disposal or the provision of sanitary water systems. Government health agencies develop facilities and programs for special groups, such as native Americans, migrant workers, and military personnel and veterans, whose health care is not the direct responsibility of any one state or locality. Many community health activities require an authoritative legal backing to ensure enforcement (another useful function of official agencies) of control in such areas as environmental pollution, highway safety practices, and harmful use of drugs. Official agencies provide important record-keeping services, which include the collection of vital statistics, research, consultation, and sometimes financial support to other community health groups.

Many different government agencies contribute to the health of a community. Most obvious are the city or county health departments, which provide a variety of direct and indirect health services, including community health nursing. Other tax-supported agencies that also give health or health-related services are the welfare department, department of public works, public schools and hospitals, police department, county agricultural service, and local housing authority.

LOCAL HEALTH AGENCIES

At the grass-roots level, community health agencies vary considerably from one locality to the next. This is due in part to variations in local needs, size, and priority setting; to differing interpretations of standards; and to the type and stipulations of funding sources. Nonetheless, each local governmental health agency shares some commonly held responsibilities, functions, and structural features.

The primary responsibilities of the local health department are (1) to assess its population's health status and needs, (2) to determine how well those needs are being met, and (3) to take action toward satisfying unmet needs (Hanlon & Pickett, 1984, p. 146). Local government also plays an important role in "coordinating inputs from the federal and state levels with those from the private sector to produce truly comprehensive health services" (American Public Health Association [APHA], 1975, p. 189). It is a critical level of health services provision because of its closeness to the ultimate recipients — health care consumers. The American Public Health Association has outlined in an official policy statement the functional areas for which local government should be responsible, either to provide services directly or by arrangement with other providers. Table 2-1 lists these areas (APHA, 1975, pp. 189–192).

The structure of the local health department varies in complexity with the setting. Rural and small urban agencies need only a simple organization while large metropolitan agencies require more complex organizational structures to support the greater diversity and quantity of work. A local board of health generally holds the legal responsibility for the health of its citizens. Health board members may be appointed by the mayor if serving a city or by a board of supervisors if serving a county. In turn, the board of health appoints a health officer, usually a physician with public health training, who employs the remaining staff of the health department. They include public health nurses, one or more environmental health workers, a health educator,

Table 2-1
The Role of Official Local Health Agencies

Community Health Services	Environmental Health Services	Mental Health Services	Personal Health Services	Processes Common to All Services
Communicable disease control	Food protection	Primary prevention of mental disorders	Personal health services, per se	Health data
Chronic disease control	Hazardous substances and product safety	Consultation	Health facilities operations	Agency program planning
Family health	Water supply sanitation	Diagnostic and treatment services	Emergency medical services	Interagency planning
Dental health	Liquid waste control		Home health services	Comprehensive state and regional health planning
Substance abuse	Water pollution control		Employee health programs	Disaster planning
Accident prevention	Swimming pool sanitation and safety		Medical care for inmates of prisons and institutions	Education of the public in health affairs
	Occupational health and safety			Health advocacy
	Radiation control			Continuing education of health personnel
	Air quality management			Involvement of health professionals
	Noise pollution control			Research and development
	Vector control			Community involvement
	Solid waste management			Organization
	Institutional sanitation			Policy direction
	Recreational sanitation			Staffing
	Housing conservation			Financing
	Environmental injury prevention			Relationships with state and federal health authorities

Source: From A.P.H.A. Position Paper, *American Journal of Public Health 65*, 189–193, 1975.

and office personnel. Others, like a nutritionist, statistician, epidemiologist, social worker, physical therapist, veterinarian, or public health dentist, may be added as needs and resources dictate. Figure 2-2 depicts the organization of one local health department serving a population of approximately 270,000.

STATE HEALTH AGENCIES

State-level health services, too, vary considerably. Each state, as a sovereign government, establishes its own state health department that, in turn, determines its goals, actions, and administrative structure. The state health department is responsible for providing leadership in and monitoring of public health needs and services in the state. It establishes statewide health policy standards, assists local communities, allocates funds, promotes state-level health planning, conducts and evaluates state-level health programs, promotes cooperation with voluntary health agencies, and collaborates with the federal government for health planning and policy development (Hanlon & Pickett, 1984, pp. 148–149).

State health department functions have been summarized in the following categories (Hanlon & Pickett, 1984, p. 149):

1. Statewide planning
2. Intergovernmental relations
3. Intrastate agency relations
4. Certain statewide policy determination
5. Standard setting
6. Regulatory functions

Each of the 50 state health departments in the United States has developed its own unique structure with no two exactly the same. All are overseen by a director of public health, but titles vary. Under the director are a number of divisions or bureaus. Those most commonly found in state health department organizational structures are disease control, local health services (which include community health nursing), hospital and technical services, laboratory services, state center for health statistics, and medical care. Figure 2-3 shows a state health department organizational chart.

FEDERAL HEALTH AGENCIES

The federal level of public health organization contains many agencies. Best known is the Public Health Service (PHS), which is concerned with a broad variety of health interests and is directed by the surgeon general. The PHS encompasses the Centers for Disease Control; the Food and Drug Administration; the National Institutes of Health; the Alcohol, Drug Abuse, and Mental Health Administration; and the Health Resources and Services Ad-

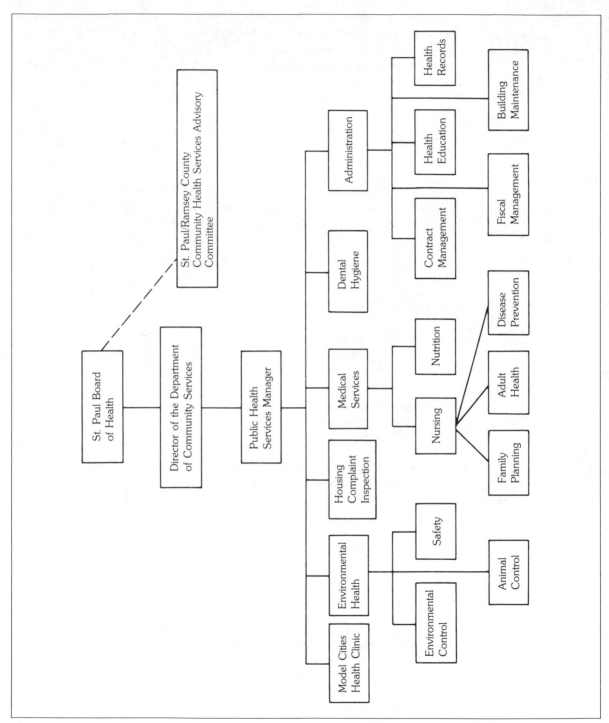

Figure 2-2
Organizational chart of the
St. Paul Division of Public
Health.

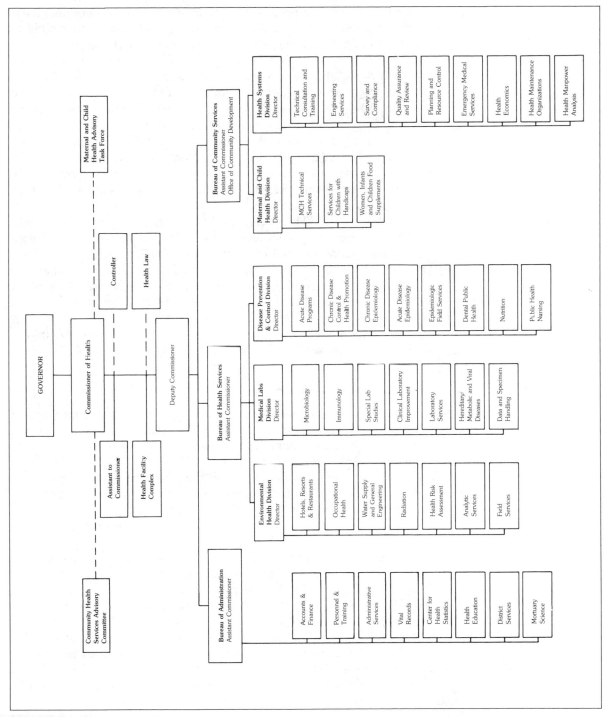

Figure 2-3
Organizational chart of a
state health organization.

ministration. Its major functions through these five branches are the administration of grants and contracts. In some instances, as with the Indian Health Service, it provides hospital and clinical services; through the Centers for Disease Control it provides epidemiologic surveillance; and through the Food and Drug Administration it monitors the safety and usefulness of various food and drug products. Figure 2-4 portrays the PHS organizational structure.

At the federal level the primary agencies concerned with health are organized under the Department of Health and Human Services. The PHS is one unit in this department. Formerly it was known as the Department of Health, Education and Welfare, established under President Eisenhower in 1953. In 1979, Education was made a separate cabinet-level department, and the department was renamed Health and Human Services. Figure 2-5 depicts this department's organization.

In addition to the PHS, a cluster of federal health agencies deals with special population groups such as the elderly (Administration on Aging), farmers (Agricultural Extension Service), Native Americans (Bureau of Indian Affairs), and the military. Another cluster addresses special programs or problems. Examples are the Bureau of Labor Standards, the Office of Education, the Bureau of Mines, and the Social Security Administration. A final cluster of federal agencies focuses on international health concerns. Two important ones are the Office of International Health, part of the PHS, and the Agency for International Development, part of the Department of State.

International Health Agencies

The health of other countries cannot be ignored. Besides important humanitarian and moral concerns, there are pragmatic reasons. We now live in an age when health, along with politics and economics, has become a global issue. The nations of the world are dependent on one another for goods and services, and like any set of interdependent systems, a problem in one has repercussions on the others. Furthermore, as the constitution of the World Health Organization states, "The health of all peoples is fundamental to the attainment of peace and security" (World Health Organization [WHO], 1971).

International cooperation in health dates back to early concerns for epidemics. In 1851, representatives from 12 countries met in Paris for the First International Sanitary Conference. They later established a more permanent organization, the Office Internationale d'Hygiène Publique in 1907. Epidemics on the American continent prompted representatives from 21 American republics also to meet for the First International Sanitary Conference in Mexico City in 1902. In that same year they formed the International Sanitary Bureau, later renamed the Pan American Health Organization. After World War I, the League of Nations in 1921 formed a health organization with which the Office Internationale d'Hygiène Publique merged.

36

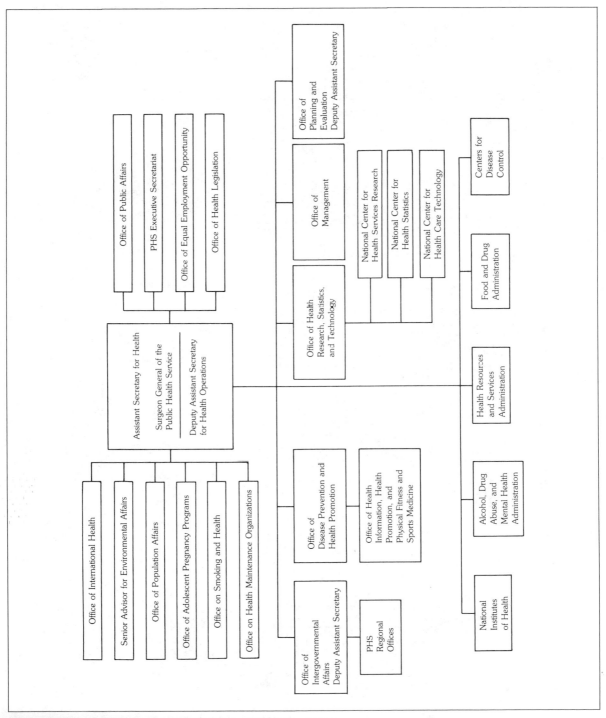

Figure 2-4
Public Health Service.

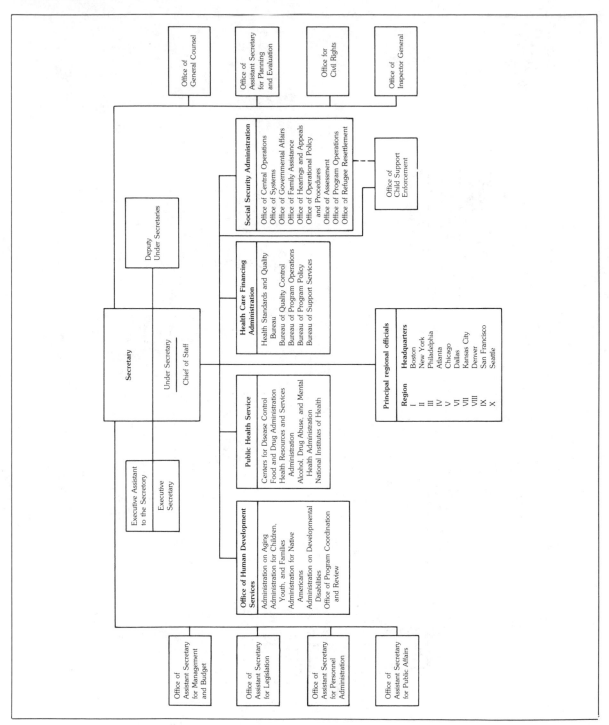

Figure 2-5
Department of Health and
Human Services.

WORLD HEALTH ORGANIZATION

The World Health Organization (WHO) was formed in 1948 and assumed the functions of the League of Nation's Health Organization. The Pan American Health Organization remained separate but became WHO's regional office for the Americas. An agency of the United Nations, WHO began its existence with 61 member nations, one of which was the United States. Its membership now numbers 158.

The responsibility or mission of WHO is to serve as "the one directing and coordinating authority on international health work" (Hanlon & Pickett, 1984, p. 79). From its inception, WHO has influenced international thinking with its classic definition of health as "a state of complete physical, mental, and social well-being and not merely the absence of disease or infirmity" (WHO, 1971). WHO's primary function is to help countries improve their health status and services by helping them to help themselves and each other. To accomplish this, it provides technical services and information from epidemiology and statistics to member countries plus advisory and consulting services and demonstration teams.

In addition to its headquarters in Geneva, Switzerland, WHO has six regional offices. The office for the Americas (the Pan American Health Organization) is located in Washington, D.C. Its funding comes from member countries and from the United Nations. It holds an annual World Health Assembly (Fig. 2-6) to discuss international health policies and programs (Hanlon & Pickett, 1984, p. 78.)

PAN AMERICAN HEALTH ORGANIZATION

The Pan American Health Organization serves as the central coordinating organization for public health in the Western Hemisphere. Founded in 1902, it is the oldest continuously functioning international health organization in the world. As WHO's regional office for the Americas, it disseminates epidemiologic information, provides technical assistance, finances fellowships, and promotes cooperative research and professional education.

UNITED NATIONS CHILDREN'S FUND

Organized in 1946, the United Nations Children's Fund, now the United Nations International Children's Emergency Fund (UNICEF), was initially established to assist children of war-torn countries. That focus has broadened. Now it promotes child and mental health and welfare globally through a variety of programs and activities. Some include provision of food and supplies to underdeveloped countries, immunization programs in cooperation with WHO, and promotion of family planning. Its International Children's Center, opened in 1940, has made a significant international impact with

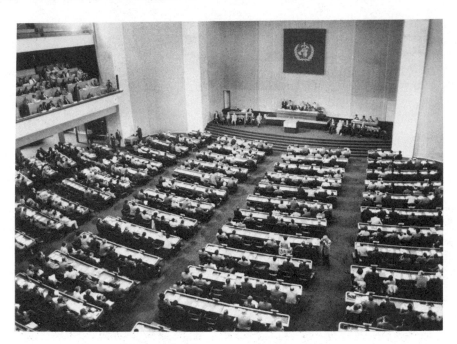

Figure 2-6
The thirty-seventh world
health assembly meets in
Geneva, Switzerland in
1984.

its teaching, research, publications, and cooperation on projects related to the health and welfare of children.

Private Health Services

The unofficial arm of the health care delivery system includes many types of services. Voluntary nonprofit health and welfare agencies make up one large group. Privately owned (proprietary) and for-profit agencies are another as well as private professional health care practice. They are the nontax-supported dimension of community health care.

Private health services are complementary and supplementary to government health agencies. They often meet the needs of special groups, such as those with cancer or heart disease; they offer an avenue for private enterprise or philanthropy; they are freer from restrictions than government agencies to develop innovations in health care; and they have been spurred to development, in part, by impatience or dissatisfaction with government programs. Their financial support comes from voluntary contributions, bequests, or fees.

Voluntary health agencies are nonprofit organizations, established and administered by private citizens for some specific health-related purpose. Often this purpose is seen as a special need either not addressed or served inadequately by government. An example is visiting nurse associations that were formed to provide care for the sick in their homes. The contribution of the voluntary health agency then becomes complemental to official health services.

Many types of voluntary agencies exist. The largest number of them has very specialized interests. Some such as the American Cancer Society and the American Diabetes Association are concerned with specific diseases. Some like the National Society for Autistic Children and the National Council on Aging focus on the needs of special populations. Others such as the American Heart Association and the National Kidney Foundation are concerned with certain body organs. These organizations are funded through private contributions.

Another group of voluntary health agencies includes the many foundations that support health programs, research, and professional education. Some agencies like the United Way, whose support comes from charitable contributions, exist to fund other voluntary efforts. Still another group includes professional associations that work to improve the public's health through the promotion of standards, research, information, and programs. Examples are the American Public Health Association, the National League for Nursing, the American Nurses Association, and the American Medical Association. These organizations are funded primarily through membership dues.

Hanlon and Pickett (1984, p. 160) describe the general functions of voluntary agencies:

1. Pioneering — detecting unserved needs or exploring better methods for meeting needs already addressed
2. Demonstration — piloting or subsidizing demonstration projects
3. Education — promoting public knowledge
4. Supplementation of official actions — assisting official agencies with innovative programs not otherwise possible
5. Guarding citizen interest in health — evaluating official programs and assuming a public advocacy role
6. Promotion of health legislation
7. Planning and coordination — promoting collaboration among voluntary services and between voluntary and official agencies
8. Development of well-balanced community health programs seeking to make services relevant and comprehensive

Significant Legislation

During the twentieth century, an ever-widening sense of responsibility for health in the public sector led to passage of an increasing amount of health-related legislation. Some acts are of particular significance to the delivery and financing of community health services.

The Shepard-Towner Act of 1921 provided federal funds for state administration of programs to promote the health and welfare of infants. The act expired in 1929. However, it had set a pattern for maternal and child health programs that was later revived and strengthened through the successful and far-reaching efforts of the Children's Bureau, housed in the Department of Labor (Hanlon & Pickett, 1984, p. 40). The Children's Bureau maintained its impact through several administrative changes (moved to the Federal Security Agency in 1946 and to the Department of Health, Education and Welfare in 1953 and became the Office of Child Development) but was phased out in 1972. Since that time federal advocacy for child health per se has considerably weakened.

The Social Security Act of 1935 had tremendous consequences for public health. In addition to its revolutionary welfare insurance and assistance programs, which particularly benefited high-risk mothers and children, Title VI of the act financially assisted states and localities in providing public health services. These funds were and still are allocated on the basis of population, public health problems, economic need, and need for training public health personnel. Many of the grants had to be matched by the states or localities serving to increase their knowledge of and commitment to health programs. The act strengthened local health departments and health programs in nearly all the states (Hanlon & Pickett, 1984, p. 37).

The Hill-Burton Act (Hospital Survey and Construction Act) of 1946 was an important breakthrough in nationwide health facilities planning. It marked the first real effort to link health planning with population need on a comprehensive basis. The act provided federal funds to states for hospital construction. Allocation of funds, however, was contingent upon the states forming planning councils to survey and document needs for new facilities and other capital expansion. The Hill-Harris Amendments in 1954 shifted the emphasis from purely construction to broader health planning based on needs assessment (Hyman, 1982, p. 11).

The Heart Disease, Cancer, and Stroke Amendments of 1965 (Pub. L. 89-239) are noteworthy for their establishment of regional medical programs, one of the first real efforts at comprehensive health planning. Fifty-six regions in the United States were designated, each charged with the responsibility to evaluate the overall health needs of its region and cooperate with other regions for program development. Although the amendments were initially categorical in nature (limited to heart disease, cancer, and stroke), amendments in 1970 expanded the focus. The act was important for two additional reasons. It encouraged local participation in health planning, previously done at federal and state levels, and it funded program operations as well as planning.

The Social Security Act Amendments of 1965 produced two pieces of legislation that attempted to address a concern for some type of national health insurance. Title XVIII, Medicare, still provides federal health insurance to persons over 65 years of age on Social Security, to the disabled, and to persons with end-stage renal disease needing dialysis. Part A of this law covers hospitalization. Part B, which is supplementary, pays for physician care and other related health services. Both parts of Medicare are financed by trust funds. Title XIX, Medicaid, is a joint federal-state assistance program; it serves low-income persons and their families as well as the medically indigent (those with high medical expenses). It is administered on a state-by-state basis. These two pieces of legislation have enabled many of the poor and elderly to gain access to high-quality health care. (Davis, 1983).

The Comprehensive Health Planning and Public Health Service Amendments Act (Partnership for Health Act) of 1966 (PL. 89-749) promoted further advances in comprehensive health planning. It established comprehensive health planning agencies and attempted to coordinate the many categorical health and research efforts into an integrated system. It emphasized comprehensive health planning at local, state, and regional levels and cost containment. Its goals were improved efficiency and effectiveness of health care. Many problems, including unclear expectations, uncertain funding, and limited authority prevented full accomplishment of these goals.

The Health Manpower Act of 1968 (PL. 90-490) sought to increase the supply of health personnel by providing federal monies to educational institutions for construction, training, special projects, student loans, and scholarships. The act replaced several previous acts with similar goals but whose efforts were fragmentary in addressing the problem. Among them were the Nurse Training Act (1966) and the Allied Health Professions Personnel Training Act (1966). In 1976, Congress passed the Health Professions Education Assistance Act (PL. 94-484) to effect a better balance between the country's health needs and the supply of available health professionals. One of its major emphases was to address the problem of physician maldistribution between underserved (rural) and overserved (urban) areas through educational incentive programs.

The Occupational Safety and Health Act of 1970 (PL. 91-956) provides protection to workers against personal injury or illness resulting from hazardous working conditions. This and other acts affecting the working population, such as workers' compensation, toxic substance control, access to employee exposure and medical records, and "right-to-know" legislation are discussed in the chapter on occupational health.

The Professional Standards Review Organization Amendment to the Social Security Act of 1972 (PL. 92-603) had two goals: cost containment and improved quality of care. Professional Standards Review Organization (PSRO) legislation created autonomous organizations, external to hospitals and ambulatory care agencies, to monitor and review objectively the quality of care delivered to Medicare and Medicaid patients. The PSRO review boards, composed mostly of physicians, examined such things as need for care, length of stay, and quality of care against predetermined standards developed locally. Failure to meet standards could mean denial of federal funding. The PSRO concept has created considerable controversy, partly because the two mandated goals, cost containment and quality of care, are potentially incompatible. The federal government's primary emphasis on costs frequently clashed with local concerns for quality. Also there were no common criteria or standards for review so that evaluation of the program's success has been difficult. Preliminary studies, however, indicate a substantial cost saving in Medicare expenditures (Hyman, 1982, p. 279).

The Health Maintenance Organization Act of 1973 (PL. 93-222) added federal support to the concept of prepayment for medical care. Congress authorized funding for feasibility studies, planning, grants, and loans to stimulate growth among qualifying health maintenance organizations (HMOs). In addition, this act requires a business employing 25 or more people to offer an HMO health insurance option, if such an option is available locally (Somers & Somers, 1977, p. 11).

The National Health Planning and Resource Development Act of 1974 (PL. 93-641) was a major breakthrough in comprehensive health planning. Replacing the Partnership for Health Act, it combined Hill-Burton, comprehensive health planning agencies, and regional medical programs into a single new program. It fostered not only comprehensive health planning, but regulation and evaluation, and promoted collaborative efforts among regional, state, and federal governments. An important contribution of this act was its emphasis on consumer involvement in health planning. The act was divided into two titles. Title XV, National Health Planning and Development, established national health priorities and assisted the development of area-wide and state planning through health systems agencies and state health planning and development agencies. Title XVI, Health Resources Development, coordinated health facilities planning with health planning, replacing Hill-Burton (Hyman, 1982, p. 63).

The Social Security Amendments of 1983 (PL. 98-21) became law in response to accelerating health care costs. The act represents a major reform in health care financing from retrospective to prospective payment. Most Medicare-participating hospitals now receive payment from Medicare on the basis of a fixed rate set in advance for each patient by diagnosis. A billing classification system has identified 23 major diagnostic categories and 467 diagnosis-related groups with prospective payment made based on hospital case mix (Joel, 1983; Shaffer, 1983). The fixed payment cannot be increased if hospital costs for care exceed that amount. Conversely, if costs are less than the paid amount, the hospital may keep the difference (Davis, 1983, p. 15). Thus a positive incentive has been introduced to reduce hospital costs.

Health Care Financing

Health care economics encompasses an intricate and complex set of interacting variables including the analysis of supply and demand, costs and benefits, and the allocation of scarce resources. It is a field of study in and of itself. Issues such as cost containment, accessibility, and need for accountability have become targets of major concern and action in recent years. We can facilitate our understanding of some of these issues and their impact on community health through examination of types of health care financing, trends influencing health care economics, and the effects of current financing patterns on community health practice.

Types of Health Care Financing

Financing of health care significantly affects community health practice. It influences the quality of services offered as well as the way those services are utilized. Methods of health care financing fall into three categories: third-party payers, direct consumer payment, and voluntary support.

Third-party payers are so called because they are a third party, or external, to the consumer-provider relationship. It is a broad term that covers four types of payment sources: private insurance companies, independent health plans, government health programs, and claims payment agents (Rapoport, Robertson, & Stewart, 1982, p. 292).

Private insurance companies market and underwrite policies aimed at decreasing consumer risk of economic loss because of health services utilization. None actually delivers health services. They are composed of three types. First are commercial stock companies that sell health insurance, generally as a sideline. They are private stockholder-owned corporations, such as Aetna, Travelers, and Connecticut General, that sell insurance nationally. Mutual companies are a second type that operates in the national marketplace, but they are owned by their policyholders. Examples are Mutual of Omaha, Prudential, and Metropolitan Life. The third type, nonprofit insurance plans, include Blue Cross, Blue Shield, and Delta Dental. These operate under special state enabling laws that give them an exclusive franchise to the whole state (or some part of it) and to a specific type of insurance. Blue Cross, for example, in most instances sells only hospital coverage, Blue Shield only medical insurance, and Delta Dental only dental insurance. Because they are nonprofit, they are tax-exempt and at the same time subject to tighter state regulation than the commercial health insurance companies. Combined, the nonprofit and commercial carriers sell 90 percent of the private health insurance in the United States (Rapoport et al., 1982, p. 293).

Independent health plans underwrite the remaining 10 percent of private health insurance in the nation. These are offered through several hundred smaller organizations such as businesses, unions, consumer cooperatives, and medical groups. HMOs and various company self-insurance plans are included in this category. They may only sell health insurance or, in some cases, may also provide health services; they focus on a very localized population. As a group, they generate a large amount of premium revenues but only one-tenth of the amount generated by the nonprofit and commercial health insurance companies.

Government health programs make up the largest source of third-party reimbursement in the country. The government's four largest third-party programs are Medicare, Medicaid, the Federal Employees Health Benefits Plan, and the Civilian Health and Medical Program of the Uniformed Services. Combined they "account for more than 50 percent of the nation's hospital revenues and nearly a quarter of physician incomes" (Rapoport et al., 1982, p. 294). A third of the government's total third-party expenditures go for direct public medical services by the military, state hospitals, the Veterans Administration, public health activities, and other "socialized" health services. Their primary target is what Health and Human Services Secretary Margaret Heckler called "the most fragile Americans" ("Known Welfare Fraud," 1983, p. 42) — the elderly, the disabled, the poor, the very young, and the unemployed. A recent federal health insurance program — this one designated to be self-financing — protects the unemployed who have lost their benefits. Another, workers' compensation, is a state-administered program that protects workers from illness or injury associated with their jobs.

In addition to third-party reimbursement, the government offers some direct health services to selected populations. They include native Americans, military personnel, veterans, merchant marines, and federal employees.

Claims payment agents administer the claims payment process of government third-party payments. That is, the government contracts with private agents to handle the claims payment process. More than 80 percent of the government's third-party payments are handled by these private contractors who are sometimes known as fiscal intermediaries (when processing Medicare hospital claims), carriers (when dealing with insurance under Medicare), or fiscal agents (as applied to Medicaid programs). As an example, Blue Cross Plans, in addition to being private insurance companies, are also claims payment agents for Medicare.

Direct consumer reimbursement is a second major type of health care financing. This refers to individual out-of-pocket payments made for several different reasons. One is payments made by individuals who have no insurance coverage so that direct payment must be made for health and medical services. Another is for limited coverage and exclusions (services for which the consumer must bear the entire expense). For example, many individuals carry only major medical insurance and must pay directly for physician office visits, prescriptions, and dental care. In other instances, the insurance contract may include a deductible amount that must be paid by the insuree before reimbursement begins. The contract may be established on a copayment basis that determines a percentage to be paid by the insurer and the rest by the individual. Or the individual may pay the remainder of a health service bill after the insurer has paid a previously agreed upon fixed amount such as a fixed coverage for labor and delivery. Direct consumer payment accounts for approximately one-third of total personal health care expenditures in the United States (Wilner, Walkley, & O'Neill, 1978, p. 138).

Voluntary support, the third type, contributes both directly and indirectly to health care financing. Many voluntary agencies, as discussed earlier in this chapter, fund programs and provide benefits for individuals who would otherwise go without services. Volunteerism, the efforts of numerous individuals who donate their time and services, provides a tremendous cost-saving to health care institutions. It also enables many individuals to receive services, such as home-delivered meals or transportation to health care facilities, at no charge. Continued voluntary support is essential, particularly during an era when large amounts of federal monies for social programs have been withdrawn (Hanlon & Pickett, 1984, p. 166).

Issues and Trends

FEDERAL REGULATION

Between the 1950s and 1970s the federal government assumed a much stronger role in the financing and regulation of health services. First, federal subsidy of health care costs increased. There was greater federal control of state programs. Health services became regionalized and more comprehensive. Federal appropriations supported operational as well as capital and planning costs. There was greater federal support for health research. Federal support for health manpower training increased. Group medical practice multiplied as a cost-saving measure. Over 60 percent of the population was covered by some form of prepaid health insurance, largely because of the effects of Medicare and Medicaid. There was an increase in interagency health planning cooperation and improved health program evaluation. Neighborhood health centers, community mental health centers, and other programs developed to improve health care access for everyone. It was a period of economic prosperity that emphasized quality of care, and during it the federal government assumed a major role in the regulation of planning, use, and reimbursement of health care services.

COST ESCALATION

Accompanying these trends, however, was an insidious escalation in health care costs. The early national effort to increase health resources, in the form of facilities, programs, and manpower, concomitantly increased the public's demand for health care. An even greater contribution to cost increases occurred through the system of third-party reimbursement. Third-party payment shielded consumers from the real costs of health care, encouraging consumer demand. More important, third-party reimbursement created a mood of unlimited spending because someone else was paying the bill. Hospitals and other providers could rely on payment regardless of what they spent, adding to the incentive to spend even more.

Government-financed programs, often unwieldy and expensive, fell prey to these escalating costs and to the pressures of inflation. Medicare, for example, which is financed through government trust funds has so depleted its resources that its insolvency was predicted for the late 1980s ("Known welfare fraud," 1983, p. 43). Recent measures in the form of prospective payment legislation and Social Security recommendations were taken to extend the solvency of Medicare funds until 1990. (Davis, 1983, p. 13).

Current health care costs have been growing at a rate of 19 percent per year (Davis, 1983, p. 13). In the period from 1950 to 1980, real per capita health care spending tripled, and total health care spending (government, insurance companies, and private individuals) was well over 10 percent of the gross national product in the early 1980s (Davis, 1983, pp. 11–12). The Department of Health and Human Services has grown exponentially to the point that today it administers the third largest budget in the world, behind only the budgets of the United States and the Soviet Union (Davis, 1983, p. 10), and it accounts for 34 percent of all federal spending ("Known welfare fraud," 1983, p. 43).

HMOs

In recent years traditional fee-for-service practice has experienced serious competition in the form of prepaid group practice. The concept of prepayment, or consumers paying in advance of health care, has existed for many years. As far back as 1933, prepaid medical groups were advocated to reduce costs and make services more accessible (Hyman, 1982, p. 13). This pattern of prepayment and group practice has continued ever since in a variety of forms. Examples of early plans were the Health Insurance Program of greater New York City and the Kaiser Plan. The success of these two plans, in particular, helped influence the growth of HMOs.

From 1930 to 1965, the HMO movement, supported initially by the private sector, gradually gained federal backing. Group plans were a part of Medicare and Medicaid bills and the Partnership for Health Act. The HMO Act of 1973 demonstrated stronger federal support. Amendments to this act in 1976 lifted restrictions and further encouraged HMOs.

Today the chief characteristics of an HMO are the following (Rapoport et al., 1982, p. 257):

1. There is a contract between the HMO and the consumers (or their representative) who are the "enrolled population."
2. A regular (usually monthly) premium to cover specified (and typically broad) services is paid for or by each enrollee to the HMO; few additional charges are levied because the payment mechanism is not basically fee-for-service.
3. The HMO contracts with professional providers to deliver the services due the enrollees; the basis for reimbursing those providers varies among HMOs.

Despite official encouragement and government subsidies, the growth of HMOs has been slow and on a relatively small scale. Yet they are still strongly endorsed as an alternative delivery system because of their potential for conserving costs owed to their greater emphasis on good health and ambulatory care with a concomitant reduction in hospital and medical care utilization (Somers & Somers, 1977, p. 467).

Figure 2-7
A community health nurse works collaboratively with another health team member to promote client health in a health maintenance organization.

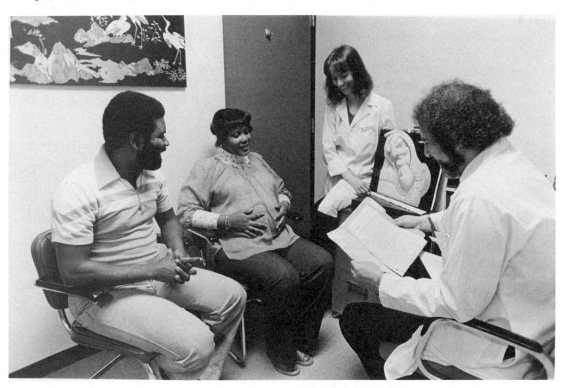

NATIONAL HEALTH INSURANCE

Growing concern over the cost and accessibility of health services led in the 1960s and again in the mid-1970s to a renewed focus on national health insurance (NHI) as a solution. NHI, as an issue, had been debated since 1912, its proponents seeking comprehensive health care protection for the aged and needy, in particular. Numerous attempts to pass some form of NHI resulted in piecemeal legislation adding various benefits for Social Security recipients. The Kerr-Mills bill (1960) set a precedent of public financing for elderly persons who were "medically needy" but not on public assistance. Medicare (1965) was the first compulsory NHI program in the United States. However, it reached only 10 percent of the population (Somers & Somers, 1977, p. 181).

In the 1970s the debate over NHI revived in full force. Many proposed NHI bills were considered by Congress. The seeming consensus over the need for government to assure access to needed health services for the total population was misleading. A multitude of divergent interests and conflicting philosophies led to heated debate. Four issues emerged as core areas of controversy. First was the public-private mix. What should the amount and nature of private health insurance involvement be in the public program? Second was the cost-sharing issue. To what extent, if any, should consumers share in the cost of the coverage? Third, What should be the amount and nature of cost and quality controls built into the program? And fourth, Should the NHI program be used as a vehicle for reform of the health care provision system (Somers & Somers, 1977, p. 182). Resolution, to date, has not been reached, and experts are predicting that a viable NHI program is not likely in the near future. (Somers & Somers, 1977, p. 189). First, we must reconcile the major roles of our large private health insurance industry, hospitals, and the medical profession along with our nation's inherent aversion to direct government intervention.

In the decade of the 1980s, study of NHI as an important concept continues. Somers & Somers (1977) recommend that NHI in its ideal form include the following:

1. Universal coverage regardless of income
2. Equitable financing using multiple sources but channeled through one mechanism
3. Comprehensive and balanced benefit structure
4. Incentives for efficient and effective use of resources and discouragement of health care price inflation
5. Controlled competition in the underwriting and administration of the program
6. Appropriate and feasible consumer options
7. Administrative simplicity

8. Flexibility
9. Acceptability to providers and consumers

COMPETITION AND REGULATION

Dramatic changes affecting health care occurred in the early 1980s. The federal government, failing to contain health care costs, shifted responsibility for the public's health and welfare back to state and local governments, emphasizing a decentralized system. Large amounts of federal support for health research, health manpower training, and public health programs were withdrawn. Continued escalation of health care costs prompted a concentrated effort among public and private providers alike to find cost-containment measures. Competition, encouraged by passage of the Budget Reconciliation Bill, was seen as a solution. Out of all this grew the competition versus regulation debate.

Competition, its proponents say, offers wider consumer choice and positive incentives for cost containment. That is, consumers have freedom to select among various health plans on the basis of cost, quality, and range of services. Competing providers must develop efficient production and distribution methods to stay in business, and consumers, because of required cost sharing that is part of the competition model, are more likely to use only necessary services. Ideally, then, competition offers the best service for the least cost.

Regulation advocates, on the other hand, point out some of the problems associated with the competition model. Consumers often don't know how to make proper choices because they have limited knowledge of health services. Competition, they argue, leads to discriminate selection of consumers, especially low-risk, low-cost patients, thus excluding those who may need services the most. The competition model may not encourage teaching and research, because these tend to be expensive elements of our present system. And because of its concern with costs, competition could likely sacrifice quality (Weiss, 1982, p. 655). Regulation, they say, is needed for standardization and controls, especially for quality and equal access. Leaders in the field have concluded that both are needed (Ehlinger, 1982, p. 520; Somers & Somers, 1977, p. 259). According to McNerney (1980, p. 1091), "It is rapidly becoming apparent that what we need is a proper balance between competition and regulation with more effective links . . . regulation [should be] used as a force to keep the market honest."

PROSPECTIVE PAYMENT

Prospective payment has evolved within the past ten years in response to the health care system's desperate need for cost containment. Under this concept, rate setting is done prospectively rather than retrospectively. That is, providers receive payment for services according to fixed rates set in advance (Shaffer, 1983, p. 389). To correct unlimited reimbursement patterns and counteract disincentives to contain costs, the concept involves four steps (Dowling, 1979, p. 34):

1. An external authority is empowered (by statute, market power, or voluntary compliance by providers) to set provider charges, third-party payment rates, or both.
2. Rates are set in advance of the prospective year during which they will apply and are considered fixed for the year (except for major, uncontrollable occurrences).
3. Patients, third-parties, or both pay the prospective rates rather than the costs actually incurred by providers during the year (or charges adjusted to cover these costs).
4. Providers are at risk for losses or surpluses.

Prospective payment, then, imposes constraints on spending and gives incentives for cutting costs. For these reasons the federal government enacted into law its diagnosis related group (DRG) prospective payment plan in 1983 in an effort to curb Medicare spending in hospitals and to extend the program's solvency period.

Although prospective payment offers some solutions, it also raises some questions. What will its effect be on quality of care? Will the use of DRGs promote premature discharge of hospitalized patients, and what effect may that have on their health and on the delivery of services outside of the hospital?

Effects on Community Health Practice

Health care financing has significantly affected community health and community health practice by advancing (1) disincentives for efficient use of resources, (2) incentives for illness care, and (3) conflict with public health values.

DISINCENTIVES FOR EFFICIENT USE OF RESOURCES

Disincentives for efficient use of resources include all the system structures that promote cost escalation and prevent cost containment. For example, retrospective financial reimbursement, with its lack of limit setting, encourages spending and drives costs up. Tax-deductible employer contributions for health care coverage and nontaxable employee health benefits encourage unnecessary use of services and raise costs. Lack of cost sharing by consumers and no financial risk for provider decision making create further disincentives to keep costs down.

Community health is affected in several ways. Abuse of resources in some parts of the system means a depletion in other areas. Community health programs have suffered greatly in recent years with diminished federal and state allocations and severe budget cuts affecting even basic community health services. Competition from the private sector in home care and other community services, such as health education programs, has forced traditional public health agencies to reexamine their programs and seek new avenues for service and new revenue sources. Costs indirectly even affect appropriate use of nursing personnel in community health. Failing to recognize the differences in skills of community health nurses and less prepared personnel, the proliferating agencies in community health often hire persons underqualified to give the high-caliber and comprehensive care needed in many instances. Finally, the advent of prospective payment and payment by DRGs is encouraging early hospital discharge and an increasing number of more acutely ill people needing home care. The immediate effect is to increase the demand for home care services of a highly skilled and more costly nature requiring changes in community health care provision patterns. The long-range effects of this phenomenon on family stress and care-giver health, on community health care reimbursement, and on the nature and structure of community health services provision has yet to be determined.

INCENTIVES FOR ILLNESS CARE

Because of its financial incentives, the traditional American health care system tends to promote illness. Health care providers are primarily rewarded for treating problems, not for preventing them. The surgeon who advises a patient who is a potential candidate for hemorrhoidectomy to increase the fiber in his diet may be losing a surgical fee. Hospitals have more income when their beds stay full of sick or injured people. The bulk of most reimbursable health services centers around hospital, physician, nursing home, ambulatory care, and skilled nursing care in the home. These services are mostly illness oriented; the individual must play the role of patient in these settings. Health promotional activities such as comprehensive prenatal, maternal, and infant care; health education; childhood immunizations; and home services to enable the elderly to live independently are not covered by many insurers.

A system that financially supports illness care affects community health practice in several ways. The number and severity of health problems in a community increase when individuals postpone care because visits to the doctor or clinic mean greater expense — expense that they often cannot afford. Illness-oriented incentives create a basic societal valuing of illness care that, conversely, devalues wellness care. Health promotion and disease prevention efforts become second-ranked priorities in competition for scarce resources. In response to increased illness care, a greater proportion of community health practice is spent on treatment of disorders and rehabilitation, thus limiting the time and resources for prevention and health promotion. Prepayment methods and the growth of HMOs are a positive move in the direction of a more wellness-oriented financial incentive structure. An HMO has the incentive to offer preventive and health-promoting services such as early detection and treatment of symptoms, regular physical examinations, and health teaching.

CONFLICT WITH PUBLIC HEALTH VALUES

Competition in health care is a reality with which community health practice must cope. Although competition offers a number of benefits, it poses some dilemmas for community health that are not easily resolved. Values underlying the competition model are in direct conflict with several basic public health values (Ehlinger, 1982). Competition, for example, encourages service providers to be adversarial, to win. Public health operates on the basis of collaboration and cooperation (Ray & Flynn). Competition serves a selected market determined, in part, by those able to purchase products or services. Public health is committed to serving all persons in need, regardless of ability to pay (Beauchamp, 1975). The competition model focuses on individuals and is present oriented; public health is concerned with aggregates and is future oriented, emphasizing prevention. Competition establishes relatively fixed limits for service, while public health must remain flexible to be responsive to the total population's health needs.

The effect of these philosophical differences plus the constraints, such as civil service restrictions and political influences, under which most public health agencies must operate, make it very difficult for them to compete. They must still remain committed to providing the health promotion and disease prevention services to aggregates, which is their public trust. Yet competition seems necessary if they are to stay in business. Exclusion from health care competition, freedom from constraints, or some kind of special support may be needed to keep many of these programs alive. Competition may also serve as a stimulus for new and innovative community health services and the possible introduction of new roles and revenue sources for traditional public health agencies.

Summary

Many factors and events have influenced the current structure, function, and financing of community health services. Understanding these gives the community health nurse a stronger base for planning for the health of community populations.

Historically health care has progressed unevenly, marked by numerous influences. Primitive practices of early centuries were replaced with more advanced sanitary measures by the Greeks and Romans. The Middle-Ages saw a serious health decline with raging epidemics followed by extensive nineteenth century reform efforts in England and later in the United States.

Organized health care in the U.S. developed slowly. Public health problems, such as need for isolation of communicable disease and control of environmental pollution, prompted the gradual development of official interventions. For example, quarantines to control the spread of communicable disease, were imposed in the late 1700s. Sanitary reform was pursued more vigorously by the mid 1800s. Local, then state, health departments were formed starting in the late 1700s. By the early 1900s the federal government had assumed a more active role in public health with a proliferation of health, education, and welfare services.

For many centuries efforts to address community health needs have been undertaken by private individuals as well as public agencies. These two arms of service have not been coordinated in the past and only gradually during this century have begun to work together to form an emerging health care system.

The public arm of health services includes all government, tax-supported health agencies and occurs at four levels: local, state, national, and international. Each level concerns itself with the health needs of the population that its boundaries encompass. Each level has a different structure and set of functions.

Private health services are the unofficial arm of the community health system. They include voluntary nonprofit agencies as well as privately owned (proprietary) and for-profit agencies. Their financial support comes from voluntary contributions, bequests, or fees. Private health organizations often supplement and complement the work of official agencies.

The delivery and financing of community health services has been significantly affected by various legislative acts. These acts have prompted such innovations as health insurance and assistance for the poor, monies to train health personnel and conduct health research, standards for health planning and delivery, health protection for workers on the job, and prospective health care reimbursement.

Health care financing falls into three categories: third-party payers, direct consumer payment, and voluntary support. Several issues and trends have influenced community health care financing and delivery. They include early federal regulation, escalating health care costs, the HMO movement, attempts to institute national health insurance, increased competition in health care, and prospective reimbursement.

Changing health care financing has affected community health and its practice in three important ways. It has created disincentives for efficient use of resources; it has promoted incentives for illness care; and it has generated a conflict with basic public health values.

Study Questions

1. Debate the pros and cons of a strong federal role in health care provision as opposed to decentralized (state and local) control.
2. Describe three ways that escalating health care costs are influencing community health practice.
3. How does prospective reimbursement affect health care provision from the hospital's perspective? From a community health perspective?
4. Why does the competition model of health care provision pose problems for community health? Discuss the potential impact of competition on the poor and medically indigent.

References

American Public Health Association. (1975). The role of official local health agencies. *American Journal of Public Health, 65,* 189–192.

Beauchamp, D. E. (1975). Public health: Alien ethic in a strange land? *American Journal of Public Health, 65,* 1338–1339.

Davis, C. K. (1983). The federal role in changing health care financing. *Nursing Economics, 1*(1), 10–17.

Dowling, W. L. (1979). Prospective rate setting: Concept and practice. *Topics in Health Care Financing, 3*(2), 35–42.

Ehlinger, E. (1982). Implications of the competition model. *Nursing Outlook, 30,* 518–521.

Hanlon, J. J., & Pickett, G. E. (1984). *Public health: Administration and practice* (8th ed.). St. Louis: Times Mirror/Mosby.

Hyman, H. (1982). *Health planning: A systematic approach* (2nd ed.). Rockville, MD: Aspen Systems.

Joel, L. A. (1983). DRGs: The state of the art of reimbursement for nursing services. *Nursing and Health Care 4,* 560–563.

Known welfare fraud is only "tip of the iceberg." (1983, November). *U.S. News & World Report,* pp. 42–43.

Lewis, R. A. (1952). *Edwin Chadwick and the public health movement, 1832–1854.* New York: Longmans.

McNerney, W. J. (1980). Control of health care costs in the 1980s. *New England Journal of Medicine, 303,* 1088–1095.

Rapoport, J., Robertson, R. L., & Stewart, B. (1982). *Understanding health economics.* Rockville, MD: Aspen Systems.

Ray, D. & Flynn, B. (1980). Competition vs. cooperation in community health nursing. *Nursing Outlook, 28*(10), 626–630.

Roemer, M. I. (1984). The value of medical care for health promotion. *American Journal of Public Health, 74,* 243–248.

Shaffer, F. (1983). DRGs: History and overview. *Nursing and Health Care, 4,* 388–396.

Somers, A., & Somers, H. (1977). *Health and health care: Policies in perspective.* Germantown, MD: Aspen Systems.

Weiss, R. J. (1982). Competition in health care. *American Journal of Public Health, 72,* 655.

Wilner, D. M., Walkley, R. P., & O'Neill, E. J. (1978). *Introduction to public health* (7th ed.). New York: Macmillan.

World Health Organization. (1971). *Basic documents* (22nd ed.). Geneva: WHO.

Selected Readings

American Public Health Association. (1975). The role of official local health agencies. *American Journal of Public Health, 65,* 189–192.

Beauchamp, D. E. (1975, December). Public health: Alien ethic in a strange land? *American Journal of Public Health, 65,* 1338–1339.

Clark, E. J. (1981). The role of the states in the delivery of health services. *American Journal of Public Health, 71*(Suppl.), 59–69.

Davis, C. K. (1983). The federal role in changing health care financing. *Nursing Economics, 1*(1), 10–17.

Dowling, W. L. (1979). Prospective rate setting: Concept and practice. *Topics in Health Care Financing, 3*(2), 35–42.

Donabedian, D. (1980). What students should know about the health and welfare systems. *Nursing Outlook, 28,* 122–125.

Ehlinger, E. (1982). Implications of the competition model. *Nursing Outlook, 30,* 518–521.

Enthoven, A. C. (1978). Consumer-choice health plan: Inflation and inequity in health care today. Alternatives for cost control and an analysis of proposals for national health insurance. *New England Journal of Medicine, 298,* 650–658.

Farley, L., & Farley, B. (Eds.) (1980). *1980–1981 National directory of health/medicine organizations.* Bethesda, MD: Science and Health Publications.

Freeland, M., Calat, G., & Schendler, C. (1980). Projections of national health expenditures, 1980, 1985, and 1990. *Health Care Financing Review, 1*(3), 17.

Greenberg, W. (Ed.). (1978). *Competition in the health care sector: Past, present, and future.* Germantown, MD: Aspen Systems.

Hanlon, J. J., & Pickett, G. E. (1984). *Public health: Administration and practice* (8th ed.). St. Louis: Times Mirror/Mosby.

Hyman, H. (1982). *Health planning: A systematic approach* (2nd ed.). Rockville, MD: Aspen Systems.

Jain, S. C. (1981). Introduction and summary: Role of state and local governments in relation to personal health services. *American Journal of Public Health, 71*(Suppl.), 5–8.

Joel, L. A. (1983). DRGs: The state of the art of reimbursement for nursing services. *Nursing and Health Care, 4,* 560–563.

Known welfare fraud is only "tip of the iceberg." (1983, November). *U.S. News & World Report,* pp. 42–43.

Lewis, R. A. (1952). *Edwin Chadwick and the public health movement, 1832–1854.* New York: Longmans.

Luft, H. B. (1982). Health maintenance organizations and the rationing of medical care. *Milbank Memorial Fund quarterly/Health and society, 60,* 268.

McNerney, W. J. (1980). Control of health care costs in the 1980s. *New England Journal of Medicine, 303,* 1088–1095.

Moran, D. W. (1982). HMOs, competition, and the politics of minimum benefits. *Milbank Memorial Fund quarterly/Health and society, 59,* 190.

Morris, R. (1983). Will the growth of health and welfare services be resumed? *American Journal of Public Health, 73,* 732–733.

Powell, P. (1983). Fee-for-service. *Nursing Management, 14*(3), 13–15.

Rapoport, J., Robertson, R. L., & Stewart, B. (1982). *Understanding health economics.* Rockville, MD: Aspen Systems.

Ray, D. & Flynn, B. Competition vs. cooperation in community health nursing. *Nursing Outlook, 28*(10), 626–630.

Roemer, M. I. (1984). The value of medical care for health promotion. *American Journal of Public Health, 74,* 243–248.

Shaffer, F. (1983). DRGs: History and overview. *Nursing and Health Care, 4,* 388–396.

Somers, A., & Somers, H. (1977). *Health and health care: Policies in perspective.* Germantown, MD: Aspen Systems.

Torrens, P. R. (1978). *The American health care system.* St. Louis: C. V. Mosby.

Wasserman, P. (Ed.). (1981). *Health organizations of the United States, Canada, and the World: A directory of voluntary associations, professional societies, and other groups concerned with health and related fields* (5th ed.). Detroit, MI: Gale Research.

Weiss, R. J. (1982). Competition in health care. *American Journal of Public Health, 72,* 655.

Wilner, D. M., Walkley, R. P., & O'Neill, E. J. (1978). *Introduction to public health* (7th ed.). New York: Macmillan.

3

The Nature of Community Health Nursing

Within the family of nursing specialties, community health nursing sometimes seems like a young adult experiencing a developmental crisis. It has undergone an identity change from "public" to "community" health nursing that is not yet complete or clear in the minds of some. With practitioners involved in so many different roles and settings, its professional character is still evolving, yet surely the current debates about this field suggest a growing, dynamic profession. This chapter examines the emerging nature of community health nursing. After defining the field, it traces historic development, examines several influential factors in that development, and then discusses the major characteristics of contemporary community health nursing.

Defining Community Health Nursing

Any nursing specialty combines nursing theory with knowledge and skills germane to the specialty area (National League for Nursing, 1980). Community health nursing combines nursing with public health (American Nurses Association, 1980). It "synthesizes the body of knowledge from the public health sciences and professional nursing theories" (American Public Health Association, 1982). The purpose of this synthesis is to improve the health of the entire community. Thus, community health nursing can be defined as a field of practice that synthesizes knowledge and skills from nursing and public health and applies them toward the promotion of optimal health for the total community.

Contrary to the popular image, community health nursing does not serve only clients in the community (those outside the acute care setting). As we shall see, nurses with other specialties have moved into the community, while some community health nurses work in hospitals. Community health nursing makes its unique contribution to health care by the nature of its practice, which combines basic concepts from nursing and public health. Increasingly it is being recognized as a subspecialty of both these fields (Ruth & Partridge, 1978).

Historic Development

Community health nursing as practiced today is the product of growth and adaptation. It has amended its structure to accommodate the needs of a changing society, yet it has always maintained its initial goal of improved community health. Its development, which has been influenced by changes in nursing, public health, and society, can be traced through several stages. This chapter examines these stages and their societal causes.

Stages of Development

The history of public health nursing in the United States portrays continuing change and adaptation. Corresponding to fluctuations in national events, that change has been marked by sensitivity and responsiveness. The historical record reveals a professional nursing specialty that has been on the cutting edge of innovations in public health practice and has provided leadership to public health efforts. William Welch has been quoted as saying, "America's two greatest contributions to public health were the Panama Canal and the public health nurse" (cited in Hanlon & Pickett, 1984, p. 533).

We can identify three general stages in the development of community health nursing: (1) the district nursing stage, (2) the public health nursing stage, and (3) the emergence of community health nursing.

DISTRICT NURSING (1860–1900)

Organized home nursing care started as a voluntary service for the poor. In 1859, William Rathbone, an English philanthropist, became convinced of the value of home nursing as a result of private care given to his wife (Kalisch & Kalisch, 1978). He was the first to promote the establishment of a visiting nurse service for the sick poor in Liverpool. In the United States, the first community health nurse, Francis Root, pioneered home visits to the poor in New York City. Immediately following this, the first visiting nurses were employed by the New York City Mission in 1877. In 1885, district nursing associates were founded in Buffalo and, in 1886, in Boston and Philadelphia. These district associations served the sick poor exclusively, because patients with enough money had private home nursing care. Before their establishment, care of the sick poor had fallen to various religious and charitable groups that delivered sporadic and limited health care.

Although district nurses primarily cared for the sick, they also taught cleanliness and wholesome living to their patients, even in that early period. Florence Nightingale, who assisted William Rathbone by training home visiting nurses, referred to them as health nurses. Her ideas and methods helped influence home nursing practice in England and the United States. The work of district nurses focused almost exclusively on the care of individuals. They recorded temperatures and pulse rates and gave simple treatments under the immediate direction of a physician. They also instructed family members in personal hygiene, healthful living habits, and the care of the sick. Nursing educational programs at that time did not truly prepare nurses for these functions.

The early district nursing services were formed by voluntary organizations (Fig. 3-1). Funding came from contributions and, in some instances, from fees charged to patients on an ability-to-pay basis. The nursing services were administered by lay boards; even the actual nursing care was supervised by lay persons. In 1893, Lillian Wald initiated a district nursing service in New York City that, in contrast, provided nursing care under the supervision of nurses. Her service was associated administratively with the health department, an official agency, although most district nursing services at that time remained voluntary.

PUBLIC HEALTH NURSING (1900–1970)

By the turn of the century, district nursing began to broaden its focus to include the health and welfare of the public, not just of the poor. This new emphasis was part of a more general consciousness about public health. A growing sense of urgency about improving the health of all people led to an increase in the number of voluntary health agencies. These agencies supplemented the often ineffective work of government health departments. Specialized programs such as infant welfare, tuberculosis clinics, and venereal disease control were developed, causing a demand for nurses in establishments that included factories and schools. In 1902, the first school nurse in the United States was employed by the New York City Board of Education. By 1910, new federal laws made states and communities accountable for the health of their citizens.

The role of the district nurse expanded during this stage. Lillian Wald, a leading figure in this expansion, was the first to use the term *public health nursing* (Bullough & Bullough, 1979). District nursing had pioneered in

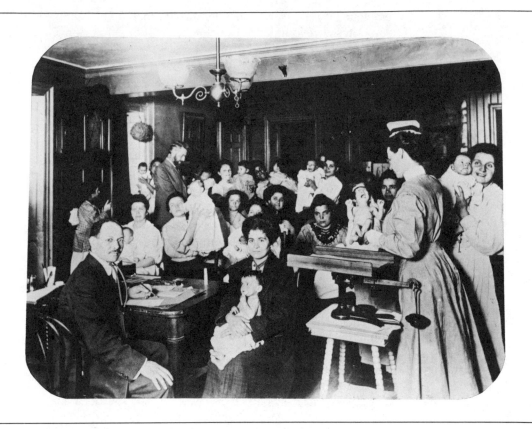

Figure 3-1
Examination of infants was part of early health department programs in which district nurses played a major role.

health teaching (Brainard, 1922, p. 208), disease prevention, and promotion of good health practices. Now, with a growing recognition of familial and environmental influences on health, public health nurses broadened their practice even more. Nurses working outside the hospital setting increased their knowledge and skills in specialized areas such as tuberculosis, school health, and mental disorders.

Then the family began to emerge as the unit of service. The multiple problems faced by many families started the trend toward nursing care generalized enough to meet a diversity of needs and provide continuity of care. By the 1920s public health nursing was acquiring more professional stature, in contrast to its earlier linkage with charity. It assumed greater leadership in improving and expanding health services and in increasing the standards of nursing education and practice. Public health nurses gradually gained more autonomy in such areas as bedside care and instruction of good health practices to families and community groups. Their collaborative relationships with other community health groups grew as the need to avoid gaps and duplication of services became apparent. Public health nurses also started to keep better records of their care giving.

During this stage, the institutional base for public health nursing shifted to the government. Public health nursing services, which emphasized health guidance but also provided care for the ill, were offered through local health departments. As a result, rural public health nursing also expanded. Some of the district nursing services, now known as visiting nurse associations (VNAs), remained under the direction of voluntary agencies and offered their own nursing services of bedside care. In some places, city or county health departments joined administratively and financially with VNAs to provide a combination of services, such as bedside care and health guidance to families.

The public health nursing stage was characterized by service to the public, although the family was recognized as the primary unit of care (Fig. 3-2). Official health agencies, which placed greater emphasis on disease prevention and health promotion, provided the chief institutional base.

Figure 3-2
The public health nurse, carrying her bag of equipment and supplies, made regular home visits to provide physical and psychological care as well as health teaching to families.

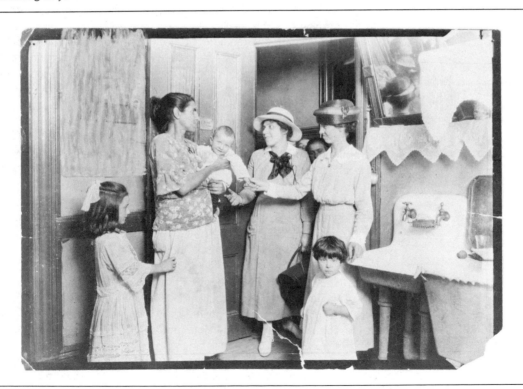

EMERGENCE OF COMMUNITY HEALTH NURSING (1970–PRESENT)

The emergence of community health nursing heralded a new era. The strengths of traditional public health nursing combined with a new consciousness of service to the total community. By the mid-1960s a number of events had occurred to cause concern about the nature of public health nursing.

First, nursing education, recognizing the importance of public health content, began to require course work in public health for all baccalaureate graduates. This prerequisite meant that graduates were expected to incorporate public health principles into nursing practice, regardless of their sphere of service. Consequently, some people questioned whether public health nursing retained any unique content.

A second source of confusion over the definition of community health nursing arose from the fact that hospital nurses followed community cases and public health nurses followed hospital cases. Hospital walls seemed permeable, for community health nurses were not the only nurses practicing in the community.

Third, many new kinds of community health services appeared, and demands on community health nurses expanded their role. Furthermore, other community health professionals assumed responsibilities that had traditionally been the domain of public health nursing. Some school counselors in Oregon, for example, began coordinating home visits previously done by school nurses, and health educators, who are part of a new discipline that has developed in the last decade, took over large segments of client education (Chavigny & Kroske, 1983, p. 312). Social workers, too, provided services that appeared to overlap with community health nursing roles. Health educators, counselors, social workers, and others working in community health came prepared with different backgrounds and emphases in their practice. Their contributions were and still are important. Their presence, however, forced community health nurses to reexamine their own contribution to the public's health and incorporate stronger interdisciplinary and collaborative approaches into their practice. These developments raised several important questions. Should community health nursing, which had become generalized in practice, carve out a new specialization? Should it incorporate more specialized skills, such as physical assessment, into its generalized practice?

Fourth, accelerated changes in health care provision, technology, and social issues made increasing demands on community health nurses' ability to adapt to new patterns of practice. By the mid-1970s various community health nursing leaders had identified knowledge and skills needed for more effective community health nursing practice (Roberts & Freeman, 1973); this information had only begun to be incorporated in nursing school curricula.

Still, the direction in which community health nursing was moving had become clear — to care for, not simply in, the community (Freeman, 1973).

Its primary responsibility was the health of aggregates; thus its focus turned to more comprehensive health care and diversity of programs. This shift made the term *community health nursing* more functional than the term *public health nursing;* this text, however, uses the two interchangeably. Community health nursing meant population-oriented nursing of problems along the entire range of the wellness-illness continuum, although health promotion was increasingly emphasized. Community health nurses were carving out new roles for themselves, including independent practice. Collaboration and interdisciplinary teamwork were recognized as crucial to effective community nursing. Practitioners served in many kinds of agencies and institutions, such as senior citizen centers, ambulatory services, mental health clinics, and family planning programs, as well as in many nonhealth settings; they followed clients before, during, and after hospitalization. Documentation of nursing care, program evaluation, peer review, and definitive community nursing research were of high priority. This field of nursing had begun to assume its responsibility as a full professional partner in community health.

Table 3-1 summarizes the most important changes that have occurred during community health nursing's three stages. It shows these changes in terms of focus, nursing orientation, service emphasis, and institutional base.

Societal Influences

Many factors influenced the growth of community health nursing. To understand better the nature of this field, we must recognize the forces that began and continue to shape its development. Five are particularly significant: advanced technology, progress in causal thinking, changes in education, the changing role of women, and the consumer movement.

Table 3-1
Development of Community Health Nursing

Stages	Focus	Nursing Orientation	Service Emphasis	Institutional Base (Agencies)
District nursing (1860–1900)	Sick poor	Individual	Curative; beginning of preventive	Voluntary; some government
Public health nursing (1900–1970)	Needy public	Family	Curative; preventive	Government; some voluntary
Emergence of community health nursing (1970–present)	Total community	Population	Health promotion; illness prevention	Many kinds; some independent practice

Advanced Technology

Advanced technology has contributed in many ways to shaping the practice of community health nursing. For example, technological innovation has greatly improved health care, nutrition, and life-style and caused a concomitant increase in life expectancy. Consequently, community health nurses direct much of their effort toward meeting the needs of older persons and working with chronic conditions. Advanced technology has also been a strong force behind industrialization, large-scale employment, and urbanization. We are now primarily an urban society; health planners project that 80 percent of the U.S. population will live in urban areas by the year 2000 (Matek, 1973). Population density leads to many health-related problems, particularly the spread of disease and increased stress. Community health nurses are learning how to combat these urban health problems. In addition, changes in transportation and high job mobility have affected the health scene. As people travel and relocate, they are separated from families and traditional support systems; community health nurses frequently help people cope with the accompanying stress. New products, equipment, methods, and energy sources in industry have also increased environmental pollution and industrial hazards. Community health nurses have become involved in related research, occupational health, and preventive education. Technological innovation has helped promote medicine's complex diagnostic and treatment procedures, thus making illness-oriented care more dramatic and desirable, as well as more costly. Community health nurses face a challenge to demonstrate the physical and economic value of wellness-oriented care.

Finally, innovations in communications and computer technology have shifted America from an industrial society to an "information society" (Naisbitt, 1982). Our economy is now built on information — the production and marketing of knowledge. Community health nurses, now more than ever, are in the business of information distribution and use new computer technologies to enhance the efficiency and effectiveness of their services. Associated with high use of technology, societal needs for "high touch" (greater human contact), stress management, and treatments for other technology-induced health problems will continue to shape the role of community health nursing in the future (Powell, 1984).

Progress in Causal Thinking

Progress in causal thinking in the health sciences and in epidemiology in particular has significantly affected the nature of community health nursing. The germ theory of disease causation, established in the late 1800s, was the first real breakthrough in control of communicable disease. Nurses incorporated the teaching of cleanliness and personal hygiene into basic nursing care. A second advance in causal thinking was initiated by the tripartite view that called attention to the interactions between a causative agent, a susceptible host, and the environment. This information offered community health nursing new ways to control and prevent health disorders. For example, nurses could decrease the vulnerability of an individual (host) by teaching the person a healthier life-style. They could instigate measles vaccination programs as a means of preventing the organism (agent) from infecting children. They could promote proper disinfection of a school's swimming pool (environment) to prevent disease. Further progress in causal thinking led to the recognition that not just one single agent but many factors — a multiple causation approach — contribute to a disease or health disorder. A food poisoning outbreak that is associated with a restaurant is caused not only by the salmonella organism but also by improper food handling and storage, lack of adherence to minimum food preparation standards, and lack of adequate health department supervision and enforcement.

Community health nurses can control health problems by examining all possible causes and then attacking strategic causal points. Current causal thinking has led to a broader awareness of unhealthy conditions; in addition to disease, problems such as accidents and environmental pollution are major targets of concern. As a result, work-related stress, environmental hazards, chemical food additives, and alcohol and nicotine consumption during pregnancy are all examples of concerns in community health nursing practice.

Changes in Education

Changes in education, especially those in nursing education, have had an important influence on community health nursing practice. Education, once an opportunity for a privileged few, has become widely available; it is now considered a basic right and a necessity for a vital society. When people's understanding of their environment grows, an increased understanding of health is usually involved. For the community health nurse, health teaching has steadily assumed greater importance in practice. For the learner, education has led to much more responsibility. As a result, people feel that they have a right to know and question the reasons behind the care they receive. Community health nurses have had to shift from planning *for* clients to collaborating *with* clients.

Education has had other effects. The scientific approach, considered basic to progress, has created a dramatic increase in knowledge. The wealth of information relevant to community health nursing practice means that nursing students have more content to assimilate, and practicing community health nurses have to make greater efforts to keep abreast. In contrast to earlier times when nurses worked as apprentices in hospitals or health agencies and perfunctorily followed orders, now educational programs, including many in continuing education, prepare nurses to think for themselves in the application of theory to practice. Community health nursing has always required a fair measure of independent thinking and self-reliance; now community health nurses need skills in such areas as family and community assessment, decision making, and collaborative functioning. As the result of expanding education, community health nurses have had to reexamine their practice and clarify their roles.

Changing Role of Women

The changing role of women has profoundly affected nursing and community health nursing. In the past century, the women's rights movement has made considerable progress. Women have achieved the right to vote and have gained greater economic independence by entering the labor force. Women today have more education and consequently more influence than did women in the past. The percentage of women in professions such as medicine, law, or engineering has increased, although it is proportionately smaller than that of men. Many women are managing the dual careers of job and family. These gains have increased the number of women entering nursing, a profession whose responsibilities and recognition have also improved.

Changes resulting from the women's rights movement continue to occur. Nurses still struggle for equality — equality of job selection, equal pay for equal work, and equal opportunity for advancement outside the nursing hierarchy. If community health nurses are to influence the field of community health, they need status and authority equal to that of their colleagues. This step will require nurses to demonstrate their competence and learn to be assertive in assuming roles as full professional partners. In community health, as in society generally, women hold very few administrative or policy-making positions. Although the majority of nurses are female, a much higher proportion of male than female nurses serve in leadership capacities. The women's movement has contributed to community health nursing's gains in assuming leadership roles, but a need for much greater influence and involvement remains.

Consumer Movement

The consumer movement has also affected the nature of community health nursing. Consumers have become more militant, as evidenced in various boycotts and tax revolts. They are demanding their rights in many areas, including health care, regardless of sex, race, color, or socioeconomic level. Consumers now assert their right to be informed about and to participate in decisions that affect them. This movement has stimulated some basic changes in the philosophy of community health nursing. Health care consumers are viewed as active members of the health team, rather than as passive recipients of care. They may contract with the community health nurse for personal or family care, represent the community on the local health board, or act as ombudsmen, for example, investigate complaints and report findings in order to protect the quality of care in the local nursing home. This assumption of consumers' responsibility for their own health means that the community health nurse supplements more often than supervises the client's care.

The consumer movement has also contributed to increased concern for the quality of health services. Quality assurance programs, peer review, and tighter evaluation are now part of most health care accreditation requirements. Community health nursing has been led to improve its evaluation of services and programs. Many community health nursing agencies have begun to implement forms of peer review.

The consumer movement has increased the demand for more humane, personalized health care. Dissatisfied with fragmented services offered by impersonal health workers, consumers now seek holistic care. A group of senior citizens living in a high-rise apartment building need more than a series of social workers, nutritionists, recreational therapists, nurses, and other callers ascertaining a variety of specific needs and starting a proliferation of programs. Community health nurses, as members of the health team, increasingly aim to provide coordinated, comprehensive, and personalized services — a case management approach.

Characteristics of Community Health Nursing

Thus far this chapter has defined community health nursing and examined events and influences that have shaped its present practice. Now the nature of community health nursing can be observed more closely. Six characteristics of community health nursing are especially salient: (1) it is a field of nursing; (2) it combines public health with nursing; (3) it is population oriented; (4) it emphasizes health; (5) it involves interdisciplinary collaboration; and (6) it promotes client participation.

Field of Nursing

Community health nursing is a field of nursing; its basic knowledge and skills are those of professional nursing practice. It seeks to give humanistic, accessible, and holistic care. For instance, community health nurses are nursing when they express concern for a group of mothers and tired children sitting on hard chairs for three hours in a clinic hallway, or when they consequently change the appointment scheduling policy and establish a comfortable waiting area. They engage in nursing when they institute a discharge planning system with local hospitals to provide continuity of care. When they visit older clients in their homes to give personal care, instruction, and comfort, they are again nursing.

Community health nursing is a nursing speciality; nursing theory forms its foundation and the nursing process is one of its basic tools, but community health nursing adds concepts, knowledge, and skills from other disciplines to become a distinctive practice.

Elements of Public Health

In addition to nursing theory, community health nursing incorporates public health content. Knowledge of the following elements of public health is essential to community health nursing (Hanlon & Pickett, 1984; Milbank Memorial Fund Commission [MMFC], 1976; White, 1982; Williams, 1977; 1983):

1. The history and philosophy of public health, including the emphasis on the greatest good for the greatest number
2. The concept of aggregates — assessing needs, planning and providing services, and evaluating services' impact on population groups — including aggregate-level decision making
3. Priority of preventive and health-promoting strategies over curative strategies
4. The means for measurement and analysis of community health problems, including epidemiologic concepts and biostatistics
5. Influence of environmental factors on aggregate health
6. Principles underlying management and organization for community health, since the goal of public health is accomplished through organized community efforts
7. Public policy analysis and development

There are many ways in which community health nursing incorporates public health knowledge into its practice. For example, some school nurses in Cincinnati, who were working with city health authorities, were concerned with the failure of many children to receive adequate immunization. They used health statistics, specifically a review of school immunization records, to determine immunization needs of school children. Next they set up an immunization program that successfully met the needs of the community (Anthony, Reed, Leff, Huffer, & Stephens, 1977). They effectively combined biostatistics with a community focus to carry out their goals.

Another nurse, working in a city jail emergency room and inpatient ward (Chavigny, 1976), noticed that prisoners (most of whom were alcoholics) appeared to have very low self-esteem, which consequently impeded their health progress. She designed an experimental program in which staff (nurses, physicians, and police officers) treated the patients with greater respect. The results were improved care and increased patient self-respect. By studying these patients' needs through an epidemiologic approach, she combined public health with nursing.

As community health nurses carefully analyze their caseloads, assess group and community needs, establish priorities, and plan, implement, and evaluate services, they are utilizing public health management and organization principles. For example, one community health nurse discovered a concern in the community whose needs she was assessing about the high incidence of dental decay among its school children. Because of the relationships she had already established within the community, she was able to help form a committee that studied the problem and initiated in one school a pilot dental health program that was to be evaluated a year later. She continues to assist this committee in its efforts (Flynn, Gottschalk, Ray, & Selmanoff, 1978).

Each of the nurses mentioned here has demonstrated an important characteristic of community health nursing — the combination of fundamental public health concepts and nursing.

Population Emphasis

The central mission of public health practice is to improve the health of population groups (Kark, 1974, p. 319). Community health nursing shares this essential feature: it is population oriented, concerned with the personal and environmental health of population groups. A population may consist of a community health nurse's caseload or all the patients in a clinic. It may be a scattered group with common characteristics, such as people at high risk of developing coronary heart disease or all the unwed mothers in the county. It may include all the people living in a district, census tract, city, or nation. In fact, the terms *population* and *community* (as defined in chapter 1) can be used interchangeably.

Working with individuals and families is also a part of community health nursing; however, such work must incorporate a population-oriented focus, a feature that distinguishes it from other nursing specialties. The difference is in degree. Basic nursing focuses on individuals and community health nursing focuses on aggregates (Williams, 1977), but the many variations in client needs and nursing roles inevitably cause some overlap. Figure 3-3 shows these distinctions between basic and community health nursing.

A population-oriented focus requires the observation of relationships. When working with individuals, families, or groups, the community health nurse does not consider them separately but rather in relationship to the rest of the community. When a case of hepatitis is diagnosed, for example, the community health nurse does more than simply treat it. The nurse tries to stop spread of the infection, locate the possible source, and prevent its reoccurrence in the community. As a result of their population-oriented focus,

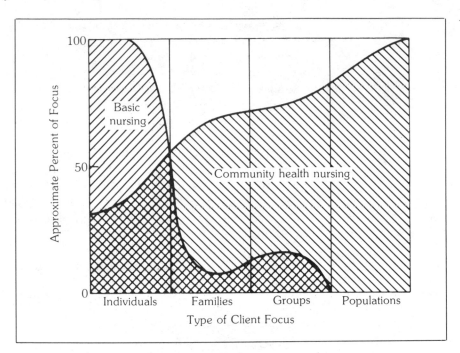

Figure 3-3
Difference in client focus
between basic nursing and
community health nursing.

community health nurses seek to discover possible groups with a common health need, such as expectant mothers, or groups at high risk of developing a common health problem, such as potential diabetics or child abuse victims. Community health nurses continually look for ways to increase environmental quality. They work to prevent health problems by, for example, promoting safety measures in school playgrounds or offering more nourishing, easily prepared meals for nursing home residents. A population-oriented focus involves a whole new outlook and set of attitudes. The community is the client; service is provided to multiple and overlapping groups.

Wellness Emphasis

Another distinguishing characteristic of community health nursing is its emphasis on positive health, or wellness. Chapter 1 discussed the wellness-illness continuum. Acute care nursing and medicine deal primarily with the illness end of that continuum because they treat health problems. In contrast, community health nursing has a primary charge to prevent health problems from occurring and to promote a higher level of health. For example, although a community health nurse may assist a woman at home with postpartum fatigue and depression, the nurse also works to *prevent* such problems among other mothers by establishing a prenatal class and encouraging proper rest, nutrition, adequate help, and reduction of stress (see Fig. 3-4). Indi-

72

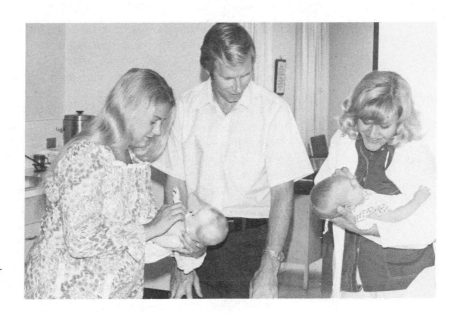

Figure 3-4
This prenatal class offers
couples an opportunity to
gain skill in caring for a
new baby. The nurse dem-
onstrates while the parents
practice with a doll.

vidualized care is important, but prevention of aggregate problems in community health practice reflects more accurately its philosophy and benefits a larger number of people.

Community health nurses concentrate on the wellness end of the wellness-illness continuum in a variety of ways. They teach proper nutrition or family planning, demonstrate aseptic technique for home care of a wound, encourage regular physical and dental checkups, start exercise classes or physical fitness programs, and promote healthy interpersonal relationships. Their goal is to help the community reach its optimal level of wellness.

This emphasis on wellness changes the community health nursing role from a reactive to a proactive stance. It places a greater responsibility on community health nurses to search for cases that require their intervention. In clinical nursing and medicine, the patients seek out professional assistance because they have health problems. As Williams (1977) puts it, "Patients select themselves into the care system, and the providers' role is to deal with what the patients bring to them." Community health nurses, in constrast, seek out potential health problems. They identify high-risk groups and institute preventive programs. They watch for early signs of child neglect or abuse and intervene when any occur, often long before a request for help is made. They look for possible environmental hazards in the community, such as smoking in public places, and work with appropriate authorities to correct them. A wellness emphasis requires taking initiative and making sound judgments, which are characteristics of an effective community health nurse.

Interdisciplinary Collaboration

Community health nurses work as full members of a health care team. Such coordination and cooperation are required in a practice that deals with population groups. Individualized efforts and specialized programs, when planned in isolation, can lead to fragmentation and gaps in health services. For example, without collaboration, a well-child clinic may be started in a community that already has a strong early and periodic developmental screening and testing program; at the same time, community prenatal services may be nonexistent. Interdisciplinary collaboration is also important in individualized practice, since nurses need to plan with the physician, social worker, physical therapist, or other involved health professional and keep them informed of clients' health status; however, it is an even greater necessity in working with population groups.

Effective collaboration requires team members who are strong individuals. A variety of expertise and ideas, together with a commitment to team goals, leads to the best solutions. Community health nurses who think and act independently make a great contribution to the team effort. In appropriate situations, community health nurses function autonomously, making independent judgments. They also function interdependently, working with members of other disciplines, for example, serving on community advisory boards or health planning committees.

Interdisciplinary collaboration requires clarification of each team member's role, a primary reason for community health nurses to understand the nature of their practice. When planning a citywide immunization program with a community group, for example, community health nurses can explain the ways they might contribute to the program's objectives. They can offer to contact key lay individuals, with whom they have established relationships, in order to help influence community acceptance of the program. They can share their knowledge of the public's preference about times and locations to offer the program. They can help organize and give the immunizations, thus assuring humanistic service, as well as influence planning for follow-up and continuity of care.

Consumer Participation

A characteristic of community health nursing that is sometimes overlooked is the encouragement of consumer participation in health care. Our examination of the consumer movement discussed consumers' rights to health care and to involvement in health care's decision making. However, consumers are frequently intimidated by health professionals and uninformed about health and health care. They do not know what information to ask for and are hesitant to act assertively. A Mexican-American woman brought her two-year-old son, who had symptoms resembling those of scurvy, to a clinic.

Recognizing a vitamin C deficiency, the physician told her to feed the boy large quantities of orange juice but gave no explanation. Several weeks later, she returned; the child was much worse. After questioning her, the nurse discovered that the mother had been feeding the child large amounts of an orange soft drink, not knowing the difference between that and orange juice. Obviously, the quality of care is affected when the consumer does not understand and cannot participate in the health care process.

The goal of public health, "to protect, promote, and restore people's health" (Sheps, 1976, p. 3), requires a partnership effort. Just as learning cannot take place in schools without student participation, the goals of public health cannot be realized without consumer participation. Community health nursing's efforts toward health improvement can go only so far. Client's health status and health behavior will not change unless they accept and apply community health nurses' proposals.

Community health nurses encourage consumer participation in several ways. They can promote the client's autonomy. Without realizing it, health professionals can easily cause their clients to depend upon them. Although providing nurturance and guidance sometimes meets the professional's needs, it may prove a great disservice to clients who need to be self-reliant. An elderly couple had been receiving three visits a week from a community health nurse for assistance with the wife's surgical dressing changes and bath. During the visits the nurse taught the husband how to perform these procedures. She also showed him how to prepare simple, nutritious meals, and together they arranged with a Meals on Wheels service to bring the couple's dinners for a few weeks. She encouraged them to contact other community resources for assistance with shopping, housework, and transportation to the doctor's office. She reduced her visits to one a week, then to one a month, and, when the couple agreed that they were able to manage on their own, the relationship ended. Independence and feelings of self-worth are closely related. By treating people as independent adults, with trust and respect, community health nurses help promote self-reliance and the ability to function independently.

Community health nurses encourage consumer participation by promoting clients' sense of responsibility for their own health. When consumers feel that their health and that of the community are their, and not the health professionals', responsibility, they will take a much more active interest in promoting it (Watkin, 1978). The process of taking responsibility for developing one's own health potential is called *self-care* (Levin, 1978; Norris, 1979), a concept that has gained considerable prominence in recent years. Nurses foster self-care by treating clients as adults capable of managing their own affairs, not, as Norris puts it, "as weak, needy, unintelligent, . . . bad, irresponsible, children" (1979, p. 486). Nurses can encourage clients to negotiate health care goals and practices, make their own appointments, contact their own resources, and learn ways to monitor their own health.

Consumer participation is promoted when clients are treated as partners on the health care team. The goal is collaborating with clients rather than working for clients. As consumers are treated with respect and trust and, as a result, gain confidence and skill in self-care — promoting their own health and that of their community — their contribution to health care services will become increasingly valuable. The consumer perspective in planning and delivering health services makes those services relevant to consumer needs. Community health nurses encourage the involvement of health care consumers by soliciting their ideas and opinions, by inviting them to participate on health boards and committees, and by using contracts for care that give them equal authority in choosing services.

Conceptual Framework for Community Health Nursing

As we have seen throughout this chapter, community health nursing combines many concepts and principles to form the basis for its practice. We shall summarize them to evince a conceptual framework for understanding the nature of community health nursing.

Practice Priorities

Three fundamental concepts are evident: prevention, protection, and promotion. Prevention includes the activities aimed at avoiding the occurrence of illness, as in enforcement of seat belt use, or minimizing its effect to the greatest extent possible, as with worker rehabilitation programs. Protection involves efforts to shield the public from elements in the environment that are harmful to health. These elements can range from obvious harmful physical agents, like cigarette smoke or lead in furniture paint that may be ingested by teething toddlers, to less obvious agents, like work stress and bereavement. Promotion refers to activities that maintain and enhance the community's level of wellness. These, too, cover a wide range from such efforts as a community-wide parks improvement program to family planning. White describes these concepts as "practice priorities" (White, 1982, p. 528). They make up one aspect of community health nursing's distinctive emphasis, the long-range goal and priority of moving people ever nearer wellness on the wellness-illness continuum.

Practice Interventions

To accomplish the practice priorities, we can identify three categories of interventions: education, engineering, and enforcement (White, 1982). They provide varying degrees of "persuasion" for enhancing the accomplishment of public health goals. By *education* we mean the nursing actions of providing information to encourage people to voluntarily modify their behavior in health-promoting ways. Typical is encouraging proper diet and exercise. *Engineering* is a stronger form of persuasion. Nursing actions directly or indirectly manage the variables in the environment to reduce health risks. That is, specific actions are taken, like immunization against disease, to prevent health problems. *Enforcement* uses more coercive measures, such as laws prohibiting child abuse or intake of harmful chemicals. Community health nursing employs these regulations and all three interventions to protect the public, prevent illness or disability, and promote health. These varying levels of persuasion are discussed in chapter 20 as three types of strategies for community health nursing management of change.

Scope of Practice

The extent of community health nursing's activity and influence still needs to be clarified. What does it encompass? The scope of community health nursing practice can be understood by answering the questions, What is practiced? and For whom? We have addressed the first question, What? as protection from health-endangering agents, prevention of illness and disability, and promotion of wellness. These practice priorities represent a trend, as we have seen in our historical review of community health nursing, away from a curative emphasis to a strong emphasis on the preventive and promotive end of the scale. The "For whom?" dimension covers a broad range from individuals to worldwide aggregates. Community health nursing, drawing on its public health foundations, maintains a conscious aggregate commitment. Wherever the nurse is engaged in practice along the individual-to-aggregate scale, the nurse still asks, What populations are affected or at risk? What are their needs? How can those needs best be served? For example, a community health nurse working with a day care center, when truly aggregate oriented, does not limit practice to the individuals in that center. Instead, the nurse considers the day care staff, its children, and their parents as three related population groups for assessment and intervention. Furthermore, the nurse with an aggregate orientation looks beyond the single day care center to clusters of day care centers in the community as potential populations for service. It is the goal of public health to reduce premature death, disease, disability, and discomfort and to protect, restore and promote people's health for the good of the entire community (MMFC, 1976, p. 3).

Figure 3-5 describes the scope of community health nursing practice on two axes. The horizontal axis shows the range from individuals to aggregates. The vertical axis exhibits the curative-preventive range. Placement of basic nursing, medicine, epidemiology, and public health—community health nursing in their respective quadrants evinces a clearer picture of the various disciplines' practice fields. Nursing and medicine both emphasize interventions at the individual end of the horizontal axis. Medicine is mostly curative; nursing

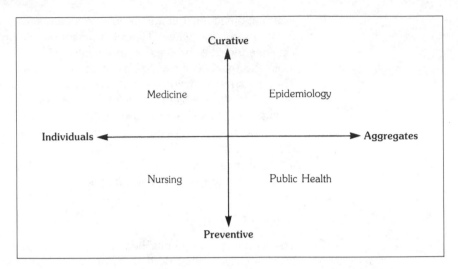

Figure 3-5
The scope of community
health nursing practice.

ranges along the vertical axis to include curative, restorative, and preventive services. Epidemiology, originally a branch of medicine, shifted its focus from acute disease to chronic and disabling conditions and preventive efforts, thus moving down the vertical axis. Its concern is always with aggregates. Public health and community health nursing emphasize aggregates and the promotion of high-level wellness.

Health Determinants

We have discussed community health nursing's practice priorities, interventions, and scope. A further set of variables in our conceptual framework must be considered — the factors that influence health positively or negatively. Four contributing elements were identified by the Canadian government in 1974 and studied in the United States (Public Health Service, 1979, p. 8). They form the basis for the health determinants in our conceptual framework (White, 1982). First are human biologic factors, those physiological defenses and vulnerabilities that influence who is at risk. Second are environmental factors, any external agents or conditions (including economic ones) capable of enhancing or inhibiting health. Third are the adequacies and inadequacies of the health care system, the medical-technological-organizational determinants. Finally, there are social factors, such as behaviors and life-styles, that influence health. A 1976 study of these variables suggested that the largest contributor to death in the United States (based on the then ten leading causes was unhealthy behaviors or life-style (accounting for about 50 percent of deaths). The other determinants were environmental factors

(20 percent), human biologic factors (20 percent), and inadequacies in the health care system (10 percent) (Public Health Service, 1979, p. 9).

Community Health Nursing Dynamics

There are two dynamics, or driving forces, energizing community health nursing practice. They are the nursing process and the valuing process (White, 1982). The nursing process, which includes assessment, diagnosis, planning, implementation, and evaluation, provides the means for analyzing healthy needs and solving health problems. Chapter 7 explores it in greater depth as a tool for enhancing community health. Its application to community health problem solving and management of community health nursing practice can be seen throughout the book.

The valuing process, a second dynamic, guides community health nursing actions. To value something is to judge it worthy. What we value determines our priorities, commitments, and behavior. Public health holds to several significant values, some of which were discussed in chapter 2. For example, public health subscribes to the greatest good for the greatest number, a concept that conflicts with our society's emphasis on individualism (Beauchamp, 1976). It bases its practice on collaboration and cooperation and believes in advocacy for the underserved and disadvantaged (Ehlinger, 1982). Values also influence consumers' attitudes and behaviors and dictate their responses to health care interventions. Chapter 5 examines values and health.

We now have the variables needed to describe the nature of community health nursing practice. Figure 3-6 exhibits them in a conceptual model that incorporates the practice priorities, interventions, scope, and health determinants with the nursing process and valuing dynamics.

Summary

Community health nursing works to promote optimal health for aggregates. It achieves this goal by applying knowledge and skills from nursing and from public health.

Historically, the specialty of community health nursing developed through three stages. The district nursing stage began in 1860 with voluntary home nursing care for the poor. Sometimes called *health nurses,* these specialists treated the sick and taught wholesome living to patients. The public health nursing stage began in 1900 and lasted until about 1970. It was characterized by a consciousness of the general public and its health care. The institutional base shifted to the government. The family became the primary unit of care. The community health nursing stage began around 1970 and has continued to the present. Nursing schools began to require course content in public

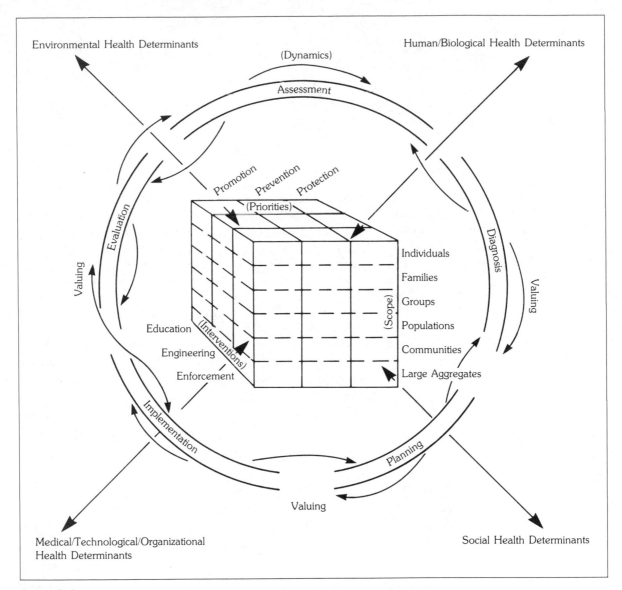

Figure 3-6
A conceptual model of
community health nursing.

health for all baccalaureate graduates. This stage made it clear that community nursing involved more than merely working in the community. Roles expanded in many different directions.

Five major societal influences have shaped the development of community health nursing. Advanced technology has solved some health care problems and created others; thus nurses' practice has focused greater attention on aging, chronic illness, and prevention. Progress in causal thinking has broadened the nurses' perspective to multiple causes, including stress, environmental hazards, and the community structure. Changes in education have led community health nurses to emphasize collaborating with clients rather than planning for clients. The changing role of women has helped to open new avenues of leadership for nurses in community health. Finally, the consumer movement has increased the public's concern for quality health service. As consumers have assumed responsibility for their own health, the community health nurse has become, in many instances, a catalyst to assist clients toward autonomy in health.

There are six important characteristics of community health nursing:

1. It is a field of nursing, a specialty within the larger discipline.
2. It combines the specialized knowledge of public health with nursing practice.
3. It has a population-oriented focus.
4. It emphasizes wellness rather than disease or illness.
5. It involves interdisciplinary collaboration, that is, teamwork, with other professionals.
6. It promotes client participation by fostering a sense of responsibility among people for their own health.

A conceptual framework for community health nursing includes five sets of variables. Its practice priorities are prevention, protection, and promotion. Its interventions are education, engineering, and enforcement. Its scope of practice encompasses the range from individuals to aggregates, emphasizing the aggregate end of the individual-to-aggregate scale and the preventive end of the curative-prevention scale. Four health determinants are factors to be considered in designing practice interventions. They are human biologic determinants, environmental determinants, medical-technological-organizational determinants, and social-behavioral determinants. Finally, two essential dynamics, the nursing process and the valuing process, guide community health nursing practice.

Study Questions

1. What is one area of public health knowledge that makes community health nursing a nursing specialty? Describe how you might use it in actual practice.
2. Select one societal influence on the development of community health nursing and discuss its continuing impact. What other events are occurring today that shape community health nursing practice?
3. Describe a situation in community health nursing practice in which use of the practice intervention of education would be most appropriate. Do

the same with engineering and enforcement. Discuss what made you match each situation with that intervention.

4. Assume you have received a referral to make a home visit to a 75-year-old man living alone whose wife recently died. Besides assessing his individual needs, what additional factors might you consider for assessment that would indicate an aggregate orientation?

References

American Nurses Association, Community Health Nursing Division. (1980). *A conceptual model of community health nursing* (Pub. No. CH-10 2M 5/80). Kansas City, MO: Author.

American Public Health Association. (1982). Definition and role of public health nursing in the delivery of health care (Policy Statement No. 8132). *American Journal of Public Health, 72,* 210–212.

Anthony, N., Reed, M., Leff, A., Hoffer, J., & Stephens, B. (1977). Immunization: Public health programming through law enforcement. *American Journal of Public Health, 67,* 763–764.

Beauchamp, D. E. (1976). Public health as social justice. *Inquiry, 13,* 3–14.

Brainard, A. M. (1922). *The evolution of public health nursing.* Philadelphia: W. B. Saunders.

Bullough, V., & Bullough, B. (1979). *The care of the sick: The emergence of modern nursing.* New York: Neale, Watson.

Chavigny, K. (1976). Self-esteem for the alcoholic: An epidemiologic approach. *Nursing Outlook, 24,* 636–639.

Chavigny, K. H., & Kroske, M. (1983). Public health nursing in crisis. *Nursing Outlook, 31,* 312–316.

Ehlinger, E. (1982). Implications of the competition model. *Nursing Outlook, 30,* 518–521.

Flynn, B., Gottschalk, J., Ray, D., & Selmanoff, E. (1978). One master's curriculum in community health nursing. *Nursing Outlook, 26,* 633–637.

Freeman, R. (1973). The dilemma of public health nursing today. In D. Roberts and R. Freeman (Eds.), *Redesigning nursing education for public health: Report of the conference.* (Pub. No. [HRA] 75-75) (pp. 9–17) Bethesda, MD: U.S. Department of Health, Education and Welfare.

Hanlon, J. J., & Pickett, G. E. (1984). *Public health: Administration and practice.* (8th ed.) St. Louis: Times Mirror/Mosby.

Kalisch, P., & Kalisch, B. (1978). *The advance of American nursing.* Boston: Little, Brown.

Kark, S. L. (1974). *Epidemiology and community medicine.* New York: Appleton-Century-Crofts.

Levin, L. (1978). Self-care: An emerging component of the health care system. *Hospital & Health Services Administration, 23,* 17.

Matek, S. J. (1973). Some key features in the emerging context for future health policy decisions in America. In D. Roberts and R. Freeman (Eds.), *Redesigning nursing education for public health: Report of the conference.* (Pub. No. [HRA] 75-75). Bethesda, MD: U.S. Department of Health, Education and Welfare.

Milbank Memorial Fund Commission. (1976). *Higher education for public health: A report.* New York: Prodist.

Naisbitt, J. (1982). *Megatrends.* New York: Warner Books.

National League for Nursing. (1980). *Community health nursing: Education and practice* (Pub. No. 52-1834). New York: Author.

Norris, C. M. (1979). Self-care. *American Journal of Nursing, 79,* 486–489.

Powell, D. J. (1984). Nurses — "High touch" entrepreneurs. *Nursing Economics, 2*(1), 33–36.

Public Health Service. (1979). *Healthy People: The surgeon general's report on health promotion and disease prevention* (DHEW Publication No. PHS 79–55071). Washington, DC: U.S. Government Printing Office.

Roberts, D., & Freeman, R. (Eds.). (1973). *Redesigning nursing education for public health: Report of the conference* (Pub. No. [HRA] 75-75). Bethesda, MD: U.S. Department of Health, Education and Welfare.

Ruth, M. V., & Partridge, K. (1978). Differences in perception of education and practice. *Nursing Outlook, 26,* 622–628.

Sheps, C. G. (1976). *Higher education for public health: A report of the Milbank Memorial Fund Commission.* New York: Neale, Watson.

Watkin, D. (1978). Personal responsibility: Key to effective and cost-effective health. *Family and Community Health, 1*(1), 1–7.

White, M. S. (1982). Construct for public health nursing. *Nursing Outlook, 30,* 527–530.

Williams, C. A. (1977). Community health nursing — What is it? *Nursing Outlook, 25,* 250–254.

Williams, C. A. (1983). Making things happen: Community health nursing and the policy arena. *Nursing Outlook, 31,* 225–228.

Selected Readings

American Nurses Association. (1974). *Standards: Community health nursing practice.* Kansas City, MO: Author.

American Nurses Association, Community Health Nursing Division. (1980). *A conceptual model of community health nursing* (Pub. No. CH-10 2M 5/80). Kansas City, MO: Author.

American Public Health Association. (1982). Definition and role of public health nursing in the delivery of health care (Policy Statement No. 8132). *American Journal of Public Health, 72,* 210–212.

Anderson, E. (1983). Community focus in public health nursing: Whose responsibility? *Nursing Outlook, 31,* 44–49.

Archer, S. (1982). Synthesis of public health science and nursing science. *Nursing Outlook, 30,* 442–446.

Archer, S. E., & Fleshman, R. P. (1975). Community health nursing: A typology of practice. *Nursing Outlook, 23,* 358.

Beauchamp, D. E. (1976). Public health as social justice. *Inquiry, 13,* 3–14.

Brainard, A. M. (1922). *The evolution of public health nursing.* Philadelphia: W. B. Saunders.

Chavigny, K. H., & Kroske, M. (1983). Public health nursing in crisis. *Nursing Outlook, 31,* 312–316.

Davis, A. J., & Underwood, P. (1976). Role, function, and decision making in community health nursing. *Nursing Research, 25,* 255–258.

Deloughery, G. L. (1977). *History and trends of professional nursing* (8th ed.). St. Louis: C. V. Mosby.

Dolan, J. A. (1978). *Nursing in society: A historical perspective.* Philadelphia: W. B. Saunders.

Freeman, R. (1973). The dilemma of public health nursing today. In D. Roberts and R. Freeman (Eds.), *Redesigning nursing education for public health: Report of the conference* (pp. 9–17). Bethesda, MD: U.S. Department of Health, Education and Welfare.

Freeman, R. (1974). The nurse practitioner in the community health agency. *Journal of Nursing Administration, 4,* 21–24.

Freeman, R., & Heinrich, J. (1981). *Community health nursing practice* (2nd ed.). Philadelphia: W. B. Saunders.

Fromer, M. J. (1983). *Community health care and the nursing process* (2nd ed.). St. Louis: C. V. Mosby.

Gardner, M. S. (1919). *Public health nursing* (3rd ed.). New York: Macmillan.

Goeppinger, J., Lassiter, P. G., & Wilcox, B. (1982). Community health is community competence. *Nursing Outlook, 30,* 464–467.

Goodson, J. (1978). Demonstrating excellence in a community nursing service. In A. Warner (Ed.), *Innovations in community health nursing* (pp. 16–22). St. Louis: C. V. Mosby.

Grissum, M., & Spangler, C. (1976). *Womanpower and health care.* Boston: Little, Brown.

Hanlon, J. J., & Pickett, G. E. (1984). *Public health: Administration and practice.* (8th ed.) St. Louis: Times Mirror/Mosby.

Hays, B. J., & Mockelstrom, N. R. (1977). Consumer survey. An approach to teaching consumer participation in community health. *Journal of Nursing Education, 16,* 30.

Heide, W. S. (1973). Nursing and women's liberation: A parallel. *American Journal of Nursing, 73,* 824–827.

Highriter, M. E. (1977). The status of community health nursing research. *Nursing Research, 26,* 183–192.

Kalisch, P., & Kalisch, B. (1978). *The advance of American nursing.* Boston: Little, Brown.

Kinlein, M. L. (1978). Point of view/On the front: Nursing and family and community health. *Family and Community Health, 1*(1), 57–68.

Leahy, K., Cobb, M., & Jones, M. (1982). *Community health nursing* (4th ed.). New York: McGraw-Hill.

Levin, L. (1978). Self-care: An emerging component of the health care system. *Hospital and Health Services Administration, 23,* 17.

Milbank Memorial Fund Commission. (1976). *Higher education for public health: A report.* New York: Prodist.

Naisbitt, J. (1982). *Megatrends.* New York: Warner Books.

National League for Nursing. *Community health nursing: Education and practice* (Pub. No. 52-1834). New York: Author, 1980.

Norris, C. M. (1979). Self-care. *American Journal of Nursing, 79,* 486–489.

Novello, D. J. et al. (1978). *Consumerism and health care.* New York: National League for Nursing.

Public Health Service. (1979). *Healthy people: The surgeon general's report on health promotion and disease prevention* (DHEW Publication No. 79–55071). Washington, DC: U.S. Government Printing Office.

Rathbone, W. (1890). *History and progress of district nursing.* New York: Macmillan.

Roberts, D., & Freeman, R. (Eds.). (1973). *Redesigning nursing education for public health: Report of the conference.* Bethesda, MD: U.S. Department of Health, Education and Welfare.

Ruth, M. V., & Partridge, K. (1978). Differences in perception of education and practice. *Nursing Outlook, 26,* 622.

Scott, J. M. (1974). The changing health care environment: Its implications for nursing. *American Journal of Public Health, 64,* 364.

Tinkham, C., & Voorhies, E. (1977). *Community health nursing: Evolution and process* (2nd ed.). New York: Appleton-Century-Crofts.

Wald, L. (1934). *Windows on Henry Street.* Boston: Little, Brown.

Wales, M. (1941). *The public health nurse in action.* New York: Macmillan.

Watkin, D. (1978). Personal responsibility: Key to effective and cost-effective health. *Family and Community Health, 1*(1), 1–7.

Werner, J. R. (1976). Effective community health nursing: A framework for actualizing standards of practice. *Nursing Forum, 15,* 265–276.

White, M. S. (1982). Construct for public health nursing. *Nursing Outlook, 30,* 527–530.

Williams, C. A. (1977). Community health nursing — What is it? *Nursing Outlook, 25,* 250–254.

Williams, C. A. (1983). Making things happen: Community health nursing and the policy arena. *Nursing Outlook, 31,* 225–228.

Winslow, C. E. A. (1946). Florence Nightingale and public health nursing. *Public Health Nursing, 38,* 330–332.

4

Roles and Settings for Practice

There was a day when uniformed public health nurses and home visits summed up the roles and settings of community health nursing, but that day is gone. In its place we find professional community health nurses practicing in a wide variety of settings, such as family planning clinics, industrial plants, and elementary schools, and these nurses are no longer restricted to giving treatment. Instead their roles range from educators and organizers to agents of change. The last chapter discussed the nature of community health nursing — how it developed and the characteristics that form a conceptual foundation for its practice. Now we shall consider the specific application of these concepts in the form of various roles assumed by community health nurses, as well as the kinds of settings in which these roles are practiced.

Roles

Community health nursing incorporates a variety of roles; one could say that community health nurses wear many hats while conducting day-to-day practice. At times, one role is primary. For example, a community health nurse may assume a set of responsibilities in a specialized role such as full-time researcher. More often, however, a number of roles are assumed simultaneously. Several factors influence the roles played by community health nurses. The organization with which the nurse is affiliated usually has policies that govern nursing activity. Consumers use community health nursing services differently, depending on their perceptions of nursing. Sociocultural norms, which vary from one group to another, will affect certain community health nurse functions. For example, some groups' values about acceptable female behavior will influence role choices. Political and legal restrictions also set limitations and determine directions for community health nursing practice. Perhaps the most important factor in determining roles will be the community health nurse's own values and ability to adapt to changing health needs. To clarify and expand our understanding of the way community health nursing is practiced, we shall examine seven major roles: (1) care provider, (2) educator, (3) advocate, (4) manager, (5) collaborator, (6) leader, and (7) researcher.

Care Provider

The most familiar role is provider of care; however, giving nursing care takes on new meaning in the context of community health. The target of service expands beyond the individual to include families, groups, and communities. Nursing care is still designed for the special needs of the client; however, when that client is a group of people, care takes different forms. It requires different skills to assess collective needs and tailor service accordingly. For instance, a community health nurse receives a referral to visit a family with multiple problems. The call is triggered by the 11-year-old son's frequent absence from and misbehavior at school. Together, the nurse and family design a plan of care that includes counseling for the whole family. It is a response to consideration of the family's resources and problems and the family members' perceptions of the situation.

HOLISTIC CARE

We recognize that nursing care is holistic, but in community health this approach means viewing the client as a larger system. The client, most often a family or group, is a composite of people whose relationships and interactions with each other must be considered in totality. Holistic care must emerge from this perspective. For example, a community health nurse may be working with a group of pregnant teenagers living in a juvenile detention center. The nurse would consider the girls' relationships with each other, their parents, the fathers of their unborn children, and the detention center staff. The nurse would evaluate their age level; developmental needs; peer influences; and knowledge of pregnancy, delivery, and issues related to the choice of keeping or giving up their babies. The girls' reentry into the community and their future plans for school or employment would also be considered. Holistic care would go far beyond the physical condition of pregnancy and childbirth.

FOCUS ON WELLNESS

The role of care provider in community health is also characterized by its focus on wellness. As we discussed in chapter 1, the community health nurse provides care along the entire range of the wellness-illness continuum but especially emphasizes promotion of health and prevention of illness. Nursing care includes seeking out clients in order to offer preventive services, rather than waiting for them to come for help after problems arise. Community health nurses identify people who are interested in achieving a higher level of health and work with them to accomplish that goal. They may help a family or group learn how to shop for and eat more nutritious foods or work with a group that wants to quit smoking. They may hold seminars at a men's club on handling stress. They may assist a family with a terminally ill member at home in developing healthier attitudes toward dying and death.

NECESSARY SKILLS

The community health nurse uses many different skills in the care provider role. In nursing's early years, the skills most often used were those associated with physical care. Such skills are still very important as a result of earlier hospital discharges and a growing number of elderly persons in the population. As time went on, skills in observation, listening, communication, and counseling became integral to the care provider role. There was an increased emphasis on psychological and sociocultural factors. Most recently, environmental considerations, for example, awareness of problems caused by pollution or of emotional stress related to urban congestion, have created a need for new skills such as assessment and intervention at the community level.

Educator

It is widely recognized that health teaching is part of good nursing care and one of the major functions of the community health nurse. Health education is especially significant for two major reasons. First, the clients in the community are usually not in an acute state of illness and are better able to absorb and act on health information. For example, a class of expectant parents, unhampered by significant health problems, can grasp the relationship of diet to fetal development. They will understand the value of specific exercises to the childbirth process and then perform those exercises. Second, the health educator role is significant because people in the community have acquired a higher level of health consciousness. Through plans ranging from the president's physical fitness program to local antismoking campaigns, people are recognizing the value of health and are increasingly motivated to achieve higher levels of wellness. When a middle-aged businessman, for example, is discharged from the hospital following a heart attack, he is likely to be more interested than he was before in learning how to prevent occurrence of an attack. He can learn how to reduce stress, develop an appropriate and gradual exercise program, and alter his eating habits. Families with young children are often interested in learning about normal child growth and development; many young parents want to raise happier, healthier children. An increasing number of businesses and industries are promoting the health of their employees through active wellness programs. They recognize that healthy workers mean less absenteeism and higher production levels. Some companies even provide exercise areas and equipment for employee use.

All nurses teach patients about personal care, diet, and medications. Community health nurses, however, go beyond these topics to educate people in a great many areas. People in the community need and want to know about a wide variety of topics. How do you toilet train a two-year-old? What foods should you avoid when you have coronary atherosclerosis? How do you manage an alcoholic spouse? What do you do with adolescent rebellion? What is the best way to lose weight and keep it off? How can you organize the community to work for clean air? What are health consumers' rights? The range of topics taught by community health nurses extends from personal health care and management of leisure to environmental health and community organization.

As educators, community health nurses seek to facilitate client learning. They share information with clients informally, often in the clients' homes (Fig. 4-1). They act as consultants to individuals or groups. They may hold formal classes to increase people's understanding of health and health care. Community health nurses utilize established community groups in their teaching. For example, they may teach parents at a PTA meeting about signs of drug abuse, discuss safety practices with a group of industrial workers, or give a presentation on the importance of early detection of child abuse to a health planning committee considering the funding of a new program. At times, the community health nurse facilitates client learning through referral to more knowledgeable sources or through use of experts on special topics. The community health nurse also facilitates clients' self-education; in keeping with the concept of self-care, clients are encouraged and helped to use appropriate health resources and to seek out health information for themselves. The emphasis throughout the health teaching process continues to be placed on illness prevention and health promotion. Health teaching as a tool for community health nursing practice is discussed in chapter 11.

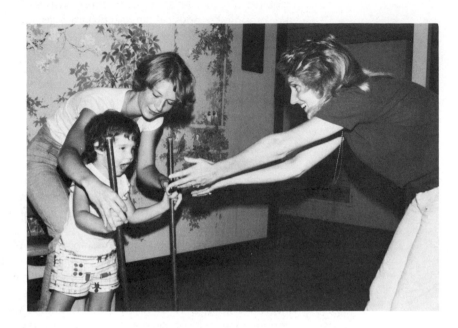

Figure 4-1
Teaching this mother how to help her child is one of the many ways that community health nurses serve as health educators.

Advocate

Patients' rights are an important issue in health care today. Every patient has the right to receive just, equal, and humane treatment. In our present society, the health care system is often characterized by fragmented and depersonalized services. Clients, especially poor ones, are frequently unable to achieve their rights. They become frustrated, confused, and degraded, unable to cope with the system on their own.

GOALS

Kosik (1972) has described two underlying goals in client advocacy. One is to help clients gain greater independence. The community health nurse shows clients what services are available, which they are entitled to, and how to obtain them until they can discover this information for themselves. A second goal is to make the system more responsive and relevant to the needs of clients. By calling attention to inadequate or unjust care, the community health nurse can influence change.

Consider the experience of a family that shall be called the Martins. Gloria Martin and her three small children had gone to the Westside Clinic on Wednesday. On Tuesday morning, the baby, Tony, had suddenly started to cry. Nothing would comfort him. Gloria called the clinic and was told to come in the next day. The clinic did not take appointments and was too busy to see any more patients that day. The rest of that day and night Tony cried almost incessantly. On Wednesday there was a 45-minute bus ride and a wait of three and a half hours in the crowed reception room, a wait punctuated by intake workers' interrogations. The children were restless, and the baby was crying. Finally they saw the physician. Tony had an inguinal hernia that could be gangrenous. The doctor admonished the mother that the baby should have been brought in sooner. Now immediate surgery was necessary. Someone at the clinic told Gloria that Medicaid would pay for it. Someone else told her that she was ineligible because she was not a registered clinic patient. By now all the children were crying. Gloria had been up most of the night. She was frantic, confused, and felt that no one cared. This family needed an advocate.

ACTIONS AND CHARACTERISTICS

As an advocate, the community health nurse pleads the cause of another by speaking and acting on that person's or group's behalf. There are times when health care clients need someone to explain what services to expect and which they ought to receive. They need someone to guide them through the complexities of the system and someone to assure the satisfaction of their needs.

The advocate role requires at least four important characteristics. First, advocates must be assertive. In the Martins' dilemma, a community health nurse took the initiative to identify their needs and find appropriate solutions. She contacted the right people and helped them establish eligibility for coverage of surgery and hospitalization costs. She helped Gloria make arrangements for the baby's hospitalization and the other children's care. A second characteristic of the advocate role is willingness to take risks, to go out on a limb if need be, for the client. The community health nurse was outraged at the kind of treatment that the Martins had received — the delays in service, the impersonal care, and the surgery that could have been prevented. She wrote a letter describing the details of the Martins' experience to the clinic director, the chairman of the clinic board, and the nursing director. It resulted in better care for the Martins and a series of meetings aimed at changing clinic procedures and providing better initial screening. A third characteristic of advocates is their ability to communicate well, to bargain thoroughly and convincingly. The community health nurse helping the Martins was able to state the problem clearly and argue for its solution. Finally, the advocate role requires the ability to identify sources of power and tap them for the client's benefit. By contacting the most influential people in the clinic and appealing to their desire for quality service, the nurse concerned with the Martins was able to facilitate change.

Manager

Community health nurses, like all nurses, are managers of client care. In community health this role may involve such activities as supervising family care, managing a caseload, administrating a clinic, or conducting a community health planning project.

PLANNING

The manager role in community health nursing utilizes three functions in particular: planning, organizing, and coordinating. Planning, the first and most basic function, enables the manager to decide on an objective (client care goals) and to achieve it (nursing process). The nurse begins by studying the situation and drawing up a detailed plan. Community health nurses, as managers, need time for planning, which involves determining client concerns and needs, establishing objectives, and deciding on an appropriate course of action. When starting a therapy group with recovering drug addicts, for example, the nurse sits down with the entire group to discuss the members' present situation and ambitions. What would they like to accomplish in group therapy? What topics would they like to cover? How would they like to approach them — through discussion or role playing? When and where would they like to meet? In the process of making these decisions, nurses are planning, that is, mapping out a course of action based on predetermined goals.

ORGANIZING

The second function of the community health nurse manager role is organizing. Organizing means structuring activities and placing people into a functioning whole aimed at attaining stated objectives (Longest, 1976). A manager must arrange matters so that the job can be done. People, activities, and relationships have to be assembled in order to put the plan into effect (Plachy, 1976, p. 60). In the process of organizing, the nurse provides a framework for the various aspects of service so that each will run smoothly and accomplish its purpose. The framework is a part of service preparation. When a community health nurse manages a well-baby clinic, for instance, the organizing function involves making certain that all equipment and supplies are present, required staff are hired and on duty, and staff responsibilities are clearly designated.

COORDINATING

Coordinating, the third function of the community health nurse manager role, means bringing people and activities together so that they function in harmony while pursuing desired objectives. Like the matching of a movie film's sound track with its pictures, coordination involves assembly and synchronization. It occurs during planning and implementation of service. On a nurse-patient or nurse-family level, some coordination is almost always necessary (Fig. 4-2). The nurse may arrange an early demonstration of walking on crutches by the physical therapist, time a home health aide's visit to coincide with an older woman's preferred bath schedule, or bring an eight-year-old boy and his parents together with his teacher and the learning disabilities specialist to discuss ways to approach his learning problems.

Coordinating becomes a more complex activity at the community level. Consider a community health nurse working with a group of citizens and health professionals who are interested in starting a mobile health center for a two-county area. Their objective is to make health service more accessible to residents. The nurse will need to contact many individuals, arrange meetings, explore funding sources, tap community leaders, and help maintain the group's focus on its objective. Once the project is in operation, the nurse, as manager, will have a continuing responsibility to coordinate it.

The manager role, at times, involves other functions, such as leading, staffing, supervising, motivating, and controlling service activities. While performing all these functions, community health nurses most often are participative

Figure 4-2
As a manager, the nurse coordinates client care so that needed resources are available at the right time.

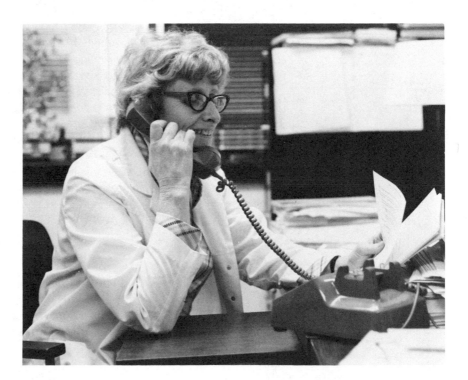

managers; that is, they participate with clients, staff, or both, in planning and carrying out services.

Collaborator

Community health nurses seldom practice in isolation. Their work involves many other people, including other nurses, physicians, social workers, physical therapists, nutritionists, attorneys, and secretaries. As a member of the health team, the community health nurse assumes the role of collaborator. To collaborate means to work jointly with others in a common endeavor, to cooperate as partners. Successful community health practice depends on this collegiality. Everyone on the team, including the community health nurse, has an important and unique contribution to make to the health care effort. As on a championship football team, the better each member plays his position and cooperates with other members, the more likely the health team is to win.

Interdisciplinary collaboration has been discussed in chapter 3 as a vital characteristic of community health nursing. The collaborator role is simply an application of that concept. For example, one family needed to find a good nursing home for their 83-year-old grandfather. The community health nurse and family, including the grandfather, made a list of desired features that included a shower. He did not like baths. The daughter, son-in-law, and community health nurse, working with a social worker, located and visited several homes. The grandfathers' physician was contacted for medical consultation, and the grandfather made the final selection. In another situation, the community health nurse collaborated with the city council, police department, neighborhood residents, and manager of a senior citizens' high-rise apartment building to help a group of elderly people organize and lobby for safer streets. In a third example, a school nurse noticed a boy with a high absentee record and low grades. Counseling was started after joint planning with his parents, teacher, school psychologist, and family physician.

The community health nurse collaborator role requires skills in communicating, in interpreting the nurse's unique contribution to the team, and in acting assertively as an equal partner. The collaborator role may also involve functioning as a consultant (Fig. 4-3).

Leader

The leadership role is not always obvious in community health nursing, but community health nurses are increasingly becoming active leaders. When they guide decision making, stimulate interest in health promotion, initiate therapy, direct a preventive program, or influence health policy, they are assuming a leadership role. It tends to be a role of influence and persuasion more than of directorship.

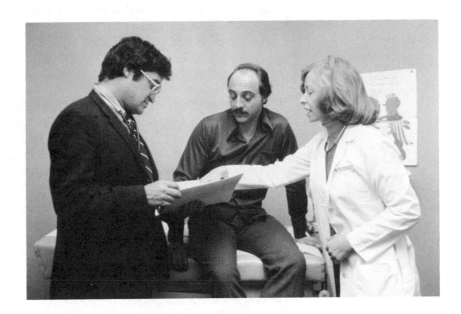

Figure 4-3
The nurse often has unique knowledge about clients that as a collaborator she shares with other health team members.

The leader role, as distinguished from the manager role, serves a unique purpose. Its main function is to effect change; thus, the community health nurse becomes an agent of change. (Chapter 20 elaborates on this role.) The nurse in the leader role influences people to think and behave differently about their health and the factors contributing to it. For example, a community health nurse who made home visits to a young mother suggested that the mother invite her neighbors over for coffee and discussion about health topics of interest. The group met once a month and grew as the community health nurse increased their desire for more information.

The leader role assumes a different form in another situation. A community health nurse was eager to start a mental health program, which she and her nursing colleagues felt was needed, through the agency for which she worked. But certain individuals on the health board were opposed to adding any new programs because of cost. Her approach was to gather considerable supportive data to demonstrate the program's need and cost-effectiveness. She lunched individually with key board members in order to convince them of the need. She prepared written summaries, graphs, and charts and, at a strategic time, presented her case at a board meeting. The mental health program was approved and implemented.

In the leader role, the community health nurse also exerts influence through health planning (McLemore, 1980). The need for coordinated, accessible, cost-effective health care services creates a challenge and an opportunity for community health nurses to become more involved in health planning at all levels — organizational, local, state, national, and even international. Nurses need to exercise their leadership responsibility and assert their right to share in health decisions (Edwards, 1983, p. 324).

Researcher

The researcher role is an integral part of community health nursing practice. But, it may be asked, how can research be combined with practice? It is true that research in the strictest sense involves a complex set of activities conducted by persons with highly developed and specialized skills. But there is another way to view research — that is, as an investigative process. From this perspective, all community health nurses are researchers, or investigators.

Research literally means to search — to investigate, discover, and interpret facts. All research in community health, from the simplest inquiry to the most complex epidemiologic study, uses the same fundamental process. Most simply put, the steps are (1) identify the question or problem to be addressed, (2) formulate an hypothesis for testing, (3) design the method for studying it, (4) collect data, (5) analyze the data, and (6) draw conclusions. The investigation builds on the nursing process, that essential dynamic of community health nursing practice, using it as a problem-solving process (Treece & Treece, 1977, p. 48). That is, the nurse identifies a problem or question, collects and analyzes data by making an investigation, suggests and evaluates possible solutions, and selects a solution or rejects them all and starts the investigative process over again. In one sense the nurse is a health planner, investigating health problems in order to design wellness-promoting and disease-preventing interventions for community populations.

ATTRIBUTES OF THE RESEARCHER ROLE

A questioning attitude is a basic prerequisite to good nursing practice. There have probably been many times when a nurse revisited a patient and noticed some change in his condition such as restlessness or skin color. Consequently, the nurse wondered what was causing this change and what could be done about it. In everyday practice, community health nurses encounter numerous situations that challenge them to ask questions. Consider the following examples:

"Mr. Hansen is still very weak on his right side since his CVA [cerebrovascular accident]. I wonder if he really understands how to do his exercises?"

"Little Marc seems unusually quiet, and I see another bruise on his left arm. Could this possibly be the beginning of child abuse?"

"This prenatal class is dragging; am I going too fast, is there some conflict in the group, or do the members need more opportunity for expressing themselves?"

"While driving through this part of the city, I haven't seen a single playground for miles. I wonder where the kids play?"

Each of these questions places the community health nurse in the role of investigator. They express the fundamental attitude of every researcher — *a spirit of inquiry*.

A second attribute, careful *observation*, is also evident in the examples just given. The community health nurse develops a sharpened ability to notice things as they are, including deviations from the norm and even subtle changes that suggest the need for some nursing action.

Coupled with observation is *open-mindedness*, another attribute of the researcher role. After observing Mr. Hansen's weakness, the community health nurse postulates that Mr. Hansen may not understand how to do his exercises but keeps an open mind to other possibilities. He can demonstrate his exercises, and if that is not the problem, perhaps he needs some different activities to strengthen the weak muscles. In the case of little Marc, the community health nurse's observations suggest child abuse as the possible cause. But open-mindedness requires consideration of other alternatives, and as a good investigator, the nurse explores these as well.

The community health nurse also uses *analytic* skills in this role. In the prenatal class example, the nurse has already started to analyze the situation by trying to determine its cause-and-effect relationships. Successful analysis depends on how well the data have been collected. Insufficient information can lead to false interpretations, so the community health nurse is careful to seek out the needed data. Analysis, like a jigsaw puzzle, involves studying the pieces and fitting them together until the meaning of the whole picture can be described.

Finally, the researcher role involves *tenacity*. The community health nurse persists in an investigation until facts are uncovered and a satisfactory answer is found. Noticing an absence of playgrounds and wondering where the children play is only a beginning. The nurse, concerned about the children's safety and need for recreational outlets in the district, gathers data about location and accessibility of play areas as well as felt needs of community residents. A fully documented research report may result. If the data support a need for additional play space, the report can be brought before the proper authorities.

LEVELS IN THE RESEARCHER ROLE

Community health nurses practice the researcher role at many levels. Up to this point we have focused primarily on simple kinds of investigations to emphasize that research is an essential and integral part of community health nursing practice; however, the attributes that have been described are basic to research practice at any level. In addition to everyday inquiries, community health nurses often participate in agency or organizational studies to determine such matters as the effectiveness of a screening program or the need for a new family planning clinic. Some community health nurses also initiate more complex research of their own or in collaboration with other health professionals, perhaps a full-scale epidemiologic study. The researcher role, at all levels, helps to determine needs, evaluate effectiveness of care, and develop theoretical bases for community health nursing practice. Chapter 7 explains community health research in greater detail.

Settings for Practice

We have just examined community health nursing from the perspective of its major roles. Now we can place the roles in context by viewing the settings in which they are practiced. The numbers and kinds of places for community health nursing practice are too varied to make it practical to examine them all. For purposes of discussion, however, they can be grouped into six categories: (1) homes, (2) ambulatory care settings, (3) schools, (4) occupational health settings, (5) residential institutions, and (6) the community at large.

Homes

One of the most frequently used settings for community health nursing practice is the home. In the home setting all of the community health nursing roles, to varying degrees, are performed. Clients discharged from acute care institutions, such as hospitals or mental health facilities, are regularly referred to community health nursing for continued care and follow-up. Here the nurse can see the client in a family and environmental context, and service can be individualized to the client's particular needs. For example, Mr. White, 67 years of age, was discharged from the hospital after undergoing a colostomy. Doreen, the community health nurse from the county public health nursing agency, immediately started home visits. She met with Mr. White and his wife to discuss their needs as a family and to plan for Mr. White's care and adjustment to living with a colostomy. Practicing the care provider and educator roles, she reinforced and expanded on the teaching started in the hospital for colostomy care, that is, bowel training, diet, exercise, and proper use of equipment. As part of a total family care plan, Doreen provided some forms of physical care for Mr. White as well as counseling, teaching, and emotional support for both the Whites. In addition to consulting with the physician and social services, she arranged and supervised home health aide visits that gave personal care and homemaker services. She thus utilized the manager, leader, and collaborator roles.

The home is a setting for health promotion as well. Many community health nursing visits focus on assisting families in understanding and practicing healthier living. They may, for example, include instruction in parenting, infant care, child discipline, eating right, getting proper exercise, coping with stress, or managing grief and loss.

The character of the home setting is as varied as the clients whom the community health nurse serves. In one day a community health nurse may visit an elderly well-to-do widow in her luxury home, a middle-income family in their modest bungalow, and a transient in his one-room fifth-story walk-up apartment. In each home situation, community health nurses can view their clients in perspective and, therefore, better understand their limitations, capitalize on their resources, and tailor health services to their needs. In the home, unlike most other health care settings, clients are on their own turf. They feel comfortable and secure in the familiar surroundings and are thus often better able to understand and apply health information. Client self-respect can be promoted since the client is host while the nurse is a guest.

Ambulatory Care Settings

Ambulatory care settings include a variety of places in which community health nurses practice. Each is a place where clients *come* for day service; in other words, they seek out or are referred to these health services for care that does not include overnight stays. Clinics are an example of an ambulatory setting. Sometimes multiple clinics, offering medical, surgical, orthopedic, dermatologic, and many other services, are located in the outpatient department of hospitals or medical centers. They may also be based in a comprehensive neighborhood health center. A single clinic, such as a family planning or well-child clinic, may be found in a location more convenient for clients, for example, a church basement or empty storefront. Some kinds of day care centers, such as those for physically handicapped or emotionally disturbed adults, utilize community health nursing services. Additional ambulatory care settings include health departments and community health nursing agencies where clients may come for assessment and referral or counseling.

Offices are another type of ambulatory care setting. Some community health nurses provide service in conjunction with medical practice; for example, a community health nurse associated with a HMO sees clients in the office and undertakes screening, referrals, counseling, health education, and group work. Others establish their own independent practice by seeing clients in their offices as well as making home visits (Goodson, 1978; Greenidge, Zimmern & Kohnke, 1973).

Another type of ambulatory care setting includes places where services are offered to selected groups. For example, community health nurses practice in migrant camps, Native American reservations, prisons, children's day care centers, churches, and remote mountain and coal-mining communities. Again, in each ambulatory care setting all the community health nursing roles are utilized to varying degrees.

Schools

Schools of all levels make up a major group of settings for community health nursing practice. Nurses from community health nursing agencies frequently serve private schools of elementary and intermediate levels. Public schools are served by the same agencies or by community health nurses hired through the public school system. Community health nurses may work with groups of children in preschool settings, such as Montessori schools, as well as in vocational or technical schools, junior colleges, and college and university settings. Specialized schools, such as those for the handicapped, are another setting for community health nursing practice.

Community health nurse roles in school settings are expanding. School nurses, whose primary role was initially care provider, are widening their practice to include much more health education, collaboration, and client advocacy. For example, one school had been accustomed to utilizing the nurse as a first-aid giver and record keeper, her duties were handling minor problems, such as headaches and cuts, and keeping track of such events as immunizations. This nurse determined to expand her practice and, after planning and preparation, implemented a series of classes on personal hygiene, diet, and sexuality; started a drop-in health counseling center in the school; and established a network of professional contacts for consultation and referral. Community health nurses in school settings are also beginning to assume manager and leader roles and recognize that the researcher role should be an integral part of their practice. The nurse's role with preschool and school-age populations is discussed in greater detail in chapter 14.

Occupational Health Settings

Business and industry provide another group of settings for community health nursing practice. Employee health has long been recognized as making a vital contribution to individual lives, productivity of business, and the well-being of the entire nation. Organizations now are expected to provide a safe and healthy work environment in addition to offering health insurance for health care. An increasing number of companies, recognizing the value of healthy employees, go beyond offering traditional health benefits to supporting health promotional efforts. Some businesses, for example, encourage healthy snacks like fruit instead of coffee at breaks and jogging during the noon hour. A few larger corporations have built exercise facilities for their employees, provided health education programs, and offered financial incentives for staying well.

Community health nurses in occupational health settings practice a variety of roles. Early industrial nursing, which started in 1895 when the first nurse was hired by an industry, mostly involved visiting sick workers in their homes (Freeman & Heinrich, 1981). The care provider role was primary for many years as nurses continued to care for sick or injured employees at work. However, recognition of the need to protect employees' safety and later to prevent their illness led to inclusion of health education. Now industrial nurses also act as employee advocates, assuring appropriate job assignments for workers and adequate treatment for job-related illness or injury. They collaborate with other health care providers and company management to offer better services to their clients and act as leaders and managers in developing new health services in the work setting, endorsing programs such as hypertension screening or weight control. Occupational health settings range from industries and factories, such as an automobile assembly plant, to business corporations and even large department stores. The field of occupational health offers a challenging opportunity, particularly in smaller businesses where nursing coverage usually is not provided. Chapter 17 more fully describes the role of the nurse serving the working population.

Residential Institutions

Facilities where clients reside form a fifth group of settings in which community health nursing is practiced. Clients may be housed temporarily in these institutions, as in a halfway house for recovering alcoholics, or on a relatively permanent basis, as in an inpatient hospice program for the terminally ill. Some of these institutions, for example, hospitals, exist solely to provide health care. Community health nurses based in a community agency maintain continuity of care for their clients by collaborating with hospital personnel, visiting clients in the hospital, and helping plan care during and following hospitalization. As part of their caseloads, some community health nurses serve one or more hospitals on a regular basis by providing a liaison with the community, consultation for discharge planning, and periodic in-service programs to keep hospital staff updated on community services for their clients. Other community health nurses with similar functions are based in the hospital and serve the hospital community. A nursing home staffed with skilled nurses is another example of a residential facility providing health care that may utilize community health nursing services. In this kind of setting, where residents are usually elderly with many chronic health problems, community health nurses function particularly as advocates and collaborators to improve care. They will coordinate available resources to meet the needs of residents and their families and help safeguard the maintenance of proper nursing home operating standards. Sheltered workshops and group homes for mentally retarded adults are other examples of residential institutions.

Community health nurses also practice in settings where residents are gathered for purposes other than receiving care. Health care is offered as an adjunct to the primary goals of the institution. One example is the many camping programs for children and adults offered by churches and other community agencies, such as the Boy Scouts, Girl Scouts, or the YMCA. As camp nurses, community health nurses practice all available roles, often under interesting and challenging conditions.

Residential institutions provide a unique kind of setting for community health nurses to practice health promotion. Their clients are a "captive" audience whose needs can be readily assessed and whose interests can be stimulated. These settings offer community health nurses the opportunity to generate an environment of caring and optimal-quality services.

Community at Large

Unlike the five already discussed, the sixth setting for community health nursing practice is not confined to a specific location or building. When nurses work with groups, populations, or the total community, they may practice in many different places. For example, a community health nurse, as care provider and health educator, may work with a parenting group in a church or town hall. Another nurse, as client advocate, leader, and researcher, may study the health needs of a neighborhood's elderly population by collecting data throughout the area and meeting with resource people in many places. Again, the community at large becomes the setting for practice of a nurse who serves on health care planning committees, lobbies for health legislation at the state capitol, or runs for a school board position.

Although the term *setting* implies place, it is important to remember that community health nursing practice is not limited to a specific arena. Community health nursing is a specialty of nursing that can be practiced anywhere.

Summary

Community health nursing incorporates many roles and is practiced in many settings. Seven major roles, when combined, describe community health nursing practice: care provider, educator, advocate, manager, collaborator, leader or initiator of change, and researcher. The types and number of roles that are practiced vary depending on the nurse, clients, and demands of the situation.

The settings of community health nursing practice are also many and varied, but they can generally be grouped into six categories: homes, ambulatory care settings, schools, occupational health settings, residential institutions, and the community at large.

Study Questions

1. What are some ways that a community health nurse can make care holistic and focused on wellness with a group of chemically dependent adolescents?
2. Select one community health nurse role and describe its application in meeting your next-door neighbor's needs.
3. Describe a hypothetical or real situation in which you, as a community health nurse, would combine the roles of leader, collaborator, and researcher (investigator). Discuss how each of these roles might be played.
4. If your community health nursing practice setting is the community at large, will your practice roles be any different from those of the nurse whose practice setting is the home? Why? What determines the roles played by the community health nurse?

References

Edwards, L. (1983). Health Planning: Opportunities for nurses. *Nursing Outlook, 31* (6), 322–325.

Freeman, R., & Heinrich, J. (1981). *Community health nursing practice.* Philadelphia: W. B. Saunders.

Goodson, J. (1978). Demonstrating excellence in a community nursing service. In A. Warner (Ed.), *Innovations in community health nursing* (pp. 16–22). St. Louis: C. V. Mosby.

Greenidge, J., Zimmern, A., & Kohnke, M. (1973). Community nurse practitioners — A partnership. *Nursing Outlook, 21,* 228–231.

Kosik, S. H. (1972). Patient advocacy or fighting the system. *American Journal of Nursing, 72,* 694–696.

Longest, B. (1976). *Management practices for the health professional.* Reston, VA: Reston Publishing.

McLemore, M. (1980). Nurses as health planners. *Journal of Nursing Administration, 1,* 13–17.

Plachy, R. (1976). Delegation and decision-making. In S. Stone, M. Berger, D. Elhart, S. Firsich, & S. Jordan (Eds.), *Management for nurses: A multidisciplinary approach.* St. Louis: C. V. Mosby.

Treece, E. W., & Treece, J. W. (1977). *Elements of research in nursing* (2nd ed.). St. Louis: C. V. Mosby.

Selected Readings

American Nurses Association. (1973). *Standards: Community health nursing practice.* Kansas City, MO: Author.

Archer, S., & Fleshman, R. (1975). Community health nursing: A typology of practice. *Nursing Outlook, 23,* 358–364.

Bernal, B. (1978). Levels of practice in a community health agency. *Nursing Outlook, 26,* 364–369.

Brown, M. L. (1981). *Occupational health nursing.* New York: Springer.

Davis, M. Z., Kromer, M., & Strauss, A. L. (1975). *Nurses in practice: A perspective on work environments.* St. Louis: C. V. Mosby.

Fromer, M. J. (1983). Functions of the community health nurse. In M. J. Fromer (Ed.), *Community health care and the nursing process* (2nd ed.) (pp. 155–172). St. Louis: C. V. Mosby.

Goodson, J. (1978). Demonstrating excellence in a community nursing service. In A. Warner (Ed.), *Innovations in community health nursing* (pp. 16–22). St. Louis: C. V. Mosby.

Greenidge, J., Zimmern, A., & Kohnke, M. (1973). Community nurse practitioners — A partnership. *Nursing Outlook, 21,* 228–231.

Hitchcock, J. (1970). Working in a nonhealth-oriented setting. *Nursing Clinics of North America, 5–12,* 251.

Igoe, J. B. (1975). The school nurse practitioner. *Nursing Outlook, 23,* 381–384.

Keller, M. J. (1979). Health needs and nursing care of the labor force. In M. J. Fromer (Ed.), *Community health care and the nursing process.* St. Louis: C. V. Mosby.

Kosik, S. H. (1972). Patient advocacy or fighting the system. *American Journal of Nursing, 72,* 694–696.

Levin, L. S. (1978). Patient education and self-care: How do they differ? *Nursing Outlook, 26,* 170–175.

Lysaught, J. P. (1974). Distributive nursing practice: Development and fusion of roles. In J. P. Lysaught (Ed.), *Action in nursing.* New York: McGraw-Hill.

Oda, D. (1979). Community nursing in schools: Developing a specialized role. In S. Archer and R. Fleshman (Eds.), *Community health nursing: Patterns and practice* (2nd ed.). North Scituate, MA: Duxbury Press.

Pacifico, P. B. (1977). The dynamic and expanded role of nurses in community health nursing. *Philippine Journal of Nursing, 46,* 86.

Peznecker, B., Draye, M. A., & McNeil, J. (1982). Collaborative practice models in community health. *Nursing Outlook, 30,* 298–302.

Quinn, M., & Reinhardt, A. (1973). Community health nursing: New directions for practice. In A. Reinhardt & M. Quinn (Eds.), *Family-centered community nursing: A sociocultural framework* (pp. 5–18). St. Louis: C. V. Mosby.

Skrovan, C., Anderson, E. J., & Gottschalk, J. (1974). Community nurse practitioner: An emerging role. *American Journal of Public Health, 64,* 847–849.

Vance, C. (1979). Women leaders: Modern-day heroines or societal deviants? *Image, 11,* 33–36.

Warner, A. (Ed.). (1978). *Innovations in community health nursing.* St. Louis: C. V. Mosby.

Williams, C. A. (1977). Community health nursing — What is it? *Nursing Outlook, 25,* 250–254.

Williams, C. A. (1983). Making things happen: Community health nursing and the policy arena. *Nursing Outlook, 31,* 225–228.

5

Values and Health

Sara T. Fry

Community health nurses encounter value differences every day. Consider, for example, the dilemma one nurse faced on her first home visit to an elderly man whom we shall call Mr. Bates. Referred by concerned neighbors, this 78-year-old gentleman was homebound and living alone with severe arthritis under steadily deteriorating conditions. Overgrown shrubs and vines covered the yard and house, making access impossible except through the back door. A wood-burning stove in the kitchen was the sole source of heat and that room plus a corner of the dining room were his living quarters. The remainder of the once lovely three-bedroom house, including the bathroom, was layered with dust, unused. His bed was a cot in the dining room, his toilet a two-pound coffee can placed under the cot. Unbathed, unshaven, and existing on the food and firewood brought in by neighbors, Mr. Bates' situation seemed deplorable and unsafe. Yet he valued his independence so highly that he adamantly refused to leave.

Values and the valuing process strongly shape the nature of community health nursing practice. Values determine nurses' as well as clients' decisions and responses. The concept of value is a familiar topic to nurses. The function and meaning of values and value systems have been a part of their educational preparation in the humanities and the sciences. They are widely discussed in history, philosophy, and literature. Theoretical consideration and empirical studies about values and value systems are also well documented in the literature of sociology, psychology, and the applied sciences such as nursing.

106

Values serve as the criteria or standards by which evaluations are made. In order to understand the relationship between values and health it is necessary to describe the nature or function of values and value systems in human behavior. Once it is clear how values and value systems function in human behavior, then we can understand the role of values in choices related to health. In this chapter, we will explore (1) the nature and function of values and value systems, (2) the role of values and value systems in decision making in general, (3) the central values related to health care choices and their potential conflicts, and (4) the implications of values for community health nursing practice.

Values and Value Systems

Social psychologist Milton Rokeach has defined values and value systems in a particularly useful manner. According to Rokeach (1973, p. 5), a value is "an enduring belief that a specific mode of conduct or end-state of existence is personally or socially preferable to an opposite or converse mode of conduct or end-state of existence." In the same work (p. 5), he defines a value system as "an enduring organization of beliefs concerning preferable modes of conduct or end-states of existence along a continuum of relative importance." With these definitions in mind, it is possible to explore the nature and function of values and value systems and their relationship to health.

The Nature of Values

The nature of values can be described according to five value qualities: endurance, relativity, belief, reference, and preference.

ENDURANCE

Values endure in the sense that they are sufficiently stable to provide continuity to personal and social existence. Religious beliefs, for example, offer stability to many people. For Mr. Bates independence was a long-term value. This is not to say that values are completely stable over time, because we know that values do change throughout one's life. Yet social existence requires standards within the individual as well as an agreement on standards among groups of individuals. As Kluckhohn (1951, p. 400) points out, without values, "the functioning of the social system could not continue to achieve group goals; individuals . . . could not feel within themselves a requisite measure of order and unified purpose." Thus, by adding an element of collective purpose in social life, values guarantee endurance and stability in social existence.

RELATIVITY

Isolated values are usually organized into a hierarchic system. As an individual confronts social situations throughout life, isolated values learned in early childhood come into competition with other values, requiring a weighing of one value against another (Fig. 5-1). Concern for others' welfare, for instance, competes with self-interest. Through experience and maturation, the individual integrates values learned in different contexts into systems in which each value is ordered relative to other values.

BELIEF

Rokeach (1973) defines values as a subcategory of beliefs. He argues that some beliefs are descriptive — capable of being true or false; other beliefs are evaluative — judging whether an object is good or bad; and still other beliefs are prescriptive-proscriptive — determining whether an action is desirable or undesirable. Values, he says, are prescriptive-proscriptive beliefs. They are concerned with what ought to be. Parents' values about child behavior, for example, determine their choices for disciplinary measures. Sharing the characteristics of all beliefs, values have cognitive, affective, and behavioral components. Rokeach (1973, p. 7) writes: "(1) A value is a cognition about the desirable. . . . To say that a person has a value is to say that cognitively he knows the correct way to behave or the correct end-state to strive for. (2) . . . he can feel emotional about it, be affectively for or against it. . . . (3) A value has a behavioral component in the sense that it is an intervening variable that leads to actions."

Figure 5-1
Values are learned and endure as they are reinforced by the significant people around us. This girl is learning values related to her appearance as a female.

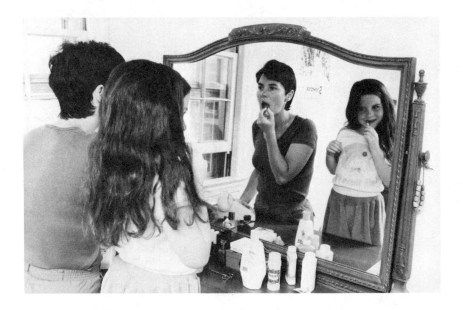

REFERENCE

Values also have a reference quality. That is, they may refer to end-states of existence called *terminal values* (e.g., religious salvation, peace of mind, world peace). Or they may refer to modes of conduct called *instrumental values* (e.g., confidentiality, promise-keeping, and honesty). The latter can have a moral focus or a nonmoral focus and these values may conflict. For example, a nurse may experience a conflict between two moral values such as whether to act honestly or to act respectfully. Similarly, she or he can experience conflict between two competence (nonmoral) values such as whether to plan logically or to plan creatively. The nurse can also experience conflict between a competence value and a moral value such as whether to act efficiently or to act fairly.

PREFERENCE

A value is something preferred over other alternatives. It is a preference for one mode of behavior over another, such as exercise over inactivity, or for one end state over another, such as trimness over obesity. We simply prefer one over the other, like Mr. Bates' preference for independence over personal comfort. The preferred end state or mode of behavior is located higher in our personal value hierarchy.

The qualities of values — endurance, relativity, belief, reference, and preference — indicate that values have the potential for an extensive range of application in human existence. Unfortunately, very little is known about the conditions under which people employ values. Theorists can only suggest that values enjoy a central place of importance within people's value-additude-belief systems. Thus, an exploration of value systems and the priority of values within those systems is the next step in understanding how values are ultimately related to individual and aggregate-level choices concerning health.

Nature of Value Systems

Contrasting value systems may be seen in many community health nursing practice settings. One nurse experienced such a contrast on her first home visit to a family. Referred by a social worker for recurring problems with head lice and staphylococcal infections, the family was living in the worst conditions the nurse had ever seen. Papers, moldy food, soiled clothing, and empty beer cans literally covered the floors. The nurse recoiled in horror. The children, home from school, were clustered around the television. Their mother, a divorced, single parent, unkempt and obese, sat smoking a cigarette with a can of beer in her hand. She had been unable to earn enough money waitressing to support herself and the children so was now on welfare. Her main pleasure in life was television soap operas. The nurse was interpreting the situation through the framework of her own value system — as we all do — yet the family clearly had its own value system as well.

Value systems are generally considered organizations of beliefs that are of relative importance in guiding individual behavior (Rokeach, 1973). Instead of being guided by single or isolated values, however, behavior at any point in time or sequence of behaviors is influenced by multiple or changing clusters of values. Thus it is important to understand how values like those of the family above are integrated into a person's attitude-value-belief system, how values assume a place in a hierarchy of values, and how this hierarchical system changes over time.

As mentioned previously, Rokeach (1973) indicates that learned values are integrated into an organized system of values and that each value has an ordered priority with respect to other values. For the welfare family, television entertainment was apparently a higher value than order and cleanliness. This system of ordered priority is stable enough to reflect the continuity of one's personality and behavior within culture and society, yet it is sufficiently flexible to allow a reordering of value priorities in response to changes in the environment, social setting, or personal experiences. Behavior change would, of course, be regarded as the visible response to a reordering of values within an individual's hierarchical value system.

Adults generally possess only a few, perhaps a dozen and a half, *terminal values,* such as peace of mind or achievement. These are influenced by complex physiological and social factors. Human needs, such as physiological needs, security, love, self-esteem, and self-actualization, proposed by Maslow (1969), are believed to be the greatest influences on terminal values. While a person may have only a few terminal values, the same person may possess as many as five or six dozen *instrumental values.* The latter, singly or in combination with other instrumental values, also help determine terminal values. For example, instrumental values of acceptance, taking it easy, living one day at a time, or not being concerned about the future, can help to shape the terminal value of peace of mind. Or instrumental values of hard work, driving oneself to compete, or not letting anyone get in one's way, can influence the terminal values of achievement. Figure 5-2 illustrates the influence of instrumental values as well as human needs on the development of terminal values.

Functions of Values and Value Systems

Values and value systems have different functions. Values primarily function as standards for behavior, and value systems function as plans for conflict resolution and decision making.

110

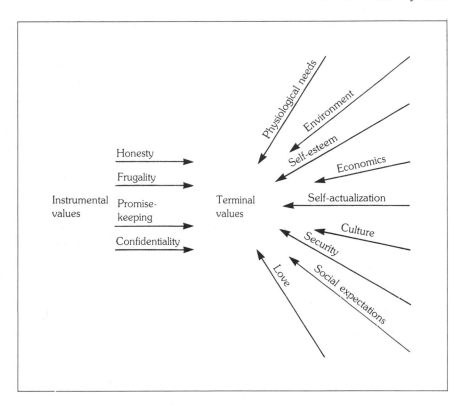

Figure 5-2
Factors influencing personal values.

STANDARDS FOR BEHAVIOR

In general, values function as standards that guide actions and behavior in daily situations. Once internalized by an individual, a value such as honesty becomes a criterion for that individual's personal conduct. Values may function as criteria for developing and maintaining attitudes toward objects and situations or for justifying one's own actions and attitudes. Values may also serve as the standards by which we pass moral judgment on ourselves and others (Rokeach, 1968).

Values have a long-term function in giving expression to human needs. According to Rokeach (1973), the strong motivational component of a value helps a person adjust to society, defend ego against threat, and test reality. In addition, values are employed as standards to guide presentation of the self to others, to ascertain whether we are as moral and as competent as others, and to persuade and influence others by indicating which beliefs, attitudes, and actions of others are worth trying to reinforce or change.

PLANS FOR CONFLICT RESOLUTION AND DECISION MAKING

When an individual encounters a social situation, several values within his or her value system are activated rather than just a single value. For example, the nurse entering Mr. Bates' home applied her values of health protection, safety, cleanliness, and respect for the individual and his right to autonomy. Clearly, all the activated values will not be compatible with one another. Thus conflict between values is inevitable in social existence, depending on the situation and the specific values activated.

Obviously, some values will triumph over others when conflicting values are activated. It is not known why some values consistently triumph over others and are stronger directives for individual behavior. Even though a value system is a hierarchy of values that slowly changes and adjusts to social existence over time, some values seem to consistently remain in higher positions than other values. Other values do, of course, lose their positions of importance in a value hierarchy. It is this changing arrangement of values in a hierarchical system that determines, in part, how conflicts will be resolved and decisions will be made. Thus an individual's value system functions as a learned organization of principles and rules that helps him or her choose between alternative courses of action and reach decisions (Fig. 5-3).

Figure 5-3
Our hierarchical value system helps us choose between alternative courses of action. This boy's love of fishing is clearly more important to him than getting his schoolwork done.

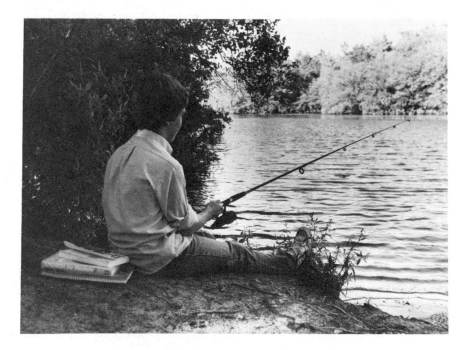

Values and Decision Making

One way to understand the influence and priority of values in our own as well as clients' behavior is to employ various values clarification techniques in decision making. According to Steele and Harmon (1983, p. 13), values clarification is a process of discovery that "attempts to bring to conscious awareness the values and underlying motivations that guide one's actions." Since individuals are largely unaware of the motives underlying their behavior and choices, values clarification is potentially important to the kind of decisions individuals make. Only by understanding our own values and their priority or importance can we be certain that our choices are more the result of rationality and less the result of other influences — cultural, social, or other kinds of previous conditioning. Values clarification by itself does not yield a set of rules for future decision making and does not indicate the right or wrong of alternative actions. Values clarification does, however, help guarantee that any course of action chosen by an individual is consistent and in accordance with one's own personal beliefs and values.

Approaches to Values Clarification

Although there are several approaches to values clarification, all aproaches seem to agree on (1) the process of valuing, and (2) strategies used in values clarification (Simon & Clark, 1975; Simon & Kirschenbaum, 1972; Steele and Harmon, 1983; Uustal, 1977a, 1977b, 1978).

PROCESS OF VALUING

Before values clarification can take place, an understanding of the process of valuing is necessary. Uustal (1977b) lists seven steps in this process:

1. A value must be freely chosen and be an individual choice.
2. A value is chosen among alternatives.
3. A value exists only after the consequences of a choice have been carefully considered.
4. A value is that which is cherished or prized.
5. A value is capable of public affirmation.
6. A value is incorporated into behavior (becomes a standard).
7. A value is consciously employed in decision making.

These steps provide specific actions for the discovery and identification of individual values. They also assist the decision-making process by explicating the process of valuing itself.

STRATEGIES IN VALUES CLARIFICATION

Uustal (1978) offers several strategies of values clarification that are ultimately useful to the decision-making process in community health nursing practice. Strategy 1 is a means by which nurses can come to know themselves and their values better (see Fig. 5-4). Strategy 2 assists in discovering value clusters and the priority of values within personal value systems (see Fig. 5-5). Strategy 3 can be used to examine one's responses to selected issues in nursing practice. Each response helps establish priorities of values by asking the nurse to choose among the alternatives presented or by indicating the degree of agreement or disagreement (see Fig. 5-6).

Other values clarification strategies are included in the study questions at the end of this chapter to assist nurses in understanding their ordering of values and to help them consider directions for change.

All of these strategies can be used to analyze and understand how values are meaningful to people and ultimately influence their choices and behavior. Clarification of one's values is the first step in the decision-making process and affects the ability of individuals to make ethical decisions. Values clarification is also important to the understanding and respect of values held by others such as patients and other health care providers. As pointed out by Uustal (1977b, p. 10), "Nurses cannot hope to give optimal, sensitive care to any patient without first understanding their own opinions, attitudes, and values." With this process in mind, it is now possible to explore the role of values in ethical decision making.

Ethical Decision Making

Values are central to any consideration of ethics or ethical decision making. Yet it is not at first obvious what counts as an ethical problem in health care or in the practice of nursing. Most nurses easily recognize the moral

Figure 5-4
Values clarification strategy 1.

> Name Tag
>
> Take a piece of paper and write your name in the middle of it. In each of the four corners, write your responses to these four questions:
>
> 1. What two things would you like your colleagues to say about you?
> 2. What single most important thing do you do (or would you do) to make your nurse-client relationships positive ones?
> 3. What do you do on a daily basis that indicates you value your health?
> 4. What are the three values you believe in most strongly?
>
> In the space around your name, write at least six adjectives that you feel best describe who you are.
> Take a closer look at your responses to the questions and to the ways in which you described yourself. What values are reflected in your answers?

Patterns

Which of the following words describe you? Draw a circle around the seven words that best describe you as an individual. Underline the seven words that most accurately describe you as a professional person. (You may circle and underline the same word.)

ambitious   reserved   assertive   opinionated

    concerned   generous   independent

easily hurt   outgoing   reliable   indifferent

    capable   self-controlled   fun-loving

suspicious   solitary   likable   dependent

    intellectual   argumentative   dynamic   unpredictable

compromising   thoughtful   affectionate   obedient

    logical   imaginative   self-disciplined

moody   easily led   helpful   slow to relate

Reflect on the following questions:

1. What values are reflected in the patterns you have chosen?
2. What is the relationship between these patterns and your personal values?
3. What patterns indicate inconsistencies in attitudes or behavior?
4. What patterns do you think a nurse should cultivate?

Figure 5-5
Values clarification strategy 2.

Figure 5-6
Values clarification strategy 3.

Forced Choice Ranking

How do you order the following alternatives by priority? (There is no correct set of priorities.) What values emerge in response to each question?

1. With whom on a nursing team would you become most angry? The nurse who
   _____ never completes assignments.
   _____ rarely helps other team members.
   _____ projects his or her own feelings on clients.

2. If you had a serious health problem, you would rather
   _____ not be told.
   _____ be told directly.
   _____ find out by accident.

3. You are made happiest in your work when you use
   _____ your technical skills in caring for clients with complex needs.
   _____ your ability to compile data and arrive at a nursing diagnosis.
   _____ your ability to communicate easily and skillfully with clients.

4. It would be most difficult for you to
   _____ listen to and counsel a dying person.
   _____ advise a pregnant adolescent.
   _____ handle a situation of obvious child abuse.

crisis in decisions, for example, to let an abnormal newborn infant die, to terminate a pregnancy resulting from rape, or to help a terminally ill client in pain end his life. These decisions clearly seem to involve ethical components, yet it is not immediately evident why we call these decisions ethical while others that are faced in the routine practice of community health nursing are not ethical in nature.

MORAL AND NONMORAL EVALUATIONS

A key requirement is distinguishing between evaluative statements and statements presenting nonevaluative facts. Ethics necessarily involves making evaluative judgments. Moving from the judgment that we *can* do something to the judgment that we *ought* to do something involves incorporating a set of norms — of judgments of value, right, duties, and responsibilities. Thus, in order to be ethically responsible in the practice of nursing, it is important to develop the ability to recognize evaluative judgments as they are made in nursing practice.

One approach is to reflect upon one's recent experiences. Select an experience that, at first, seems to involve no particular value judgments. Begin describing what occurred and watch for evaluative words. Among the words to watch for are verbs such as *want, desire, prefer, should,* or *ought.* The evaluations may also be expressed in nouns such as *benefit, harm, duty, responsibility, right,* or *obligation.*

Sometimes the evaluations are expressed in terms that are not direct expressions of evaluations but are clearly functioning as value judgments. For example, the American Nurses Association (ANA) *Code for Nurses* (1976, p. 4) states that "the nurse provides services . . . unrestricted by considerations of social or economic status, personal attributes, or the nature of health problems." In this statement the ANA could be describing the facts about the way all nurses behave. However, it is not the case that all nurses do behave in this manner. Rather, this statement prescribes that nurses *ought* to provide services without discrimination and that the ethical nurse does provide services in this manner.

Another approach to ethical decision making is to distinguish between moral and nonmoral evaluations (Veatch, 1977). Moral evaluations are prescriptive-proscriptive beliefs having certain characteristics that separate them from other evaluations such as aesthetic judgments, personal preferences, or matters of taste. The differences between the evaluations lies in the grounds on or the reasons for which the evaluations are being made (Frankena, 1973).

Moral evaluations are evaluations of human actions, institutions, or character traits rather than inanimate objects such as paintings or architectural structures. Moral evaluations also have distinctive characteristics. First, the evaluations

116

are ultimate. They have a preemptive quality, meaning that other values or human ends cannot, as a rule, override them (Beauchamp & Childress, 1983; Fried, 1978). Second, they possess universality or reflect a standpoint that applies to everyone. They are evaluations that everyone in principle ought to be able to make and understand, even if some individuals, in fact, do not (Baier, 1958; Rawls, 1971). Third, moral evaluations avoid giving a special place to one's own welfare. They have a focus that keeps others in view or, at least, considers one's own welfare on a par with that of others (Beauchamp & Childress, 1983; Rawls, 1971).

Judgments possessing the above characteristics are moral judgments. Because these judgments involve moral values, however, conflicts among them are inevitable. Hence, it is easy to see that any clinical decision in nursing practice that involves a conflict over values potentially involves a moral conflict. The nurse may be faced with the choice between preserving the client's welfare or the welfare of someone else. The nurse may have to choose whether to keep a promise of confidentiality or to provide needed assistance for a client even though a confidence would have to be broken. The nurse may have to decide to protect the interests of colleagues or the interests of the employing institution, whether to serve future clients by striking for better conditions or to serve present clients by refusing to strike. Each decision involves a potential conflict between moral values and creates a decision-making problem in quite ordinary nursing situations.

DECISION-MAKING FRAMEWORKS

In attempts to resolve the conflict between moral values in community health nursing practice and to provide morally accountable nursing service, several frameworks for ethical decision making have been proposed. In each framework, the role of values is a key element in the decision-making process. For example, the list of questions below from Stanley (1980) demonstrates the use of values clarification techniques as a preliminary step to decision making:

1. What is going on in this case situation?
   Separate scientific facts from questions of values and morals
   Identify the nurse's value system
2. By what criteria should decisions be made?
   Professional codes
   Religious perspectives
   Philosophical reasoning or works
3. Who should decide?
4. For whose benefit is the decision made?
5. How should professionals decide and act?
   Alternative actions
   Response to ethical principles

The separation of questions of fact from questions of value and the identification of the nurse's value system are considered fundamental to the choosing of alternative courses of action.

The identification of clients' values and those of other persons involved in conflict situations is also an important part of ethical decision making. For example, what are Mr. Bates' values, what are the neighbors' values who are concerned but feel they can no longer care for him, and what are the nurse's values? An ethical decision-making framework that includes the identification and clarification of all values impinging on the making of ethical decisions is outlined below (Thompson & Thompson, 1981):

1. Review the situation
   - What health problems exist?
   - What decisions need to be made?
   - Separate ethical components of the decisions from those decisions that can be made solely on a scientific knowledge base.
   - Identify all individuals/groups affected by the decision.
2. Decide what further information is needed before decision can be made.
3. Identify ethical issues. Discuss historical, philosophical, and religious bases for these issues.
4. Identify your own values and beliefs. Identify professional responsibilities dictated by the ANA *Code for Nurses*.
5. Identify values and beliefs of other people involved in situation.

Figure 5-7
Ethical decision-making framework 3.

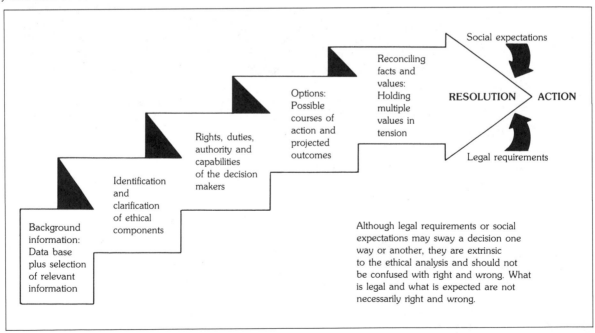

Background information: Data base plus selection of relevant information

Identification and clarification of ethical components

Rights, duties, authority and capabilities of the decision makers

Options: Possible courses of action and projected outcomes

Reconciling facts and values: Holding multiple values in tension

Social expectations

RESOLUTION > **ACTION**

Legal requirements

Although legal requirements or social expectations may sway a decision one way or another, they are extrinsic to the ethical analysis and should not be confused with right and wrong. What is legal and what is expected are not necessarily right and wrong.

6. Identify value conflicts, if any.
7. Decide who should make the decision. Determine nurse's role in making the decision.
8. Identify range of decisions or actions that are possible. Determine implications for all people involved. Identify how suggested actions conform to the *Code for Nurses*.
9. Decide on a course of action and follow through.
10. Evaluate the results of the actions or decisions. Generalize for future situations.

In a different consideration of values, the framework in Figure 5-7 advocates keeping multiple values in tension before resolution of conflict and action on the part of the nurse. This framework apparently does not view value conflict as capable of resolution until all possible alternative actions have been explored. Final resolution of the ethical conflict would then occur through conscious choice of action even though some or even many values would be overridden by stronger, presumably moral values. The triumphant values would apparently be those values located higher in the decision maker's hierarchy of values.

Values and Health Care

The relationship between values and health has been extensively studied by the President's Commission for the Study of Ethical Problems in Medicine and Biomedical and Behavioral Research. Created by the U.S. Congress in November 1978, the President's Commission had the responsibility to study and report on the ethical and legal implications of a number of issues in medicine and research. Between 1981 and 1983, the Commission published most of its findings and conclusions in a series of nine reports on the following topics: definition of death, informed consent, genetic screening and counseling, access to health care, life-sustaining treatment, privacy and confidentiality, genetic engineering, compensation for injured research subjects, and whistle-blowing.

In all of its reports, the Commission discussed the importance of three basic human values — self-determination, well-being, and equity (President's Commission, 1983b). These values are considered the key values that ought to guide decision making in the provider-client relationship and are the criteria by which the success of a particular interaction is judged.

Self-determination

The value of self-determination or individual autonomy is defined by the Commission (1983a, p. 44) as "an individual's exercise of the capacity to form, revise, and pursue personal plans for life." Self-determination is instrumentally valued because self-judment about one's goals and choices is conducive to an individual's sense of well-being. Thus respecting self-determination is based on the belief that better outcomes will result when self-determination is respected and encouraged. Those outcomes that apparently will be maximized by respecting self-determination seem to include enhanced self-concept, enhanced health-promoting behaviors, and enhanced quality of care.

Yet self-determination is also intrinsically valued. It is valued (1) for the freedom from outside control it provides, and (2) because it indicates that the individual chooses his own actions or the actions that affect him. To not respect this value of self-determination is to demonstrate disrespect to persons or to fail to provide them with adequate protection against arbitrary domination by others. Those desiring to be self-determining express the desire to be instruments of their own acts of will, not the will of other persons.

The Commission noted that in health care contexts this desire was of such high ethical importance that self-determination actually overrides practitioner determinations in most situations. This position was supported by the results of a survey undertaken by the Commission (1982): 72 percent of those surveyed said they would prefer to make decisions jointly with their physicians after treatment alternatives had been explained. Physician responses in the same survey, however, indicated that the majority of physicians (88 percent) believe that patients want doctors to make decisions for them. The wide difference between patient expectations regarding self-determination and physician beliefs indicates that self-determination on the part of patients is at high risk in most health care contexts. Physicians and possibly other health practitioners simply fail to recognize the high value attributed to self-determination by patients.

The Commission (1982) also noted that respect for self-determination promotes personal integration within a chosen life-style and is important for creative self-agency. Thus, the value of self-determination is a value that should be nourished in the provision of health care. Noting that "personal responsibility for decision-making is one of the wellsprings of a democracy," the Commission (1983a, p. 46) said the concept of health care decision making includes informing patients of alternative courses of treatment and of the reasoning behind all recommendations.

Yet it is important to note that self-determination cannot be respected at all times and in all situations. There are times when self-determination is impermissible or even impossible. For example, there are times when society must impose restrictions on the range of acceptable client choices; at other times, clients are not competent to exercise self-determination. Thus the Commission recognized two instances in which restrictions might be put on self-determination: (1) when some objectives of individuals are contrary to the public interest or the interests of others in society and (2) when a person's

120

decision making is so defective or mistaken that the decision fails to promote the person's own values or goals. As an example of the first instance, restriction might occur when clients request professional help in carrying out criminal activities or when a client's request entails depleting of health care resources for other individuals. As an example of the second instance, restriction might occur when clients refuse life-saving treatment for trivial reasons. In these situations, self-determination is justifiably overridden on the basis of the promotion of well-being, another important value in health care decision making.

Well-being

The Commission's reports defined the value of individual well-being in terms of health or the client's subjective preferences concerning health. It is noted that therapeutic interventions offered by health professionals are intended to improve a client's health. Health care is, therefore, considered a means of promoting clients' well-being.

Unfortunately, interventions believed to promote health, health care decisions, and an individual's sense of well-being are not necessarily causally related. Sometimes there are no objective medical criteria (or nursing criteria) for determining if some proposed intervention will promote health. In the case of alternative methods of providing health care, the proffered method may simply reflect the health professional's values or subjective choice. Thus the value of client well-being may be more a matter of professional choice rather than client choice in many situations.

Determining what constitutes health and how the client's well-being can be promoted often requires a knowledge of the client's subjective preferences. It is generally recognized that clients may be inclined to pursue different directions in treatment procedures based on individual goals and interests. Community health nurses, on the other hand, are committed to helping clients and avoiding harms to them. Thus they are obliged to understand each client's needs and develop reasonable alternatives for treatment or care from which clients may choose what they prefer. In addition, when individuals are not capable of making a choice, the nurse is obliged to make health care decisions that promote the value of well-being. This may mean that the alternatives that the nurse presents for choice are only ones that will, in fact, promote well-being. According to the Commission (1983a, p. 44), "Shared decision-making requires that a practitioner seek not only to understand each patient's needs and develop reasonable alternatives to meet those needs but also to present the alternatives in a way that enables patients to choose one they prefer." Well-being and self-determination are therefore two values that are intricately related in the provision of community health nursing service.

Equity

The third value important to decision making in health care contexts is the value of equity. It is a value of central importance to the provision of health care but poses many practical and philosophical difficulties.

Like the values of self-determination and well-being, equity has several facets. It is sometimes defined as the value that directs that like cases be treated alike. In other contexts, it is defined as the value that directs that all individuals be treated fairly. Both definitions include the notions that it is unjust to treat differently individuals who are in relevant ways alike and it is unfair (or inequitable) to treat people identically when they are in significant respects unalike. The need for health care and other goods differs among individuals. Equity means that all individuals should have access to health care according to benefit or needs. It also means that an adequate level of health care should be provided for all citizens.

Focus on an adequate level of health care for everyone makes equity a value that avoids unacceptable restrictions on individual liberty while not overcommitting resources to every citizen. The major problem with this definition of equity, of course, is that it assumes that an adequate level of health care can be economically available to all citizens. In times of limited technical resources and decreased financial resources, however, it may be impossible to respect the value of equity. In these situations, the value obligations of professional practice may well create conflicts of values that seem impossible to resolve.

In attempting to deal with the difficult problems posed by the distribution of available health goods in times of economic crisis, the Commission wisely refrained from definitive interpretations of the values of equity, well-being, and self-determination. It did, however, set terms of reference by which those who are responsible for formulating policy on health care could compare the ethical implications of alternative proposals. Considering the availability of health care services for all citizens, the justifications for claiming that health care services should, as a matter of national policy, be available to all, and the importance of the values involved, the Commission (1983b, pp. 29–30) reached several conclusions:

> 1. Society has an ethical obligation to ensure equitable access to health care for all. This obligation rests on the special importance of health care and is derived from its role in relieving suffering, preventing premature death, restoring functioning, increasing opportunity, providing information about an individual's condition, and giving evidence of mutual empathy and compassion.
>
> 2. The societal obligation is balanced by individual obligations. Individuals ought to pay a fair share of the cost of their own health care and take reasonable steps to provide for such care when they can do so without excessive burdens.
>
> 3. Equitable access to health care requires that all citizens be able to secure an adequate level of care without excessive burdens. Equitable access also

means that the burdens borne by individuals in obtaining adequate care ought not to be excessive or to fall disproportionately on particular individuals.

4. When equity occurs through the operation of private forces, there is no need for government involvement. But the ultimate responsibility for ensuring that society's obligation is met, through a combination of public and private sector arrangements, rests with the Federal government.

5. The cost of achieving equitable access to health care ought to be shared fairly. The cost of securing health care for those unable to pay ought to be spread equitably at the national level and not allowed to fall more heavily on the shoulders of particular practitioners, institutions, or residents of different localities.

6. Efforts to contain rising health care costs are important but should not focus on limiting the attainment of equitable access for the least well-served portion of the public. Measures designed to contain health care costs that exacerbate existing inequities or impede the achievement of equity are unacceptable from a moral standpoint.

Considering the relationships among the values of self-determination, well-being, and equity, what are the implications of the Commission's conclusions for community health nursing? Specifically, how do these human values affect the practice of nursing and the provision of nursing services to the community?

Implications for Community Health Nursing Practice

Values and their relationship to health have many implications for community health nursing. The value of self-determination has implications for how community health nurses (1) respect the choices of clients, (2) protect privacy, (3) provide for informed consent, and (4) protect diminished capacity for self-determination. The value of well-being has implications for how community health nurses (1) reduce harms and provide benefits to client populations, (2) measure the effectiveness of nursing services, and (3) balance costs of services against real benefits. The value of equity has implications for community health nursing in terms of its priorities for (1) distributing health goods (macroallocation issues) and (2) deciding which populations obtain available health goods and nursing services (microallocation issues).

Decisions based on one value will mean, of course, that this value will come in conflict with other values. For example, deciding on the basis of well-being may conflict with deciding on the basis of self-determination or equity. How community health nurses balance these values may even conflict with their own personal values or the values of the nursing profession. In these situations, values clarification techniques and the use of values clarification in decision making may assist the community health nurse in making decisions that are not only ethical but that promote the greatest well-being for clients without substantially reducing their self-determination or ignoring equity.

Summary

Values and the valuing process strongly influence community health nursing practice. It is important that community health nurses understand the meaning of values and their relationship to health and health decisions.

A value is a lasting belief that a certain means or end state is preferable over other choices. A value system organizes these beliefs into a continuum of relative importance that guides human behavior.

One can understand the nature of values by examining their qualities — endurance, relativity, belief, reference, and preference. Multiple values form changing clusters of values, or value systems, that shape people's behavior. People generally possess multiple *instrumental* values that help to determine their *terminal* personal values, such as what they believe about love or self-determination. Values function as standards for behavior, as criteria for attitudes, as standards for moral judgments, and give expression to human needs. Value systems order values by priority, provide a plan for conflict resolution, and organize principles.

Since values and value systems guide decision making, nurses need to be aware of and understand their own underlying beliefs. The process of valuing goes through several steps from selection and prizing of a value to integration and conscious use of the value in decision making. Various strategies can be employed to accomplish values clarification.

Understanding personal values assists the nurse in making ethical evaluations in practice. Responsible ethical decision making requires an effort on the nurse's part to make moral evaluations based on moral values. That is, the moral values used should reflect high-level priority, universality, and a focus on others rather than self. Ethical conflicts in nursing practice involve a conflict between moral values. Several frameworks for ethical decision making are available to guide the nurse.

Three key human values influence client health and the nurse-client relationship — self-determination, well-being, and equity. The community health nurse must, as often as possible, respect clients' self-determination to enhance their acting responsibly on their own behalf. The nurse seeks to promote clients' sense of well-being through interventions that respect clients' subjective preferences but reduce potential harms and offer benefits. The nurse also promotes equity — the value that everyone should have access to health care as needed. The nurse must keep these values in balance, using values clarification techniques when conflicts between values arise.

Study Questions

1. Where do you stand on the following issues? For each statement, decide if you strongly agree, agree, disagree, or strongly disagree with it or if you are undecided about it.

a. Clients have the right to participate in all decisions related to their health care.
b. Nurses need a system designed to credit self-study.
c. Continuing education should be mandatory.
d. Clients should always be told the truth.
e. Standards of nursing practice should be enforced by state examining boards.
f. Nurses should be required to take relicensure examinations every five years.
g. Clients should be allowed to read their health record when they request to.
h. Abortion should be an option available to every woman.
i. Badly deformed newborns should be allowed to die.
j. There should be laws guaranteeing desired health care for each person in this country.

2. In a grid similar to the one below, write a statement of belief in the space provided and examine it in relation to the seven steps of the process of valuing. Some areas of confusion and conflict in nursing practice that you might want to examine are peer review, accountability, confidentiality, euthanasia, licensure, patients' rights, abortion, informed consent, and terminating treatment.

   To the right of your statements, check the appropriate boxes indicating when your beliefs reflect one or more of the seven steps in the valuing process. Is your belief a value according to the valuing process?

Statement	Freely chosen	Alternatives	Consequences	Cherished	Affirmed	Incorporated	Employed
	1	2	3	4	5	6	7

3. Rank in order the 12 potential nursing actions below by using 1 to indicate the choice that you feel is most important in a nurse-client relationship and 12 to indicate the choice you believe is least important.

Touching the client.

Empathetically listening to clients.

Disclosing yourself to clients.

Becoming emotionally involved with the client.

Teaching clients.

Being honest in answering client's questions.

Seeing that clients adhere to medical therapy.

Helping to decrease the clients' anxiety.

Making sure that medications and treatments are done on time.

Following doctors' orders.

Remaining "professional" with clients.

Choice. (Add an alternative of your own.)

Examine the way in which you have ordered these options. What values can you identify based on your responses in this exercise? How do these values emerge in your behavior?

References

American Nurses Association. (1976). *Code for nurses with interpretive statements*. Kansas City, MO: Author.

Baier, K. (1958). *The moral point of view*. Ithaca, NY: Cornell University Press.

Beauchamp, T. L., & Childress, J. F. (1983). *Principles of biomedical ethics* (2nd ed.). New York: Oxford University Press.

Curtin, L. (1978). A proposed model for critical ethical analysis. *Nursing Forum, 17,* 12–17.

Curtin, L. (1982). No rush to judgment. In L. Curtin & J. Flaherty (Eds.), *Nursing ethics: Theories and pragmatics* (pp. 57–63). Bowie, MD: Robert J. Brady.

Frankena, W. K. (1973). *Ethics*. Englewood Cliffs, NJ: Prentice-Hall.

Fried, C. (1978). *Right and wrong*. Cambridge, MA: Harvard University Press.

Kluckhohn, C. (1951). Values and value-orientations in the theory of action: An exploration in definition and classification. In T. Parsons & E. A. Shils (Eds.), *Toward a general theory of action* (pp. 388–433). Cambridge, MA: Harvard University Press.

Maslow, A. (1969). *Toward a psychology of being* (2nd ed.). New York: Van Nostrand.

President's Commission for the Study of Ethical Problems in Medicine and Biomedical and Behavioral Research of (1978), Pub. L. No. 95-622, 1978 U.S. Code Cong. & Ad. News (92 Stat.) 3438 (codified primarily at 42 U.S.C.A. §§ 300v.–300v.–3. [1982]).

President's Commission for the Study of Ethical Problems in Medicine and Biomedical and Behavioral Research. (1982). *Making health care decisions: Volume One Report*. Washington, DC: U.S. Government Printing Office.

President's Commission for the Study of Ethical Problems in Medicine and Biomedical and Behavioral Research. (1983a). *Securing access to health care: Volume One Report*. Washington, DC: U.S. Government Printing Office.

President's Commission for the Study of Ethical Problems in Medicine and Biomedical and Behavioral Research. (1983b). *Summing up*. Washington, DC: U.S. Government Printing Office.

Rawls, J. (1971). *A theory of justice.* Cambridge, MA: Harvard University Press.

Rokeach, M. (1968). *Beliefs, attitudes and values: A theory of organization and change.* San Francisco: Jossey-Bass.

Rokeach, M. (1973). *The nature of human values.* New York: Free Press.

Simon, S. B., & Clark, J. (1975). *More values clarifications: Strategies for the classroom.* San Diego, CA: Pennant Press.

Simon, S. B., & Kirschenbaum, H. (1972). *Values clarification: A handbook of practical strategies for teachers and students.* New York: Hart Publishing.

Stanley, T. (1980). Ethics as a component of the curriculum. *Nursing and Health Care, 1,* 63–72.

Steele, S. M., & Harmon, M. V. (1983). *Values clarification in nursing.* (2nd ed.). Norwalk, CT: Appleton-Century-Crofts.

Thompson, J. B., & Thompson, H. O. (1981). *Ethics in nursing.* New York: Macmillan.

Uustal, D. B. (1977a). Searching for values. *Image, 9 February,* 15–17.

Uustal, D. B. (1977b). The use of values clarification in nursing practice. *Journal of Continuing Education in Nursing, 8 May–June,* 8–13.

Uustal, D. B. (1978). Values clarification in nursing. *American Journal of Nursing, 78,* 2058–2063.

Veatch, R. M. (1977). *Case studies in medical ethics.* Cambridge, MA: Harvard University Press.

Williams, R. (1968). Values. In D. L. Sills (Ed.), *International Encylcopedia of the Social Sciences* (p. 283). New York: Crowell, Collier and Macmillan.

Selected Readings

Aroskar, M. A. (1979). Ethical issues in community health nursing. *Nursing Clinics of North America, 14*(1), 35–44.

Beauchamp, T. L., & Childress, J. F. (1983). *Principles of biomedical ethics* (2nd Ed.). New York: Oxford University Press.

Carlson, R. (1975). *The end of medicine.* New York: John Wiley & Sons.

Churchill, L. R., & Simon, J. J. (1982). Abortion and the rhetoric of individual rights. *The Hastings Center Report, 9,* 10–12.

Curtin, L. (1978). A proposed model for critical ethical analysis. *Nursing Forum, 17,* 117.

Curtin, L. (1982). No rush to judgment. In L. Curtin & J. Flaherty (Eds.), *Nursing ethics: Theories and pragmatics* (pp. 57–63). Bowie, MD: Robert J. Brady.

Davis, A. & Aroskar, M. (1983). *Ethical dilemmas and nursing practice* (2nd ed.). Norwalk, CT: Appleton-Century-Crofts.

Dubos, R. (1968). *So human an animal.* New York: Scribner's.

Frankena, W. K. (1973). *Ethics.* Englewood Cliffs, NJ: Prentice-Hall.

Fried, C. (1978). *Right and wrong.* Cambridge, MA: Harvard University Press.

Illich, I. (1975). *Medical nemesis: The expropriation of health.* New York, Pantheon.

Matejski, M. P. (1981). Ethical issues, nursing and the health care system. *Nursing Leadership, 27,* 33.

President's Commission for the Study of Ethical Problems in Medicine and Biomedical and Behavioral Research. (1982). *Making health care decisions: Volume One Report.* Washington, DC: U.S. Government Printing Office.

President's Commission for the Study of Ethical Problems in Medicine and Biomedical and Behavioral Research. (1983a). *Securing access to health care: Volume One Report.* Washington, DC: U.S. Government Printing Office.

President's Commission for the Study of Ethical Problems in Medicine and Biomedical and Behavioral Research. (1983b). *Summing up.* Washington, DC: U.S. Government Printing Office.

Rokeach, M. K. (1973). *The nature of human values.* New York: Free Press.

Simon, S. B. & Clark, J. (1975). *More values clarification: Strategies for the classroom.* San Diego, CA: Pennant Press.

Simon, S. B. & Kirschenbaum, H. (1972). *Values clarification: A handbook of practical strategies for teachers and students.* New York: Hart Publishing.

Stanley, T. (1980). Ethics as a component of the curriculum. *Nursing and Health Care, 1,* 63–72.

Steele, S. M. & Harmon, M. V. (1983). *Values clarification in nursing* (2nd ed.). Norwalk, CT: Appleton-Century-Crofts.

Thompson, J. B. & Thompson, H. O. (1981). *Ethics in nursing.* New York: Macmillan.

Uustal, D. B. (1978). Values clarification in nursing. *American Journal of Nursing, 78,* 2058–2063.

Veatch, R. M. (1977). *Case studies in medical ethics.* Cambridge, MA: Harvard University Press.

6

Culture and Community

For most health professionals, individual differences are a treasured value. We are delighted to see children grow and develop in unique ways. We applaud someone's creative achievement. We each have preferences about the kind of food we eat, the way we dress, and how we decorate our living quarters. The right to be ourselves and different from others is highly valued. But although individuality is part of our culture, we recognize limits to the range of acceptable differences. People whose behavior falls outside that range become deviants or misfits. Our culture approves moderate social drinking but not alcoholism. Why are some behaviors acceptable and others not? Why do so many health professionals have difficulty trying to convince their clients to accept new ways of thinking and acting? Explanations can be found by examining the concept of culture and its application to community health nursing practice.

The Meaning of Culture

Culture refers to the ideas, values, and behavior that are shared by members of some social group. It is a design for living, a way of life. More than simply custom or ritual, culture is a way of organizing and thinking about life. It gives people a sense of security about their behavior; without having to consciously think about it, they know how to act. Culture also provides the underlying values and beliefs upon which this behavior is based. For example, culture determines the value we place on achievement, independence, work, and leisure. It forms the basis for our definitions of male and female roles and determines our responses to authority figures. As anthropologist Edward Hall says, "Culture controls our lives" (1959, p. 38).

Influence on Behavior

Every community, every social or ethnic group, has its own culture. Furthermore, all the individual members behave in the context of that specific culture. Each of us belongs to a group or set of overlapping groups that influences our thoughts and actions. Even very small elements of everyday living are influenced by our culture. For instance, culture determines the distance we stand from another person while talking. A comfortable talking distance for Americans is at least two and a half feet (Fig. 6-1), while Latin Americans prefer a shorter distance, often only 18 inches for dialogue. Consider how culture influences our perception of time. When we make an appointment to see someone, we expect to be on time or not more than a few minutes late. To keep a person waiting (or to be kept waiting) for 45 minutes or an hour is insulting and intolerable. Yet there are other cultures and subcultures, including Native American and Asian groups, whose response to time is much more flexible; their members think nothing of waiting or keeping someone else waiting for an hour or two. Clearly, culture, as Benjamin Paul puts it, "is a blueprint for social living" (cited in Landy, 1977, p. 233).

Figure 6-1
Culture influences every-day behavior by giving people a prescribed set of norms for their conduct. It has taught these people how far apart to stand during a casual conversation.

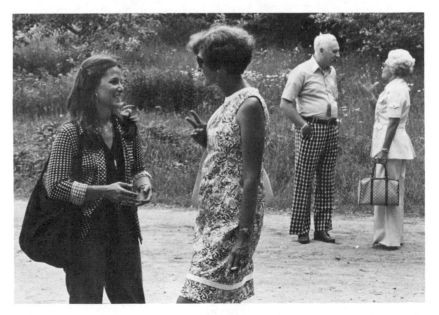

Relationship to Health Care

Culture, because it so profoundly influences thinking and behavior, is an essential dimension of health care. Just as physical and psychological factors determine clients' needs and attitudes toward health and illness, so too does culture. Kark emphasizes that "culture is perhaps the most relevant social determinant of community health" (1974, p. 149). Culture influences diet and eating practices and determines how children are reared. How people react to pain, cope with stress, deal with death, respond to health practitioners, and value the past, present, and future are all affected by culture, yet the concept of culture is not always clearly understood or incorporated into health care. Many nursing care plans omit consideration of clients' cultural and social needs. Others may include them only after some painful experience at the client's expense, as is shown in the following illustration.

Maria Juárez, a 53-year-old Chicano widow, was referred to a community health nursing agency by a clinic. Her married daughter reported that Mrs. Juárez was having severe and prolonged vaginal bleeding and needed medical attention. The daughter had made several appointments for her mother at the clinic, but Mrs. Juárez had refused at the last minute to keep any of them.

After two broken home visit appointments, the community health nurse made a drop-in call and found Mrs. Juárez at home. The nurse was greeted courteously and invited to have a seat. After introductions, the nurse explained that she and the others were only trying to help. Mrs. Juárez had caused a lot of unnecessary concern to everyone by not cooperating, she scolded in a friendly tone. Mrs. Juárez quickly apologized and explained that she had felt fine on the days of her broken appointments and saw no need "to bother" anyone. Questioned about her vaginal bleeding, Mrs. Juárez was evasive. "It's nothing," she said, "it comes and goes like always, only maybe a little more." She listened politely, nodding in agreement, as the nurse explained the need for her to see a physician. Her promise to come to the clinic the next day, however, was not kept. The staff labeled Mrs. Juárez unreliable and uncooperative.

Mrs. Juárez had been brought up to be a traditional Chicano woman. Her role was to be submissive and interested primarily in the welfare of her husband and children. She had learned long ago to ignore her own needs and, in fact, found it difficult to identify any personal wants. Her major concern was to avoid causing trouble for others. To have a medical problem, then, was a difficult adjustment. The pain and bleeding had caused her great apprehension. Many Chicanos have a particular dread of sickness and especially hospitalization (Herrera & Wagner, 1977). Furthermore, Mrs. Juárez's culture had taught her the value of modesty. "Female problems" were not discussed openly. This cultural orientation meant that the sickness threatened her modesty and created intense embarrassment. Conforming to Chicano cultural values, she had first turned to her family for support. Often it is only under dire circumstances that Chicanos seek help from others; to do so means sacrificing pride and dignity (Murillo, 1971). Mrs. Juárez agreed to go to the clinic because refusal would have been disrespectful, but her fear of physicians as well as her extreme reluctance to discuss such a sensitive problem kept her from going. Mrs. Juárez was being asked to take action that violated a number of deeply felt cultural values. Her behavior was far from unreliable and uncooperative. With no opportunity to discuss and resolve the conflicts, she had no other choice.

Cultural Differences

A major barrier to meeting Mrs. Juárez's needs was a failure by the nurse to recognize cultural differences. In fact, many of the health care system's failures result from this shortsightedness (Branch, 1976). It is most obvious that every group has its own culture when we contrast our way of life with a vastly different one, for example, that of a New Guinea tribe. We easily recognize culture when we see people sleep on the floor together in large extended family groups, eat monkey meat with their fingers from a common bowl, or seldom discipline young children.

Cultural differences, however, are equally strong in the United States. Although broad cultural values are shared by many of us, a rich diversity of subcultures also exists. Immigration patterns in recent years have changed the United States' population composition. During the 1970s, roughly half a million immigrants legally entered the United States. The *Harvard Encyclopedia of American Ethnic Groups* (S. Thernstrom et al., eds., 1980) lists one hundred different ethnic groups living in the United States, 50 of which are significant in size. Two of the largest minorities include Spanish-speaking Americans, numbering fifteen million officially (with many more entering illegally), representing approximately 6.4 percent of the population, and Asian-Americans numbering 3.5 million, or approximately 1.5 percent of the United States population. The largest minority group continues to be blacks, numbering 26 million and equal to about 10 percent of the United States population.

The increase in and great variety of cultural groups reinforces the need to understand and appreciate cultural differences. It also presents a significant challenge to community health nurses, requiring, among other things, new communication skills to cross language barriers and exploration of traditional ethnic health and curing practices to determine their effectiveness and safety.

The members of each subculture retain some of the characteristics of the society from which they came or in which their ancestors lived (Mead, 1960). Some of their beliefs and practices, such as the food they eat, the language they speak at home, the way they celebrate holidays, or their ideas about sickness and healing, remain an important part of their everyday life (Fig. 6-2). Native American groups have retained some aspects of their traditional

132

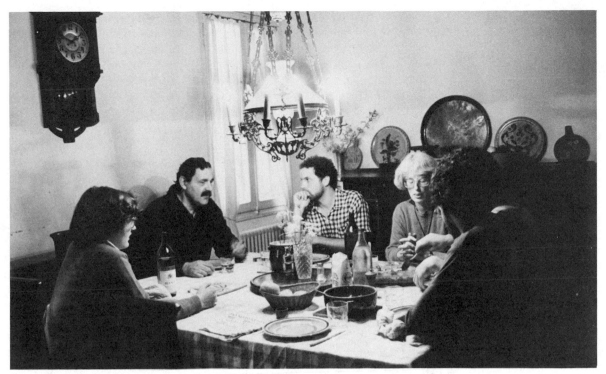

Figure 6-2
This Italian-American family enjoys a traditional Italian meal.

cultures. Mexican-Americans, Irish-Americans, Swedish-Americans, Italian-Americans, Afro-Americans, Puerto Ricans, Chinese-Americans, and many other ethnic groups have their own subcultures. Furthermore, certain customs, values, and ideas are unique to the poor, the rich, the middle class, women, men, youth, and the elderly. Many deviant groups, such as narcotic addicts, criminals, and skid row alcoholics, have developed their own subcultures. Regional subcultures, for instance, that of the Kentucky mountain people, also have distinctive ways of defining the world and coping with problems. Even occupational and professional groups develop their own special languages and outlooks. Nurses, for example, have a special culture with unique vocabulary, values, clothes, and customs. Recognizing such cultural differences is a first step toward cultural understanding.

Ethnocentrism

Another barrier to effective care for Mrs. Juárez was judging her behavior by a middle-class standard. Good patients, many people believe, appreciate help from health professionals and comply with their requests. This kind of thinking is based on the assumption that "my way is right." It is easy to view one's own way of life as the best and to reject those whose ideas differ as inferior, ignorant, or irrational. Such a belief is called *ethnocentrism* (Leininger, 1970; MacGregor, 1960). Ethnocentrism creates biases and misconceptions about human behavior that can cause irreparable damage to interpersonal relationships. Ethnocentrism, as Gagnon (1983, p. 127) points out, "interferes with [nurses'] perception of the knowledge received from others." Mrs. Juárez was labeled unreliable and uncooperative because she failed to conform to prescribed patterns of correct behavior, yet these same patterns contradicted Mrs. Juárez's value system. From her perspective, American health culture must have seemed equally strange and irrational. It is one thing to believe that your way is good for you, and it is another to insist that everyone else conform to it. Here lies the distinction between healthy cultural identification and ethnocentrism. Here also is another clue to the mystery of bridging cultural gaps; rather than apply moral judgments, one should understand and appreciate cultural differences.

Overcoming ethnocentrism requires a concerted effort on the nurse's part to see the world through the eyes of clients. It means learning to set aside, as much as possible, the nurse's own biases and preconceptions. It means attempting to understand the meaning of other people's culture for them, and it means appreciating their culture as equally important and useful.

Characteristics of Culture

In their study of culture, anthropologists and sociologists have made significant contributions to the field of community health. Five characteristics of culture are especially pertinent to consider in the effort to improve community health.

Culture Is Learned

Patterns of cultural behavior are acquired, not inherited. As Murdock explains, "cultural behavior is socially rather than biologically determined" (1972, p. 258). Each of us learns a cultural heritage through the process of socialization, sometimes called *enculturation*. As a little girl grows up in a given society, she acquires certain attitudes, beliefs, and values. She learns how to behave in ways appropriate to that society's definition of the female role. She is learning that culture (Fig. 6-3). Benedict summarizes this learning process (1934, p. 2):

> The life-history of the individual is first and foremost an accommodation to the patterns and standards traditionally handed down in his community. From the moment of his birth the customs into which he is born shape his experience and behavior. By the time he can talk, he is the little creature of his culture, and by the time he is grown and able to take part in its activities, its habits are his habits, its beliefs his beliefs, its impossibilities his impossibilities.

134

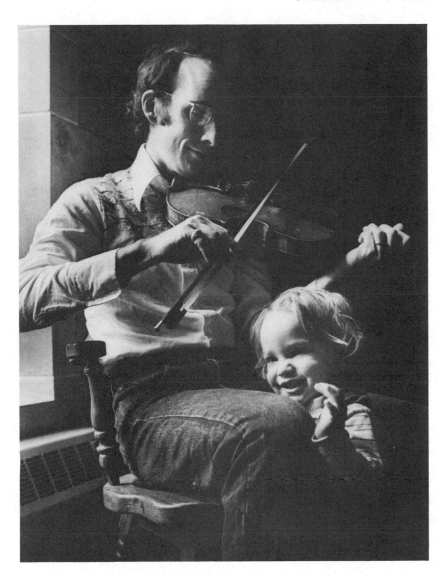

Figure 6-3
This child at her father's knee learns early to enjoy and value music.

Although culture is learned, the process and results of that learning are different for each person. Each individual has a unique personality and experiences life in a singular way; both these factors influence acquisition of culture. Families, social classes, and other groups within a society differ from one another, and this social variation has important implications for planned change. Since culture is learned, it is possible for parts of it to be relearned. People might change some cultural elements or adopt some new behaviors or values. In addition, Foster points out, "There will be differences in the ease and ability with which [people] continue to learn and in their flexibility in casting off old forms of behavior that conflict with new forms" (1962, p. 18). Some individuals and groups will be more willing to try new things than others and thus potentially influence change.

Culture Is Integrated

Rather than an assortment of various customs and traits, a culture is a functional, integrated whole. As in any system, all the parts of a culture are interrelated and independent. Benedict, who first examined the systemic nature of culture, says, "A culture, like an individual, is a more or less consistent pattern of thought and action" (1934, p. 46). The various components of a culture, such as its social mores or religious beliefs, perform separate functions that depend upon and articulate in relative harmony with each other to form an operating whole. Benedict emphasizes that this cultural whole is greater than the sum of its individual parts (1934, p. 47). In other words, to understand culture, one cannot simply describe single traits. Each part must be viewed in terms of its relationships to the other parts and to the whole.

Our own culture is an integrated web of ideas and practices. For example, we promote three balanced meals a day, a practice tied to our belief that nutrition leads to good health and that prevention is better than cure. These cultural traits, in turn, are related to our values about health. Health, we say, is essential for, among other conditions, maximum energy output and productivity at work. Productivity is important because it enables us to compete effectively. These values are linked to religious beliefs about hard work and taboos against laziness. Nutrition, health, economics, religion, and family are the fibers of a web whose design and usefulness depends upon their integration.

Another person's culturally determined behavior can be understood, therefore, by considering it in the context of that person's larger culture. For example, when parents who are Jehovah's Witnesses refuse blood transfusions for their child, their action is neither irrational nor ignorant. Rather, it represents behavior consistent with the couple's cultural values and beliefs and, in regard to their child's health, results from deeply held religious convictions. The single behavior of refusing blood transfusions, when viewed in context, is part of a larger religious belief system and a basic component of their culture.

The recognition that culture is integrated, that introducing a change in one part of a cultural system will affect other parts, influences community health nursing practice. Mrs. Juárez's cultural beliefs about modesty and self-effacement were related to her culture's definition of the woman's role that, in turn, influenced her interpersonal relationships. To change one practice was to affect many others. Likewise, the request from a nurse to submit to a physical exam with a male physician was equal to saying, "Stop behaving like a woman!" Asking certain Native American groups to accommodate rigid appointment scheduling means requiring them to reframe their concept of time. It also violates their values of patience and pride. Before nurses attempt a change in a person's or group's behavior, they need to ask how that change will affect the clients through its influence on other parts of their culture. Extra time and patience or different strategies may be needed if change is still indicated. Nurses may often find that their system can be modified to preserve the client's cultural values.

Culture Is Shared

Culture is the product of aggregate behavior, not individual habit. Certainly, individuals practice a culture, but customs are phenomena shared by all members of the group (Fig. 6-4). Because it is collectively shared, culture has been called *superindividual*. Murdock explains (1972, p. 258):

> Culture does not depend on individuals. An ordinary habit dies with its possessor, but a group habit lives on in the survivors, and is transmitted from generation to generation. Moreover, the individual is not a free agent with respect to culture. He is born and reared in a certain cultural environment, which impinges upon him at every moment of his life. From earliest childhood his behavior is conditioned by the habits of those around him. He has no choice but to conform to the folkways current in his group.

Knowing that culture is shared helps us to understand human behavior. For example, a community health nurse tried unsuccessfully to convince an American mother to stop heavily oiling her infant's skin (Taylor, 1973). She discovered that the mother was acting in a tradition of her subculture that held that oil promoted good health. The fact that all the other mothers in that religious group also used oil on their babies proved a powerful deterrent to the change requested by the nurse. Individual health behavior is always influenced by other people of the same culture. Thus, it becomes very difficult for one person to ignore some cultural practice when it will continue to be reinforced by other group members. In fact, group acceptance and a sense of membership almost always depend on conforming to shared cultural practices.

EFFECT ON COMMUNITY HEALTH NURSING

Community health nursing practice with groups and communities takes on added significance when it recognizes that culture is shared. Attempting to provide health care to one individual at a time limits community health nurses' effectiveness. Once a nurse leaves, the client must face all the informal cultural pressures that come from friends and family. On the other hand,

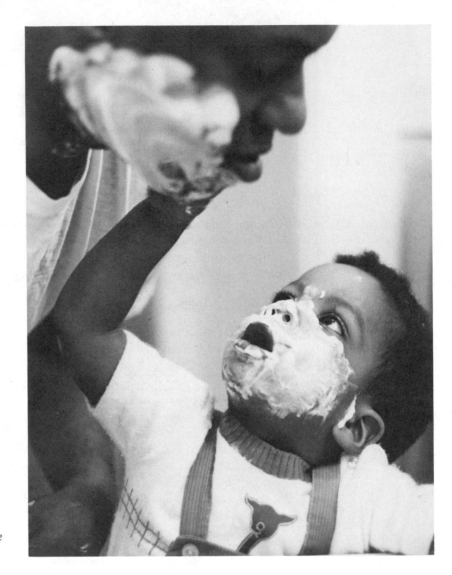

Figure 6-4
Children learn much of
their culture and future
roles through observation
and imitation of adult behavior. The little boy imi-
tating his father shaving is
learning to identify with the
male sex role.

focus on an entire group can change that group's health behavior positively and thus affect individual practices. The pattern of oiling young infants, for instance, ceased when the nurse worked with the entire church group. She began with a well-recognized cultural strategy, that is, work through formal or informal leaders. She contacted the minister and discussed the cultural practice. He admitted that anointing with oil, a Biblical teaching, was one of their beliefs. When she explained her concerns, he agreed that a drop of oil on the head was all that was needed. He clarified this teaching in his

138

next sermon, and as a result, additional health problems also cleared up when other members of the group stopped rubbing oil into wounds and infections (Taylor, 1973).

In another example, a community health nursing instructor with several groups of nursing students successfully developed a series of health classes for a group of Indian women who lived on the northwest coast of Washington state (Aichlmayr, 1969). As the group accepted teaching on subjects such as child care, treatment of burns, and prevention of colds, individual behavior was affected. A group focus also gives the nurse a broader picture of the culture being served and a better understanding of its health needs. Respect and trust of the entire group can be won, thus increasing the chance to improve health practices.

SHARED VALUES

One of the most important elements shared by a culture is its values. Each culture classifies phenomena "into good and bad, desirable and undesirable, right and wrong" (Foster, 1962, p. 18). When people respond in favor of or against some practice, they are reflecting their culture's values about that practice. One man may eagerly anticipate eating a steak for dinner. Another, who believes that eating meat is sacrilegious, will experience revulsion at the idea. Some American subcultures think that loud, vocal expressions are a necessary way to deal with pain. Others value silence and stoicism. Either way, values serve a purpose. Shared values give a culture stability and security; they provide a standard for behavior. Members know what to think and how to act. Values are more deeply rooted than behaviors and consequently change more slowly.

Culture Is Tacit

Culture provides a guide for human interaction that is mostly unexpressed, or tacit. Members of a cultural group, without the need for discussion, know how to act and what to expect from one another. Culture provides an implicit set of cues for behavior, not a written set of rules. It "may be thought of as a memory bank where knowledge is stored, available immediately and usually without conscious effort, to guide us in the situations in which we routinely find ourselves" (Foster, 1962, p. 18). Culture teaches us the proper tone of voice to use for each occasion. It tells us how close to stand when talking with someone (see Fig. 6-1). We learn to make the responses appropriate to our sex, role, and status. We know what is right and wrong. All of these attitudes and behaviors are so ingrained, so tacit, that we seldom, if ever, need to discuss them. We know. The same is true for each culture.

The difficulty comes when we cross cultural boundaries. No longer does our culture provide a guide for behavior. The cues given by a person in another culture may mean something entirely different. Silence in a group meeting with Native American women was uncomfortable for some nurses but enjoyed by the Indian women, who valued patience and listening (Foster, 1962). Offering food to a guest, in many cultures, is not merely a social gesture but an important symbol of hospitality and acceptance. To refuse, for any reason, is insulting and rejecting. Thus our behavior, albeit completely well intentioned and appropriate for our own culture, can cause misunderstanding and damage to relationships in another.

Because culture is tacit, it is difficult to realize the number and types of behaviors of ours that may be offensive to people from other groups. It is also difficult to know the meaning and significance of their practices. Consequently, community health nurses have a twofold task in developing cultural awareness; not only is it necessary to understand the clients' culture but also the nurses' culture. Effective practitioners maintain awareness of the aspects of their own culture they take for granted. Cross-cultural conflict can be resolved through conscious efforts at developing awareness, patience, and acceptance of cultural differences.

Culture Is Dynamic

Every culture experiences constant change; none is entirely static. Within every cultural group are individuals who generate innovations. More important, there are members who see advantages in other people's ways and are willing to adopt new practices. Each culture, then, becomes an amalgamation of ideas, values, and practices from a variety of sources. This process depends, of course, on the extent of exposure to other groups. Nonetheless, every culture is in a dynamic state of adding or deleting components. Functional aspects are retained; less functional ones are eliminated. When we tend toward ethnocentrism, saying, "Our way is best," we should remind ourselves that our culture is largely a collection of borrowed traits. We owe much of our beliefs, actions, and possessions to other cultures.

The dynamic nature of culture is useful to community health nursing for several reasons. Cultures and subcultures do indeed change over time. Patience and persistence are probably key attributes to cultivate when working toward improvement of health behaviors. Another point to remember is that cultures change as their members see greater advantages in the "new ways." Convincing them of these advantages will have to be done in a language they understand and in the context of their own cultural value system. This is an important reason for nurses to develop an understanding of their clients' culture (Leininger, 1977). Furthermore, change within a culture is usually brought about by certain key individuals who are receptive to new ideas and able to influence their peers. Tapping this resource becomes imperative for successful change. Finally, the health culture can change, too. Consider its changes in the past. Nurses can learn a great deal from their clients and

140

their cultures. And as practitioners discover more effective ways of working with clients, they can and should modify their own practices.

Culture and Nursing Practice

Our examination of the meaning and nature of culture has shown the need to recognize cultural differences and understand clients in the context of their cultural backgrounds. Practically speaking, however, how can the concept of culture be applied to everyday community health nursing practice? The following case studies give some insights.

Culture of the Poor

This first case study represents a community of people whose way of life is not often considered as a separate subculture (Fig. 6-5).

The Jacksons came to the city health center through a welfare referral. Albert, 42 years of age, had left each of his last three jobs only after a few days of employment. The caseworker made a home visit and found Vera Jackson, a shy, thin, 38-year-old woman, with three of her children. The

Figure 6-5
The poor have values, attitudes, and practices that give them a separate culture of their own. This Tennessee family enjoys the stability and security that its culture provides.

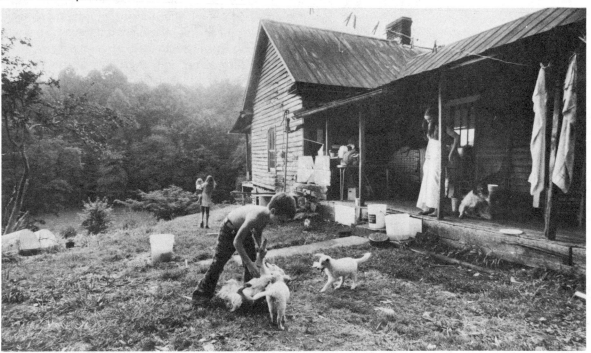

other three were in school. The small, two-bedroom apartment, part of a multiracial, low-income housing project, was "shabby, dirty, and cluttered," according to the referral. Albert seldom came home. Vera held the family together, supplementing the welfare checks through occasional day housework and a night cleaning job in an office building. She didn't know where Albert was, maybe somewhere drunk again. They had been in the city for eight months. Before that, Albert had done itinerant farm labor. Neither had finished high school. "We ain't stayed long anywheres, I guess," Vera told the caseworker. Two of the children had bad colds, one of which was complicated by a deep, chesty cough. The boy felt feverish, and the caseworker, concerned, arranged for Vera to take him to the health center.

The center's waiting room was crowded and noisy; staff hustled impatiently through the hallways. Vera's neighbor at the housing project had warned her, "That place don't like us poor folks." She and the children waited anxiously and then started when the loudspeaker blared out "Jackson." The nurse was friendly but brisk. "Mrs. Jackson," she inquired, "how are you?" There was no time for Vera to reply as the nurse launched into an explanation of the care and prevention of colds while checking the boy and taking his temperature. The physician, too, had many instructions. "These children should be on vitamins all the time," he commented. "Are they eating well-balanced meals?" Vera was confused. "Do you have any questions?" the nurse asked, handing her the antibiotics and some pamphlets on child growth and development. Vera shook her head. She felt too stupid to say anything, too embarrassed to admit she did not understand. A well-balanced meal, she thought, must mean not overfeeding the kids. That was no problem, considering the little they had to eat. She saw no point in vitamins. Why did they need to take something when they were well? She could not afford them anyway. She guessed that giving her son the medication at supper, their one "meal" a day, was what the doctor meant when he directed that the boy take it with each meal. Several days later the Jackson boy was hospitalized with pneumonia. Although he recovered, the Jacksons never returned to the health center.

Cultural Differences

The culture of the low-income population is an enigma to most health professionals. It is seldom considered a separate subculture; consequently, the poor are assumed to have the same values and attitudes as middle-class professionals. On the contrary, low-income people in our country are distinctive. Compared to health professionals, they think and respond in terms of sharply contrasting values, customs, and life-styles. Most important, their ideas about wellness and illness differ from those of health professionals, yet our system of health care tends to ignore this fact.

The economically disadvantaged differ from middle-class professionals in a variety of ways. For example, many poor people "live strictly and whole-heartedly in the present" (Strauss, 1967, p. 10). Much of the health practitioner's emphasis, on the other hand, is preventive and thus future-oriented. Taking vitamins, eating right, and preventing colds all involve a future-orientation, a value conflicting with values in Mrs. Jackson's realm of understanding. Economically disadvantaged persons may have an orientation to the present because frequently they must meet immediate needs at the expense of long-term gains.

Another difference is that the lives of the poor "are uncertain, dominated by recurring crises" (Strauss, 1967, p. 10). Middle-class professionals espouse a value of ordered, controlled, and well-planned lives. They advocate crisis prevention. For the lower socioeconomic class, the demands of daily living with limited resources require adaptation on a day-to-day and even moment-by-moment basis. In many instances, positive health may be valued by this group but unattainable; thus they learn to live with illness and crisis.

Many of the poor have learned to accept their life conditions and to make the most of them. Despite limited resources and education, many have positive health practices (Pratt, 1971). Differences in life-style, dress, and behavior can easily lead the nurse to make assumptions about this group that are not necessarily correct. For instance, the poor are often characterized as having low self-esteem (Robertson, 1969). While this may be true in some classes, it is not fair or accurate to make such a generalization. Mrs. Jackson's behavior was less likely owed to low self-esteem than to the confusing, depersonalized atmosphere of the health center.

Mrs. Jackson's cultural differences needed recognition and acceptance. Her point of view needed to be explored, her questions and concerns discussed. She required a relationship of trust with a caring person who understood and appreciated her culture and who offered health assistance within the context of that culture.

Culture of International Clients

This case study involves clients transplanted from one culture to an entirely different culture; it presents an interesting challenge to the community health nurse (Fig. 6-6).

Armed with enthusiasm and pamphlets on pregnancy and prenatal diet, the community health nurse began home visits to the Kim family. Her initial plan was to discuss pregnancy and fetal development, teach diet, and prepare the mother for delivery. Mr. Kim, a graduate student, was present to interpret since Mrs. Kim spoke very little English. Their two boys, three years and one and one half years of age, played happily on the kitchen floor. The family offered tea to the nurse and listened politely as she explained her reasons for coming and added, "How can I be most helpful to you? What would you like from my visits?"

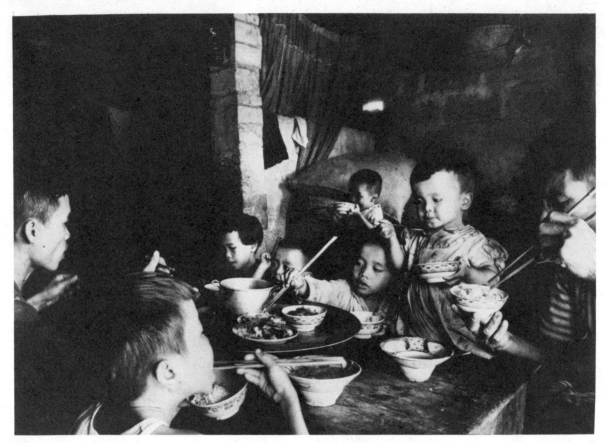

Figure 6-6
Clients transplanted from completely different cultures will continue to adhere to their own beliefs and practices. This Vietnamese family enjoys eating a traditional meal with chopsticks — one of many customs it will maintain until selected aspects of the new culture are gradually absorbed.

The Kims were grateful for this approach. Hesitant at first, they hinted at Mrs. Kim's fears of American doctors and hospitals; her first two children had been born in Korea. None of the family had any experience with Western medicine. They shared some concerns about adjustment to living in the United States. It was difficult to shop in American food stores with their overwhelming variety of foods, many of which the Kims found unfamiliar. Mrs. Kim, who had come from a family whose servants prepared the food, was an inexperienced cook. Servants had also cared for the children, and her role had been that of an aristocrat in hand-tailored silk gowns.

Listening carefully, the nurse began to realize the striking differences between her own and her clients' culture. Her care plans changed. In subsequent visits she determined to learn about Korean culture and base her nursing intervention on that knowledge. She learned about their traditional ways of raising children, male and female roles, and practices related to pregnancy and lactation. She respected their value of ''saving face'' and attempted

144

never to offend their pride or dignity. As time went on, her interest and respect for their way of life won their trust. She inquired about their cultural practices before attempting any intervention. As a result, the Kims were receptive to her suggestions. Appropriate changes were made in Mrs. Kim's diet, for example, that were still compatible with her food preferences and cultural eating patterns. Because she was not accustomed to drinking milk, she increased her calcium intake by learning to prepare custards (which disguised the milk flavor) and to eat more green, leafy vegetables. After five months, a strong, positive relationship had been established between this family and the nurse. Mrs. Kim delivered a healthy baby girl and looked forward to continued supportive visits from the community health nurse.

Although she had not initially considered the possibility of cultural barriers, the nurse soon recognized that subtle but important differences existed and thus changed her objectives. She proceeded to gain understanding and respect of this family's culture as a means toward improving their health. Whenever possible, she adapted her teaching and suggestions to comply with the Kims' culture. Implicitly, her message was, "Your culture is valuable and necessary for you. The parts of that culture that can continue to be useful, I will help preserve. The parts that are not functional for you in this new society, I will help you change, over time."

Culture of a Native American Group

A third case study portrays another distinct culture. Its members live in the United States, assume many American values and practices, yet preserve large aspects of their own culture (Fig. 6-7).

As she drove up the dirt road and parked her car next to the community hall, Sandra felt apprehensive. She had been warned by the previous community health nurse that these Indian people were hard to work with: "They're all lazy and unappreciative. You can't get anywhere with them." It was only through the urging of an Indian community aide, Mrs. Brown, that a group of the women had reluctantly agreed to meet with the new nurse. They would see what she had to say.

Sandra's steps echoed hollowly as she walked across the wooden floor of the large room to the far corner where a group of women sat silently in a circle. Only their eyes turned; their faces remained impassive. Mrs. Brown rose slowly, greeted the nurse, and introduced her to the group. Swallowing her fear, Sandra smiled. She told them of her background and explained that she had not worked with Indian people before. There was a long silence. No one spoke. Sandra continued, "I'd like to help you if I can, maybe with problems about care of your children when they are sick or questions about how to keep them healthy, but I don't know what you need or want." Silence fell again. She would like to learn from them, she repeated. Would they help her? Again an uncomfortable silence ensued.

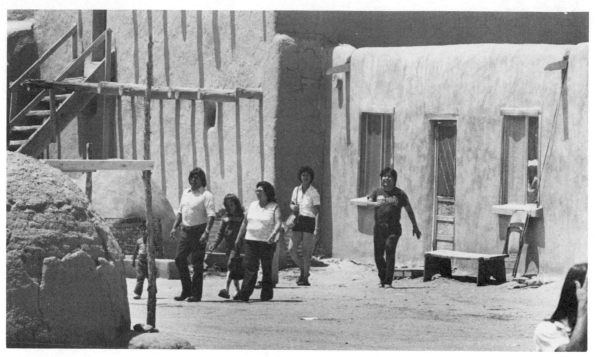

Figure 6-7
Many Americans, such as these Native Americans, come from culturally diverse backgrounds and retain many aspects of their original culture.

Then one woman began to speak. Quietly, but with deep feeling, she described several bad experiences with the previous nurse and the county social worker. Then others spoke up: "They *tell* us what we should do. They don't listen. They say our way is not good." Seeing Sandra's interest and concern, the women continued. One of their main concerns was their children's health. Another was the high incidence of accidents and injuries on the reservation. They wanted to learn how to give first aid. Other concerns were expressed. The group agreed that Sandra could help them by teaching a first-aid class.

In the weeks that followed, Sandra taught several classes on first aid and emergency care. She then began a series of sessions on child health. Each time she would ask the women to choose a topic or problem for discussion and elicit from them their accustomed ways of dealing with each problem, for example, how they handled toilet training or taught their children to eat solid foods. Her goal was to learn as much as she could about their culture and incorporate that information into her teaching, which preserved as many of their practices as possible. Sandra also visited informally with the women in their homes and at community gatherings. She learned about their way of life, their history, and their values. For example, patience was highly valued. It was important to be able to wait patiently, even if a scheduled

146

meeting was delayed as much as two hours. It was also important for others to speak, which explained the Indian women's comfort with silences during a conversation. Other values influenced their way of life. Courage, pride, generosity, and honesty were all important determinants of behavior. These were also values by which they judged Sandra and other professionals. Sandra's honesty in keeping her promises enabled the women to trust her. Her generosity in giving her time, helping them occasionally with some household task, and arranging for child care during classes won their respect.

The women came to accept her, and Sandra was invited to eat with them and share in tribal get-togethers. The women criticized and advised her on acceptable ways to speak and act. Her openness and patience to learn and her respect for them as a people had paved the way to improving their health. At first, Sandra felt that her progress was very slow, but this slowness was actually an advantage. She had built a solid foundation of cross-cultural trust, and in the months that followed, she saw many changes in their health practices.

Principles for Practice

In the context of these cases and our earlier discussion of culture, several principles for nursing practice can be identified.

Recognize and Appreciate Cultural Differences

Our beliefs and ways of doing things frequently contrast with those of our clients. A first step toward bridging cultural barriers is recognition of those differences. Mrs. Jackson's values and health practices sharply contrasted with those of the center's staff. Failure to recognize these differences led to a breakdown in communication and ineffective care. Once differences in culture are recognized, it is important to accept and appreciate them. A nurse's ways are valid for the nurse; clients' ways work for them. The nurse visiting the Kims avoided the dangerous trap of assuming that her way was best and consequently developed a fruitful relationship with her clients.

Understand Cultural Basis for Client Behavior

Each of the client's actions, like our own, is based on underlying culturally learned beliefs and ideas. Mrs. Kim did not like milk because her culture had taught her that it was distasteful. The Indian women's response to waiting or keeping someone else waiting was influenced by their value of patience. Instead of making assumptions or judging client behavior, first learn about the culture that guides that behavior (Aichlmayr, 1969). Some culturally based reason is causing clients to engage in (or avoid) certain actions. The nurse can collect data about clients' culture through questioning, observation, and reading. Conducting a "community cultural assessment" (Gagnon, 1983, p. 128) is one way to enhance understanding of a cultural group. Two other methods proven effective for study in greater depth of cultural groups are ethnographic interviewing and participant observation (Spradley, 1979, 1980).

Listen and Learn Before Advising

We do not change people's behavior by just giving suggestions or instructions. For Mrs. Jackson as well as the Native American women, this approach had, in fact the opposite effect. Health teaching must be geared to the client's level of understanding and frame of reference. We accomplish this by finding out about the client first. Asking questions, listening, and observing help us to understand clients and their culture. Consequently, nursing intervention can be tailored to their needs.

Empathize with Culturally Different Clients

In addition to learning their culture or subculture, we need to understand clients' points of view. We need to stand in their shoes, to identify with them. The ability to show interest, concern, and compassion enabled Sandra to win the affection and respect of the Native American women. It told the Kims that their nurse cared about them. These nurses participated in the feelings and ideas of their clients. Empathizing with clients gives them needed reassurance and often provides the motivation to adopt new health behaviors (Robertson, 1969).

Show Respect for Clients and Their Culture

Respect is shown in many ways. When Sandra involved the Native American women in decisions and gave them choices, she was showing respect. When the nurse gave positive recognition to the importance of the Kims' culture, she was showing respect. Within the United States, people of different cultures and subcultures particularly need respect. Their ways are in contrast to the dominant culture. It is difficult for them to retain pride in their life-styles, or in themselves, when constantly reminded that their ways are inferior. The message may be only implied or even unintentional. Such was the case for Mrs. Jackson. The health center's routine and the manner of the staff were certainly not meant intentionally to show disrespect. They did, nevertheless, and Mrs. Jackson was intimidated and unable to receive the help she needed. Everyone needs respect to enhance pride, dignity, and self-esteem; it is an important contributor to good mental health. Showing respect is also an important means for breaking down barriers in cross-cultural communication.

Be Patient

It takes time to build trust and effect culture change. It can be difficult to establish the nurse-client relationship when it involves two different cultures. Trust must be won, and winning it may take weeks, months, or even years. Patience is essential. Time must be allowed for both the nurse and the client to learn how to communicate with one another, to test each other's trustworthiness, and to learn about each other. Change in behavior (learned aspects of the culture) occurs gradually. Some aspects of both the nurse's and the client's cultures can, and probably will, change. The Kims' nurse, for example, modified some of her usual practices and adapted them to the Kims' culture and needs. They, in turn, began to assume some American practices and values. However, the process took several months. Time and patience help to break down cultural barriers.

Analyze Your Behavior

Self-awareness is crucial for the nurse working with people from other cultures (Leininger, 1970). Remember your culture is different from theirs. Are you aware of your own values, habits, and typical responses? How would you appear to clients? The nurse who assisted Mrs. Jackson probably thought she was being friendly, efficient, and helpful. In terms of her own culture, this nurse's behavior was intended to reassure clients and meet their needs. Unaware of the negative consequences of her behavior, she caused damage rather than met needs.

To gain skill in analyzing your behavior, nurses should keep in mind two points. First, knowledge of the clients' culture helps nurses to know how clients will interpret various behaviors. It tells nurses what responses are most appropriate to make. Second, establishing a relationship of trust with clients of different cultures opens doors of communication. As in Sandra's experience, trust creates a willingness to share reactions and constructively criticize behavior.

Summary

In community health, each client, whether a family, group, or community, has its own culture. A culture is a design for living, and every culture is different. The unique culture of each group is essential for the functioning of that group. It serves as a guide for behavior, a map telling the people of that group how to live. Culture provides a set of norms and values, which are the threads holding together the fabric of a society. It offers stability and security.

Several characteristics of culture are significant for community health nursing practice. It is *learned*, not acquired. Thus some elements can be relearned, and some practices changed. It is *integrated*. All of the many traits making up a culture work together as a functioning whole. Specific cultural practices must be considered in the context of the client's larger culture. Changing one set of traits will affect other aspects of the culture. It is *shared*. Culture is a group phenomenon; it controls all the members' values and behavior. Attempts to change individual behavior may be ineffective; a group approach might be more productive. It is *tacit*. Culture tells people how to behave without the need for conscious thought. A collision between two different cultures can create considerable conflict and misunderstanding. Conscious effort is required to understand and accept cultural differences. It is *dynamic*. Every culture preserves its integrity by deleting nonfunctional practices and acquiring new components that will better serve the group. Consequently, it is possible to introduce improved health practices that are presented in a manner consistent with the clients' cultural values.

Some principles, drawn from an understanding of the concept of culture, can guide community health nursing practice:

1. Recognize and appreciate the differences between your clients' culture and your own.
2. Understand the cultural basis for your clients' behavior.
3. Listen and learn before giving advice.
4. Empathize with clients of different cultural backgrounds.
5. Show respect for clients and their culture.
6. Be patient. It takes time to build trust and effect cultural change.
7. Analyze your behavior in the context of the clients' culture.

Study Questions

1. Based on your own cultural background, how would you feel and what behaviors would you exhibit if you were:
   a. A client sitting in a clinic waiting room in a foreign country whose language you didn't know?
   b. Part of a nutrition class being told to eat foods you had never heard of before?
   c. Visited in your home by a nurse who told you to discipline your child in a way that contradicted everything you had been reared to believe about parenting?
2. Describe three tacit cultural rules that govern your own behavior. How might these affect your interaction with clients from another culture?
3. What does the term *ethnocentrism* mean to you? Have you ever ex-

perienced someone else being ethnocentric in their attitude toward you? If so, describe that experience.

References

Aichlmayr, R. H. (1969). Cultural understanding: A key to acceptance. *Nursing Outlook, 17,* 20–23.

Benedict, R. (1934). *Patterns of culture.* Boston: Houghton Mifflin.

Branch, M. (1976). Models for introducing cultural diversity in nursing curricula. *Journal of Nursing Education, 15,* 7–13.

Foster, G. M. (1962). *Traditional cultures and the impact of technological change.* New York: Harper & Row.

Gagnon, A. (1983). Transcultural nursing: Including it in the curriculum. *Nursing and Health Care, 4*(3), 127–131.

Hall, E. T. (1959). *The silent language.* Garden City, NY: Doubleday.

Herrera, T., & Wagner, N. (1977). Behavioral approaches to delivering health services in a Chicano community. In A. Reinhardt & M. Quinn (Eds.), *Current practice in family-centered community nursing.* St. Louis: C. V. Mosby.

Kark, S. L. (1974). *Epidemiology and community medicine.* New York: Appleton-Century-Crofts.

Landy, D. (1977). *Culture, disease and healing: Studies in medical anthropology.* New York: Macmillan.

Leininger, M. (1970). *Anthropology and nursing: Two worlds to blend.* New York: Wiley.

Leininger, M. (1977). Transcultural nursing: A promising subfield of study for nurses. In A. Reinhardt and M. Quinn (Eds.), *Current practice in family-centered community nursing* (pp. 36–50). St. Louis: C. V. Mosby.

MacGregor, F. C. (Ed.). (1960). *Social science in nursing.* New York: Wiley.

Mead, M. (1960). Cultural contexts of nursing problems. In F. C. MacGregor (Ed.), *Social science in nursing.* New York: Wiley.

Murdock, G. (1972). The science of culture. In M. Freilich (Ed.), *The meaning of culture: A reader in cultural anthropology* (pp. 252–266). Lexington, MA: Xerox College Publishing.

Murillo, N. (1971). The Mexican-American family. In N. Wagner and M. Haug (Eds.), *Chicanos: Social and psychological perspectives.* St. Louis: C. V. Mosby.

Pratt, L. (1971). The relationship of socioeconomic status to health. *American Journal of Public Health, 61,* 281–291.

Robertson, H. R. (1969). Removing barriers to health care. *Nursing Outlook, 17,* 43–46.

Spradley, J. P. (1979). *The ethnographic interview.* New York: Holt, Rinehart and Winston.

Spradley, J. P. (1980). *Participant observation.* New York: Holt, Rinehart and Winston.

Strauss, A. L. (1967). Medical ghettos. *Trans-Action, 4*(62), 7–15.

Taylor, C. (1973). The nurse and cultural barriers. In D. Hymovich and M. Barnard (Eds.), *Family health care* (pp. 119–127). New York: McGraw-Hill.

Thernstrom, S., et al. (Eds.). (1980). *Harvard encyclopedia of American ethnic groups.* Cambridge, MA: Harvard University Press.

Selected Readings

Aichlmayr, R. H. (1969). Cultural understanding: A key to acceptance. *Nursing Outlook, 17*, 20–23.

Asian Americans: The neglected minority. (1973). *Personnel Guidance Journal, 51*, 385–416.

Bauwens, E. (Ed.). (1978). *The anthropology of health*. St. Louis: C. V. Mosby.

Bello, T. A. (1976). The third dimension: Cultural sensitivity in nursing practice. *Imprint, 23*, 36.

Benedict, R. (1934). *Patterns of culture*. Boston: Houghton Mifflin.

Blackwell, J. E. (1975). *The black community: Diversity and unity*. New York: Dodd, Mead.

Brinton, D. (1972). Value differences between nurses and low-income families. *Nursing Research, 1*, 3–15.

Brownlee, A. T. (1977). *Community, culture, and care*. St. Louis: C. V. Mosby.

Bullough, B., & Bullough, V. (1972). *Poverty, ethnic identification and health care*. New York: Appleton-Century-Crofts.

Davis, M. Z. (1975). The public health nurse: Some aspects of work. In M. Z. Davis, M. Kramer, & A. L. Strauss (Eds.), *Nursing in practice* (pp. 223–233). St. Louis: C. V. Mosby.

Davitz, L. J., Sameshima, Y., & Davitz, J. (1976). Suffering as viewed in six different cultures. *American Journal of Nursing, 76*, 1296–1297.

DeGracia, R. (1979). Cultural influences on Filipino patients. *American Journal of Nursing, 79*, 1412–1414.

Dubos, R. (1974). The dangers of tolerance. *Journal of School Health, 44*, 182–186.

Fire, M., & Baker, C. (1976). A smile and eye contact may insult someone. *Journal of Nursing Education, 15*, 14–17.

Foster, G. M., & Anderson, B. G. (1978). *Medical anthropology*. New York: Wiley.

Freeman, H. E., Levine, S., & Reeder, L. G. (1972). *Handbook of medical sociology* (2nd ed.). Englewood Cliffs, NJ: Prentice-Hall.

Gagnon, A. J. (1983). Transcultural nursing: Including it in the curriculum. *Nursing and Health Care, 4*(3), 127–131.

Gordon, V., Matousek, I. M., & Lang, T. A. (1980). Southeast Asian refugees. *American Journal of Nursing, 80*, 2031–2036.

Hall, E. T. (1959). *The silent language*. Garden City, NY: Doubleday.

Hodgson, C. (1980). Transcultural nursing: The Canadian experience. *Canadian Nurse, 6*, 23–25.

Kane, R. L., Kasteler, J., & Gray, R. (Eds.). (1976). *The health gap: Medical services and the poor*. New York: Springer.

Kerr, L. (1975). The poverty of affluence. *Amercan Journal of Public Health, 65,* 17–20.

Kneip-Hardy, M., & Burkhardt, M. (1977). Nursing the Navajo. *American Journal of Nursing, 77,* 95–96.

Koshi, P. T. (1977). Symposium on cultural and biological diversity and health care. *Nursing Clinics of North America, 12,* 1.

Kramer, M., & Schmalenber, C. (1977). *Path to biculturalism.* Wakefield, MA: Contemporary Publishing.

Leininger, M. (1970). *Anthropology and nursing: Two worlds to blend.* New York: Wiley.

Leininger, M. (1973). The culture concept and its relevance to nursing. In M. Auld & L. Birum (Eds.), *The challenge of nursing: A book of readings.* (pp. 36–50). St. Louis: C. V. Mosby.

Leininger, M. (Ed.). (1975). *Barriers and facilitators to quality health care.* Philadelphia: Davis.

Leininger, M. (1978). *Transcultural nursing.* Somerset, NJ: Wiley.

Mackie, J. B. (1974). The father's influence on the intellectual level of black ghetto children. *American Journal of Public Health, 64,* 615–616.

Martinez, R. A. (Ed.). (1978). *Hispanic culture and health care.* St. Louis: C. V. Mosby.

Mays, R. M. (1979, November/December). Primary health care and the black family. *Nurse Practitioner,* pp. 13, 15, 20–21.

Mead, M. (1960). Cultural contexts of nursing problems. In F. C. MacGregor (Ed.), *Social science in nursing,* (pp. 74–78). New York: Wiley.

Mei-Li, L. (1976). Folk beliefs of the Chinese and implications for psychiatric nursing. *Journal of Psychiatric Nursing, 14,* 38–41.

Milio, N. (1973). Values, social class and community health services. In A. Reinhardt and M. Quinn (Eds.), *Family-centered community nursing: A sociocultural framework* (pp. 187–197). St. Louis: C. V. Mosby.

Mitchell, A. C. (1978). Barriers to therapeutic communication with black clients. *Nursing Outlook, 26,* 109–112.

Paul, B. D. (1955). *Health, culture and community.* New York: Russell Sage Foundation.

Pratt, L. (1971). The relationship of socioeconomic status to health. *American Journal of Public Health, 61,* 281–291.

Primeaux, M. (1977). Caring for the American Indian patient. *American Journal of Nursing, 77,* 91–94.

Primeaux, M. H. (1977). American Indian health care practices. *Nursing Clinics of North America, 12,* 55–65.

Spector, M. (1979). Poverty: The barrier to health care. In R. E. Spector (Ed.), *Cultural diversity in health and illness.* New York: Appleton-Century-Crofts.

Spector, R. E. (1979). *Cultural diversity in health and illness.* New York: Appleton-Century-Crofts.

Spradley, J. P. (1975). Public health services and the culture of skid row bums. In *Proceedings: Seminar on public health services and the public inebriate* (pp. 1–19). Rockville, MD: National Institute on Alcohol Abuse and Alcoholism.

Spradley, J. P. (1979). *The ethnographic interview*. New York: Holt, Rinehart and Winston.

Spradley, J. P. (1980). *Participant observation*. New York: Holt, Rinehart and Winston.

Stanley, S., & Wagner, N. (Eds.). (1973). *Asian-Americans: Psychological perspectives*. Ben Lomond, CA: Science and Behavioral Books.

Strasser, J. A. (1978). Urban transient women. *American Journal of Nursing, 78*, 2076–2079.

Stumpf, P. S. (1983). The culture of poverty: An overused conceptual model. In P. L. Chinn (Ed.), *Advances in nursing theory development*. Rockville, MD: Aspen Systems.

Taylor, C. (1973). The nurse and cultural barriers. In D. Hymovich & M. Barnard (Eds.), *Family health care*. New York: McGraw-Hill, 119–127.

Wagner, N., & Haug, M. (Eds.). (1971). *Chicanos: Social and psychological perspectives*. St. Louis: C. V. Mosby.

Weaver, J. L. (1976). *National health policy and the underserved*. St. Louis: C. V. Mosby.

Weeks, H. A. (1977). Income and disease — The pathology of poverty. In L. Corey, M. Epstein, & S. E. Saltman (Eds.), *Medicine in a changing society* (2nd ed.). St. Louis: C. V. Mosby.

two

Tools for Practice

7

The Nursing Process in Community Health

Underlying all community health nursing practice flows one of its essential dynamics — the nursing process (White, 1982, p. 529). Defined as a systematic purposeful set of interpersonal actions (Mauksch & David, 1972), the nursing process provides the active, driving force for change that is the first and most important tool employed by the community health nurse.

Three characteristics emphasize the importance of this tool for community health nursing. First, the nursing process is a problem-solving process that addresses community health problems at all aggregate levels and aims to prevent illness and to promote the public's health. Second, it is a management process that requires analysis of a situation, decision making, planning, organizing, directing and controlling service efforts, and evaluating outcomes. As a management tool the nursing process addresses all aggregate levels. Third, it is a change process that works to improve various levels of health-related systems and the way people behave within those systems.

In this chapter we shall examine the nursing process: its components and dynamics for solving problems, managing nursing actions, and improving community health nursing practice.

The Nursing Process

Process, the moving element of this tool, means forward progression in an orderly fashion toward some desired result. In community health it involves a series of actions that enable the nurse to work with clients toward achieving their optimal health.

Components

The nursing process incorporates several components or steps. Nursing theorists attach different labels to these components but all agree on the basic sequence of actions. The five major components are assessment, diagnosis, planning, implementation, and evaluation. All of these depend on a sixth component — interaction. Current literature and practice give increasing emphasis to this element of the nursing process (Brill, 1973; Daubermire & King, 1973; Langford, 1978). Nurse-client interaction is often an implied or assumed element in the process; for community health nursing, particularly, it is an essential first step.

INTERACTION

Community health nursing practice involves helping clients to help themselves. Listening to an elderly couple, teaching a class of expectant mothers, lobbying in the legislature for the poor, or working with parents to set up a dental screening program for children — all involve relationships. The nurse may establish an initial relationship, maintain an existing one, or redefine a previous one. Whatever its stage of development, a relationship involves reciprocal influence and exchange — in a word, interaction. This mutual give and take between nurse and clients, whether a family, a group of mothers on an Indian reservation, or school children, is the first step in the nursing process.

Need for Communication
Interaction requires communication. When a community health nurse initially contacts a family, for example, any information she may have in advance can give only partial clues to that family's needs and wants. Unless they begin by talking and listening, the later steps in the nursing process will go awry. By open, honest sharing, the nurse will begin to develop trust and establish lines of effective communication. For instance, she will explain who she is and why she is there. She will encourage the family members to talk about themselves. Nurse and family together will discuss their relationship and clarify the desired nature of that alliance. Does the family want help to identify and work on its health needs? Would its members like this nurse to continue regular contacts? What will their respective roles be? Effective

communication, as a part of interaction, is essential to develop understanding and facilitate a free exchange of information between nurse and clients.

Interaction is reciprocal. Nurses must avoid the temptation either to do all the talking or merely to listen while a father or mother monopolizes the conversation. There is a dynamic exchange between two systems: the community health nurse represents one system, and the client the other. Whether the client is a handicapped family, a parent group, or an entire community, this exchange involves a two-way sharing of information, ideas, feelings, concerns, and ultimately self. There are mutuality and cooperation.

Consider the following example: A dozen junior high school boys, most of whom were on the football team, met for several weeks with the school nurse to discuss physical fitness, nutrition, and other health topics. After their agreed-upon goals had been accomplished, the nurse wondered whether further meetings were needed. She raised the question and offered several topics, such as taking drugs and preventing injuries, for possible future sessions. The boys were not interested in these suggestions but, after more discussion, said they did want help with talking to girls. Renewed interaction was necessary as a first step in reapplying the nursing process.

Interaction paves the way for a helping relationship. As nurse and client interact, each is learning about the other. There is a period of testing before trust can be fully established. For the school nurse, establishing interaction had been more difficult at the time of her initial contact with the boys. They had been reluctant to talk, felt embarrassed to discuss personal subjects with a woman, and yet had strong interests in bodybuilding and personal appearance, strong enough to attract them to these optional sessions. Interaction began with a friendly exchange on nonthreatening topics and gradually deepened as the boys seemed ready to discuss personal subjects. Now it was relatively simple to talk about a new "problem" (to start the nursing process over again) because a helping relationship had already been developed. The nurse had a track record. The boys trusted, respected, and liked her, so they were happy to interact around a new need.

Group Level

Because community health practice focuses largely on the health of population groups, interaction goes beyond the one-to-one approach of clinical nursing (Williams, 1977). The challenge that faces the community health nurse is a one-to-group approach. A family, a group of concerned neighbors, and a group of handicapped persons are all collections of people with different concerns and opinions. Each person in a group is influenced by the thinking and behavior of the other group members. Nursing interaction with a group as the client demands an understanding of group behavior and group-level decision making and requires interpersonal communication at the group level. Thus, the task of interacting becomes more complex with a group than with an individual, but it also can be challenging and rewarding. Once community health nurses address themselves to understanding aggregate behavior, they can capitalize on the potential of group influence in order to make a far-reaching impact on the health of the total community. During this phase of the nursing process, however, the challenge lies with learning to interact effectively at the aggregate level. Later chapters will deal more specifically with communicating and working with groups.

Not only the first step, interaction is an integral, ongoing part of the nursing process (see Fig. 7-1). It is central to the process because nurse-client interaction forms the core of the relationship and information exchange. The effectiveness of each successive step — assessment, diagnosis, planning, implementation, and evaluation — depends on nurse-client interaction.

ASSESSMENT

After establishing ongoing interaction, the community health nurse is ready to determine client needs; therefore, assessment is the next phase of the nursing process. According to Webster, *assessment* means judgment of the

Figure 7-1
Nursing process compo-
nents. Nurse-client interac-
tion, a permeable structure,
forms the core of the pro-
cess. As nurse and client
maintain a reciprocal ex-
change of information and
trust through interaction,
they can effectively assess
client needs; diagnose
needs; and plan, imple-
ment, and evaluate care.

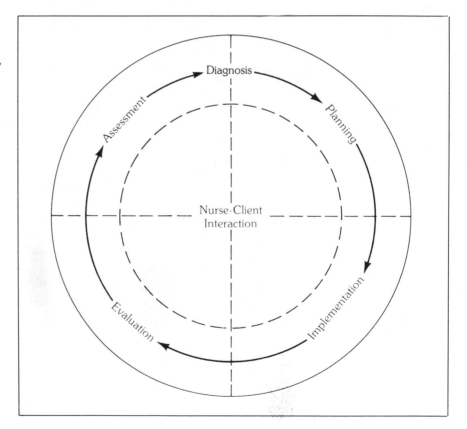

importance, size, or value of something; it is an act of appraisal. Nurses judge client health status to discover existing or potential needs as a basis for planning future action.

Assessment involves two major activities: (1) collection of pertinent data and (2) interpretation of data. These actions overlap and are repeated constantly throughout the assessment. Thus, while assessing a family's need for counseling, the nurse may simultaneously collect data on a persistent cough in a child and interpret previously collected data about nutritional deficiencies.

Collection of Data

The nurse can collect a wide range of data in the process of assessing community clients. What information and how much to collect depend, in the first place, on the initial reason for nurse-client contact. A specific health problem, such as Down's syndrome in the family, obesity among a group of teenagers, or widespread pediculosis in a grade school, focuses the data collection on information related to the present problem and its resolution. If the initial reason for nurse-client contact is health promotion, as for a normal postpartum family, data collection can be broadened to include information such as family history, constellation, present health status, coping abilities, support systems, and parenting skills.

A second consideration in data collection involves actual versus potential needs. Assessment of clients with multiple problems may force the community health nurse to focus only on existing (actual) needs because of limited time and resources. When possible, however, the community health nurse collects data aimed at uncovering potential needs in order to prevent problems from occurring (Fig. 7-2). Early and periodic screening of children or health screening for hypertension, glaucoma, and diabetes are examples of preventive assessment.

Community health nurses utilize many sources in data collection. They begin with clients because clients are closest to their own situation and can frequently offer the most accurate insights and comprehensive information. This is primary data because it is obtained directly from the client. A secondary source of data is people who know the client group well. In working with a family, the extended family members, friends, neighbors, and work associates may all be potential sources of information, pending client permission. Additional secondary sources include health team members, client records, community agencies, reference books, research reports, and community health nurses themselves. Secondary data may not accurately describe the client or reflect client self-perceptions. Thus, secondary data may need further validation.

Data collection in community health requires the exercise of sound professional judgment, effective communication techniques, and special investigative skills. Observation is a basic method for gathering primary data. Seeing the family and its home environment tells the nurse something about its socioeconomic level and ability to cope using present resources. Hearing inter-

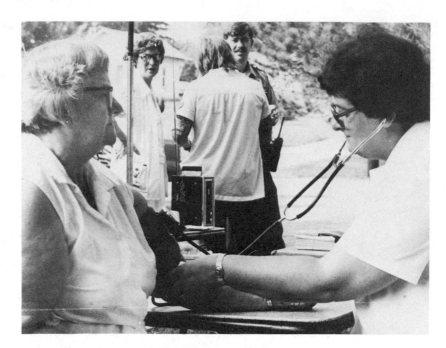

Figure 7-2
The nurse assesses individual, family, and community health through data collection. Here a free health screening program for hypertension gives the nurse important information on which to base future plans.

personal conflict among the members of a weight control group can give the nurse clues about possible client concerns and stress levels. Noticing the absence of a caring atmosphere in a nursing home may suggest a need for intervention. Observation, as a data-gathering method, depends largely on nonverbal communication. The tone of a conversation may be friendly, hostile, or passive. A family may fail to keep appointments. A group's body language or a neighborhood's appearance conveys a message. All offer information about clients.

Another method for data collection is the interview. The interview involves a series of questions designed to elicit needed information. The community health nurse may conduct a formal interview during an early encounter to gather a health history and to encourage client expression. Informal directed questioning can sometimes provide even more data about client health status and needs. Communicating with clients serves as an important follow-up observation. If you observe children with bruises that suggest possible abuse, a carefully planned informal interview may be useful. You may discover a mother who is isolated and under emotional stress. Then you can undertake cooperative nurse-client planning for dealing with the problem.

Listening is an important data collection method. It is a skill that must be acquired through discipline and concentration. Too often we listen inattentively while we formulate our next question or allow our minds to wander. Good listening involves eye contact. It assures clients of sincere interest and encourages greater expression of ideas and feelings. The community health nurse who is a good listener can gain a wealth of information about clients.

Direct examination is still another method for collecting data. When working with individuals we think of percussion, auscultation, palpation, inspection, and measurement as means of direct examination. Applied to community groups and aggregates direct examination assumes different forms such as surveys, screening instruments, epidemiologic research, or environmental testing for pathological determinants. Surveys, like interviews, provide specific information in response to selected questions. They can be especially useful for gathering data such as patterns of behavior among teenage alcoholics or battered women. Community health nurses also use surveys to assess neighborhood and community needs. Many kinds of standard screening instruments, including blood pressure apparatus, audiometers, scales, neurologic appraisal guides, and developmental tests, are useful for collecting data about clients. Epidemiologic research and environmental measurements add further data for community health analysis.

Interpretation of Data

This stage of assessment is analytic. Interpretation of data means analyzing the information gathered, drawing inferences or possible conclusions about the data's meaning, and validating those inferences to determine their accuracy. First, the nurse separates the data into categories such as physical, mental, social, and environmental. In many instances, data base sheets used in community agencies provide a structure for gathering and analyzing data. Second, the nurse examines each category to determine its significant meaning. At this point the nurse may need to search for additional information to clarify the meaning of the present data. Next, inferences are made. The nurse has analyzed the data base and come to a tentative conclusion about its meaning. But before making a diagnosis, the nurse must validate those assumptions. Are they accurate? Are they sound? The client should participate actively in data interpretation by clarifying feelings, explaining the circumstances surrounding the situation, and acting as a sounding board for testing assumptions. The nurse also uses other resources, such as other health team members, to check out and confirm inferences. An example of data interpretation follows.

A community health nurse had been collecting data about a group of mothers who regularly attended a well-child clinic. Their responses to child health information and parenting classes had been considerably less than enthusiastic, yet when questioned, they expressed no dissatisfaction with the teaching program. After examining all the data, the nurse concluded that their social and supportive needs were far greater than their need for child care information. Merely gathering weekly at the clinic served an important function for them. She sat down with the mothers and discussed her findings.

All agreed that they needed to get out of the house and be with people who had similar kinds of problems and interests.

In the situation just cited, data analysis led to drawing an inference, which was then validated. These are the important activities in interpretation of data. There is an ever-present danger in data interpretation, however, of making inaccurate assumptions and diagnoses. Many nursing care plans and activities have been based on false ideas of clients' needs, resulting in wasted and sometimes detrimental efforts. Thus, the importance of validation cannot be overemphasized. Data collection and data interpretation are sequential activities with validation serving as a bridge between them (see Fig. 7-3). When performed thoroughly, these steps lead to an accurate diagnosis.

DIAGNOSIS

Diagnosis, the next step in the nursing process, is the conclusion the nurse draws from interpretation of collected data. It is a statement of client need, sometimes called the *problem statement*. However, in community health, nurses do not limit their focus to problems; they consider the client as a total system and look for evidence of all kinds of needs that may influence the client's level of wellness. Needs cover the whole length of the health-illness continuum from a specific health problem, such as chemical dependency, all the way to opportunities for maximizing client health by filling needs such as improvement of parenting skills or development of better nutrition. Thus the statement of client need, the diagnosis, can focus on a wide range of topics.

Diagnoses differ in their scope. A *broad diagnosis,* such as the well-child clinic mothers need for emotional support, must be further broken down to

Figure 7-3
Assessment and diagnosis phases of the nursing process. Interpretation of data leads to diagnosis of client needs.

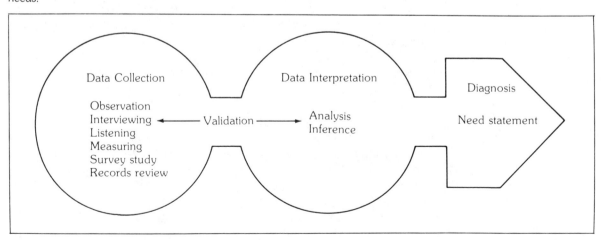

become manageable for planning care. The community health nurse in the above instance did further data collection and interpretation to develop a list of specific needs or diagnoses. Together, she and the mothers identified their feelings of inferiority as housewives, feelings of limited sexual satisfaction, and feelings of powerlessness about family decision making and spending of family money. A broad diagnosis is useful as a starting point. It can serve as a summary, as in the diagnosis of culture shock, nonsupportive parenting, or an unsafe school playground. Using the broad diagnosis as a base, the nurse can ask further questions, gather more data, and with the client develop a set of *specific diagnoses* on which to act. Diagnoses that are already specific are ready for the planning step.

The nursing diagnosis changes over time because it reflects changes in client health status; therefore, diagnoses need to be periodically reevaluated and redefined. The changing diagnosis can be a useful means of encouraging clients toward improved health because it gives them a clear standard against which to measure their progress.

PLANNING

The purpose of the planning phase is to determine how to meet client needs. Assessment discloses needs but does not prescribe the specific actions necessary to meet them. Knowing that the group of well-child mothers needed emotional support did not tell the nurse what to do about it. A diagnosis of culture shock for a family newly arrived from Cuba does not reveal what action to take. The nurse must plan.

Planning is a logical, decision-making process. It means designing an orderly, detailed program of action around specific goals. There is a systematic approach to planning that guides the community health nurse during this phase of the nursing process: (1) list needs in order of priority, (2) establish goals and objectives, and (3) write the care plan. As they do in the rest of the nursing process, community health nurses collaborate with clients in each of these planning activities.

Setting Priorities
Setting priorities means assigning rank to client needs (diagnoses). One way to order needs is to group them into three categories — immediate, inter-mediate, and long-range — and then assign a priority to those in each group. Immediate needs are more urgent but not necessarily more important. For example, a meeting place was the most immediate need identified by a community health nurse and a group of senior citizens who wanted a class on exercise for the aging. Obviously their goal, to learn about appropriate exercises, was more important than finding a place to meet; however, the immediate need was requisite to accomplishing the long-range goal. Some needs are ranked as immediate because they are potentially hazardous or

life-threatening, such as lack of eye protection in a school welding class. Other needs are ranked first because they are of the greatest concern to the client. One family could not see how they would manage to lift and move their grandfather, a man who had recently had a cerebrovascular accident (CVA). They selected his transportation as their highest priority. Other needs were identified but could not be addressed until this first concern had been alleviated.

Establishing Goals and Objectives

Goals and objectives are as crucial to planning as a target is to a missile-firing team. The nurse without planned objectives who visits a needy family cannot expect to accomplish anything. Needs must be translated into goals to give direction and meaning to the nursing care plan. Goals can first be stated broadly to give an overview of the proposed end product and then divided into subgoals or objectives that describe specific desired outcomes and target dates. Objectives, as used here, are like stepping stones to help us reach the larger goal. For the family concerned about transporting their grandfather, their need, goal, and objectives were defined in the following manner:

Need
  Family members do not know how to help the grandfather, who recently had a CVA, move around the house after his discharge from the nursing home.
Goal
  Within a week after the grandfather comes home, the family will be able to help him move about the house.
Objectives
  1. On the grandfather's first day home, the community health nurse will determine with the family their capabilities (including the grandfather's) for helping him move about the house.
  2. A physical therapist, making a joint home visit on the first day with the community health nurse, will recommend needed equipment and procedures to be used for helping the grandfather move.
  3. Recommended equipment will be installed by the end of the second day.
  4. Each day, family members will practice lifting and moving procedures under the nurse's supervision.
  5. By the end of the first week, family members will all be able to help grandfather move safely in and out of bed and to the bathroom, kitchen, and living room.

Development of objectives depends on a careful analysis of all the ways one could accomplish the larger goal. One needs to select the courses of action best suited to meeting the goals and then build objectives. For the grandfather and family, other alternatives, such as keeping him in the nursing home longer, hiring an orderly to assist him at home, or confining him to bed with a strong exercise program, were considered and rejected. The grandfather's and family's choice was to rehabilitate him as soon as possible in his normal environment.

Some rules of thumb are helpful when writing objectives. Each objective should state a single idea. When more than one idea is expressed, as in an objective to obtain equipment and learn procedures, completion of the objective is much more difficult to measure. State each objective as an outcome. In other words, write the objective so that it describes one end result. For instance, objective 5 describes what the family will be able to do to help their grandfather move. This is a behavioral objective because it describes observable behaviors that can be measured. One can more readily evaluate objectives that include specifics like what will be done, who will do it, and when it will be accomplished. Then everyone knows exactly what has to be done and within what time frame. Writing measurable objectives makes a tremendous difference in the success of planning.

Planning means thinking ahead. The nurse looks ahead toward the desired end product and then decides on all the intermediate actions necessary to meet that goal. Sometimes an objective itself describes the intermediate actions. At other times the nurse may wish to break down an objective further into several activities. For example, with objective 4, the nurse first explained the procedures, then demonstrated how they were done, and then helped each family member try them. Their ability to practice was dependent on this sequence of activities. Good planning requires this kind of detail.

Decision making is an important part of planning. Decisions must be made while establishing priorities. Selecting goals and, from a variety of possible solutions, the best courses of action to meet the goals requires decisions. Further decision making is involved in selecting objectives and, when indicated, the specific actions to accomplish the objectives.

To facilitate planning and decision making, the community health nurse involves other people. Clients, of course, must be included at every step. They, after all, are the ones for whom the planning is being done and without whose insights and cooperation the plan may not succeed. At times other nurses are important to involve. Team meetings, nurse-supervisor conferences, or nurse-expert consultant sessions are all useful resources for planning. In addition, the community health nurse will frequently wish to confer with members of other health disciplines. Interdisciplinary team conferences are valuable for gaining a broader perspective and enlisting wider support for the evolving plan.

Recording the Plan

Recording the plan comes next. Until now, the planning phase has been a series of intellectual exercises done jointly with the client and perhaps with other health team members. The nurse has probably written notes on the decisions made about priorities, goals, objectives, and actions. Now the nurse can spell these out clearly in a format that meets the needs of the particular practice setting (see Fig. 7-4 for an example). Regardless of the type of care plan form(s) used, certain items should be addressed:

1. *Data base* is all the subjective and objective information — physical, psychological, social, and environmental — collected about clients. It includes background health information (past and present); individual, family, group, and community assessment; and health history or system's review. The data base is usually kept on separate forms that allow space for ongoing entries and analysis.
2. *Needs* are the specific areas related to the client's health that have been identified for intervention. Preferably, they are areas that both client and nurse agree require action. In some settings, they are called *problems, problem list,* or *nursing diagnoses.* Goals are statements that describe the resolution of the need. For clarity in planning, both a written need statement and goal statement are helpful.
3. *Expected outcomes* are the objectives. They are specific statements that describe what the nurse and the clients hope to accomplish. It is often necessary to construct two or three expected outcomes (objectives) for each need or goal to achieve comprehensive results. These objectives provide the nurse planner with specific targets at which to aim and around which to design actions.
4. *Planned actions* are the activities or methods of accomplishing the expected outcomes. They are specific, planned interventions to meet the objectives. Plans should include appropriate actions by nurse and client.
5. *Progress and evaluation* describe the actual outcomes or results and what they mean. What happened? How was each objective met and when, and if not, why not? It is essential to include evaluation in the written care plan. Too often, progress notes become a substitute for evaluation. Progress notes are useful, periodic summaries; evaluation requires analysis and conclusions. Progress notes and evaluation may be combined if space is allowed on the care plan. Generally, it is best to enter progress notes on a separate page.

One way to record the plan is to list items 2–5 in columns with space for the nurse to record specifics (see Fig. 7-4). An increasing number of nurses find it helpful to give a copy of the plan to clients. In many instances, having a copy promotes clients' sense of being equal partners in the responsibility of meeting goals.

IMPLEMENTATION

Implementation is putting the plan into action. It means that the activities delineated in the plan are carried out, some by the nurse and some by the

NURSING CARE PLAN

Client _____ Jones Family _____

Date	No.	Need/Goal	Expected Outcomes	Planned Actions	Progress/Evaluation	Date
2/20	1.	Parents and 14-year-old daughter rarely have time to talk to each other. Goal: To increase amount and quality of communication between parents and daughter.	a. Family will eat together at least once a day on weekdays for 3 months.	a. Determine which meal will be eaten together and select appetizing menus.	a. Have eaten all but 2 dinners together since 2/26. Had breakfasts together instead on 4/6 and 4/13. Family feels objective has been accomplished. Plan to continue frequent meals together.	5/28
			b. Family conversation during meals will include discussion of everyone's activities.	b. Parents will show interest in daughter by asking questions and decreasing amount of discussion between themselves. Daughter will ask parents questions about their days.	b. Family states meal conversation is much more satisfying. All say they are learning much about each other. Conversation is free-flowing. Family interaction in front of nurse is relaxed, open. Objective accomplished.	5/28
			c. Family will have one activity together each month for next 3 months.	c. Family will go to a movie in March, eat dinner out in April, have a picnic in May.	c. Watched TV movie instead. Made popcorn. Had a good time.	3/24
					Ate at nice restaurant. Enjoyed being together.	4/21
					Daughter invited friend to picnic on 5/19. All played games together. Family is satisfied that communication goal is met and plans to continue monthly family activities.	5/28
				d. Family will meet with nurse monthly to evaluate progress.		

Figure 7-4
Partial sample of nursing care plan.

client. In community health nursing, this is a point of particular emphasis. It is not just nursing action or nursing intervention but *collaborative* implementation. Certainly, the nurse's professional expertise and judgment provide a necessary resource to the client. The nurse is also a catalyst and facilitator in planning and activating the nurse-client action plan. But a primary goal in community health is to help people learn to help themselves toward their optimal level of health. To realize this goal, the nurse must constantly involve clients in the deliberative process and encourage their sense of responsibility and autonomy. Other health team members, too, may participate in carrying out the plan. Therefore, all are partners in implementation.

Preparation

The actual course of implementation, outlined in the plan, should be fairly easy to follow if goals, expected outcomes, and planned actions have been designed carefully. Nurse and clients should have a clear idea of the who, what, why, when, where, and how. Who will be involved in carrying out the plan? What is each person's responsibilities? Do all understand why and how to do it? Do they know when and where activities will occur? As implementation begins, nurses should review these questions for themselves as well as clients. This is the time to clarify any doubtful areas and thus facilitate a smooth implementation phase.

Even the best planning, though, may require adjustments. For example, the Jones family ran into a snag when they discovered that the three of them could not agree on what constituted an appetizing menu. To solve this unexpected conflict, they elected to take turns planning the menu so that each had a regular opportunity to eat favorite foods. This solution, they decided, would contribute to feelings of good will and enhance mealtime conversation. Thus implementation requires flexibility and adaptation to unanticipated events.

Activities

Sometimes implementation is referred to as the action phase of the nursing process. In one sense, this is true because action is finally taken to solve the problem or meet the need. Up to this point, the nursing process has been largely background work. The early steps of the nursing process are much like preparing to build a bridge. Bridge construction requires initial negotiation (interaction); research on bridge construction, environmental considerations, and traffic use (assessment); and bridge design (planning). Implementation is actually building the bridge and seeing its completion.

The process of implementation requires a series of nursing actions. First, the nurse applies appropriate theories to the actions being performed. For the Jones family, the community health nurse used theories of communication and of adolescent behavior, among other theories, to guide the implementation process. Second, the nurse provides an environment that is conducive for carrying out the plan, such as a quiet room in which to hold a teaching session. Third, the nurse prepares the client for the care to be received. This step means building on the interaction established earlier so that open communication and trust are maintained. Client knowledge, understanding, and attitudes are assessed. The plan is carefully interpreted. Nurse and client form a contractual agreement about the content of the plan and how it is to be carried out. Fourth, the plan is carried out or modified and carried out by the nurse and client. Modification requires constant observation and interchange during implementation since these actions determine the success of the plan and the nature of needed changes. Finally, the nurse documents the implementation process through progress notes.

EVALUATION

Evaluation, the final component of the nursing process, is the last in a sequence of actions leading to the resolution of client health needs. The nursing process, as a professional tool for goal attainment, is not complete without measuring and judging the effectiveness of that goal attainment. Too often emphasis is placed primarily on assessing client needs and planning and implementing care. But how effective was the care? Were client needs truly met? Professional practitioners owe it to their clients, themselves, and to other health service providers to evaluate.

Evaluation is an act of appraisal. When one evaluates something, one judges its value in relation to a standard and a set of criteria. For example, when eating dinner in a restaurant, diners evaluate the dinner in terms of the standard of a satisfying meal. The criteria for their standard may include qualities such as a wide variety of choices on the menu, reasonable price, tasty food, nice atmosphere, and good service. They also evaluate the meal for a purpose. Was money and time well spent, and will they want to eat there again? Evaluation requires a purpose, standards and criteria, and judgment skills.

Purpose
The ultimate purpose of evaluating care in community health nursing is to determine whether planned actions met client needs; how well they were met; and if not, why not. In the pressure of daily practice, nurses are frequently limited to writing a quick progress note and a short final summary. This substitute for evaluation describes what occurred but does not judge its value. Evaluation is a critical component in the nursing process; without it, there is no basis for knowing whether previous actions were worthwhile and no evidence on which to base future plans. Therefore, nurses need

evaluation to complete the series of activities that help them reach their goal — client health.

Standards and Criteria

Evaluation utilizes standards and criteria. In community health nursing, the standards are the intended results of the nursing care plan — the goals. The criteria for these standards are the specific, expected client behaviors that will demonstrate accomplishment of goals — the objectives. The Jones family had a standard that was their goal to increase the amount and quality of communication between parents and daughter (Fig. 7-4). How did they and the nurse know when the goal was met? The expected outcomes (objectives) were written as specific behaviors; these became criteria for evaluation. When all of the conditions or criteria were met, they knew the goal had been accomplished.

Consider another example. Several diabetic women attending a clinic had a problem with obesity. A community health nurse working in the clinic helped them form a weight loss group. Each woman set a goal of a specific number of pounds to lose in a year and then developed objectives (expected outcomes) to help her reach that goal. One of them, Mrs. Sanders, planned the following:

Goal (Standard)
   Lose 50 pounds by the end of the year (target date).
Objectives (Criteria)
   1. Lose two pounds a week for the first 10 weeks.
   2. Lose one pound a week for the next 30 weeks.
   3. Maintain weight loss for 12 weeks.

The women planned ways to meet each of their objectives such as a specific daily calorie limit and regular exercise program. Some added hobbies or a series of personal rewards (a new dress after losing 15 pounds) to serve as motivators and pleasure substitutes. Mrs. Sanders evaluated the completion of her goal by using the standard (50 pounds in a year) and the criteria spelled out in her objectives. To maximize group support and encourage healthy behavior patterns during weight loss, the nurse suggested having a group goal. This became their standard for measuring group success:

Group Standard
   The group will stay healthy while accomplishing 90 percent of the weight loss goals.
Group Criteria
   1. By the end of the year the group will lose at least 90 percent of the sum of the expected individual weight losses.
   2. The group will have no diabetes-related infections during the year.
   3. All of the group members will be exercising at least once a week by the end of the year.

172

4. No more than 10 percent of the group will have had an illness that kept them in bed more than one day during the year.

The prepared standard and set of criteria helped the group evaluate its success.

The above examples emphasize the relationship of good planning to evaluation. When nurse and client prepare clear, specific goals and objectives, there is then no question about how or what to evaluate. It will be obvious that the goal is either met or not met (Fig. 7-5).

Judgment Skills

Evaluation requires judgment skills. The nurse compares real outcomes with expected outcomes and looks for discrepancies. When actual client behavior matches the desired behavior, then the goal, if well planned, is met. If it is not met, why not? The nurse will need to examine several possible explanations for the failure. Data collection may have been inadequate, the diagnosis incorrect, the plan unrealistic, or implementation ineffective. Circumstances,

Figure 7-5
Elderly clients in a community health education program are being interviewed to evaluate the outcomes of the program.

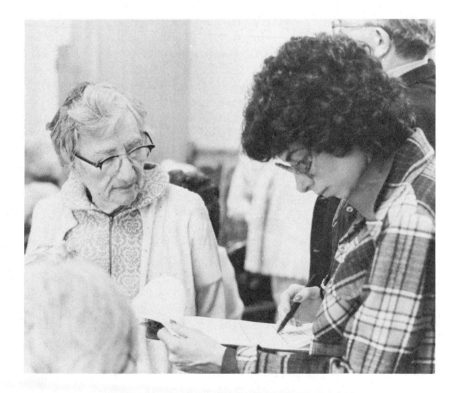

client motivation, or both may have changed. There may not have been enough client participation in one or more parts of the process. After determining the cause of the failure, the nurse can reassess, plan, and initiate corrective action.

Quality Assurance

In community health nursing, evaluation is also done to measure the quality of client care, nurse performance, and programs and services (Decker, Stevens, Vancini, & Wedeking, 1979). These measurements reflect nursing's increasing concern with quality assurance. An ideal quality assurance system includes the following (*Assessing Quality*, 1976):

1. An organizational entity created for assessing quality
2. Establishment of standards or criteria against which quality is assessed
3. A routine system for gathering information
4. Assurance that such information is based on the total population or representative sample of patients or potential patients
5. A process that provides the results of review to patients, the public, providers, and sponsoring organizations as well as methods to institute corrective actions

With the burgeoning emphasis on accountability in health care, community health nursing is being challenged to devise better ways of documenting service effectiveness and cost efficiency. A variety of methodologies and tools exists and is constantly being broadened to facilitate these evaluative processes. One method is the nursing audit, which evaluates quality of nursing care by analyzing client records. Some instruments, such as Wandelt's Quality Patient Care Scale, evaluate care while it is being given (Wandelt & Ager, 1974). All of these methods, however, operate on the same basic principle discussed earlier, that is, that evaluation requires a clear purpose, and a standard and specific criteria against which outcomes are measured.

Characteristics

The nursing process provides a framework or structure upon which community health nursing actions are based. Application of the process varies with each situation, but the nature of the process remains the same. Certain elements of that nature are important for community health nurses to emphasize in their practice (see Fig. 7-6).

The process is *deliberative* (Weidenbach, 1964). That is, it is purposefully, rationally, and carefully thought out. It requires the use of judgment. Community health nurses frequently practice in situations that demand independent thinking and difficult decision making. The nursing process is a tool to facilitate making these determinations.

174

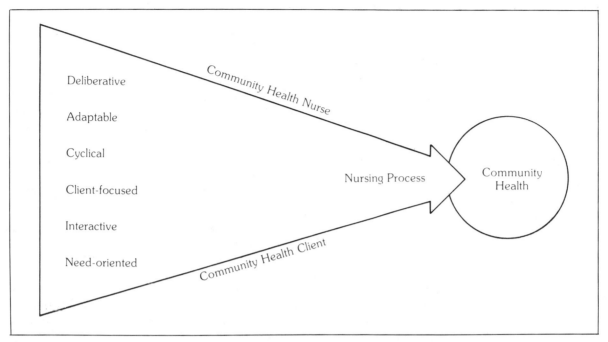

Figure 7-6
Nursing process character-istics emphasized in community health nursing practice.

The process is *adaptable* (Yura & Walsh, 1973). Its dynamic nature enables the community health nurse to adjust appropriately to each situation, to be flexible in applying the process to client needs. The nurse adapts and individualizes service for each community client.

The process is *cyclical.* Although a sequence of actions constitutes the framework of the nursing process, these actions are in constant progression (Marriner, 1979). The nurse in any given situation engages in continual interaction, data collection, analysis, intervention, and evaluation. Steps are repeated over and over in the nurse-client relationship, and as interactions between nurse and client continue, various steps in the process are used simultaneously.

The process, because it is used for and with clients, is *client focused.* Clients are nursing's raison d'être, nursing's reason for being. Nurses use the nursing process for the express purpose of helping clients, directly or indirectly, to achieve and maintain health. The client as a total system, whether a family, group, or community, is the target of the nursing process.

The process is *interactive.* Nurse and client are engaged in a process of ongoing interpersonal communication, "a communicative interaction process" (Daubenmire & King, 1973, p. 512). Giving and receiving accurate information are necessary to promote understanding between nurse and client and foster effective use of the nursing process. Furthermore, as the consumer movement, patient's rights, and the self-care concept have gained emphasis, client and nurse have increasingly jointly assumed responsibility for promoting client health. The client-nurse relationship can and should be a partnership (Yura & Walsh, 1973). Called "peer practice" by some (Bayer & Brandner, 1977, p. 86), the nursing process is shared by nurse and client.

Finally, the nursing process, as applied in community health, is *need oriented*. Long association with problem solving has tended to limit the nursing process's focus to the correction of problems. Although problem solution is certainly an appropriate use of the nursing process, its application in community health to anticipation of needs and prevention of problems assumes additional significance. This focus is needed if we are to realize the goals of community health, "to protect, promote, and restore the people's health" (Sheps, 1976, p. 3).

Summary

The effectiveness of comunity health nursing practice depends on how well the nursing process is used as a tool for enhancing aggregate health. The nursing process means appropriately applying a systematic series of actions toward helping clients achieve their optimal level of health. These actions or components of the process include interaction, assessment, diagnosis, planning, implementation, and evaluation.

Interaction is the first component because nurse and clients must establish a relationship of reciprocal influence and exchange. It requires effective communication to assess needs and establish trust between nurse and clients as partners in the process.

Assessment is a process of appraising client health status to determine existing or possible future needs. Community health nursing is not limited to identifying problems. Rather, there is a strong emphasis on exploring ways to maximize client health potential. Assessment provides the basis for future nursing action. It involves collecting and interpreting data.

Diagnosis involves analyzing the collected data and determining what needs to be corrected or changed. It is a judgment of client needs.

Planning means designing a specific course of action to meet identified client needs. To plan, one must rank client needs, establish goals and objectives, design activities to meet the objectives, and write the care plan. The plan should include a data base, statements describing client needs and goals to be achieved, specific objectives, progress notes, and finally, an evaluation of each objective.

Implementation is activating the plan and seeing it through to completion. During implementation, the nurse applies appropriate theory; provides a facilitative environment; prepares the client for care; with the client, carries out or modifies and carries out a plan; and documents the implementation.

Evaluation measures and judges the effectiveness of the plan. Were client needs met? If not, why not? To evaluate, nurses need to understand clearly why they are evaluating. What is the purpose? They also need a standard (goal) and a specific set of criteria (objectives) for each goal to use in measuring the outcomes. There is an important relationship between good planning and evaluation, because well-prepared goals and objectives are essential for adequate evaluation. If goals are not met, the failure may result from inadequate assessment or planning. Determining the cause of the failure can lead to corrective action. Evaluation does not end the nursing process; rather, it documents what has been accomplished and what yet needs to be done in order that the process, a continuing cycle, can start again.

Certain characteristics of the nursing process should be emphasized by community health nurses in their practice. The process is *deliberative*, requiring and aiding the exercise of judgment in decision making. It is adaptable, encouraging flexibility in practice. It is *cyclical*, fostering a constant, ongoing use of the process. It is *client focused*, helping the nurse to keep the proper target of client health in view. It is *interactive*, promoting nurse-client communication and client participation. Finally, it is *need oriented*, encouraging identification of ways to maximize client health potential.

Study Questions

You have been practicing the nursing process with individuals to effect change in their health status. Now consider how you can expand that application to aggregates. Select a population group in your community, such as preschoolers, unwed mothers, Southeast Asian refugees, or elderly homebound persons.

1. As potential clients, how might you start the interaction phase with them?
2. What specific areas would you want to assess? Make a list of hypothetical symptoms that indicate a need.
3. Invent a diagnosis for this group that would be supported by the data you collected in your assessment.
4. What alternative courses of action should you consider for addressing this need? Select the most appropriate one.
5. Start a plan for implementation including an overall goal and at least one objective.
6. List the activities needed to meet your objectives(s), and describe how you might carry them out.
7. How would you evaluate your nursing interventions with this population group?

References

Assessing quality in health care: An evaluation (Final Report). (1976). Washington, DC: Institute of Medicine, National Academy of Sciences.

Bayer, M., & Brandner, P. (1977). Nurse/patient peer practice. *American Journal of Nursing, 77,* 86–90.

Brill, N. I. (1973). *Working with people: The helping process.* Philadelphia: Lippincott.

Daubenmire, M. J., & King, I. M. (1973). Nursing process models: A system approach. *Nursing Outlook, 21,* 512–517.

Decker, F., Stevens, L., Vancini, M., & Wedeking, L. (1979). Using patient outcomes to evaluate community health nursing. *Nursing Outlook, 27*(4), 278–282.

Langford, T. (1978). Establishing a nursing contract. *Nursing Outlook, 26*(5), 386–388.

Marriner, A. (1979). *The nursing process* (2nd ed.). St. Louis: C. V. Mosby.

Mauksch, I. G., & David, M. L. (1972). Prescription for survival. *American Journal of Nursing, 72,* 2189–2193.

Sheps, C. G. (1976). *Higher education for public health: Report of the Milbank Memorial Fund Commission.* New York: Neale, Watson.

Wandelt, M., & Ager, J. (1974). *Quality patient care scale.* New York: Appleton-Century-Crofts.

Weidenbach, E. (1964). *Clinical nursing: A helping art.* New York: Springer.

White, M. S. (1982). Construct for public health nursing. *Nursing Outlook, 30,* 527–530.

Williams, C. A. (1977). Community health nursing — What is it? *Nursing Outlook, 25,* 250–253.

Yura, H., & Walsh, M. B. (1973). *The nursing process: Assessing, planning, implementing, evaluating.* New York: Appleton-Century-Crofts.

Selected Readings

Assessing quality in health care: An evaluation (Final Report). (1976). Washington, DC: Institute of Medicine, National Academy of Sciences.

Bayer, M., & Brandner, P. (1977). Nurse/patient peer practice. *American Journal of Nursing, 77,* 86–90.

Bloch, D. (1975). Evaluation of nursing care in terms of process and outcome: Issues in research and quality assurance. *Nursing Research, 24,* 256–259.

Blum, H. (1981). *Planning for health: Generics for the eighties* (2nd ed.). New York: Human Sciences Press.

Bohm, S. M. (1978). Toward 2002: A community perspective. *New Zealand Nursing Journal, 71,* 24–28.

Brill, N. I. (1973). *Working with people: The helping process.* Philadelphia: Lippincott.

Browning, M. H. (1974). *The nursing process in practice.* New York: American Journal of Nursing.

Cordes, S. M. (1978). Assessing health care needs: Elements and processes. *Family and Community Health, 1*(2), 1–16.

Daubenmire, M. J., & King, I. M. (1973). Nursing process models: A system approach. *Nursing Outlook, 21,* 512–517.

Davidson, S. V. (1978). Community nursing care evaluation. *Family and Community Health, 1*(1), 37–55.

Decker, F., Stevens, L., Vancini, M., & Wedeking, L. (1979). Using patient outcomes to evaluate community health nursing. *Nursing Outlook, 27,* 278–282.

Donabedian, A. (1978). *The quality of medical care: Methods for assessing and monitoring the quality of care for research and for quality assurance programs in health.* Washington, DC: U.S. Government Printing Office.

Evaluation of quality of public health nursing. (1976). Washington, DC: American Public Health Association, Public Health Nursing Section.

Flynn, B., & Ray, D. (1979). Quality assurance in community health nursing. *Nursing Outlook, 27,* 650–653.

Gilman, S., & Nader, P. (1979). Measuring the effectiveness of a school health program — Methods and preliminary analysis. *Journal of School Health, 49,* 10–13.

Gordon, M. (1976). Nursing diagnosis and the diagnostic process. *American Journal of Nursing, 76,* 1232–1234.

Hadley, R. D. (1978). Nurses develop quality assurance program in community health setting. *American Nurse, 10,* 3–6.

Januska, C. (1976). *Status of quality assurance in public health nursing.* Washington, DC: American Public Health Association, Public Health Nursing Section.

Keeler, J. D. (1972). The process of program evaluation. *Nursing Outlook, 20,* 316–319.

Kleffel, D. (1972). *A utilization review program for home health agencies* (No. HSM 72-6502). Washington, DC: U.S. Government Printing Office.

Knight, J. H. (1974). Applying nursing process in the community. *Nursing Outlook, 22,* 708–711.

Langford, T. (1978). Establishing a nursing contract. *Nursing Outlook, 26,* 386–388.

Marram, G. (1973). Patients' evaluation of their care — Importance to the nurse. *Nursing Outlook, 21,* 322–324.

Marriner, A. (1979). *The nursing process* (2nd ed.). St. Louis: C. V. Mosby.

Mauksch, I. G., & David, M. L. (1972). Prescription for survival. *American Journal of Nursing, 72,* 2189–2193.

Mayers, M. G. (1972). A search for assessment criteria. *Nursing Outlook, 20,*323–326.

Mayers, M. G. (1972). *A systematic approach to the nursing care plan.* New York: Appleton-Century-Crofts.

National League for Nursing. (1975). *Accreditation of home health agencies and community nursing services* (No. 21-1306). New York: Author.

Parzick, J., & Nolan, M., Sr. (1978). POMR at work in a home health agency. *Family and Community Health, 1*(1), 101–113.

Phaneuf, M., & Wandelt, M. (1974). Qualilty assurance in nursing. *Nursing Forum, 4,* 328–345.

Ramphal, M. (1974). Peer review. *American Journal of Nursing, 74,* 63–67.

Scutchfield, F. D. (1975). Alternate methods for health priority assessment. *Journal of Community Health, 1*(3), 29–38.

Shaffer, M. K., & Pfeiffer, I. L. (1978). Home visit: A gray zone in evaluation. *American Journal of Nursing, 78,* 239–241.

Simmons, D. A. (1980). *A classification scheme for client problems in community health nursing* (DHEW 80-16, HRP 0501501). Springfield, VA: National Technical Information Services, Nurse Planning Information Series No. 14.

Wandelt, M., & Ager, J. (1974). *Quality patient care scale.* New York: Appleton-Century-Crofts.

Wray, J. G. (1977). Problem-oriented recording in community nursing — A new experience in education. *Journal of Nursing Education, 16*(9), 12–15.

Yura, H., & Walsh, M. B. (1973). *The nursing process: Assessing, planning, implementing, evaluating.* New York: Appleton-Century-Crofts.

Zimmer, M. (1974). Quality assurance for outcomes of patient care. *Nursing Clinics of North America, 6,* 305–315.

8

Epidemiology

Shirley Jean Thompson
Sara Louise Turner

Community health nursing is based on a synthesis of nursing science and the public health sciences applied to promoting and preserving the health of populations. The clients of the community health nurse include individuals, families, groups, communities, and populations at risk who need to have their health monitored as well as their problematic characteristics identified. Much of the information on health and illness characteristics of groups comes from epidemiology, a public health science and specialized form of scientific research.

Definition

Epidemiology is the study of the distribution and determinants of health, health conditions, and disease in human population groups. Epidemiologists are concerned with such questions as, What is the occurrence of health and disease in a population? Is there an increase or decrease in a health state over the years? Does one geographical area have a higher frequency of disease than another? Do certain characteristics of persons with a particular condition distinguish them from those without the condition? Is one treatment or program more effective than another in changing the health of individuals? Why do some people recover from a disease and others do not? The ultimate goal of epidemiology is to search for causes of health problems and identify solutions to prevent disease and improve the health of the entire population. In its search for causes, epidemiology provides health workers with a body of knowledge on which to base their practice, and methods for studying new and existing problems. This chapter focuses on methods of study. On pages 184–185, you will find a glossary of terms most often used in epidemiology.

Epidemiology differs from other disciplines by the nature of the questions asked and the use of population approaches to answer these questions. Notice in the questions above that the focus is always on a health state or change in a health state. The more precisely and specifically the health state can be defined, the better able we are to describe and study it epidemiologically. For example, the epidemiologist studies the occurrence of a specific disease, such as influenza, or a health condition such as hypertension. In contrast to other disciplines, the epidemiologist focuses on identifying possible causes of the influenza or high blood pressure; the sociologist focuses on the relationship between social phenonoma such as the relationship between socioeconomic status and clients' compliance with taking hypertensive medications; clinical nursing deals with the diagnosis and treatment of the clients' response to the health problem of hypertension. Community health nurses must be concerned with each of these aspects as they make decisions about screening, education, and service programs that are intended to reduce the high blood pressure in the particular client population.

A broad array of environmental (i.e., physical, chemical, pathogenic, social, cultural) and personal (i.e., psychological, biologic, behavioral, genetic) factors are considered by the epidemiologist as potential causes or determinants of a health state. For our purposes, the term *health state* refers to a disease, health condition, health outcome, or dependent variable. A *causal* or *putative causal factor* may also be referred to as factor, exposure variable, risk factor, characteristic, precursor, or independent variable. Examples of exposure factors include herpes virus, radiation, oral contraceptives, chemicals such as hair dyes, crowding, personality types, cholesterol level, use of tobacco, physical exercise, and blood group.

Although epidemiologists observe individuals, their interpretations and conclusions are based on combined results from many people. They are concerned with people who are well and people at risk of ill health as well as those who are sick. The basic strategy in epidemiology is the comparison of groups. This population approach is required to make causal inferences about relationships between factors and disease. The group as the unit of concern helps to distinguish epidemiology from biomedical sciences, which typically focus on tissues and organs, or from clinical nursing and clinical medicine, which typically involve the care of a small number of persons who present themselves individually for service.

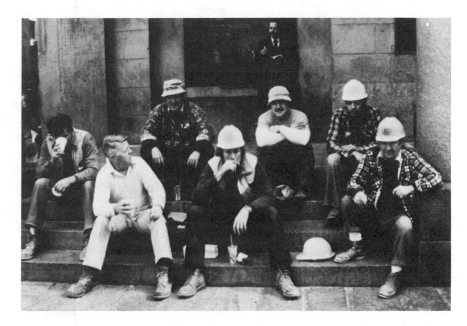

Figure 8-1
Epidemiology is concerned with the health of groups. The study of populations, such as this group of workers, is necessary to make causal inferences about relationships between factors and disease.

Historical Roots

The roots of epidemiology can be traced back to antiquity. The term, derived from the Greek words *epi* (upon), *demos* (the people), and *logos* (knowledge), thus means the knowledge or study of what is experienced by and burdens the people. Prevailing theories about disease causation, statistical developments, and social and sanitary reforms have greatly influenced the development of epidemiology. Hippocrates (460–377 B.C.), known as the first epidemiologist, believed that disease not only affected individuals but was a mass phenomenon. Furthermore, unlike other leaders of his day, he recognized that epidemics of disease did not appear by chance but indeed showed patterns in their occurrence. He was one of the first to differentiate health from disease and to associate disease and health occurrence with life-style and environmental factors.

One of the great burdens on communities in the past has been the epidemics of disease, discussed also in chapter 2. Cholera, bubonic plague, and smallpox swept through community after community, killing millions and altering the life-style of masses of people. In 1348, the Black Death moved through Europe and England, decimating the population. In England alone, approximately one-fourth of the population died. This dread disease

Glossary of Terms

Agent: Refers to a putative cause of a health problem, particularly a biological infecting organism such as Hepatitis A virus. Often used of other specific physical and chemical entities such as carbon monoxide, vitamin C.

Analytic studies: Investigations designed to identify associations between a particular human disease or health problem and its possible cause(s).

Association: Events are associated when they appear together more often than they would by chance alone. These events may include risk factors or other characteristics and disease or health states.

Attack rate: The proportion of a group or population that develops a disease among all those exposed to a particular risk. This term is used frequently in investigations of outbreaks of infectious diseases. See incidence rate.

Causal relationship/association: Inferred if the incidence of disease increases when the putative cause is present and decreases in the absence of this same putative cause or risk factor.

Case series: A complete description of persons considered disease cases. No comparison group is present; no conclusion can be drawn.

Cohort: A group of people who share a common experience in a specific time period.

Descriptive studies: Investigations describing groups of people with regard to certain characteristics (for example, time, place or person) as these relate to disease occurrence.

Epidemiology: The study of the distribution and determinants of health, health conditions, and disease in human population groups.

Endemic: "The habitual presence of a disease or infectious agent within a geographical area . . . or the usual prevalence of a given disease within such area"(Berenson, 1980).

Environment: Everything outside of human individuals — physical, chemical, biological, and social factors, including other people, social customs and codes, etc.

Epidemic: "The occurrence in a community or region of a group of illnesses . . . of similar nature, clearly in excess of normal expectancy" (Berenson, 1980).

Experimental study: A study design in which the investigator actually controls or changes the factors suspected of causing the health condition under study and observes what happens to the health state. Experiments to test the cause of disease in human populations are rarely ethical. However, this approach can be used in trials to prevent disease or to treat established disease processes (clinical trials).

Incidence: All new cases of a disease or other health conditions appearing during a given time.

Incidence rate: All new cases appearing during a given time is the numerator; the denominator is the population at risk during the same period of time.

Pandemic: Epidemics which are worldwide in distribution.

Population at risk: Persons with one or more characteristics in common, to whom a health or disease event could have happened whether or not it did. The denominator for vital rates, and for incidence or prevalence rates. Sometimes called referent population.

Prevalence: All people with a health condition existing in a given population at a given time. The condition may be new or have affected some for many years.

Prevalence rate: All new and old cases of a health condition prevailing at a particular place and time is the numerator; the total population for the same time and place is the denominator.

Prospective study: (From the words "looking forward"). The study group consists of persons free of the health condition in question (e.g., lung cancer). Persons are initially classified on the basis of their exposure characteristics (e.g., smoking vs. non-smoking), are followed longitudinally (forward over periods of time), and are observed for new development of the health condition/disease. Also called cohort and incidence study.

Rate: A statistical way of expressing the proportion of persons with a given health problem (or who develop a given health problem) among a population at risk. A rate is a quotient, or a fraction (e.g., prevalence rates, incidence rates, attack rates, and vital rates). A true rate exists when the numerator is a part of the denominator, and the denominator represents the entire population at risk. Compare with ratio.

Ratio: A statistical way of expressing the size or magnitude of one condition or occurrence in relation to the size of another. A ratio (e.g., sex ratio) need not be a rate.

Relative risk (RR): The comparison of disease occurrence in a group of people when a certain factor is present with the occurrence of the same disease in persons when that certain factor is absent.

Retrospective study: (From the words "looking back"). A design whereby the investigator begins by identifying cases of a disease and controls without the disease, and looks backward in time to identify exposures or precursor factors. Also called case-control study.

Risk factor: When the presence of a particular factor increases the likelihood that a disease will occur. Then, for that disease the factor is a risk factor, and people with that factor are at high risk for that disease.

Sensitivity: Refers to a screening test or set of criteria which detects a very high percentage of persons with the specific disease or condition tested for — detects true positives. (Compare with "Specificity.")

Specificity: Refers to a screening test or set of criteria which accurately indicates a very high percentage of persons who do not have the disease or condition tested for — indicates true negatives. (Compare with "Sensitivity.")

continued in Europe, but with less force, until the plague bacillus was identified in 1896.

Contagium, Miasma, and Germ Theories

By the early 1700s two theories were emerging to explain these epidemics. According to the contagium theory, disease was caused by living seeds of disease capable of reproducing their kind after an incubation period. There is some evidence that the contagium theory was the scientific basis for filtration of the water supply of London in 1829. When this theory failed to explain all epidemic diseases and lead to their control, an alternative explanation, the miasma theory, developed. This theory suggested that disease was caused by bad air, noxious vapors associated with decaying organic matter. Attempts were made to reduce disease by eliminating the sources of the miasma. With the discovery of bacteriology in the eighteenth century, the germ theory evolved and the study of disease became more or less restricted to infectious agents. It was a generally held belief that a specific germ or agent outside the body caused disease.

Multicausal Theory

As the threat of the epidemics slowly declined epidemiologists discovered that disease causation was much more complicated than at first suspected. Soon it was clear that not only the presence of the germ but the characteristics of the people could determine the occurrence of new diseases brought on by industrialization. Gradually, the multicausal theory of disease emerged to better elucidate both infectious and chronic disease etiologies and to guide epidemiologists in deciding what factors needed to be studied and controlled in order to reduce such problems as heart disease and cancer. According to multicausal disease theory, disease onset usually requires many factors to exist simultaneously. These factors may derive from man's external environment, from personal characteristics, or a combination thereof (see Figure 8-2). The same factors may cause more than one disease by occurring in different combinations under different circumstances. Many complex behaviors, environmental situations, or both probably need to be changed in order to control the problem and the origins of health and disease states may slowly evolve beginning at birth. Recognizing multiple causes offers many different strategies and points of prevention, health promotion, and treatment for health practitioners. Also, as the concept of disease etiology has expanded, the definition of health outcome has broadened to include wellness and health conditions as well as disease.

During the late 1600s and early 1700s, mathematical principles developed and were used to describe, analyze, and understand the epidemics. Epi-

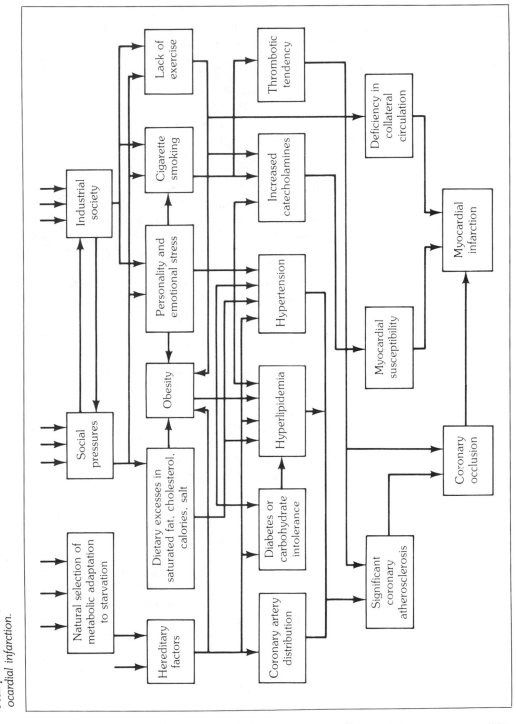

Figure 8-2
Multiple causation for myocardial infarction.

demiology began to flourish with the use of mortality rates, incidence and prevalence rates of disease, vital statistics, rules of probability, and methods employing comparison groups. Only recently have advances in statistical theory and computer technology allowed multicausal theories of health and disease to be tested in such a manner as to show the effect of a given risk factor when studied with many other factors and to describe how factors interact with each other to produce disease. For example, today we can say that the heavy alcohol user is about eight times more likely to develop esophageal cancer than a nonuser of alcohol of the same age, and we can say that a heavy smoker is about four times more likely to develop esophageal cancer than his nonsmoker counterpart. More important, those persons who are both heavy drinkers and heavy smokers may be as many as 90 times more likely to have esophageal cancer than the nonsmoker-nondrinker.

A significant influence on the development of epidemiology is social reform, a reflection of the concerns of the poeple at any given time in history. During the eighteenth and nineteenth centuries, sanitary reforms seeking to improve the needs and living conditions of the poor also stimulated the study of infectious diseases. The industrial revolution resulted in increased interest in occupational health problems and their control. Today environmentalists are focusing epidemiology on the health effects of toxic agents such as asbestos in our daily living space, nuclear wastes in the atmosphere from power plants, and chemicals such as ethylene dibromide in our food chain.

Florence Nightingale's Influence

The roots of epidemiology in nursing can be traced back to Florence Nightingale (1820–1910) (Cohen, 1984). Miss Nightingale often obtained advice on issues related to hospital statistics and disease classification from her close friend William Farr, who was chief statistician of England's General Register Office for health and vital statistics. Her detailed and careful description of the health conditions among the military in the Crimea represents one of the first systematic descriptive studies of the distribution and patterns of disease in a population. Changes made according to her suggestions brought dramatic proof of the authenticity of her observations and knowledge. Forty out of every 100 British troops were dying in the Crimea before Miss Nightingale instituted environmental and nutritional changes in the hospital and field. When her work in the Crimea was finished, the death rate was only 2 percent. Florence Nightingale's imaginative use of the numerical approach and her commitment to environmental reform in caring for the sick strongly influenced nursing to expand into a profession whose service addressed public health problems as well as hospital care. As nursing has evolved, the community health nurse has continued to deal with both the personal and environmental health of people, entering the environment in which people live and thinking in terms of groups at risk within the total population. This wellness as well as illness orientation to populations requires that the community health nurse think quantitatively as well as qualitatively.

Quantitative Measurements — Rates and Proportions

In order to predict and control health and disease occurrences that can affect a community, epidemiologists have learned to describe precisely what is happening. This requires, first, information about the number of times a disease event has happened (count of affected persons). In order for this information or count of events to be descriptive of a group or community it must be viewed in proportion to the total size of the group or community of concern (commonly known as the population at risk). Usually this proportion, instead of being expressed as a percentage, is called a *rate*. A rate includes the numerator (number of events) and the denominator (number of persons whom these types of events might have affected — those at risk of this event). Additionally, because such proportions frequently turn out to be very small, they are multiplied by a constant such as 1,000, 10,000, or 100,000, and thus become both more readable and more easily discussed:

Numerator: Events (counts of sick people)

Denominator: All those to whom the event could have happened (and did not) and all those to whom the event did happen (population at risk)

For example, the school nurse who screens third-graders for vision and hearing difficulties may find two students whose hearing appears faulty and whom she will refer for diagnostic workup. If the nurse works in a rural school in which there are 60 third-graders, the proportion affected is 2/60 = .03, 3 percent, or a rate of 3/100 or 30/1,000 of all the third-graders at risk of hearing impairment. If the nurse works in a metropolitan area and finds two cases among 500 third-graders screened, the rate is 2/500, 0.004, 0.4 percent or 4/1,000. Obviously in comparing these two rates the likelihood of hearing difficulties appears far greater in the rural area. A difference of this degree would stimulate an investigation of *why*. We discuss comparing rates later in the section on measure and the meaning of risk. Thus a rate, whether used to compare communities or a description of the current situation within one community or group, is a statement that estimates the frequency of occurrence of some event within the target population.

Rates readily available to community health nurses are those that describe mortality (death), natality (birth), and morbidity (illness). Some rates are actually indices. That is, they are the best available approximation to a true rate, an approximation used when the obvious population at risk or denominator cannot be counted (see the example of maternal mortality under "Vital Rates").

Ratios are also used in community health. The sex ratio of a given group, for example, is the proportion of males to females. If there are 105 males to every 100 females at birth, the ratio is 1.05. Or if there are 45 males to every 100 females among persons 85 years and older, the ratio is expressed as 0.45. The number of males (numerator) is divided by the number of females (denominator) to calculate the ratio. In a ratio the numerator and denominator may each be a count of events or people that do not necessarily overlap. That is, the numerator count is not necessarily a part of the denominator, and the denominator is not necessarily a population at risk.

Morbidity Rates

Events of illness, which can begin, continue, and end, obviously differ from events like births and deaths, which can best be thought of as occurring or becoming obvious at one particular point in time. The term incidence refers to an initial occurrence or event. In epidemiology, *incidence* means the new appearance of a disease over time in a population. Incidence rates of illness are those that refer to the frequency with which people newly acquire a specific health problem (such as measles, rabies, diabetes, or arthritis) during a given period of time. Prevalence, on the other hand, refers to all conditions in existence, whether newly acquired or not. *Prevalence,* in epidemiology, refers to all existing (specific) disease (whether old or new, continuing, or about to end) at a point or period in time. Prevalence rates measure the number of persons in a population who have the disease or condition of interest at any given point in time. For example in Figure 8-3, the cases of disease that would be counted in the numerator of an incidence rate during 1983 would include case numbers 2, 3, 7, 8 and 9. For measuring period prevalence from January 1 to December 31, case numbers 1, 2, 3, 4, 5, 6, 7, 8, 9, 10 would be included.

Reportable infectious diseases like measles or rabies are primarily spoken of in terms of incidence or attack rates. *Attack rates* are incidence rates expressed as percentages for particular populations, as in food poisoning outbreaks when the population at risk is exposed to a contaminated food product and the time period is limited. When illness is self-limiting, short-lived, and there are no old cases (i.e. food poisoning), prevalence is the same as incidence. Describing prevalence in that situation adds no new or useful information. On the other hand, for conditions like diabetes or arthritis, it may be difficult to determine time of onset, and thus difficult to gather incidence data except through specific study designs (see "Prospective Studies" below). It is generally easier to estimate prevalence by means of surveys.

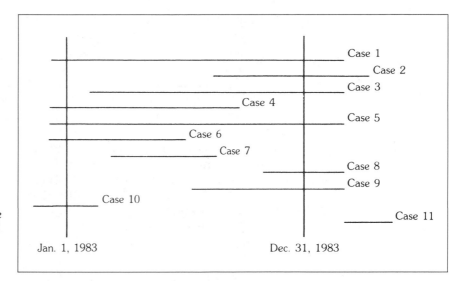

Figure 8-3
Number of cases of disease beginning, developing, and ending during the period of time January 1, 1983– December 31, 1983.

Prevalence rates are extremely helpful to those who plan services for persons with chronic disease and those who develop professional educational programs. Incidence rates are not helpful for these purposes when dealing with long-term illness because the rates of new occurrences or incidence will be much smaller than the prevalence rates. At times in the literature the term *incidence* is used when *prevalence* is meant. The concept of incidence as the rate of new development of disease is too valuable to confuse in this way because it is from incidence rates that we are able to assess risk to population groups and evaluate risk factors (as will be discussed later under measures and meaning of risk).

Vital Rates

Vital events such as births and deaths, as well as other legal changes in civil state (adoptions, marriages, divorces, separations, and annulments), are registered locally in the vital statistics office as a part of the state's responsibility for keeping track of its people. These events form the numerators for birth and death rates. When population counts are used as denominators, these are based on estimates from the decennial U.S. Census enumerations.

Thus birth and death rates, based on routinely collected data, express relationships between these vital events and the population in which they occur. Birth and death rates are called *crude* when the numerator events describe the midyear population. The midyear estimate of the population is used on the assumption that deaths, or births, will be evenly distributed throughout the year and thus the July first population indicates the size of the average population at risk.

191

In contrast to crude rates, death rates may be specific when the numerator (in the case of specific causes of death) or the numerator and the denominator (in the case of specified age, sex, or racial groups) are more clearly delineated. In similar fashion, natality data may be specified to compare white and nonwhite populations (black, Oriental, Native American, and others). When live births are related to the population of women aged 15–44 years the rate is called a *fertility* rate because it refers to the childbearing years. Live births are used not only as numerators (in birth rates and in fertility rates), but as denominators. For example, to understand the community impact of deaths of women from puerperal (childbirth-related) causes, one should ideally use the population at risk — the number of pregnancies occurring during the year — as the denominator. Because this denominator is not available, the maternal mortality rate is based on the number of live births occurring during the year. Infant mortality, a crucial public health index of unmet needs for health care, nutrition, education, and sanitation, is based on live births, as are abortion rates. There are data available on fetal deaths from fetal death certificates. These data are not as complete as data for other mortality events or as data on live births. However, one of the uses of counts of fetal death events is measuring perinatal mortality. This is a measure of the vulnerability of the very young to environmental effects, hygiene, and health care. This rate estimates loss in late fetal life and the first week of extrauterine life. Table 8-1 illustrates the composition and calculation of rates using data from the United States vital statistics of 1978. In it are examples of crude rates; of cause-, sex-, and/or race-specific mortality rates; and of race-, sex-, and age-specific rates using both natality and mortality events. Table 8-1 lists the numerators and the denominators as well as the initial proportions calculated, the usual factors or bases (which may be 1,000 or 100,000), and the actual death rates.

Mortality rates are also used to calculate life expectancy. Given the age-specific death rates occurring, for example, among 11 or 12 groupings during 1980, an estimate of how long an infant born in 1980 will live can be calculated. This is the usual meaning of the term *life expectancy*. However, average years of life remaining for persons reaching age 20, age 50, age 65, or age 85 can be projected and calculated by sex and race as well. Insurance rates are set by these actuarial or life table methods. Other uses of these types of calculations are for demonstrating survival rates from special diseases — the cancers, for example. Calculations like these show how survival rates improve over time.

Mortality (and natality) rates may also be *adjusted* to take into account the age structure of the population or a number of other characteristics that may differ from one area to another or from country to country (or race, economic status, or other like variable). Obviously, an older population such as one might anticipate in St. Petersburg, Florida, is at a higher risk of death than the population of space technicians that might dominate the population

Table 8-1
Composition and Calculation of Rates Illustrated with Data from the 1978 Vital Statistics of the United States

Crude Rates

Crude death rate:
$$\frac{\text{Number of deaths during year (1978)}}{\text{midyear (July 1, 1978, estimated) population}} = \frac{1,927,788}{218,228,000} = .008834 \times \text{usual base of } 1,000 = 8.8 \text{ deaths per } 1,000 \text{ population}$$

Crude birth rate:
$$\frac{\text{Number of live births during year (1978)}}{\text{midyear (July 1, 1978, estimated) population}} = \frac{3,333,279}{218,228,000} = .01527 \times \text{usual base of } 1,000 = 15.3 \text{ births per } 1,000 \text{ population}$$

Cause, Sex and/or Race-Specific Mortality Rates

Cause-specific:
$$\frac{\text{Number of deaths from a stated cause in a year (myocardial infarction in 1978)}}{\text{midyear (July 1, 1978, estimated) population}} = \frac{302,664}{218,228,000} = .0013869 \times \text{usual base of } 100,000 = 138.9 \text{ deaths per } 100,000 \text{ population}$$

Cause- and sex-specific:
$$\frac{\text{Number of deaths from myocardial infarction among males in 1978}}{\text{midyear (July 1, 1978, estimated) male population}} = \frac{184,121}{106,120,000} = .0017350 \times \text{usual base of } 100,000 = 173.5 \text{ deaths per } 100,000 \text{ males}$$

Cause-, sex-, and race-specific:
$$\frac{\text{Number of deaths from myocardial infarction among white males in 1978}}{\text{midyear (July 1, 1978, estimated) white male population}} = \frac{171,122}{92,035,000} = .0018953 \times \text{usual base of } 100,000 = 185.9 \text{ deaths per } 100,000 \text{ white males}$$

Race-, Sex- and Age-Specific Rates Using Natality and Mortality Events

Race-specific birth rate:
$$\frac{\text{Number of white live births in 1978}}{\text{July 1, 1978, white population}} = \frac{2,681,116}{188,657,000} = .01421 \times \text{usual base of } 1,000 = 14.2 \text{ births per } 1,000 \text{ whites}$$

Fertility rate:
$$\frac{\text{Number of live births in 1978}}{\text{July 1, 1978 population of females aged 15–44}} = \frac{3,333,279}{50,024,000} = .0666 \times \text{usual base of } 1,000 = 66.6 \text{ births per } 1,000 \text{ females aged 15 to 44}$$

Infant mortality:
$$\frac{\text{Number of deaths of children less than 1 year of age in 1978}}{\text{Number of live births in 1978}} = \frac{45,945}{3,333,279} = .01378 \times \text{usual base of } 1,000 = 13.8 \text{ infant deaths per } 1,000 \text{ live births}$$

Perinatal mortality:
$$\frac{\text{Number of fetal deaths of 28 weeks or more gestation and deaths of infants under 7 days of age in 1978}}{\text{Number of live births and fetal deaths of 28 weeks or more in 1978}} = \frac{18,033 - 26,607}{3,333,279 + 18,033} = \frac{44,640}{3,359,886} = .01328 \times \text{usual base of } 1,000 = 13.3 \text{ perinatal losses per } 1,000 \text{ perinatal events}$$

Maternal mortality:
$$\frac{\text{Number of deaths from puerperal causes in 1978}}{\text{Number of live births in 1978}} = \frac{321}{3,333,279} = .0000963 \times \text{usual base of } 100,000 = 9.63 \text{ maternal deaths per } 100,000 \text{ live births}$$

Source: National Center for Health Statistics, 1982.

at Cape Canaveral, Florida. When age-specific death rates are used to compare these two communities, differences found will be due to factors other than age. When one summary comparison is desired, the crude death rate is always affected by the age distribution, so adjustment for age should be calculated. Adjusted or standardized rates are fictitious; that is, they do not mirror the mortality experience of a community. They do allow for the unbiased comparison of diverse communities and allow for an interpretation of mortality that is not possible with crude rates.

The data in Table 8-2 demonstrate more clearly how community health nurses can make use of contrasting data for descriptive purposes. Table 8-2 is, of course, a comparison over time, reflecting the change in economic conditions, advances in sanitation and in health care, and the revolution in clinicians' understanding and ability to control infections. The life expectancy prediction in 1901 is based on the high rates of death during infancy, preschool, and school age, which occurred before the introduction of pure water and milk and the immunizations available today. It is clear, however, that if a person born in the 1900s survived through the 1960s, he or she would then have a life span similar to that projected for 65-year-olds today

Table 8-2

Comparison of Vital Statistics Rates and Indexes in the United States, 1900 and 1980

Variable	1900	1980
Life expectancy	49.24 years (1901)	73.7 years
Life expectancy at age 65	77.86 years (1901)	81.4 years
Crude death rate[a]	1719.1	878.3
Heart disease		
Death rate	137.4	336.0
Age adjusted (direct)		220.0
Influenza and pneumonia		
Death rate	202.2	24.1
Age adjusted (direct)		12.4
Maternal mortality[b]	610.0 (1915)	9.2
Infant mortality[c]	99.0 (1916)	12.6
Nonwhite infant mortality[c]	184.9 (1916)	21.4
Crude birth rate[a]	250.0	159.0

[a] Per 100,000 population.
[b] Per 100,000 live births.
[c] Per 1,000 live births.
Sources: For 1900 death rates, Linder & Grove (1943); for 1901 life expectancy data, Glover (1976); for 1980 data, National Center for Health Statistics (1982a, 1983).
Note: Mortality statistics collection began in 1900 with a national death registration area of ten states, the District of Columbia, and a number of cities in other states. By 1933 all of the U.S. continental states were included. National natality statistics began in 1915 with a registration area of ten states and the District of Columbia. As with mortality statistics, by 1933 all of the states were included. The 1940 census enumeration of the population of the United States is used as the standard for age-adjusted rates.

194

on the basis of current death rates. The age structure of the U.S. population today, with the increasing proportion of elderly (compared with earlier times), is suggested by the 1980 age-adjusted rates for heart disease and influenza mortality.

Although this table does not provide evidence of the changes in styles of diagnosing diseases and in potential accuracy of diagnosis that has occurred over this 80-year period, we realize that this has happened. Consider the technologies and tests available to clinicians today that were unknown even thirty years ago. We know that deaths frequently attributed to "indigestion" in the Victorian years would more reasonably today be considered a result of myocardial infarction. These issues can only be suggested by Table 8-2.

Most mortality and morbidity rates do vary according to time and place and according to the many personal characteristics of the population. In practice, health problems are most often described by age, sex, race, ethnic group, social class, occupation, marital status, and other physical and emotional characteristics of the people involved. When this is done, we are using epidemiological data descriptively in order to specify issues and highlight problems in the population. In researching infant health, community health nurses may find that the highest death rates in the first year of life are among nonwhite babies, among male babies, and among those babies born to unmarried mothers, teenage mothers, or mothers living in low socioeconomic conditions. Nurses may also learn that in their state the infant death rate has dropped from 35.3/1,000 live births in 1955 to 18.5/1,000 live births in 1982 and that the rate is much higher in the eastern area of the state than in the western area. Although this pattern does not identify the cause of infant mortality, it describes facets of the problem important to the community health nurse. This information can be used to plan, provide, and evaluate health services to vulnerable women and children, and to identify areas that need further study. Community health nurses can systematically examine the mortality data for the community of interest using existing state and local statistics.

Quality and Sources of Data

Quality Issues

All consumers of health data need to carefully obtain and use the best, most precise, reliable (reproducible), and valid (correct) information. Only in this way can clinical conclusions relative to clients' care be made and feasible policy established for community health needs.

Epidemiologists use the term *bias* to indicate that crucial aspects of information or data are systematically slanted and thus in error. When errors occur in a systematic fashion, the evidence for useful scientific or clinical inference is obscured or reversed. Measurements or observations of events can often be unreliable. For example, when a sphygmomanometer leaks pressure, clinicians are tired, or interviewers skip questions, information becomes unreliable. Clients may also exhibit variability, such as diurnal changes in mood, or blood pressure variations, that cause information to be unreliable or not reproducible when checked again. Finally, there is the concept of validity, that is, producing the correct measurement or description of what is really there. Epidemiologists must determine whether or not the subjects or events (births, deaths, and illness, for example) called *cases* really are cases of the disease, health state, or problem being investigated.

Issues of bias, reliability, and validity will be discussed frequently in the written sources community health nurses turn to for information on their community or a special target population. When nurses are gathering firsthand information — interviewing a community group, reviewing a community agency's health records, or planning and carrying out other research — they should seek advice to avoid the pitfalls caused by bias, unreliable measures, and invalid labeling.

Sources of Information

A variety of information is available nationally, by states, and by sections, such as counties or urbanized areas. It includes vital statistics, census data, and morbidity statistics on certain communicable or infectious diseases. Local health departments can often provide this data upon request. Community health nurses seeking information on their own localities may also find the health system agencies most helpful. These agencies work to collect health information for groups of counties within states and interact with health planning authorities at the state level. They have access to many types of information and can additionally give advice on specific problems raised by nurses.

VITAL STATISTICS

We have already discussed mortality and natality rates, but more can be learned. Obtain blank copies of your state's birth and death certificates and examine them. As you will see, a lot of information is recorded beside the fact and cause of death on the death certificate. Birth certificates also provide helpful information. The weight of the baby and the amount of prenatal care received by the mother have been examples of information used to identify high-risk mothers and babies.

THE CENSUS

The national census, conducted every ten years for governmental functions other than health, is a valuable aid in assessing communities. Localities usually project population estimates year by year on the basis of the national

196

data. Populations within counties and within census tracts in urbanized areas can be analyzed by age, sex, race, ethnic background, type of occupation, income gradient, marital status, educational level, as well as by other standards, for example, housing.

REPORTABLE DISEASES

Each state has developed laws or regulations that require hospitals, clinics, and clinicians to report when they find certain communicable and infectious diseases that can be spread through the community. The purpose, of course, is to enable the health department to take the most appropriate and efficient action. All states require that the six diseases covered by international quarantine regulations be reported immediately. Among these are diseases unknown now in developed countries (plague, cholera) as well as "dead" diseases such as smallpox. (The World Health Organization announced the eradication of smallpox in 1979 after more than ten years of international cooperation and commitment [Henderson, 1980]. The disease remains on the list on the chance that it may reappear and because the virus is being maintained in laboratories to ensure vaccine availability if needed.) The other reportable diseases (varying between 20 and 40 by state) are usually classified according to the speed with which the health department should be notified. Some should be reported by phone or telegraph, others by mailing information weekly. They vary in potential severity from chicken pox to rabies and may include AIDS (acquired immune deficiency syndrome), encephalitis, syphilis, and toxic shock syndrome. Community health nurses should get the list of reportable diseases from their health department offices. Following up on occurrences of these diseases is a task frequently assigned to community nursing services.

REGISTRIES

In some areas or states there are disease registries or rosters for conditions with major public health impact. Tuberculosis and rheumatic fever registries were more common in the past years when these diseases were more frequent. Cancer registries and psychiatric registries are useful for providing incidence, prevalence, and survival data.

ENVIRONMENTAL MONITORING

State governments, sometimes through health departments, sometimes through other agencies, have begun to monitor hazards to health found in the environment. Pesticides, industrial wastes, radioactive or nuclear materials, chemical additives in food, and medicinal drugs have joined the list of pollutants. Concerned community members and leaders view these as risk factors that on the community and individual level affect health. Community health nurses can also obtain data from federal agencies such as the Food and Drug Administration, the Consumer Product Safety Commission, and the Environmental Protection Agency.

NATIONAL CENTER FOR HEALTH STATISTICS HEALTH SURVEYS

On the national level (published data are frequently also available for regions), the National Center for Health Statistics (NCHS) furnishes valuable health prevalence data from surveys of Americans. The Health Interview Survey reports interviews of a sample of 40,000 U.S. households each year for information on many health topics. The Health Examination Survey reports physical measurements on smaller samples of the population and augments the information provided by interviews. This survey provides prevalence information on conditions, diseases, and disabilities that appear frequently in the population. A third type of NCHS survey is of health records. This survey samples institutional records of hospitals and nursing homes primarily. This survey provides information on who is served along with diagnoses and other characteristics. Other NCHS surveys focus on fertility and family planning, follow-back studies on vital statistics events, and characteristics of ambulatory patients in physicians' community practices.

Each of these nationally sponsored efforts suggests ways in which community health nurses can examine health problems or concerns affecting their communities. Interviews, physical examinations of samples of community members, and surveillance of institutions, clinics, and private physicians' practices can be carried out locally when needs are identified and funds made available. Other sources may be found in data kept routinely but not centrally on the health problems of school children or of workers in local industry.

Measures and Meaning of Risk

Epidemiology is concerned with identifying factors that are thought to be causally related to a disease outcome. Identifying associations is the first step toward inferring causality. An association is said to exist between a factor and a disease when changes in the factor are accompanied by changes in the disease. An observed association may or may not be causal. Stated in probability terms, epidemiology seeks to identify those factors that increase the risk of disease. Risk simply means the chance, or the probability, of developing a disease or health condition. By the laws of nature there is a great deal of individual variation. The range of normal for most of our biologic, psychological, and social variables is wide. What is normal for one individual may not be normal for another. Everyone in the population can be thought of as carrying some chance of experiencing a given health condition. Some individuals, because of unusual exposure to a given factor, carry additional risk. It is this additional risk or chance of developing disease that epidemiology attempts to identify.

The most frequently used measure of the association between exposure to a factor and risk of disease or health outcome is the *relative risk*. The relative risk expresses the chance of developing the disease or condition for the group of individuals with the factor compared with (or "relative" to) the chance of developing the disease or condition for the group without the factor. Thus, the relative risk is not a rate but a ratio of two incidence rates, a conditional probability:

$$\frac{\text{Incidence rate of disease among exposed}}{\text{Incidence rate of disease among nonexposed}}$$

It is frequently expressed as $\dfrac{a}{a+b} \bigg/ \dfrac{c}{c+d}$ when the population is expressed as proportions in a fourfold table as in Table 8-3. The incidence rate of disease among the exposed is represented by $a/a + b$, and the incidence rate of disease among the nonexposed is shown as $c/c + d$. For example, the relative risk indicates how much the risk of a certain disease (benign breast disease) is increased or decreased by a factor (use of oral contraceptives) compared with the risk of the nonexposed (nonusers of oral contraceptives). Conversely, it measures the decrease or increase in risk to be anticipated if the factor or behavior such as use of oral contraceptives is changed. A relative risk of 1 indicates there is no association between the factor and the disease; the factor does not increase or decrease the risk of the problem. Any value higher than 1 means there is a positive association or increased risk relative to the reference group having no exposure. Keep in mind that the reference group (expressed as the denominator of the ratio of the two rates) must be stated to allow interpretation of the relative risk. For example, if the relative risk associated with the exposure factor is 4, this means that the probability for disease is four times higher in someone with the exposure factor than in someone without the factor. A value lower than 1, or a negative association, suggests that the factor of interest may have a protective effect.

Table 8-3
Cross-classification of a Population by Risk Factor and Disease as a Basis for Relative Risk

Risk factor classification	Disease	No Disease	Total
Exposed to factor	a	b	$a + b$
Not exposed to factor	c	d	$c + d$

A relative risk of 0.90 indicates that the probability of disease for those with the factor is 10 percent lower than for those without the factor. For example, one study has shown that women using oral contraceptives have a relative risk of 0.80, or a 20 percent reduction, of having fibroadenosis of the breast compared with women who never used oral contraceptives (Royal College of General Practitioners, 1974). Other studies have shown that high-density lipoprotein cholesterol and moderate intake of alcohol have a protective effect or reduce the chances of developing coronary heart disease. Identifying factors that offer a protective effect emphasize improvement of the health state of individuals. These factors are of particular importance to the community health nurse because they suggest direct interventions that may prevent disease in a population.

Relative risk measures the strength of the association or the relative importance of the presumed etiologic factor in producing disease. Since our multicausal disease theory reflects the fact that most diseases have many causes, a one-to-one correspondence between a factor and disease would not be expected. Therefore, it is necessary to be satisfied with a degree of association that is somewhat less than perfect. The higher the relative risk, the stronger the association; the stronger the association, the more likely it is causal. The greater the number of causal factors producing a given disease or condition, the weaker will be the association between any one of them and the disease (the smaller the relative risk). For many of the chronic conditions such as benign breast disease, heart disease, cancer, and low birth weight, relative risks of 2 to 6 indicate strong associations. Consider the example of coronary heart disease. Studies have repeatedly shown the relative risk for coronary heart disease for sedentary as opposed to active people to be about 2.2, for smokers of one pack or more cigarettes per day compared with nonsmokers to be 3.3, and for persons with high total serum cholesterol compared with those who have low cholesterol to be from 2.0 to 4.0.

Because we believe that many factors account for the onset of most disease or health conditions and we know that many of the factors of interest are highly correlated with each other, we may observe an association (a high relative risk) that is biased or noncausal (a third factor causes both risk factor and disease). When a health outcome is affected by many factors, to examine the influence of a single factor one must make adjustments for the effects of the others. The simplest technique for looking at the effect owed to one variable is cross-classification. This technique allows one to examine the incidence rates of the conditions at several levels of the factor while holding the other variables constant. More sophisticated statistical approaches involve the use of multiple regression or multiple logistic analyses. Relative risks derived from these analyses are called *adjusted relative risks,* whereas an unadjusted risk is called a *crude relative risk.* This concept is similar to that of age adjustment used with mortality and natality rates discussed previously.

A given factor may increase the risk for several conditions, being a stronger risk factor for some diseases than others. For example, for oral contraceptive users compared with nonusers the relative risk for acute myocardial infarction has been reported to be 3.2, for nonrheumatic heart disease and hypertension to be 4.7, and for subarachnoid hemorrhage to be greater than 10.0 (Lilienfeld & Lilienfeld, 1980). Smoking is a very common behavior that has been shown to be associated with many diseases. Women who smoke heavily are 5–29 times as likely to develop lung cancer as nonsmokers, 1.3–2.2 times as likely to have myocardial infarctions as nonsmokers, 1.6–2.7 times as likely to develop bladder cancer, 2.0–7.2 times as likely to develop cervical cancer, and 2.0–2.6 times as likely to be delivered of low birth weight babies as nonsmokers (U.S. Department of Health, Education and Welfare [US-DHEW], 1980).

Being able to determine the relative risk of disease conferred by a factor is very important because it tells which factors may be causal, and thus, what needs to be changed to prevent the disease or condition. It should be remembered that the relative risk is a probability statements: it does not measure the chance that someone with the factor will have the disease but merely that the chance for the disease is higher in someone with the factor than someone without the factor. All of those exposed to the factor will not develop the disease; and some who are not exposed to the factor will develop the disease. Although a factor may have a high relative risk for a disease or condition, the impact can be small if the factor is found only rarely in the population or if the disease is rare. Adenocarcinoma of the cervix is a relatively rare disease; however, daughters exposed in utero to diethylstilbestrol have increased risk of cervical cancer, although the number of young women so affected by DES is fairly small (Herbst, Ulfelder, & Poskanzer, 1971).

Methods of Study

The epidemiologist develops theories about disease etiology by first confirming observations that attribute the development of a disease to one or more risk factors and then synthesizing results from many epidemiological and non-epidemiological studies to derive causal inferences. Epidemiologists confirm associations by employing two basic study methods, *observational* and *experimental*. They apply established criteria to assess the extent to which the available evidence supports a causal interpretation. Both the methods of study and criteria for judging causality have relevance for community health nursing.

Generally speaking, one may take either an experimental or observational approach to investigating the relationship between potential risk factors and disease. Each of these strategies is appropriate for investigating certain health problems or aspects of these problems. In experimental studies, the investigator actually intervenes, changing factors suspected of altering the health condition under study and observing what happens in relation to the health outcome. In observational studies there is no deliberate human intervention; nature is allowed to take its course and changes and differences in environmental, psychological, social, or biologic factors are observed and related to changes in the health state. It is often difficult or unethical to perform well-controlled experiments on human populations; therefore, epidemiologists tend to concentrate on observational studies, controlling for extraneous variables by their study designs and methods of data analysis.

Epidemiologic studies may be further classified as *descriptive* or *analytic*, depending upon the aims of the investigations. Descriptive studies describe the occurrence of disease and health phenomena in populations as discussed above. Analytic studies attempt to explain the observed pattern of occurrence of the health phenomena or to identify etiologic factors. An analytic investigation is designed to test a specific hypothesis concerning a cause or causes of the disease in question. Experimental strategies are usually analytic in nature. Observational studies fall into both categories — descriptive and analytic. Observational studies may be further divided into *cross-sectional, prospective,* and *retrospective* designs. This final categorization relates to the time sequence of the occurrence of exposure variables or potential risk factors and the occurrence of disease. In actual practice, the various types of studies (cross-sectional, retrospective, and prospective) are frequently mixed, depending upon the nature of the variables under study and the data available.

Many terms are used in the literature today to indicate the type of study design employed. For our purpose, cross-sectional will refer to any studies called *prevalence* or *correlational* surveys. Prospective studies may be referred to in the literature as cohort, historical prospective, historical cohort, retrospective cohort, synthetic retrospective, incidence, longitudinal, concurrent, or non-concurrent prospective. Retrospective designs are frequently described as case-control or case-history studies, and experimental studies are referred to as clinical trials, controlled intervention trials, and community trials. Table 8-4 provides an overview of the major studies by the time dimension inherent in the design.

Cross-sectional Studies

Cross-sectional studies, although primarily descriptive, examine the relationship between disease and factors thought to be causal as they exist in a defined population at a particular time. The basic question that a cross-sectional study poses is, Do the characteristics or exposure factors coexist with the health problem? Cross-sectional studies provide prevalence data; therefore, they are important for identifying the extent of a problem in a given community so that programs can be planned to prevent or treat the problem.

The cross-sectional study begins by clearly defining a question for study in terms of the relationship between some possible risk factor and the disease of interest. Next a referent population or study group is identified. If this population is small, the entire population can be included in the study. If the target population is large, ideally a representative sample is selected. Once the sample is defined, the necesssary data are collected. Each subject in the sample is contacted, and measurement of the characteristics of interest are made at the same time that cases and noncases of disease are identified. Most often disease is detected by special examination of each person in the sample. The presence of or exposure to the possible risk factors is determined by asking the subject specific questions or by taking appropriate measurements such as blood pressure readings or weight.

The data are tabulated by subdividing the population according to the suspected factor or factors and comparing the disease prevalence rates in each subgroup. If the group of individuals with the suspected factors is found to experience a higher rate of disease than those individuals without the factor, an association between the characteristic and disease is said to exist. However, one should interpret data from prevalence or cross-sectional studies with caution. First, there is the antecedent-consequent problem. Because the information about the characteristics of interest and the health condition is obtained simultaneously, one does not know which occurred first, the presumed cause or the disease (effect). Second, a cross-sectional study deals with survivors. Individuals with the suspected characteristic may have died or migrated out of the study area at a different rate from those without the characteristic. This is known as selective survival and may lead to an unknown overestimate or an unknown underestimate of the association between the factors of interest and disease. Third, the disease process itself may change the biochemical, psychological, or physiological, responses of those found to have the disease. (For example, there is some evidence that cholesterol is lower after an acute myocardial infarction than before; one might expect anxiety in cancer patients to be higher than in unaffected members of the population.) Because of the problems cited above, risk cannot be calculated from cross-sectional data.

Cross-sectional studies are often the only source of information about chronic disease for the community health nurse and other health workers. If the community health nurse is interested in knowing what proportion of the population she serves has needs related to diabetes, high blood pressure, arthritis, cancer, or heart disease and what the characteristics are of individuals experiencing such problems, the data must be obtained by survey because complete registries of chronic diseases are rarely available. The well-designed Health and Nutrition Examination Survey conducted by the National Center for Health Statistics (1981) is an example of this type of study.

From an analytic standpoint, cross-sectional studies also serve a very useful purpose. Associations observed in prevalence studies often suggest etiologic hypotheses that can then be tested using more rigorous study methods.

Table 8-4
Types of Studies by Time Dimension: Summary of Advantages and Disadvantages

Past	Present

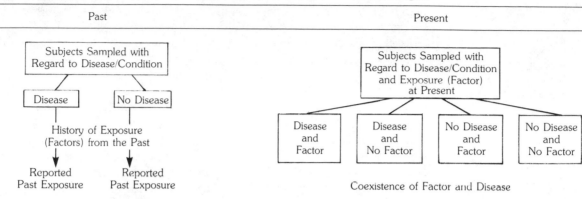

Coexistence of Factor and Disease

Retrospective		Cross-sectional	
Advantages	Disadvantages	Advantages	Disadvantages
Well suited to study of rare conditions or diseases with long latency period.	Relies on recall or records for exposure information — subject to bias.	Quick to mount and conduct.	Risk estimates are not possible with prevalence data.
Requires fewer subjects than prospective design.	Selection of control group difficult.	Relatively inexpensive compared with prospective study.	Temporal sequence of factor and outcome unknown.
Allows estimation of risk of disease with odds ratio.	Rates of disease cannot be calculated.	Gives a quick idea about whether an association between factor and disease may exist.	
Possible to study multiple factors presumed related to a given disease.		Provides prevalence data needed for planning health services.	
Relatively inexpensive and quick to conduct compared with prospective study.			
No risk to subjects.			

Table 8-4 Continued

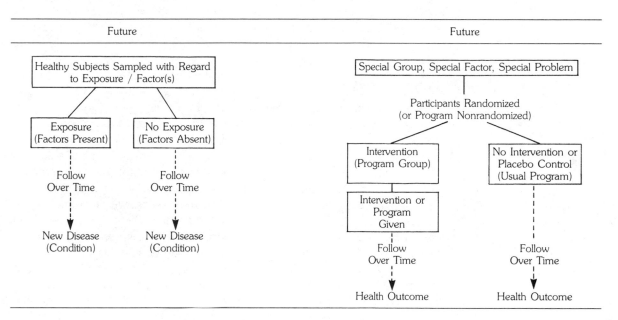

Prospective		"Experimental" or Intervention	
Advantages	Disadvantages	Advantages	Disadvantages
Allows calculation of incidence of disease rates and relative risk.	Long follow-up period.	With randomization, gives confidence that outcome is due to treatment or intervention and not other unknown factors.	Often impractical and unethical to conduct in human populations.
Antecedent factors precede disease/condition.	Large numbers of subjects needed.		Increased risk may occur to some subjects in unanticipated ways.
Reduces bias in the exposure (factors).	Problem of attrition and maintaining follow-up of all subjects.	Provides strong evidence that a factor is causal when an effect is seen.	Requires relatively long time to conduct and factors and/or disease may change.
Possible to study multiple effects (outcomes) of a given exposure.	Exposure to factors may change, making findings less relevant.		
	Relatively expensive.		
	Possible bias in diagnosing disease over time.		

Frequently, a cross-sectional study is a preliminary to a prospective study. When a representative sample is employed with a cross-sectional study, those individuals defined as noncases or healthy become the study population for a prospective study.

Prospective Studies

Prospective studies, rather than measure the relationship of factors as they coexist with a health condition, address the question, Do persons having the exposure factor or characteristic have the disease or condition more frequently than those who are not exposed to the factor? The prospective study focuses on the initial or new development of the disease or health problem. In order to show that a problem develops, it must, of course, be absent initially. Thus the study population must be shown, in some way, to be free of the health problem to be studied. That is, the group studied must be a population at risk for the development of the disease or problem. As previously mentioned, the study population may be identified from a cross-sectional survey. More often in practice, the study population is a special group such as volunteers or all the workers in an occupation who are examined and shown to be free of the problem. Framingham, Massachusetts, has become famous as the site for the classic Framingham heart disease prospective studies (Gordon & Kannel, 1970; Haynes & Feinleib, 1980).

Once the population is defined, information is obtained to determine which persons have or do not have a particular characteristic (or have or have not been exposed to a factor) that is suspected of being related to the development of the health problem being investigated. All individuals are then followed over a period of time to observe who becomes affected by and who dies from that disease or problem. Follow-up to detect new cases needs to be complete and may require several different procedures, including periodic reexaminations, regular correspondence with the participants, surveillance of deaths, and continual monitoring of disease registeries and hospital or doctor visits. The duration of follow-up is often long, perhaps 20 to 30 years, depending on the number of new disease or health events that occur. Follow-up is often complicated because subjects move out of the geographic area or decide they do not wish to continue to participate. However, to obtain the incidence rates of interest, the epidemiologist must account for each person in the original study group throughout the study.

In prospective studies, the data are analyzed at predetermined periodic intervals, say every three or five years. The population is subdivided according to the characteristics or exposure factors measured at the onset of the study. The disease or condition incidence rate is determined for each subgroup. The disease incidence rate for those with the characteristic of interest is compared with the disease incidence rate for those without the characteristic of interest. If these rates are different, an association is said to exist between the characteristic and the disease. The prospective investigation clearly demonstrates that factors associated with a disease or health condition precede the onset of the disease. An association based on data indicating the presumed cause precedes its consequences (health outcome) in time is more likely to be causal (given that other extraneous variables are controlled) than associations based on prevalence data.

Retrospective Studies

The retrospective study begins by selecting individuals with a particular condition or disease (the cases) for comparison with a group of individuals in whom the condition or disease is absent (the controls). From these individuals, a history of current and past exposure to the factor or characteristic of interest is obtained by personal interview, by review of existing records or by both. Although the goal is the same as that of the study of prospective design, the actual question posed by the retrospective approach is, Do persons with the health condition or disease (cases) have the exposure characteristic more frequently than those without the condition (controls)?

Definite criteria for defining a person as having the disease must be established and rigorously applied in selecting subjects. Cases should consist of all persons diagnosed with the condition during a specified time period. Incident or newly diagnosed cases are preferred to prevalent cases during this time period for several reasons. For new cases, the time of disease onset is closer to the time of exposure to the factor than at any later time. Individuals newly diagnosed can recall past events better than individuals diagnosed in the distant past. The characteristics of incident cases are less likely to have been changed by the determinants of survival than those of prevalent cases. Controls are selected in such a manner to be representative of persons without the disease or to be comparable with the cases in as many ways as possible. For instance, the case and control groups will often differ in age, sex, and color, because many diseases differ according to these factors. To avoid biases in comparing groups that might differ in their composition, the epidemiologist must initially select similar controls or the analysis must adjust for these factors. Most often, instead of matching each case to each control on a factor such as age, statistical adjustment is performed in the analysis of the data. Even so, careful consideration must be given to the selection of the control group. Cases and controls may be selected from a variety of sources, but the source should be the same for both. A method commonly used in conducting retrospective studies is to select all cases of the study disease admitted to one or more hospitals during a specified period of time. The control group in this instance usually consists of persons admitted to the same hospital for conditions other than the study disease.

Once the study individuals with and without the disease are identified, information about the characteristics and exposure factors of interest must be obtained by interviewing the subjects or reviewing past records, such as past chemical exposures documented in industry files. Bias may distort the findings from retrospective studies when the interviewer's awareness of who is a control and who is not influences the individual's response. This knowledge may change the interviewer's manner or structuring of the questions, which in turn may influence the response given to questions. Therefore, it is best when interviews can be conducted without the interviewer having prior knowledge of the health or disease status of the subjects. Another bias, known as selective recall bias, may also affect study results. Selective recall bias occurs when the person experiencing the disease or condition is more likely (or less likely) to recall past events and exposures accurately than the person without the condition. For example, a person diagnosed with lung cancer may recall his history of smoking cigarettes differently than a person without lung cancer recalls his own history. Retrospective studies are also subject to other biases that may result from the way people enter a hosptial for treatment, that is, whether they chose the hospital or entered as an emergency, for example.

In retrospective studies the data are analyzed by subdividing the population according to disease or nondisease status and comparing the proportion of

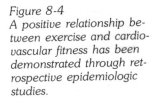

Figure 8-4
A positive relationship between exercise and cardiovascular fitness has been demonstrated through retrospective epidemiologic studies.

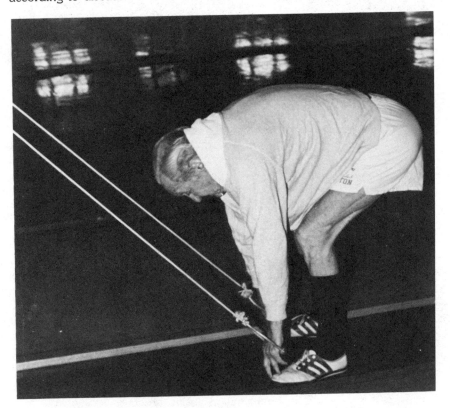

cases possessing the characteristic or factor of interest with the corresponding proportion in the control group. Thus, it is clear that this is neither incidence nor prevalence data. Even so, if a higher frequency of individuals with the characteristic is observed among the cases than the controls, an association is said to exist. We can estimate the strength of this association using the odds ratio, which allows an interpretation similar to that of relative risk.

A major difference between prospective and retrospective study methods is the time sequence between the presence or absence of the factor and the subsequent occurrence of the health event (see Table 8-4). A prospective study selects individuals who are initially free of the disease and follows them over time to determine the (incidence) rates of disease in the presence or absence of exposure. By contrast, the retrospective method selects individuals on the basis of the presence or absence of the disease under study. Both methods allow one to estimate the effect of the presumed causal factors on the risk of disease. The prospective method has the advantage of more clearly indicating that the presumed causal factor precedes the disease or condition in time than the retrospective design. However, the retrospective approach is often the only method appropriate for studying rare diseases and diseases with a long latency period such as the cancers. The study of cervical cancer by Herbst and colleagues is an example of the retrospective design (Herbst et al., 1971).

Experimental Studies

Experimental studies, perhaps more accurately termed *intervention trials*, are similar in many ways to prospective studies. The strength of the intervention study lies in the control the investigator has over the interventions or factors of interest and the random assignment of individuals to the study (experimental) and control groups. When something is done to the study group, the observed outcome is presumed to be the effect of that action, provided the same outcome did not occur in the control individuals who did not receive the action. The differences between the two groups can be ascribed to the investigator's action or the treatment because randomization assures comparability of these groups with respect to all factors except the one being studied. The analysis of the data is usually straighforward using life table methods and statistics appropriate for observational studies.

For obvious ethical reasons, studies employing the experimental method usually deal with disease prevention, health promotion, or treatment of disease. Because there are few such studies, several are discussed here. Of particular interest to public health workers are tests of the efficacy of vaccines and environmental interventions such as fluoridation of drinking water to prevent caries. A classic example is the randomized control trial of the Salk poliomyelitis vaccine by the Poliomyelitis Vaccine Evaluation Center at the University of Michigan (Francis et al., 1955). Health departments in 11 states agreed to participate and called upon their nursing services to carry out the proposed trial. All children in the first through third grades received a series of three injections, but half received the vaccine and half received an inactive placebo. The medication came from numbered vials with codes that only the evaluation center staff could identify as vaccine or placebo. In this study, 200,745 children were vaccinated and 201,229 children received the placebo. All children were closely followed for a year and uniform procedures were instituted to detect and investigate all suspected cases among first- through third-grade children. At the end of the year, the incidence of paralytic poliomyelitis was 28/100,000 in those who were vaccinated compared with 71/100,000 in those who were given the placebo. These differences were very significant statistically and clearly indicated the vaccine's effectiveness. The original reports of the polio vaccine field trials also illustrate the role of the community health nurse in large community intervention trials.

The Kingston-Newburgh caries study was a fluoride study begun about 40 years ago (Arnold, Dean, Jay, & Knutson, 1956). Observational studies had shown that children living in areas with 1 part per million (ppm) or greater fluoride concentration of drinking water had a lower incidence of tooth decay than children living in areas with virtually no fluoride in the drinking water. On the basis of these findings, two cities, Newburgh and Kingston, New York, were selected for study. Since randomized control groups were not practical, Newburgh agreed to serve as the fluoride-treated commmunity and Kingston as the control. The dental health of children in each community was assessed before the trial to allow a before-after comparison. On May 2, 1945, sodium fluoride was added to the Newburgh drinking water to raise the fluoride content from about 0.1 ppm to 1.0–1.2 ppm; Kingston's water supply was left unchanged with its fluoride concentration of about 0.1 ppm. Periodic assessments of both dental and other health measures have been made since 1945 of those individuals in the study. After the experiment had gone on almost ten years, the data showed a reduction in Newburgh of dental caries rates in all age groups compared with the Kingston rates. Six- to nine-year-olds who had used fluoridated water all of their lives in Newburgh had a 57 percent reduction in caries compared with Kingston children of the same age. Furthermore, no adverse effects of fluoridation were found on physical examination. In 1954 the Kingston water supply was fluoridated. A sample of the original study participants examined periodically since 1945 have remained free of conditions whose prevention is attributable to fluoridation. In addition, vital statistics data have shown no differences between the two communities studied and other communities in cancer and cardiovascular death rates, infant and maternal mortality, or stillbirth rates. The benefits of water fluoridation were shown by community intervention trials even when randomized control groups could not be used. Similar trials could be used today to compare the effectiveness of our health programs.

Experiments are believed to be the best test of a cause-and-effect relationship.

Because few of our findings from cross-sectional, retrospective and prospective studies can be tested in a classical experimental mode in human populations, we must search for ethical ways to mimic an experiment. One way to contrive an acceptable experiment is to remove or reduce the presumed causal factor in one group and look for a reduction in the effect, while making no change in the control group. The ten-year Lipid Research Coronary Primary Prevention Trial, which randomized men with high cholesterol levels to a drug or placebo group and showed a reduction in coronary heart disease for the drug-treated group compared with the controls provides one example (Lipid Research Clinics Program, 1984). The Multiple Risk Factor Intervention Trial (MRFIT), a community-based study of 12,866 high-risk men randomly assigned either to a special intervention of treatment of hypertension, counseling for cigarette smoking, and dietary advice for lowering blood cholesterol levels or to their usual sources of health care, was less successful in demonstrating that a reduction in the presumed factors resulted in lower coronary heart disease rates (Multiple Risk Factor Intervention Trial Research Group, 1982). Over the seven-year follow-up period, hypertension, smoking, and blood cholesterol levels declined in both groups but to a greater degree for men on the special intervention program. Nevertheless, the coronary heart disease mortality rates between the two groups was not significantly different statistically. One potential reason for finding no difference between the groups is that both groups improved on the risk factors because of awareness of hazards of cholesterol, smoking, and lack of exercise. The MRFIT demonstrates many of the problems that plague long-term community intervention programs and thus warrants reading.

The recently completed 30-month clinical trial of change in maternal smoking and its effect on birth weight is of special interest to community health nursing. Women who were smoking just before pregnancy at least ten cigarettes per day were randomized to a control group ($N = 472$) and to a treatment group ($N = 463$). Questionnaires were used to obtain a history of smoking and results from a thiocyanate saliva test (biochemical marker of smoking) were obtained at the time of randomization and again during the eighth month of pregnancy. The intervention was encouragement and assistance to stop smoking through information, support, practical guidance, and behavioral strategies. Forty-three percent of the treatment group and 20 percent of the control group reported quitting smoking by the eighth month of pregnancy. The infants born to mothers in the treatment group had a mean birth weight 92 gm heavier than infants born to mothers in the control group (a significant difference). This finding is consistent with birth weight results in both retrospective and prospective studies. Other findings from this clinical trial suggest that few women who quit in the first trimester will resume smoking during the remainder of the pregnancy, and very few women who have not quit in the first trimester will quit without special help in the second or third trimester (Sexton & Hebel, 1984).

Criteria for Judging Causality Using Epidemiologic Evidence

The major aims of epidemiology are to describe accurately the health states of populations and to search for the causes of disease or health conditions in human populations. As we have suggested in the previous sections, the assessment of causality in human health is difficult at best; no single study is adequate to establish causality. Causal inference depends on synthesizing results from many studies. Most often the accumulation of evidence begins with a clinical observation or hunch that a certain factor may be causally related to a health problem. Cross-sectional studies then show that the factor and problem coexist; retrospective studies allow a fairly quick assessment of whether or not an association exists. Nonepidemiologic animal studies may suggest a biologic mechanism whereby the factor could cause the disease or condition. At this point, prospective studies are crucial to assure that the presumed causal factor actually precedes the onset of the health problem. And finally, if ethically possible, the experimental approach is used to confirm the associations derived from the observational studies. Thus, it often requires many years to accumulate enough evidence to provide adequate information for developing a health intervention strategy or for changing a current practice.

Epidemiologically, we accept that a causal relationship may exist when two major conditions are met: (1) the factor of interest is shown to increase the probability of occurrence of the disease or condition as observed in many studies in different populations; and (2) there is evidence that a reduction in the factor decreases the frequency of the given disease. The synthesis of data begins by selecting as many as possible of all the various types of epidemiologic studies on the problem. After discarding those studies that are not methodologically sound, the studies are reviewed. The better the data meet the following six criteria, the more likely the factor of interest will be one of several causes of the disease:

1. Temporal relationship: If the factor causes the health condition, logically the factor should occur first.
2. Strength of the association: The higher the relative risk or odds ratio, the stronger the association and the more likely the association is causal.
3. Dose response between levels of the factor and the health outcome: An increase in the frequency of the condition occurs with an increase in the level of exposure to the factor.
4. Consistency: Similar associations and dose responses are observed in varying types of studies in different populations and countries.
5. Biologic plausibility and coherence of the evidence: The hypothesized cause makes sense based on current biologic knowledge.
6. Lowering of disease risk: Interventions that decrease the exposure or factor result in a lowering of disease risk (relative risk).

Consider the following epidemiologic facts summarizing the evidence regarding the causal role of maternal smoking in the outcome of pregnancy (USDHEW, 1980):

1. Many investigators have demonstrated that the fetal and neonatal mortality rate is significantly higher for infants of smokers than for infants of nonsmokers. Cigarette smoking is a common habit among women of childbearing age in the United States. In 1978, approximately one-third of American women of childbearing age were cigarette smokers. The percentage of U.S. women who smoke throughout pregnancy is not definitely known but is presumably lower, probably in the neighborhood of 20–25 percent.

2. The results from many large studies in which the relationship between smoking and birth weight was examined have demonstrated a strong association between maternal cigarette smoking and delivery of infants of low birth weight. On the average, the smoker has nearly twice the risk of delivering an infant of low birth weight as that of a nonsmoker. Babies born to women who smoke during pregnancy are, on the average, 200 gm lighter than babies born to women who do not smoke.

3. Available evidence shows that cigarette smokers' infants tend to be smaller for gestational age rather than gestationally premature; that is, infants of smokers are consistently lighter in weight during each week of gestation than those of nonsmokers.

4. Infants of smokers have lower birth weights than infants of nonsmokers, and within groups of comparable gestational age, smokers' infants experience higher mortality rates than nonsmokers' infants.

5. When a variety of known or suspected factors (age, parity, previous pregnancy history, prenatal visits, etc.) that also exert an influence upon birth weight have been controlled, cigarette smoking has always been shown to be related to low birth weight.

6. A strong dose-response relationship has been established between cigarette smoking and the incidence of low birth weight; the more cigarettes the pregnant woman smokes, the greater the reduction in birth weight.

7. The association has been demonstrated in many different countries, among different races and cultures, and in different geographical settings.

8. The infants of smokers experience an accelerated growth rate during the first six months after delivery, compared with infants of nonsmokers. This finding is compatible with viewing birth as the removal of the smoker's infant from a toxic influence.

9. Data from experiments in animals have documented that exposure to tobacco smoke results in the delivery of offspring with a low birth weight.

10. Evidence from randomized trials shows that a reduction in smoking during pregnancy improves the birth weight of the infant (Sexton & Hebel, 1984).

Recently there has been a formal attempt to synthesize the epidemiologic evidence about specific problems so that it can be readily used by researchers, practitioners, and policymakers. Several reviews that may be of interest to the community health nurse are those relating to postneonatal mortality (Pharoah & Norris, 1979), birth defects (Janerich & Polednak, 1983), rubella vaccination (Preblud et al., 1980), induced abortion (Hogue, Cates & Tietze, 1982), whooping cough (Miller, Alderslade, & Ross, 1982), breast cancer (Kelsey, 1979), and oral contraceptives and vascular disease (Sartwell & Stolley, 1982). The evidence regarding causal factors has been summarized for relatively few of our major health problems. Therefore, the practitioner must review the literature and make judgments about the relevance of specific information for the practice situation. Even when the evidence has been summarized and evaluated, new knowledge may change the significance of a given finding for practice; therefore, it is important for community health nurses to recognize the complexity of judging evidence for causality, continually update their knowledge base, and make changes in their practice accordingly.

Epidemiologic Applications in Community Health Nursing Practice

The community health nurse uses epidemiologic information and epidemiologic approaches in many aspects of practice related to primary prevention and health promotion and in secondary prevention with groups, families, and individuals. Table 8-5 summarizes the broad areas of epidemiology as they relate to levels of prevention and intervention strategies. Epidemiology is especially useful at the primary prevention level in performing the following:

1. Describing and diagnosing the state of health and changing health problems in the community in order to set program priorities. As previously described, the nurse uses mortality data and morbidity information from many sources to identify problems in the practice area. For example, if the infant mortality rate in the area is twice that of the national rate, clearly services should focus on maternal and child health concerns. By comparing the rates over time, the community health nurse can determine whether the problem is getting worse or being solved. Similarly, in a given community there may be high rates of diabetes in an area compared to the rate nationwide but low rates of hypertension. The community health nurse looks at the number of events occurring to decide which of the problems is large enough to warrant a special program.
2. Identifying high-risk groups needing attention. Once the problems have been identified as described above, the nurse asks *where* the problems are occurring and to what kinds of people. Nurses may find that most of the infant deaths or low birth weights occur in a small geographical

Table 8-5
Epidemiologic Contributions to Community Health Nursing Practice by Levels of Prevention

	Intervention Level			
	Primary Prevention			Secondary Prevention	Tertiary Prevention

Healthy State ⇢ → ⇢ → ⇢ → ⇢ → ⇢ → ⇢ → ⇢ → Risk Factors Present

Specific Protection	Health Promotion	Reduction of Known Risk Factors	Early Detection and Treatment	Reducing Severity of Condition
Typical Intervention Strategies				
Improvement in sanitation Fluoridation and chlorination of water Protection against hazards in environment such as removal of toxic waste dumps Regulations against air pollution Immunization of children and adults	Moderate, regular exercise Eating balanced diet Life-style conducive to health Health education	Changes in life-style related to identified risk factors such as cessation of smoking, increase in aerobic exercises, reduction in cholesterol intake, stress reduction	Screening programs for diseases and conditions such as high blood pressure, dental caries, cervical cancer, arthritis, etc. Teaching of breast self-examination Health programs targeted to special problems	Medication and treatment compliance Rehabilitation activities
Epidemiologic Contributions				
Assessing population immunization levels Studying health effects of specific protective measures such as water chlorination and fluoridation	Describing and diagnosing the state of health of the population Identifying and solving health problems in the community	Providing information about what factors need to be changed — risk factors and their potential impact on the population — for use in program planning Identifying high-risk groups needing attention	Investigating specific outbreaks of infectious disease Monitoring and surveillance (through regular screening programs) of the total population for new and existing chronic diseases Describing how well services are working by examining change in health problems in total population Evaluating the effectiveness of health programs in terms of improvement of health status Investigating new health problems in the community	Assessing the community's burden of disease and disability Studying factors related to recovery

area where primarily poor families with low education live. This information allows nurses to target maternal and child health services to a special group.

3. Determining what risk factors need to be changed to reduce a problem such as prematurity. The literature on the epidemiology of prematurity helps the nurse decide how to incorporate in her teaching plan strategies to reduce smoking and alcohol consumption and to improve nutrition.

Because many of the community health nurse's activities relate to primary prevention intervention strategies, the nurse needs to know the epidemiologic facts about health problems as a basis for practice. When a threat to the health of a group is identified, epidemiologic methods can be used to investigate and interpret each clue. For example, if children are injured and die from bicycle accidents, the answers to why these occur and how they can be prevented can be found by using the lessons learned from the epidemiologic investigation process. First, the nurse describes the scope of the problem — how many children are involved, their ages, what time of the day or night the accidents occur, what police records are kept about the type of accident, and in what areas of town the accidents occur. Then the nurse decides who needs to be questioned, collects the data and analyzes the findings using basic rates for comparisons. Finally, the nurse develops conclusions and applications. In other situations, the community health nurse may identify a problem such as sudden infant death syndrome (SIDS), an identification that requires a formal epidemiologic investigation by a team of workers over several years. Here it becomes important for nurses to understand the basic epidemiologic methods so that they can help in the collection of reliable and valid data that will answer the questions posed about SIDS.

In the area of secondary prevention, epidemiologic approaches are valuable in monitoring health problems in the community, in evaluating the effectiveness of health services, and in investigating outbreaks of infectious disease. In screening activities, the nurse selects and uses reliable and valid instruments, sees that all workers are consistent in collecting data, and uses rates and proportions to describe the screening results. Data derived from screening programs and the clinical follow-up are then used in replanning services for the area. Figure 8-5 is an example of data from a nurse-directed study in secondary prevention.

Evaluating to what extent a health program is improving the health of the population served offers fertile ground for applying epidemiologic methods. Suppose community health nurses in a maternal and child health service wish to know if their services make any difference. Based on the services available, they hypothesize that the more comprehensive the prenatal care, the higher will be the mean birth weights of the babies. Next, they decide on the special services that might make a difference in birth weight. They randomize some of the pregnant women into a group to receive special

216

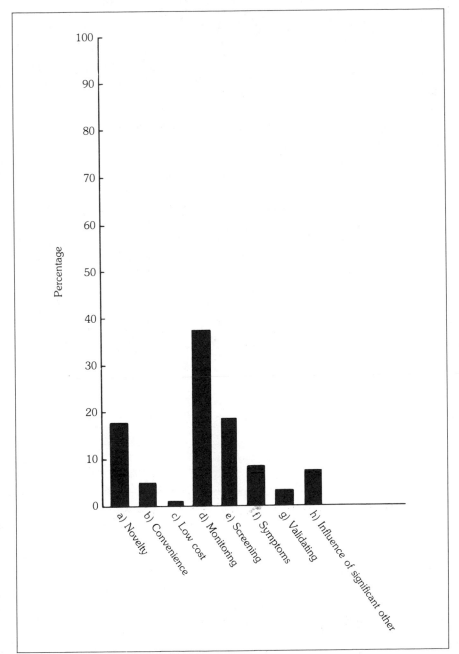

Figure 8-5
Reasons Subjects Use
Coin-operated Computer-
ized Sphygmomanometers
(N = 209). Study results
suggest that when these
machines are used in con-
junction with nurse or phy-
sician guidance, individuals
may actively participate
in control of their
hypertension.

services (individual counseling, home visits, intense service, and other special services in addition to usual services) and some of the women into a group to receive the usual clinic visits, food supplements, and group counseling.

After providing the different services, the babies born to the mothers are compared on birth weight. If the babies whose mothers received special care show a mean birth weight of, say, 2900 gm compared with a mean birth weight of 2816 gm for babies whose mothers received usual care, there is evidence that the program resulted in the higher birth weight, other things being equal.

At times the community health nurse is called upon to investigate an outbreak of infectious disease such as pediculosis in a day care center. This calls for an epidemiologic investigation of a problem with a known cause. The process begins by verifying the diagnosis and determining if there are more cases than usual occurring by calculating an attack rate or incidence rate among the children with the condition. In further steps, the community health nurse describes when the problem began, which children are involved, and to what extent it has spread. After hypothesizing about the source and manner of spread, the nurse conducts further studies by taking histories and examining family members; develops conclusions regarding source, spread, and duration of the problem; and begins control measures and teaching to cure existing cases and stop the spread of pediculosis.

Health problems of unknown cause such as pulmonary symptoms among large numbers of people may also be investigated by the nurse using epidemiologic approaches. However, a team approach is often necessary to obtain and analyze all the information required to find a solution to a problem of unknown etiology. Although factors related to recovery are appropriate for studying epidemiologically, they are most frequently investigated in acute care settings.

Summary

Epidemiology is the study of the distribution and determinants of health, health conditions and disease in human population groups. Today, epidemiology is grounded in multicausal theories of health and disease and thus focuses on identifying the many factors — genetic, environmental, personal, social-cultural — which influence health states. It shares with community health nursing the common theme of the health of groups. The use of epidemiology by nurses can be traced back to Florence Nightingale who instituted changes in Crimea based on her observations of the patterns and spread of disease in the military population. Today community health nursing incorporates epidemiology at three levels: (1) in the use of existing epidemiologic information to decide what risk factors in individuals, families or groups need to be changed; (2) in informal investigations such as those identifying high risk groups, describing changing health problems in the community, investigating outbreaks of infectious disease and in evaluating health services; (3) in carefully designed scientific studies.

Epidemiology employs two basic methods, observational and experimental; it then uses established criteria to assess the extent to which available evidence supports a causal interpretation. In experimental studies the investigator actually intervenes, changing factors suspected of altering the health condition under study and observing what happens to the health status. For obvious ethical reasons, there are few experimental studies in human populations and these usually deal with health promotion and new treatments of disease. Observational studies are used to describe health-related conditions as they naturally occur. Observational studies can be cross-sectional (prevalence), prospective (cohort) or retrospective (case-control). Prevalence data from cross-sectional studies measure the rate of all existing disease in the population and are used to describe the health of groups of people and to plan services. Prospective studies generate incidence data. Incidence rates which measure the proportion of new cases of the disease/condition in the population are the basic rates from which relative risk is derived. Relative risk expresses the chance of developing the disease for a group of individuals with a presumed causal factor compared to the chance of developing the disease for the group without the presumed causal factor. Factors which show high relative risks are known as risk factors. Although the retrospective study generates neither incidence nor prevalence data, it allows one to estimate the effect of the presumed causal factor on the risk of disease (the relative risk). Retrospective, prospective and experimental studies seek to explain causes or determinants of health conditions while cross-sectional studies primarily describe existing conditions.

Thinking epidemiologically can enhance community health nursing practice at each of the levels of prevention — primary, secondary and tertiary. Epidemiology provides both the body of knowledge — information on the distribution and determinants of health conditions — and methods for investigating health problems and evaluating services.

Study Questions

1. Define epidemiology. How does it compare or contrast with other types of research?
2. Explain the concept of the multicausal theory of health or disease. How can this concept influence your practice as a community health nurse?
3. What is "risk"? What is "relative risk"? Why are these concepts important for us to know in community health practice?
4. Explain the difference between a prospective and a retrospective study. When is it appropriate to use a prospective study? A retrospective study?

5. Describe one community health situation in which you might use epidemiologic investigation for primary-level prevention.

References

Arnold, F. A., Jr., Dean, H. T., Jay, P., & Knutson, J. W. (1956). Effect of fluoridated public water supplies on dental caries prevalence. *Public Health Reports, 71,* 652–657.

Cohen, I. (1984). Florence Nightingale. *Scientific American, 250*(3), 128, 133.

Francis, T., Jr., et al. (1955). An evaluation of the 1954 poliomyelitis vaccine trials: Summary report. *American Journal of Public Health, 45*(5), 1–63.

Glover, J. W. (1976). *United States Life Tables, 1890, 1901, 1910, and 1901–1910.* New York: Arno Press.

Gordon, T., & Kannel, W. B. (1970). The Framingham, Massachusetts, study, twenty years later. In I. I. Kessler and M. L. Levin (Eds.), *The community as an epidemiologic laboratory: A casebook of community studies* (pp. 119–148). Baltimore, MD: Johns Hopkins Press.

Haynes, S. G., & Feinleib, M. (1980). Women, work and coronary heart disease: Prospective findings from the Framingham heart study. *American Journal of Public Health, 70,* 133–141.

Henderson, D. A. (1980). Smallpox eradication. *Public Health Reports, 95,* 422–426.

Herbst, A. L., Ulfelder, H., & Poskanzer, D. C. (1971). Adenocarcinoma of the vagina: Association of maternal stilbestrol therapy with tumor appearance in young women. *New England Journal of Medicine, 284,* 878–881.

Hogue, C. J. R., Cates, W., Jr., & Tietze, C. (1982). The effects of induced abortion on subsequent reproduction. *Epidemiologic Reviews, 4,* 66–94.

Janerich, D. T., & Polednak, A. P. (1983). Epidemiology of birth defects. *Epidemiologic Reviews, 5,* 16–34.

Kelsey, J. L. (1979). A review of the epidemiology of human breast cancer. *Epidemiologic Reviews, 1,* 74–109.

Leavell, H. R., Clark, E. G. (1965). *Preventive medicine for the doctor in his community.* New York: McGraw-Hill.

Lilienfeld, A. M., & Lilienfeld, D. E. (1980). *Foundations of epidemiology* (2nd ed.). New York: Oxford University Press.

Linder, F. E., & Grove, R. D. (1943). *Vital statistics rates in the United States, 1900–1940.* Washington, DC: U.S. Government Printing Office.

Lipid Research Clinics Program. (1984). The Lipid Research Clinics coronary prevention trial results. I. Reduction in incidence of coronary heart disease. *JAMA, 251,* 351–364.

Miller, D. L., Alderslade, R., & Ross, E. M. (1982). Whooping cough vaccine: The risks and benefits debate. *Epidemiologic Reviews, 4,* 1–24.

Multiple Risk Factor Intervention Trial Research Group. (1982). Multiple risk factor intervention trial: Risk factor changes and mortality results. *JAMA, 248,* 1465–1477.

National Center for Health Statistics. (1981). *Plan and operation of the Second National Health and Nutrition Examination Survey, 1976–1980: Vital and Health*

Statistics (Pub. No. [PHS] 81-1317). Washington, DC: U.S. Government Printing Office.

National Center for Health Statistics. (1982a). *Monthly Vital Statistics Report: Vol. 31, No. 8* (Pub. No. [PHS] 83-1120). Hyattsville, MD: Public Health Service.

National Center for Health Statistics. (1982b). *Vital Statistics of the United States, 1978: Vol. I (Natality)* (Pub. No. [PHS] 83-1100); *Vol. II (Mortality), Part A* (Pub. No. [PHS] 83-1101). Washington, DC: U.S. Government Printing Office.

National Center for Health Statistics. (1983). *Monthly Vital Statistics Report: Vol. 32, No. 4* (Pub. No. [PHS] 83-1120). Hyattsville, MD: Public Health Service.

Pharoah, P. O. D., & Norris, J. N. (1979). Postneonatal mortality. *Epidemiologic Reviews, 1,* 170–183.

Preblud, S. R., Serdula, M. K., Frank, J. A. Jr., Brandling-Bennett, A. D., & Hinman, A. R. (1980). Rubella vaccination in the United States: A ten-year review. *Epidemiologic Reviews, 2,* 153–194.

Royal College of General Practitioners. (1974). *Oral contraceptives and health: An interim report from the oral contraceptive study of the Royal College of General Practitioners.* London: Whitefriars Press.

Sartwell, P. E., & Stolley, P. D. (1982). Oral contraceptives and vascular disease. *Epidemiologic Reviews, 4,* 95–109.

Sexton, M., & Hebel, J. R. (1984). A clinical trial of change in maternal smoking and its effect on birth weight. *JAMA, 251,* 911–915.

U.S. Department of Health, Education and Welfare. (1980). *The health consequences of smoking for women: A report of the surgeon general.* Washington, DC: Department of Health, Education and Welfare, Public Health Service, Office of the Assistant Secretary for Health, Office on Smoking and Health.

Selected Readings

Barancik, J. I., Chatterjee, B. F., Greene, Y. C., Michenzi, E. M., Fife, D. (1983). Northeastern Ohio trauma study: I. Magnitude of the problem. *American Journal of Public Health, 73,* 746–751.

Barkauskas, V. H. (1983). Effectiveness of public health nurse home visits to primiparous mothers and their infants. *American Journal of Public Health, 73,* 573–580.

Benenson, A. S. (1980). *Control of communicable disease in man* (13th ed.). Washington, DC: American Public Health Association.

Block, D. (1975). Evaluation of nursing care in terms of process and outcome: Issues in research and quality assurance. *Nursing Research, 24,* 256–263.

Block, G. (1982). A review of validations of dietary assessment methods. *American Journal of Epidemiology, 115,* 492–505.

Branch, L. G., & Jette, A. M. (1981). The Framingham disability study: Social disability among the aging. *American Journal of Public Health, 71,* 1202–1210.

Broadhead, W. E., Kaplan, B. H., James, S. A., et al. (1983). The epidemiologic evidence for a relationship between social support and health. *American Journal of Epidemiology, 117,* 521–537.

Butler, W. J., Ostrander, L. D., Carman, W. J., & Lamphiear, D. E. (1982). Diabetes mellitus in Tecumseh, Michigan: Prevalence, incidence, and associated conditions. *American Journal of Epidemiology, 116,* 971–980.

Cassel, J. C. (1973). Information for epidemiologic and health services research. *Medical Care, 11*(2) (Suppl.), 76–80.

Christenson, K., & Lingle, J. A. (1972). Evaluation of effectiveness of team and nonteam public health nurses in health outcomes of patients with strokes or fractures. *American Journal of Public Health, 62,* 483–490.

Derschewitz, R. A., & Williamson, J. W. (1977). Prevention of childhood household injuries: A controlled clinical trial. *American Journal of Public Health, 67,* 1148–1153.

Dever, G. E. A. (1984). *Epidemiology in health services management.* Rockville, MD: Aspen Systems.

Earp, J. A. L., Ory, M. G., & Strogatz, D. S. (1982). The effects of family involvement and practitioner home visits on the control of hypertension. *American Journal of Public Health, 72,* 1146–1154.

Frerichs, R. R., Aneshensel, C. S., & Clark, V. A. (1981). Prevalence of depression in Los Angeles County. *American Journal of Epidemiology, 113,* 691–699.

Harter, L., Frost, F., Grunenfelder, G., Perkins-Jones, K., & Libby, J. (1984). Giardiasis in an infant and toddler swim class. *American Journal of Public Health, 74,* 155–156.

Haynes, S. G., Feinleib, M., Levine, S., Scotch, N., & Kannel, W. B. (1978). The relationship of psychosocial factors to coronary heart disease in the Framingham study: II. Prevalence of coronary heart disease. *American Journal of Epidemiology, 107,* 384–402.

Johansson, S., Vedin, A., & Wilhelmsson, C. (1983). Myocardial infarction in women. *Epidemiologic Reviews, 5,* 67–95.

Kennedy, E. T., Gershoff, S., Reed, R., & Austion, J. E. (1982). Evaluation of the effect of WIC supplemental feeding on birth weight. *Journal of American Dietetic Association, 80,* 220–227.

Langford, H. G. (Ed.). (1982). Hypertension and obesity: Epidemiologic, physiologic and therapeutic considerations: Proceedings of a symposium. *Journal of Chronic Diseases, 35,* 873–919.

Levinson, S. S., Bearfield, J. L., Ausbrook, D. K. et al. (1982). The Chicago Rheumatic Fever Program: A 20 plus–year history. *Journal of Chronic Diseases, 35,* 199–206.

Lilienfeld, A. M. (Ed.). (1980). *Times, places, and persons: Aspects of the history of epidemiology.* Baltimore, MD: Johns Hopkins University Press.

Lilienfeld, A. M., & Lilienfeld, D. E. (1980). *Foundations of epidemiology* (2nd ed.). New York: Oxford University Press.

Linn, S., Schoenbaum, S. C., Monson, R. R., Rosner, R., Stubblefield, P. C., & Ryan, K. J. (1983). The association of marijuana use with outcome of pregnancy. *American Journal of Public Health, 73,* 1161–1164.

Long, G., Whitman, C., Johansson, M., Williams, C., & Tuthill, R. (1975). Evaluation of a school health program directed to children with history of high absence. *American Journal of Public Health, 64,* 388–393.

MacMahon, B., & Pugh, T. F. (1970). Epidemiology: Principles and methods. Boston: Little, Brown.

Mauser, J. S., & Bahn, A. K. (1974). *Epidemiology: An introductory text.* Philadelphia: W. B. Saunders.

McNeil, H. J., & Holland, S. S. (1972). A comparative study of public health nurse teaching in groups and in home visits. *American Journal of Public Health, 62,* 1629–1637.

Morton, R. F., & Hebel, J. R. (1979). *A study guide to epidemiology and biostatistics.* Baltimore, MD: University Park Press.

Payne, S. M. C., & Strobino, D. M. (1984). Two methods of estimating the target population for public maternity service programs. *American Journal of Public Health, 74,* 164–166.

Quick, J. D., Greenlick, M. R., & Rothmann, K. J. (1981). Prenatal care and pregnancy outcome in an HMO and general population: A multivariate cohort analysis. *American Journal of Public Health, 71,* 381–390.

Schoenbach, V. J., Kaplan, B. H., Wagner, E. H., Grimson, R. C., & Miller, F. T. (1983). Prevalence of self-reported depressive symptoms in young adolescents. *American Journal of Public Health, 73,* 1281–1287.

Selwyn, B. J. (1978). An epidemiological approach to the study of users and nonusers of child health services. *American Journal of Public Health, 68,* 231–235.

Shapiro, S., McCormick, M., Starfield, B., Krischer, J. P., & Bross, D. (1980). Relevance of correlates of infant mortality for significant morbidity at one year of age. *American Journal of Obstetrics and Gynecology, 136,* 363–373.

Thompson, S. E., & Washington, A. E. (1983). Epidemiology of sexually transmitted *Chlamydia trachomatis* infections. *Epidemiologic Reviews, 5,* 96–118.

Willett, W. C., Hennekens, C. H., Bain, C., Rosner, B., & Speizer, F. E. (1981). Cigarette smoking and non-fatal myocardial infarction in women. *American Journal of Epidemiology, 113,* 575–582.

Winkelstein, W., Jr., Shillitoe, E. J., Brand, R., & Johnson, K. K. (1984). Further comments on cancer of the uterine cervix, smoking, and herpes virus infection. *American Journal of Epidemiology, 119,* 1–8.

9

Working with Populations and Groups

Community health nursing offers us a considerable challenge: to promote the health of aggregates while continuing to serve smaller units, like families, groups, and individuals, within the community. Outside public health, no other health care discipline has aggregates as its primary concern or the entire community's health as its trust. For the community health nurse, then, the challenge lies in responding to that mandate, in adopting an aggregate orientation for practice. It is the primary emphasis on the community health nursing scope of practice continuum discussed in chapter 3.

That orientation raises an important question. How do we work with aggregates? The purpose of this chapter is to explore how the community health nurse works with populations and groups of all sizes. Because they are most familiar, we shall begin by examining how to work with small groups. Then we shall discuss applying knowledge of groups to serving subpopulations and larger aggregates in the community.

Working with Small Groups

Small groups are an important part of community health nursing service. Nurses meet the collective needs of many elements of the community population through work with groups. Each collection of people — a parenting

224

group, a mastectomy club, a group of Southeast Asian refugees learning a new culture, a school health committee, or a group of discharged mental patients — has different needs. Some groups function for the purpose of problem solving; others for sharing, support, learning, or therapy. Whatever the reason and whether the nurse serves as leader or member, basic knowledge about groups enables the nurse to facilitate group process and outcomes.

All of us have had experience with groups. Our first group encounter is with the family, which is known as a primary group because it is one of several basic, informal social groups to which we belong during our lifetimes (Tubbs & Moss, 1974). As we grow, our primary groups extend to include our childhood peer group, associations with our neighbors, friendship groups, and other social affiliations. Informal and generally social in nature, primary groups function with spontaneous and unstructured communication.

In addition to primary groups, we also experience secondary, or formal, group relationships (Sampson & Marthas, 1977). These groups usually exist for a specific purpose and include professional associations, therapeutic groups, work-related relationships, educational gatherings, and community affiliations. Examples are a student council, an exercise group, a patients' rights committee, and an assertiveness training class. These groups emphasize completing a job and accomplishing specific goals.

Although we spend much of our adult lives participating in formal and informal groups, how well do we understand such groups and how they function? With an increasing number of the community health nurse's activities taking place in and for groups — client groups, community groups, work groups, and others — the nurse's need for group skills becomes ever more important. Let us examine groups and ways in which nurses can work more effectively with them.

The framework for our discussion involves the major processes in which a community health nurse will be involved while working with small groups:

1. *Preparing for small group work* occurs before the group begins, but may continue after the group forms. Preparation involves knowing the nature of groups, types of groups, and their functions and needs.
2. *Starting a group* involves specific activities to help the group begin work.
3. *Building group cohesiveness* is essential during the early growth of a group.
4. *Working with a group* involves recognizing its developmental phases, assuming appropriate leader and member roles, and solving various sorts of problems that arise.
5. *Terminating a group* begins early in the group's life and requires specific interventions.
6. *Evaluating a group* occurs in two dimensions: we examine group process as well as the outcomes of the group's work.

Preparing for Small Group Work

A group is two or more persons engaged in repeated, face-to-face communication, who identify with each other and are interdependent. This definition suggests several characteristics found in groups. A small group is always a collection of people but never so large that members cannot maintain direct communication with one another (Homans, 1950). Because their collective social interaction influences the way they think, members assume similar values and norms and establish a sense of belonging to each other. Konopka (1954) refers to this characteristic as the development of "bonds," the links that connect individuals and create a group from a mass of loosely related people. Furthermore, the members of a group are interdependent; that is, they need and help each other. As Konopka points out (1954, p. 22), human beings need to belong to groups: "group life . . . gives the individual security and nourishment so that he can fulfill his greatest promise while helping others to fulfill theirs too." At the same time, the group molds its members' behavior and attitudes, thus developing its own personality, or "syntality" (Uris, 1964, p. 58).

Let us look at some examples of how these group characteristics influence the health of clients. Steve discovered when he was 15 years of age that he had epilepsy. The fact was difficult to accept, particularly because he had just been elected captain of his swim team. He was told that epilepsy meant an end to his future in swimming. After a seizure at work, his boss fired him. A period of several months of bitterness and frustration followed, and then he was invited to attend an epilepsy club recently formed in his high school. This group knew what it was like to be epileptic. Many of them had undergone experiences similar to Steve's and could truly empathize with him. The sense of belonging that developed for Steve soon erased his feelings of loneliness and gave him a new sense of hope. The attitudes and behavior of the group gradually shaped his own feelings to the point that he could accept his diagnosis and start developing constructive plans for his life.

A group of elderly persons started a bridge club in their retirement building. Although conversation covered many topics, several members initially were reluctant to discuss the future. "I have no future," one said. "I'm just biding my time until I die." Group comraderie and influence gradually changed this attitude to fit the group norm of having a good time together and looking forward to living a long time.

Not all groups influence people positively. Take the case of Tommy, 13 years of age, who has gone from petty theft to armed robbery as a result of gang pressure. Or consider Nancy, once a promising student, now a hard drug user. Her friends made fun of anyone who did well in school and, instead, promoted drug taking as a condition for group membership.

Groups are powerful. Although groups meet basic individual needs for

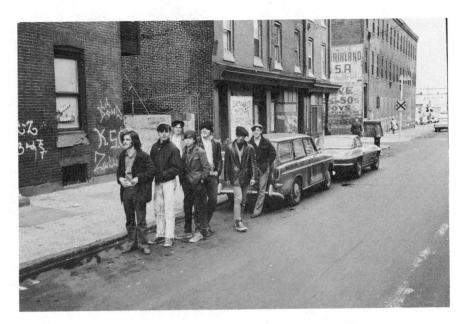

Figure 9-1
Adolescents feel strong pressure to conform to their group's standards. Acting tough and laughing at each other's jokes are some of the ways this group influences its members' behavior.

belonging, security, safety, and the opportunity to help others, they also shape their members' thinking and behavior through internal processes of acceptance and rejection (Fig. 9-1). We have seen that they can be either a constructive or destructive force in people's lives. Our concern in community health is to facilitate their constructive use for client health.

TYPES OF GROUPS

Community health nurses work with many different kinds of small groups. Since each group forms for some purpose, we shall categorize them according to their primary goal. There are five types of small groups with which community health nurses work: learning groups, support groups, socialization groups, psychotherapy groups, and task-oriented groups.

Learning Groups
The primary goal of a learning group is to have its members gain understanding in order to effect behavior change in some specified area of need. Many community health nurses lead prenatal groups. The parents-to-be have many practices to learn, such as exercises, diet, breathing techniques, and what to do during labor and delivery. For each topic, nurses leading these groups make certain that the needed information is covered and, when appropriate, demonstrate its application. The parents-to-be practice their new skills regularly at home, and the nurse-leader may ask them to display their understanding by demonstrating what they have learned to the group. This learning group

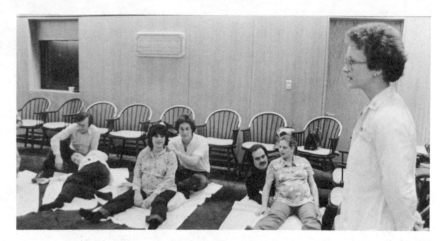

Figure 9-2
This childbirth education class enables couples to practice techniques that will facilitate the birth experience.

will have met its goals when the members have assimilated knowledge to the point that it changes their behavior (Fig. 9-2).

A class can be a learning group, but the two are not usually the same. No doubt you have sat in many classes where, other than a brief conversation or two with a neighbor, you have had little interaction with the other class members. That class is not a true group. The members of a group have repeated, face-to-face communication. They identify with each other and are interdependent. These characteristics typify a learning group, whose function is to utilize the benefits of group identity and interaction to accomplish learning and behavior change. Classes and learning groups share a common advantage of transmitting information more efficiently to a number of people than a one-to-one basis allows. However, learning groups, in contrast to most classes, use group commitment and reinforcement to produce desired behavior changes. They may actually practice natural childbirth, control hypertension, or maintain a postcoronary diet and exercise program. Individuals in these groups not only learn what to do and how to do it (the limit of most classes), but also have the advantage of group influence to promote and stabilize their practices at a healthier level.

The composition of a learning group varies with each situation and depends upon the group's goals. When a group goal is to teach assertiveness to females, for example, the membership would most likely be limited to women. A group goal aimed at preparing people for retirement would probably include members at midlife or approaching retirement. The composition of many learning groups, such as those concerned with weight loss, leadership training, or learning how to manage diabetes, is determined by its members' shared interest in the topic. The chief common denominator of most learning groups, however, is that the members are people who desire to gain information about some subject and better themselves as a result.

228

The nurse may start some learning groups; others, particularly self-help groups such as Weight Watchers or Alanon groups, will not require this kind of initiative. The nurse's role, therefore, wil vary depending upon whether she initiates and leads the group, participates as a member, or participates as an outside consultant. Nevertheless, the nurse's role in any learning group includes providing some degree of structure and focus to the group's activities. The nurse also utilizes the basic teaching-learning principles described in chapter 11 to encourage client interest in, and application of, the information presented.

Support Groups

The primary goal of an emotional support group is to maintain healthy behaviors and prevent maladaptive coping patterns among its members (Loomis, 1979). In community health, nurses encounter many people who already have good health practices but who need help during times of stress. The support of other people enables them to adapt and preserve their healthy behaviors. Support groups meet this need. A woman alone found adjustment to the ordeal of a mastectomy painfully difficult. Feelings of loss, disfigurement, changed body image, and fear of the cancer returning, in addition to her physical weakness and discomfort, were almost more than she could handle. A single woman, she was convinced that no man would ever want to touch her. She was invited to join a mastectomy club and, through this group, found the comfort and courage that she needed to face her situation. The other members had also had mastectomies. They shared a common experience and could empathize with her feelings. The support and acceptance of the group gave her the strength to put her life back together again.

Support groups, also called therapeutic groups (Marram, 1978), are composed primarily of emotionally healthy people (not needing psychiatric help) caught in some change or crisis. A laryngectomy club or a divorce support group, for example, contains people involved in situational crises who need therapeutic reinforcement. A developmental crisis, such as entering parenthood, may prompt others to form a parenting group for the purpose of reassurance and reinforcement of personal resources. The need for support during adaptation to job change prompted one church to form its Job Transition Support Group for members and others in the community. So great was the need and so successful the group that, in 1984, the group, with an evolving membership, celebrated its seventh anniversary. Groups such as this often have secondary learning goals. For instance, one week the Job Transition Support Group heard a lecture on the interview process, but its primary goal remained emotional support. The support group provides members with comfort and courage to face the difficulties of their present situation. It seeks to maintain and utilize their existing strengths; it helps them cope successfully and regain their equilibrium (Fig. 9-3).

Support groups sometimes serve an advocacy role as well. They can plead

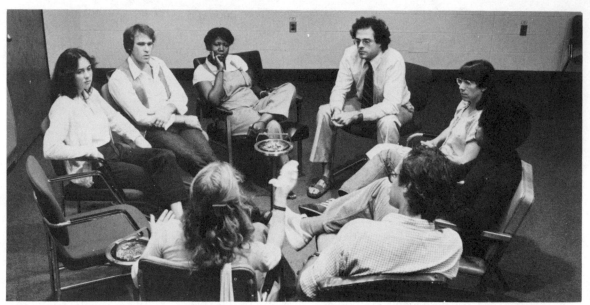

Figure 9-3
*Members of this support
group listen and share their
feelings with one another.*

the cause of their members whose physical and emotional health, job security, or social status may be threatened because of their current problem. Alcoholics Anonymous, while primarily a support group, represents a strong social force working in favor of its members' rehabilitation and constructive participation in the community. The Gray Panthers, a senior citizens' lobby group, promotes the causes of the elderly while providing them with a group with which they can identify and from which they can derive sustenance. A support group for epileptics rallied around a member who had been fired from her job when her boss discovered her diagnosis. The nurse leader of the group, accompanied by two of the group members, met with the boss, explained epilepsy, and convinced him that the woman's condition was under control. She kept her job.

Nurses working with support groups aim to facilitate group interactions, but their most important role is to model acceptance and caring. Demonstrating a warm, understanding attitude with, for example, a smoking cessation group or a group of individuals grieving the loss of spouses encourages members to assume these same caring feelings and to create a supportive climate. This approach energizes individuals to resume responsible, healthy behaviors.

Socialization Groups

Occasionally nurses encounter clients from another culture or subculture who must learn new social roles in order to achieve a positive level of health. Their old patterns of behavior are inappropriate, nonfunctional, sometimes detrimental, or at least a source of uneasiness in the larger society. Some

230

Native Americans, accustomed to living on a remote reservation, have difficulty adjusting to urban living. Southeast Asian refugees, flocking to American cities in increasing numbers, experience even greater culture shock. Contrasting patterns of eating, living, rearing children, and health practices, as well as language barriers and value differences, all call for adaptation in order for these clients to function in the new culture. Even American veterans who have served in the armed forces overseas experience some degree of culture shock upon returning to the United States. They must adjust to new values, clothing styles, social relationships, and political and economic changes. Some individuals in our society have lived in a confined subculture, such as a mental hospital, a prison, or a school for the deaf, and upon discharge must learn new ways of behaving. All of these individuals can benefit from a socialization group.

The primary goal of a socialization group is to help its members learn new social roles. A socialization group must not be confused with a purely social group. Nurses will want to be aware of social groups and their functions. For example, lonely, isolated individuals may benefit greatly from joining a bridge club, bowling league, or bird-watching group. Such groups offer friends, enjoyable activities, and support. The elderly, for instance, may need information about an activities group in their area and encouragement, even assistance, to participate. However, this chapter is concerned with groups in which the community health nurse works. Socialization groups bring together people who are adapting to a new culture or subculture. They offer the nurse an opportunity to capitalize on the benefits of group influence to help these people learn new social skills that will promote their physical and emotional health.

The nurse's role in a socialization group is first to demonstrate caring and acceptance of the group's members, to respect their present values and behaviors. The nurse also provides structure and focus to the group process. For example, with discharged mental patients or a refugee enculturation group, the nurse can encourage members to share their experiences and help them learn new ways of coping with this culture. The mental patients may discuss how to interview for a job, how to meet people, or how to behave at parties. Topics such as shopping in a supermarket, how to ride a bus, or what to expect when one goes to a health clinic would be a few of those discussed in the refugee group. The nurse uses group support to give these people courage to give up their familiar practices and group influence to help them learn new roles.

Psychotherapy Groups

Psychotherapy groups are formed for people who need treatment of an emotional disturbance. Many clients in community health have emotional problems ranging from minor neuroses to severe maladjustments. Psychotherapy groups can serve the needs of families in which child abuse or parent abuse occurs, married couples in conflict, chemically dependent persons, and those with suicidal impulses. These individuals may be referred by a family member, neighbor, professional worker, or agency. They may also refer themselves. Some receive group therapy following individual counseling; others are able to gain all the help they need from a psychotherapy group alone.

The primary goal of psychotherapy groups is to provide members insight into themselves and to help them change their behavior (Loomis, 1979). The group focuses on how its members relate to themselves and to each other; it becomes a "social microcosm" (Loomis, 1979, p. 10). That is, the group serves as a minisociety, allowing members to display their negative feelings and behaviors in an accepting and corrective milieu. An occasional group member may not be ready or willing to participate in self-change and may need to be counseled in some other setting.

Some nurses in community health have advanced training and experience in group psychotherapy and serve as therapists for these groups. More often, the community health nurse is a cotherapist working with a psychiatrist, psychologist, or psychiatric social worker. For example, a nurse and psychiatric social worker co-led a psychotherapy group for delinquent adolescent girls. They considered many behaviors, but they focused on the girls' tendency to "run away," to avoid anything perceived as unpleasant. The nurse's role included demonstrating acceptance and caring, encouraging the girls to share their feelings, helping them to understand the reasons behind their feelings and behavior, and providing structure and focus to the group process.

Task-oriented Groups

A final category of small groups with which community health nurses work includes all those groups whose primary goal is to accomplish some predetermined task. In community health there are many complex problems to solve, decisions to make, and tasks to accomplish that require a collaborative effort. Nursing staff in a public health agency disagree over the proper method for supervising home health aides. A day care center needs new health and safety policies. Community residents are concerned about a rising incidence of vandalism in their area and want to develop some constructive program to keep children and teenagers busy. The local elementary school wants help in planning a health fair. Mothers attending the well-child clinic would like to make the waiting room more pleasant and interesting. Each of these tasks will need people contributing their unique perspectives and skills and working together as a group to address the issue. Community health nurses play a significant part in this process.

Membership in task-oriented groups varies but generally encompasses clients, community residents, and health-related professionals. Client task-oriented groups often form spontaneously out of a desire to improve the current situation. With minimal assistance from their community health nurse, several elderly clients, feeling lonely and useless, established a foster grand-parents program. Volunteering their services through local churches and clubs, these retirees soon had more requests than they could handle. As foster grandparents, they met real needs of children in the community and also contributed to their own enjoyment and satisfaction. The community health nurse may work with a group of clients whose goal is to accomplish some task but whose collaboration also serves other health-related functions. One such group was the well-child clinic mothers who wanted to redecorate the waiting room. The nurse helped them plan and implement a fund-raising rummage sale and worked as a group member during the redecoration. Group cohesiveness developed as a result of the many hours spent together, and the nurse was able to form an ongoing mothers' support group with these women.

Community residents frequently initiate task-oriented groups in which community health nurses participate. A school nurse was asked to lead the elementary school task force to plan its health fair. Two community health nurses served on a local community council's planning committee to develop a hypertension screening program. In contrast, the nurse may initiate a task-oriented group involving community residents. A community health nurse influenced some concerned Native Americans to form a committee to raise the health consciousness of the people on their reserve. She met with the committee weekly for three months and accompanied its chairman when he presented the committee's recommendations to the tribal council. She assisted the woman who started the weekly health column, one element of the committee's health consciousness-raising plan, for the tribal newspaper. In another instance, a community health nurse initiated a task-oriented group in order to develop a friendly visitor program for elderly shut-ins.

Professional task-oriented groups are a frequent part of community health nursing practice (Fig. 9-4). They might include an agency team meeting, a state nursing association subcommittee, a state health planning commission, or an environmental safety task force. In these groups, the nurse, whether leader or member, works with other health-related professionals to accomplish specific tasks. For example, a community health nurse in St. Paul, Minnesota, chaired a subcommittee of the Metropolitan Health Board to study ways and means of facilitating greater collaboration between health care agencies. In addition to consumer members, the committee included health care ad-ministrators from public and private agencies, nurses, physicians, and health planners.

The nurse's role in task-oriented groups varies depending upon whether the nurse is the leader or a member of the group. This chapter will examine group leader and member roles in more detail later. In either case, however, the nurse works to facilitate group progress toward goal achievement.

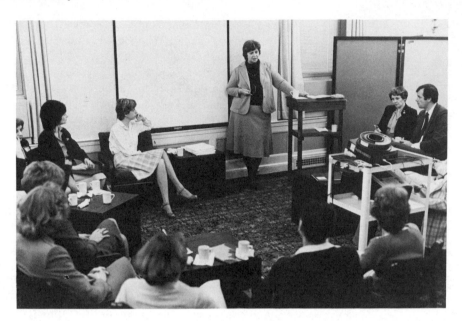

Figure 9-4
Health planning groups, such as this Visiting Nurse Association directors' meeting, form a vital link in the provision of community health services.

Table 9-1 summarizes the five types of small groups with which community health nurses work by listing each type's primary goal, membership, and nurse's role.

ESSENTIAL GROUP NEEDS

Group needs differ from individual needs. We are all familiar with various definitions of individual needs, such as those outlined in Maslow's *Hierarchy of Needs* (1954) or Erikson's *Eight Ages of Man* (1963). These needs include belonging, recognition, generativity, and self-actualization. For individuals to achieve a maximum level of functioning, their basic needs must be met. A group, as an entity, has a different set of needs that must be satisfied and maintained in order to allow optimal group functioning. Gouldner and Gouldner (1963) describe four essential small group needs.

Shared Goals
First, a group needs an agreed-upon goal and a shared understanding about the means for its achievement. No purposeful small group can function for long if its members have different ideas about what it is trying to accomplish. A group learning about family planning, for instance, can make little progress if some members define it as a sex education class, others join to help influence people against abortion, and some use it as a social outlet. The

234

Table 9-1
Types of Small Groups in Community Health

Type of Group	Primary Goal	Membership	Nurse's Role
Learning	Develop and apply knowledge	People desiring information and improvement in their lives	Provide structure and focus for group process
Support	Maintain healthy behavior and prevent maladaptive coping	Emotionally healthy people needing support during change or crisis	Present role model of acceptance and caring Facilitate group interaction
Socialization	Learn new social roles	People adapting to a new culture or subculture	Offer acceptance and caring Provide structure and focus for group process
Psychotherapy	Gain insight into self and change behavior	People needing treatment of an emotional disturbance	Offer acceptance and caring Encourage sharing of feelings Help members understand the reasons behind their feelings and behavior Provide structure and focus for group process
Task-oriented	Accomplish task	People assigned to or volunteering to complete a job	Facilitate progress toward goal achievement

group must be solidly behind the stated goals if members are to work together and accomplish desired results.

Consistent Norms

Second, a group needs consistency in its norms. That is, there must be some continuity and stability in the internal rules and policies, spoken and unspoken, that govern the group's actions (Loomis, 1979). Every group has to establish ground rules for operating. These rules govern areas such as membership eligibility, attendance requirements, whether or not new members can join after the group is in progress, what kind of participation is expected of each member, and what is expected of the leader. If rules and policies are ignored or frequently broken, the structure of the group is weakened, members do not feel secure, and the group eventually is unable to function.

Motivation

Third, a group needs members motivated to do their various jobs. Many variables influence motivation; among them are leader power and charisma, degree of member commitment to group goals and group success, how well individual needs are being met, group cohesiveness, and members' sense of belonging. Group goals can be accomplished only through collaborative effort; unless members do their share of the work, the job does not get done. Nor can the group function if members are lazy or morale is low.

Each member has a unique role to play and, as for any system, the group's viability depends on the proper functioning of all its parts.

Communication
Fourth, every group needs stable communication channels among the members. No group can function without a dependable system for giving and receiving information. The effectiveness of a divorce support group depends on members' ability to share their feelings of anger, rejection, or loneliness freely and to receive accepting, understanding responses in return. The work of a committee to study safety hazards in a summer camp cannot be done without an active exchange of ideas. Were it not for demonstrated acceptance and caring and constant two-way communication to help members gain insight into their feelings and behavior, a psychotherapy group would have minimal success. In order to function, all groups require viable lines of communication.

GROUP FUNCTIONS

Every small group serves two types of functions: a task-related function and a group maintenance function (Sampson & Marthas, 1977). The task function focuses on completing the job while the maintenance function deals with how members are interacting. The former is goal related and instrumental; the latter member related and interpersonal.

Consider how a student council operates. Part of the group's focus will be on the task dimension. Members will explore ideas, make plans, decide on jobs to be done, keep discussion on target, and make certain that members have done their delegated tasks. The other part of the group's concentration is on the maintenance dimension, which includes responsibilities such as keeping up group morale, making certain that individual members' needs are met, encouraging and praising member accomplishments, and mediating conflicts.

A well-functioning group emphasizes both task and maintenance concerns (Guthrie & Miller, 1978). You may have experienced membership in a group that focused so heavily on tasks that the interpersonal dimension was neglected. This situation happens most often in task-oriented groups, such as committees, where the job to be done becomes so important that it is accomplished at the expense of members' feelings. Internal dissatisfaction develops, resulting in poor attendance, disruptive behavior, or withdrawal. Everyone expects and needs to get something from group membership; if they do not, they will either drop out or possibly disrupt the group in some way. On the other hand, a group that concentrates too heavily on the interpersonal dimension may have happy members but not accomplish its goals. An appropriate balance between task and maintenance functions is needed.

Starting a Group

When any group is about to be formed, certain questions must be answered. First, does a group need or wish to form, and who initiates that process? In some instances, several people may get together because they have identified a reason for meeting. Their common concern prompts the group formation. Sometimes an outside person or agency, like Alcoholics Anonymous, starts a new group in the community. On other occasions, the nurse, having identified a need, may be the initiator. For example, a community health nurse with several postpartum clients in her caseload may suggest that they meet as a group for mutual support and shared information. Or the nurse may contact several local churches and offer to form a group of interested volunteers who would begin making friendly visits to shut-ins. Initial formation of a group is based on identifying a need — determining a reason or reasons for people to get together — then convening the group. Once the decision is made to form the group other questions must be addressed. Who should the members be? What is the best size for this group? What are the group's needs, and what should its goals be? Where should it meet, and what type of physical arrangements would most enhance its purpose? How can members be oriented to facilitate effective group development and group process? We shall consider the answers to each of these questions separately.

SELECTING MEMBERS

A group's members are determined by several factors. One is the group's general purpose. If it is task oriented, is members should be people who have expertise or skills pertinent to accomplishing the task. If its purpose is support, the members will be people who are experiencing change or crisis and need emotional reinforcement. In other words, the members should have something in common that relates to the group's primary goal.

Members should also exhibit similarities relative to the group's specific goals. Sometimes age- or sex-specific membership is necessary. For example, a support group for men in midlife crisis would limit its membership to middle-aged men. A preschoolers' mothers' group aiming to understand early childhood growth and development and learn appropriate mothering responses would limit its membership to young mothers. In other groups, the members may be very dissimilar in age, sex, or social role, but have some other common denominator. A weight loss group, for instance, might be composed of members of a variety of ages and both sexes since obesity is their shared concern. The epileptic support group mentioned earlier included young people from grade school through high school. Their variant ages and sexes gave a broader range of perspectives to group discussion and further enhanced the group's value. Their common denominator was epilepsy.

Members should choose to be part of the group. Any group member who does not participate willingly is not likely to benefit from or contribute positively to the group. If, for example, a client is coerced into a psychotherapy group or a professional is drafted reluctantly to serve on a health committee, we may see nonparticipation, conflict, or disruption in group process.

One should also select members on the basis of their commitment to the group's success. People who are genuinely interested in the group's goal and motivated to work for their accomplishment will gain more from the group experience and make a greater contribution to its process and outcomes. We see strong evidence of this contribution particularly in self-help groups, such as Alcoholics Anonymous, where group loyalty and commitment accomplish significant results.

Finally, leaders are helped by selecting members with whom they enjoy working and are more likely to be effective. Some leaders enjoy working with challenging groups, such as drug addicts, while groups with a strong commitment to change may be more satisfying for others. As Loomis (1979, p. 52) points out, "Therapists should be encouraged to become familiar with their own personal characteristics and preferences in the selection of clients." This factor clearly affects a group's success.

DETERMINING GROUP SIZE

Not long ago a community health nurse and seven other professionals formed a task force to study service delivery problems and make recommendations to a county board. The group met for several months and formed a good working relationship. However, its final product, a set of recommendations, met with resistance from county agencies not represented on the original task force. They insisted on expanding the task force and restudying the problems. Later composed of 22 members, the group met frequently but made almost no progress. Most of the leader's energy was spent resolving conflicts and attempting to pacify a few vocal members who dominated the discussion with lengthy diatribes defending their agencies' territory. Many members could not or chose not to participate. Attendance began to drop. As the deadline drew near, the leader, in desperation, appointed a subcommittee of five members to draft a proposal to which the larger group could respond. The draft, with minor changes, was approved, and the task force limped to its final conclusion with participation from about half of the original group.

Why was the first task force so successful and the second not? Because group size affects performance. The larger the group, the longer it takes to reach decisions, especially if consensus is required. In addition, the subgroups that almost always develop within larger groups can polarize interests, create conflicts, and impede group progress.

Group size also influences satisfaction. We have known for many years that as a group expands, the individual member's satisfaction declines (Tubbs & Moss, 1974). The larger the group, the less likely is the opportunity for all members to participate. In a large group, a few people usually do most of the talking while the rest are either intimidated, bored, or dissatisfied to the point of choosing not to participate.

Large groups do exist; examples are professional nursing groups, parent-teacher-student associations, student bodies, and older adults clubs. In order to meet specific group needs, however, formal, purposeful groups must divide into smaller units of workable size. Loomis (1969, p. 61) emphasizes: "It is not good clinical practice to remain with too large a group simply because there are not enough funds available to start a second group. Client needs and group task should be the primary consideration in determining group size."

Determining the number of members in a group varies, depending upon the situation and the group goals. To allow an appropriate mix of members and enough people to promote good interaction, a group should have at least five or six members. Ten to twelve members is considered the maximum size before subgroups start to form. The optimal size for any talk-oriented group that aims at problem solving, support, learning, insight, or behavior change is six to ten members (Loomis, 1979). The choice of seven members is often preferred for providing the best balance of variety of ideas with opportunity for all members to participate.

SETTING GROUP GOALS

We set goals and objectives on the basis of needs. That important step in the nursing process — assessment — must be taken. A community health nurse, working with an interpreter, started a socialization group for deaf high school students. These young people attended a state residential school for the deaf and would soon be graduating. The nurse's assessment showed that they were concerned about functioning in a hearing world, about getting jobs, developing a social life, applying to colleges, and planning careers. They had needs. On the basis of these needs, the group established its goals and objectives.

Every group must identify its needs before setting goals. Needs assessment involves collecting and interpreting data, and then a diagnosis can be made and a plan developed for making needed changes. A detailed discusson of needs assessment, diagnosis, and goal setting is provided in chapter 7. In order to set goals and objectives with a nursing leadership training group, for instance, a leader may ask the members what they think they need and probably evaluate their leadership knowledge and skills. On the basis of this data, the leader determines this group's specific needs, needs such as how to make decisions, how to plan, and how to delegate. Then the goals and objectives can be established.

Setting goals is a group activity involving all members. Unless members participate in this process, it is possible that their expectations for the group will differ from others. Members and leader together need to agree on the group's major goals and its specific objectives, the activities that will ensure the desired outcomes. It is often helpful to negotiate a group contract in which the nurse-leader and members mutually agree on their expectations for the group and the manner in which the outcomes will be achieved. Negotiating a fee for service with some groups is an important element in the contract and contributes to group commitment (Loomis, 1979).

MAKING PHYSICAL ARRANGEMENTS

Where, how, and when a group meets significantly influences its productivity. The meeting place must be conveniently located, perhaps near a bus line, in order to be accessible to members. It must also have appropriate facilities, such as wheelchair access or parking space, to accommodate members' needs.

Space is another consideration. Some groups, such as an exercise group or a first aid demonstration class, need a larger meeting area in order to accomplish their goals. Other groups function best in a more intimate setting that is conducive to sharing and expressing feelings; for them, a smaller room works best.

Seating arrangements can influence group process. If chairs are set in classroom style, there is a tendency for members to direct their comments only to the leader. Many task-oriented groups, such as committees, work around long tables. It is difficult for members along the sides of the tables to have eye contact with others along the same side. As a result, communication is inhibited and group cohesiveness is slower to develop. A circular seating pattern in which every member can see every other member facilitates communication in all directions.

A comfortable atmosphere, compatible with group goals, is important. A group dealing with feelings may find softer chairs or even sitting on the floor relaxing, informal, and conducive to free expression, while a "think" group may need firmer seating. Background noise, a room that echoes, distracting posters, or distasteful decorations may often detract from group productivity.

Finally, the time when a group meets is also important. Dates and times should fit members' schedules so that all can attend, and length and frequency of meetings should enhance group goals. A support group, for instance, may find it most helpful to meet weekly to receive frequent reinforcement. Other groups, such as some learning or task groups, may need more time between sessions to practice new skills or research a problem.

240

ORIENTING GROUP MEMBERS

Three points need emphasis to ensure smooth functioning as a group starts. First, members must agree on the group's goals. Members should agree as early as possible in the life of the group to erase misconceptions and to help solidify the group behind its purpose.

Second, new group members need to know how the group will function; they must begin to establish its structure and rules for operating. Structure refers to the way a group defines and regulates its members' behavior in terms of roles, communication patterns, and power relationships within the group (Sampson & Marthas, 1977). It must be clear from the beginning of any group who, if anyone, is leader and what that person is expected to do. Expectations for the members should be clearly spelled out, and special roles, such as a timekeeper in a discussion group or a referee for debates, should be assigned. More specific leader and member roles will emerge during the life of the group; we will discuss these shortly. Communication patterns evolve as group members work together, but awareness from the start of how members communicate is important. The interaction networks tend to be most effective in groups whose members are all free to communicate with each other as well as with the nurse-leader (Tubbs & Moss, 1974).

Power structure in informal groups often fluctuates, depending upon which members have the most influence, while formal groups, such as an agency's nursing organization, generally have a stable, clear-cut structure of power, influence, and authority. In any group, however, decisions can be made to designate who has power to do what. For example, the leader of a learning group may have absolute power over all decisions, or the group may choose a completely democratic format with decision-making power distributed among the members. Rules governing group action also need to be established early. The group must decide on matters such as attendance, physical arrangements, and whether smoking will be permitted.

Third, members need to hold the same expectations for the group's outcomes. The anticipated final product of the group can be restated and discussed to make certain that everyone understands and agrees that this is the outcome wanted. Part of this discussion should include how the group members will evaluate the group's final product. How will they know when their goals have been met? Some groups will find it easier to evaluate than others. A smoking cessation group or a weight loss group, for instance, will have clear standards for measuring success. An assertiveness training group for women may decide that its outcome is the ability of every member to assert herself appropriately in public and will evaluate this outcome by having each member describe one such experience. A divorce support group may have more difficulty agreeing on outcomes but perhaps will choose to measure them in terms of each member's satisfaction, feelings of comfort, or self-confidence.

Building Group Cohesiveness

Group cohesiveness is the sum of all the forces that influence members to stay in a group. These forces include whether (1) a member's needs can be met in the group, (2) group goals are consistent with member needs, (3) members expect the group to benefit them, and (4) members actually perceive that the group is benefitting them (Loomis, 1979). These are positive forces that attract members toward the group. In some instances, negative outside pressures may also promote group cohesiveness.

Cohesive groups display certain characteristics that begin early in the group's development and increase over time. There is an attraction of members to the group and a sense of pride in membership, which intensifies as the group becomes more successful. Pride is usually accompanied by an emotional commitment of the members to the group and manifests itself in increasing loyalty and high morale. The members feel good about one another and their group identification. They are loyal to each other and to the group's goals and values and, in some instances, may talk, dress, or act in similar ways. They work well together and enjoy spending time together, even outside of the regular group meetings.

During the life of every group there are times of internal problems and external threats. Group cohesiveness helps a group to weather these times. When the members of a parenting group disagreed among themselves over ways to discipline children, their closeness and unity as a group helped them over this period of conflict and prevented the group from disintegrating. The members of a chemical dependency group discovered that their funding source had been cut off and that there would be no more money for medications or consultation. Because of the members' commitment to remaining together, they sought and found new resources and continued working on their goals.

Group cohesiveness is as important to the group as the nurse-patient relationship is to individual therapy (Yalom, 1975). Research demonstrates that there is a positive correlation between group cohesiveness and positive group therapy outcomes (Loomis, 1979). Thus it becomes essential to foster group cohesiveness in the small groups with which nurses work.

Nurse-leaders build cohesiveness in a group by making certain that its four basic needs are met. First, there must be agreement among all members on the group's goals and the means by which these goals will be achieved. No group will be cohesive if members disagree on or misunderstand the goals. To avoid misunderstanding, members need to know exactly what the goals mean, have a clear (preferably written) statement of them, agree on the methods and actions to use in implementing them, and have a sense of hope that they are attainable. Second, group norms, the standards for acceptable behavior in the group, must be continuous and stable to help the group function. These norms are developed through discussion between leader and members about what is expected and acceptable behavior. Formal groups tend to define norms at the start. Norms often develop more gradually in informal groups. Third, there must be group motivation. Clarity and feasibility of goals can help members feel that working for the group is worthwhile. The leader can be a strong motivator by giving individual members recognition and positive reinforcement and by promoting each member's participation and sense of belonging. Fourth, communication channels within the group must remain viable. It is often up to the leader to monitor communication networks and make certain that they function effectively. Members, too, can help to facilitate a good exchange of information and feelings, but the group may need an outside process observer to make objective recommendations for improving its communication patterns.

Several factors can block group cohesiveness from developing or remaining (Loomis, 1979). Open membership, particularly with an unlimited number of sessions, sometimes makes it difficult for a group to stabilize its norms. Some groups, such as Alcoholics Anonymous or Weight Watchers, overcome this difficulty by having established goals and norms for the group that essentially do not change as new members join. In a less formal group with open membership, such as an ostomy club, the nurse-leader can help the founding members to develop a charter or written statement describing the group's general purpose and policies. Then, as new members enter and old ones leave, there can be some flexibility within this structure to allow specific goals and norms to reflect the changing membership's needs. That is, both goals and norms would have to be renegotiated depending on the rate of member turnover. When members move in and out of a group very rapidly, it is almost impossible to establish cohesiveness. In general, the more stable the membership, the more likely is the achievement of group cohesiveness.

Other blocks to group cohesiveness include members who do not conform to norms or agree with goals, the formation of competitive subgroups, or a leader-centered group. Deviant members can sometimes be persuaded to change their behavior or perhaps to leave the group. Strong group agreement on goals and norms prevents competition and allows the formation of positive subgroups that enhance cohesiveness. One can also minimize splintering by keeping the subgroups task-specific and time-limited. Responsible group leadership focuses on uniting the group behind its goals and maximizing its potential to meet client needs.

Some groups need cohesiveness more than others. Without a close working relationship, a support group, for example, will probably not be able to function while a learning group may be able to accomplish its goals; however, the learning group's full potential cannot be realized without group cohesiveness.

Working With a Group

Let us say you have prepared for a group by gaining an understanding of the types of small groups and their needs. Then you actually started a group and worked to build cohesiveness. The group appears to be moving along well. Between this initial period of establishing a group and the final period of terminating it, you will be working with an ongoing group. This work requires an understanding of the phases of group development, the different roles that leader and members can play, and the ways problems can be resolved.

PHASES OF GROUP DEVELOPMENT

Groups, like individuals, go through predictable growth phases. It is easiest to observe these phases in groups whose membership is constant; it is more difficult to distinguish the phases in groups whose membership or goals frequently change. The phases are dependence, counterdependence, and interdependence (Bennis & Shepard, 1956; Guthrie & Miller, 1978).

Dependence
During this first phase, members depend on the leader for guidance and direction. They are still sorting out why they are there and what their roles will be. They do not question the leader's authority. It is during this phase that members are most concerned with inclusion in the group (Schutz, 1966). It is a time of personal contact and encounter. Members want to be part of the group but still feel some conflict in giving up their personal identity. Dependence has been called the "childhood" stage of group development (Guthrie & Miller, 1978).

Counterdependence
As members become more comfortable in their roles, they also become more assertive. Conflict and power struggles develop, and acceptance of the leader's authority diminishes. The major issue in the counterdependent phase is control. Who has power and authority? Who will influence and control? Who will be controlled? It is an "adolescent" stage of group development.

Interdependence
Finally, group members learn to work out their relationships. They make decisions together, engage in open communication, manage conflict successfully, and experience satisfaction in the entire group's accomplishments. During this phase, the issues revolve around communicating and meeting individual needs to express and receive affection. Subgroups develop and members pair to handle intimacy needs. Interdependence is a "mature" phase of group development that may take weeks, months, or even years for a group to reach, depending on the stability of the membership. Some groups never achieve interdependence.

While monitoring a group's development, leaders notice that as each new issue arises the group will again progress through the developmental phases with regard to that issue. According to Sampson and Marthas (1977,

p. 184), "A particular developmental stage . . . is never fully completed for all time; rather, as circumstances change, the same developmental [stage] may crop up again and again." For example, a nursing team in a community health agency has been working on solving case problems. During the past five months the team members have worked through their dependence on the team leader and their conflicts over different ways to manage family problems; now they are communicating well and assuring everyone the opportunity to express ideas. They are experiencing the interdependent phase on this issue. Recently the team was told that it would have to redistribute members' geographic work boundaries. Feeling insecure and uncertain about how to accomplish this task, members initially looked to the team leader for suggestions (dependent phase). Soon they recognized advantages and disadvantages of various proposals for redefining work boundaries, ignored the leader, and began arguing among themselves over how to decide. Power struggles signal that they are currently in the counterdependent phase on this issue.

Knowing the phases of group development helps us recognize at what stage a group is and what to expect from the members. Groups must be allowed to progress through each phase at their own pace; this progress can be greatly enhanced by an understanding and facilitative leader.

LEADER ROLE

The group leader has a specific responsibility: to help the group achieve its goals. Sometimes a formal, designated leader assumes this role; at other times, an informal leader emerges to help focus the group's energy on its business. The nurse may be either a formal leader, an informal leader, or simply a member. All the members, including the leader, must be committed to working together to accomplish the group's goals. Leadership style influences this task. Whether the leader should assume an autocratic (leader-centered, persuasive) style, a democratic (member-centered, problem-solving) style, or a laissez-faire (noncentered) style depends on the group's needs. Each style has advantages as well as disadvantages, although the democratic style works best in most situations. Leadership styles are presented in more detail in chapter 20. During the group process, the leader exercises some unique functions and employs certain techniques.

Functions
Leader functions include a variety of activities designed to strengthen the group's ability to achieve its purpose. Important ones are the following (Sampson & Marthas, 1977):

Obtain and receive information
Help diagnose group goals, obstacles, and consequences of decisions

Facilitate communication
Help integrate varying perspectives and alternate possibilities for action
Test and evaluate proposals and decisions

Techniques
To carry out these functions, the leader needs skill in the use of certain techniques or leader interventions (Sampson & Marthas, 1977):

Support. Support means to create an encouraging climate that reinforces positive behaviors and makes members feel secure and accepted. A leader could use this technique by telling the group, "You have made real progress today. Several people shared feelings as well as ideas, and you have all listened attentively and accepted these comments without judging them."

Confrontation. Confrontation is a technique that counters negative behavior through constructive feedback. The leader may direct it toward an individual member or the group as a whole. It consists of making direct, honest, reflective statements about how behaviors appear to us. People do not always want to hear these statements, but they may be necessary to facilitate group progress. It is helpful to combine support with confrontation.

Advice and Suggestion. Offering advice and suggestion is another technique to use when leader expertise or perspective is needed. Leaders should be careful to use it only when members are unable to solve problems for themselves.

Summarizing. Summarizing means providing the group with a concise, descriptive review. The leader may wish to summarize the group's actions to date, its progress in relationship to goals, its unresolved issues, and other areas of functioning. The value of this technique is to refocus group attention for future planning.

Clarification. Clarification is used to prevent confusion or distortion of ideas. A leader could use this technique by saying, "From the comments I've heard, it seems to me that the group would like to switch to Tuesdays. Is that correct?"

Questioning. Probing or questioning is a useful technique for gaining information and greater understanding. By asking questions, leaders help members explore ideas in greater depth.

Reflection. Reflection can be used to mirror people's ideas, feelings, or behaviors. To reflect ideas, leaders repeat, paraphrase, or highlight comments in order to facilitate communication. For example, when a member says, "I don't agree," a reflective response is, "You don't agree?"; thereby the person receives an opportunity to further discuss the idea. Reflecting feelings means restating to the group or member the feelings the leader thinks are being conveyed. If a learning group complains, "We've never had to do anything like this before," the leader may reflect back, "You seem to be a little

246

frightened of doing this." To reflect behavior, leaders simply describe the behavior they see, thus allowing the group to clarify the meaning. The leader can say to the group, "I notice that you've become silent since I made that last suggestion."

Interpretation and Analysis. Interpretation and analysis may be used as a technique to uncover the underlying meaning of group comments and behaviors. In using this technique, leaders summarize observations of the group and then offer an analysis of the behavior's deeper meaning or reason. The leader might say, "I notice that several of you who are usually active have not participated in the past two sessions. I wonder if the decisions about this issue seem to be a foregone conclusion, and you feel it's useless to say anything?"

Listening. Listening attentively shows the group that the leader is interested in them and what they have to say. It also provides a positive model for group members to use with each other. Attentive listening helps sharpen the focus of the conversation by allowing specific responses to the comments being made.

MEMBER ROLES

A new mothers' group has been meeting weekly now for a month and a half. As their leader, you notice that each person's behavior is unique in some way. Susan, for instance, asks many questions and also tends to agree with whoever is speaking. Diane, on the other hand, is full of ideas and frequently offers suggestions or proposes some new plan of action. Then there is Maureen. Her friendly, warm responses seem to make the others feel better in contrast to Fran's constant complaining. Verona has been especially helpful to you by keeping the group on track, helping to smooth out differences, and encouraging others to participate in the discussion. Each of the five women has assumed different group member roles.

Every group needs its members to perform specific roles. Member roles serve one of two basic functions necessary for a viable group — task or maintenance functions. Some roles are task related: they help the group do its work. Diane, for instance, is an initiator of ideas, and Susan is both an information seeker and follower. Verona orients the group to its goals (keeps it on track). These are task roles. Other roles are maintenance related: they deal with group members' participation. Maureen encourages members by showing acceptance and support, and Verona serves as gatekeeper, keeping communication channels open and facilitating member involvement. Both women play maintenance roles.

The most common task and maintenance roles are the following (Mill & Porter, 1976, pp. 28–30):

Task Roles

Initiator — *proposes tasks, goals, or actions; defines group problems; suggests a procedure*

Information seeker — *asks for factual clarification; requests facts pertinent to the discussion*

Opinion seeker — *asks for a clarification of the values pertinent to the topic under discussion; questions values involved in alternative suggestions*

Informer — *offers facts; gives expression of feelings; gives an opinion*

Clarifier — *interprets ideas or suggestions; defines terms; clarifies issues before the group; clears up confusion*

Summarizer — *pulls together related ideas; restates suggestions; offers a decision or conclusion of the group to consider*

Reality tester — *makes a critical analysis of an idea; tests an idea against some data to see if the idea would work*

Orienter — *defines the position of the group with respect to its goals; points to departures from agreed-upon directions or goals; raises questions about the direction that the group discussion is taking*

Follower — *goes along with movement of group; passively accepts ideas of others; serves as audience in group discussion and decision*

Maintenance Roles

Harmonizer — *attempts to reconcile disagreements; reduces tension; gets people to explore differences*

Gatekeeper — *helps to keep communciations channels open; facilitates the participation of others; suggests procedures that permit sharing remarks*

Consensus taker — *asks to see if the group is nearing a decision; sends up a trial balloon to test a possible solution*

Encourager — *is friendly, warm, and responsive to others; indicates by facial expression or remark the acceptance of others' contributions*

Compromisor — *offers a compromise that yields status when his own idea is involved in a conflict; modifies in the interest of group cohesion or growth*

Standard setter — *expresses standards for the group to attempt to achieve; applies standards in evaluating the quality of a group process*

All of the roles just listed are needed for a group to function effectively (Guthrie & Miller, 1978). Some members will play several overlapping roles; others will play only one or two. A leader can determine the roles the group's members are playing by having an outside observer evaluate the group or by using one of various member participation checklists (Bradford, Stock, & Horwitz, 1976; Hill, 1962; Pfeiffer & Jones, 1974). Should a vital role, such as gatekeeper, be missing from a group, the leader and the group may wish to ask someone to assume this role.

Some roles are dysfunctional; they hinder the group from reaching its goals. Fran's constant complaining is an example of a dysfunctional role that inhibits communication and demoralizes the group. Other behaviors, such as being aggressive, blocking, dominating, distracting, or seeking recognition or sympathy, are also dysfunctional. These roles cannot be ignored. The group must identify and deal with them. If someone disrupts the group meeting, the leader may redirect the focus back to the topic by saying, for example, "I'd like to hear other people's ideas, too." When disruptive behavior is persistent, a technique such as reflection or interpretation and analysis may be a constructive way to deal with it. Confrontation should be used with discretion, particularly in front of the group, since it may be too threatening and counterproductive.

SOLVING GROUP PROBLEMS

Many difficulties arise during the life of a group. We have dealt with a few such as how to start the group, avoid blocks to group cohesiveness, and deal with dysfunctional behavior. Three group problems in particular are worthy of further discussion. They are interpersonal conflict, dominance, and nonparticipation.

Resolving Conflicts

Conflict, by itself, is neither good nor bad. It is a form of tension frequently found in groups that may be used constructively by broadening the group's outlook and sharpening its problem-solving skills, or destructively by dissolving group cohesiveness.

Conflict arises when one or more members take sides against others in the group. There is sharp disagreement, arguing, tension, and impatience. Conflict may occur because one or more members is seeking special status or making a power play, because some members have vested interests in or loyalty to another conflicting organization, or because members have overinvested in the group's productivity (Bradford et al., 1976).

Managing conflict means taking neither the extreme of flight (avoidance) or of fight (head-on confrontation), but rather a realistic attitude aimed at maximum gain for all those concerned. It is called a Win/Win approach (Guthrie & Miller, 1978; Veninga, 1973):

Lose/Lose	you lose/I lose
Win/Lose	you win/I lose
Lose/Win	you lose/I win
Win/Win	you win/I win

Using the Win/Win approach encourages people to work together to benefit all parties. Group members examine all the issues at stake and maximize the opportunity for everyone to satisfy at least some of their desires. Win/Win refocuses energy into problem solving instead of competition.

There are four steps to take to resolve conflicts. First, acknowledge that there is a conflict and reach agreement on its definition in the group. People may not be arguing different points, after all. Second, identify possible areas of agreement. There are nearly always some points that are not mutually exclusive. Third, determine the changes each party in the dispute must make to resolve the problem satisfactorily. Fourth, keep the focus of the conflict on issues rather than people. Personal attack will stalemate any attempt at resolution and may even strengthen the conflict (Tubbs & Moss, 1974).

Dealing with Excessive Participation or Nonparticipation
Most groups need a relative equality of member participation for group work to be effective. To allow a full diversity of views, to foster cohesiveness through members' self-expression, and to make best use of the group's time, each member should have a fair share of the group's attention. Either nonparticipation or excessive participation will disrupt the group.

Excessive participation of members in the form of monopolizing conversation can produce feelings of anger and frustration for the leader and the group. Dominant members may be trying to cover up anxiety or seeking attention, recognition, and approval. However, their compulsive talking and apparent insensitivity to their effect on the group only create dislike and disrespect. Other members feel cheated out of their share of the group's time. The group cannot benefit from a complete range of member contributions.

The leader copes with a dominant member by first trying supportive interruption. "Your point is well taken, but, in the interest of time, we need to allow others to express their views." If the member is not responsive to this approach, the leader may try another technique, such as reflection: "You seem to be doing most of the talking today." The leader might offer an interpretation: "I wonder if you are talking so much because you feel a little anxious about something, perhaps about how the group sees you?" Even confrontation may be necessary. It is also possible that the group is permitting the dominant member to monopolize as a way of avoiding its own responsibility. In that case, confrontation of the group may be needed.

A member may refuse to participate as a result of apathy, lack of commitment to the group's goals, anger, fear of ridicule, timidity, or poor self-image. When other members do not know why this person is quiet, they begin to feel uncomfortable (Is this person judging us, ridiculing us, or not liking us?) and resentful.(It is unfair of members not to carry their share of the group's work.) The silence of several members may indicate an angry reaction to a few who are dominating or discomfort in the presence of conflict. When the entire group is silent or apathetic, they may be responding to the leader's style or the current task, which may seem unimportant or too difficult.

Nonparticipation must be diagnosed before the leader can intervene. Diagnosis can be made by offering a reflective or interpretive statement such as, ''I've noticed that there is very little participation in the group today. Are people uncomfortable with this topic or perhaps with the way I'm leading the group?'' or ''Susan, you haven't said much in the last few sessions. Are the rest of us not giving you a chance?'' From member responses and discussion, the leader learns the reasons behind the nonparticipation and then can take appropriate action. Nonintervention is sometimes best if it appears that too much group time and energy will be spent on the problem or if nonparticipation is infrequent. Occasional silence, particularly in one individual, may only be temporary. As the group becomes increasingly supportive and accepting, such individuals may gradually feel secure enough to start participating on their own.

Terminating the Group

Termination is an extremely important phase in the life of a small group (Loomis, 1979). Like any ending, including death, termination involves a mixed set of feelings that the group must face, explore, and resolve. Members must cope with feelings of loss and grief at leaving people to whom they have become attached. They must deal with a sense of success or failure, depending on whether their goals were met. They must recognize that they will no longer experience the group's support and other benefits. Termination is important because it is a time in the group's life when members have an opportunity to analyze the meaning of the group experience, which they can build on when planning for the future. Successful termination creates a sense of completion and a positive attitude toward future group experiences.

Termination is an issue that must be dealt with in every group. Most health care groups mark a beginning to their work and an ending when that work is complete. For these groups, the entire group will terminate. Other groups have an open-ended membership; thus the group (e.g., an ongoing support group) remains while members come and go. In these instances, the individual member terminates. Leaders, too, sometimes leave a group, perhaps for health reasons or a job change. Whether it is the entire group or an individual who is terminating, all the group members are affected. Positive leader intervention can make the difference in whether or not a group terminates successfully.

PREPARING FOR TERMINATION

Ideally, criteria for termination are established at the onset of the group. If the criteria are built into individual and group goals, clients know that, upon completion of their goals, it will be time to terminate. A failure on the part of many leaders, however, is not to explain these criteria fully to clients. The subject of termination is even avoided by some leaders, which suggests they may be denying its reality because they do not want to face the pain of separation. Part of the leader's responsibility, as early as possible in the life of the group, is to clarify with the group the exact conditions and date for termination.

Termination may be defined in terms of time (number of sessions or specific target date), behavior (when specific behavior changes have occurred), or circumstances (moving, job change, health). For example, a parenting group may choose to meet for 12 sessions and then terminate. If additional needs are identified at the end of that period, the group can renegotiate for more time. The members of a psychotherapy group will most likely decide that termination is appropriate when they see the desired changes in their behavior. Circumstances, such as moving or job change, are usually known far enough in advance to allow the group time to prepare adequately for termination.

WORKING THROUGH TERMINATION

When facing termination, group members may experience a mixture of feelings, such as sadness, anger, joy, or fear. They may deny the possibility of termination altogether. Members' behavior gives the leader clues about their reactions to termination. For instance, members who were formerly open in sharing feelings may become defensive and superficial. Others may appear angry and upset for no apparent reason. People may start to make plans for getting together beyond the termination date. Some may withdraw, come late, or act as if the group were no longer important to them. Most of these are unhealthy responses and require intervention.

Leader intervention during the termination process includes the following. First, the leader helps the group to identify and acknowledge that termination is occurring. Members must accept its reality. Second, the leader assists group members in finding appropriate alternatives for meeting the needs that the group has met. Fear of having to function without the group drives some members to return to old, unhealthy behaviors such as smoking or overeating after having not smoked or gone off their diets for months. Instead, the leader should encourage members to assess what the group has been providing for them and identify other ways to meet these needs outside of the group. For instance, one woman who was leaving an assertiveness training group decided to meet weekly with a friend for continued reinforcement of her new behaviors. The leader should allow enough time before termination for members to accomplish this task. Third, the leader gives group members an opportunity to express and deal with their feelings, which need to be worked through until the group senses that its business is finished. Finally, the leader facilitates termination by having the group evaluate its progress. "Here is where we were when we started. Look how far we have come" is a message that helps people leave with a sense of accomplishment and a positive outlook on the future.

Evaluating a Group

Group evaluation includes two important areas, process measurement and outcomes measurement. The first examines ongoing group interaction, and the second looks at the group's final product.

PROCESS EVALUATION

It is important for groups to conduct periodic self-examinations. Leaders and members both need to hear reactions to their performances. Are they conducting their roles effectively? Are they making progress toward their goals? This information is vital to making improvements in the way members work together.

Process evaluation can be done in several ways. One useful method is to have an outside observer sit in on the group, watch for specific behaviors, and then give reactions to the group. The observer can use one of several guides available for this purpose (Bradford et al., 1976; Pfeiffer & Jones, 1974). Another method is to have a group member act as an impartial observer during a session in which the member only observes and refrains from participating. The group itself may diagnose its health by periodically or even regularly using some form of checklist or questionnaire, followed by discussion (Bradford et al., 1976; Guthrie & Miller, 1978; Hill, 1962). The kinds of behaviors to observe will vary with each group; generally, however, a group needs to examine all of the roles listed earlier and ask questions pertaining to areas such as communication skills and patterns, responses to leadership style, group climate, stage of group development, and progress on group objectives. Sweeney (1975) has developed a useful set of criteria that appraises the strength and effectiveness of groups in terms of their physical, interpersonal, intrapersonal, and community dimensions.

MEASURING GROUP OUTCOMES

Determining the effectiveness of any group means measuring its outcomes. Did the group accomplish its objectives? Are the group members different now from how they were when the group started? Clear goals and specific objectives are the keys to unlocking the answers to these questions. Goals spell out the overall purpose of the group; objectives narrow goals down into specific behaviors that we can measure. For example, the group's goal may be to learn the techniques of natural childbirth. Objectives should describe separate behaviors, such as specific breathing techniques or exercises, that demonstrate the accomplishment of the goal. Thus objectives that describe outcome behaviors are criteria for measuring the group's performance. If members can and do demonstrate ability in the breathing techniques and the exercises (or any other behaviors outlined in the objectives), then we can say that the group goal has been accomplished.

Some groups' goals are more difficult to evaluate than others, but all can be measured to some degree. A group of women with mastectomies may have a goal of learning to accept their own bodies. They can identify specific behaviors that will tell them when they have met this goal. The behaviors may include looking in the mirror without wincing, admitting to having undergone a mastectomy to another person outside the group, or wearing form-fitting clothing and not feeling overly self-conscious.

The group should participate equally with the leader in the evaluation process. Group members' own observations, insights, and feedback are essential to collecting the necessary data for evaluating the objectives. If specific behavior changes, such as staying on a special diet or exercising daily at home, are part of the objectives, then further supporting data can be solicited from family members or friends.

Working with Aggregates

Concern for aggregates is a basic public health value but one that tends to be foreign to our individualistic, or even small group, orientation and customary provision of health care. Enlarging that view requires adopting a new mind set, a new way of perceiving community health needs. Let us begin that process by hearing from a nurse who described her experience of broadening her focus to include these larger aggregates. She was employed by an agency we will call Wilford County Public Health Nursing Service.

I received a referral to see a family whose 15-year-old daughter, Mary Jo, had run away from home for the third time. She was obese (215 pounds) and flunking out of school. There were so many problems in that family — unemployment, poor diet, stress, family conflict, another daughter's recent delivery of a sick illegitimate baby, and the obesity of the mother and all three daughters — that I hardly knew where to begin, but the parents were willing to work with me. We discussed their concerns and started with their biggest worry — the running away of Mary Jo. We finally found her. She and another girl who was also flunking out of school had hitchhiked to the city to find jobs but had no luck and ended up at the YWCA. When they got home, we had some long talks, and she agreed to stay and give it another try.

Up to this point, I felt some success in working with this family, and Mary Jo in particular. Then, an offhand comment made by Mary Jo shifted my attention to a larger aggregate.

"I know a lot of other girls at school in the same boat as me," she said. I asked her what she meant. "Well, there's a lot of others who don't give a damn about school and feel that life is pretty worthless." I should have followed up on that remark right away, but I didn't. Then a girl committed suicide in that same school, one of *my* schools. I felt terrible. If some kind of effort had been made to reach those kids who were hurting emotionally, maybe that girl would be alive today. I had spent a lot of time with Mary Jo and her family, but it wasn't too late to work with other girls. We started to look at the needs of the whole population of adolescent girls. Then we went into both of my schools and started working with their organizations. We did something about those other students and, would you believe, we now have 35 girls coming to our Teen Topics meetings after classes on Tuesdays in one school and Thursdays in the other.

Because nurses have traditionally worked with individuals and families, it was not surprising that this nurse focused on Mary Jo. Here was a family that needed and, in fact, asked for help. The nurse understandably gave care where a need had been clearly identified. In contrast, a whole population of girls appeared to be an amorphous mass of people, too indistinct to be assessed, too nebulous to treat as a whole, and too large for one nurse to serve. But was it? Belatedly, this nurse discovered that she could assess and meet the needs of aggregates. In this case, the aggregate was a subpopulation of high school girls.

Defining Population Groups

What is an aggregate? A population group or aggregate is a large, unorganized collection of people grouped by one or more common demographic features. In contrast to a small group, a population group is a loose collection of people. As a whole they do not have direct, face-to-face contact. They may or more often may not be aware of common problems or share similar goals. Members share a set of defining criteria but do not participate in a structure. That is, when we designate a special population, we identify one or more environmental or personal characteristics that the group of people have in common (Williams, 1977). They might share the feature of age, as in a pediatric population or a population group of the elderly. The defining characteristic might involve language; consider the Spanish-, Italian-, French-, Native American-, or Vietnamese-speaking populations within our country. Some population groups, such as blue-collar, pink-collar, and migrant workers, are defined in terms of their common type of employment (Fig. 9-5). Other aggregates share a common diagnosis. We may speak of the diabetic population, or the populations of stroke or automobile accident victims. We often define aggregates in terms of their potential vulnerability to health problems; for instance, we identify populations at risk for coronary heart disease, home accidents, or family abuse. The special population groups of unwed teenage mothers in a city, managers demonstrating stress symptoms in a specific corporation, and farm workers in the state who have experienced accidents with machinery in the past year all share a clear set of defining criteria. These criteria describe the population group.

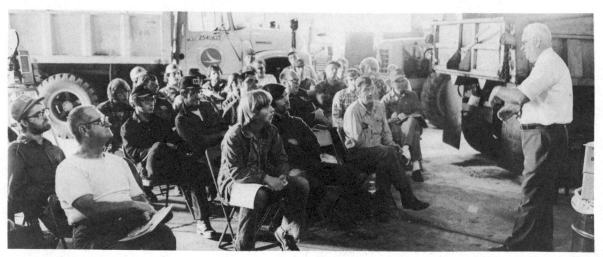

Figure 9-5
These farm workers consti-
tute a population group.
Here they meet to learn in
an agricultural training
session.

The purpose for designating a population group arises from some special need residing in that collection of people. When a number of school children in the same school district contract measles, the nurse may study all the children of that district as a population group to determine immunization levels and institute preventive immunization programs. There may be a large group of elderly people living alone in a community who are at risk of developing physical and emotional health problems because they do not utilize available resources. A significant number of employees with hypertension in an organization may attempt to function with their problem unrecognized and untreated. Community health professionals, therefore, single out population groups for the purpose of meeting health needs. The larger groups themselves become units for study and service.

Strategies for Working with Populations

Aggregates, by definition, are quite different from small groups and require new approaches on the part of the community health nurse. Still, the knowledge of groups, discussed earlier in this chapter, offers insights and strategies applicable to working with populations.

ASSESSMENT AND DIAGNOSIS

Aggregates as clients in community health have needs that are just as real as those identified for families or small groups. The community health nurse assesses those needs through a combination of various methods. Four are especially useful.

256

Observation can provide valid information about aggregates. It is often one of the best ways to begin any assessment. In the course of daily practice, nurses can watch for evidence of existing or potential problems. For example, after a community health nurse noticed symptoms of malnutrition in some migrant children, she broadened her observations to include the entire migrant community. Many of these hard-working people showed evidence of being undernourished. A nurse at an automobile manufacturing plant observed that several workers acted tense and fatigued. She began to pay attention to these symptoms when she walked through the plant.

Interviewing, a second assessment strategy, can offer detailed information about a population group. The nurse working with migrants prepared a set of questions about diet and eating practices. She interviewed several families in their shacks and discovered they ate no meat or dairy products, but only white bread, potatoes, and occasional vegetable scraps stolen from the fields. Their income was too meager to allow purchase of better foods. At the automobile plant, the nurse interviewed several selected workers and discovered that they had frequent headaches and nausea. These symptoms were most evident at the end of the day after long hours of exposure to the chemicals they were using in their work.

The nurse concerned about migrant nutrition took her initial findings to the state health department. With a team of professionals, she helped design an *epidemiologic survey,* a third assessment strategy (Dever, 1980). In an organization such as a manufacturing plant, it is also possible to conduct an epidemiologic survey. In her role as part of the company's middle management, the nurse pointed out the symptoms among workers on this unit. Others agreed that they had noticed them, too, and had seen them in workers in other units as well. She then helped develop a study to determine the plant's chemical hazards and their impact on employees' health. (Epidemiologic research as an aggregate assessment tool was discussed in the previous chapter.)

A fourth assessment strategy uses *existing data.* Nurses can learn a great deal about a population group by examining information that has already been collected for other purposes. Census records, community demographic data, or surveys done by other community organizations can often provide needed information for assessment and health planning for population groups. Statistics on infant morbidity and mortality from automobile accidents, for example, as well as records describing infant car seat use could assist in a study of the safety of the infant car-riding population. Other sources of existing data are described in chapters 7 and 8.

Thorough needs assessment at the aggregate level usually requires an interdisciplinary team effort to ensure proper data collection and analysis. Community-wide needs assessment is discussed in chapter 13.

The determination of health problems among population groups, then, depends on careful analysis and interpretation of this collected data. At the aggregate level diagnosis becomes a more complex task, and the community health nurse seldom does it alone. As during needs assessment, the nurse requires the expertise and collaborative input of other public health professionals, such as epidemiologists, statisticians, health planners, and environmentalists. There must be a clear and accurate diagnosis of the problem to be addressed.

PLANNING AND IMPLEMENTATION

Interventions at the aggregate level are on a larger scale and generally more complex than working with small groups. They are often what we know as community health programs. Nonetheless, many group principles apply. A clear goal and set of objectives are needed (Blum, 1981, p. 181). There must be agreement among the planning team members (Nutt, 1984, p. 38). Nurses cannot easily communicate with an entire aggregate to gain each person's input and cooperation; therefore, they ask representatives of that population to serve on the planning team along with an appropriate mix of health professionals. Because the planning is done by a team, the nurse can apply principles of small group interaction to enhance the group's functioning. Health planning and implementation for aggregates follow in the same general process as any kind of nursing care planning. For population groups, however, health planners must also be concerned about factors in the external environment, such as health policy, economic conditions, legislation, other programs competing for service to the same population, or funding, that may influence planning decisions. A family planning education program for Southeast Asian refugees, for example, was being considered by a local public health nursing agency. However, state funding for refugees' programs was drying up, and the nurses had to seek other sources of financial backing before the program could be implemented.

EVALUATION

Most often we evaluate aggregate level health care in terms of four types of results depending on our goals. They are outputs, outcomes, impact, and efficiency (Churgin, 1981, p. 280). *Outputs* are measured in terms of quantity. That is, if a family planning program aims to teach a certain number of people in the population, then the evaluation effort measures how many people were served. *Outcomes* are a quality measure and refer to the consequences of the program. Were the desired end results accomplished? For example, did the family planning program accomplish fewer unwanted pregnancies? *Impact* evaluation looks beyond the immediate results of the intervention and asks what effect it had on the rest of the community. Did this program meet the needs of one subpopulation but overlook other populations' needs? Should more extensive programs be developed? Finally, *efficiency* evaluation asks if the resources (costs in money, time, and personnel) were used as effectively as possible, or did the resources produce as much as could reasonably be expected (Churgin, 1981, p. 282).

Evaluation of community health programs follows five steps (Churgin, 1981, p. 284). First is criteria setting. The planning group must develop a list of criteria to be used to determine successful completion of the objectives. This is best done during the planning stage. Second, it must devise ways to measure these criteria. The measures should be objective, reliable, and valid. For example, if the group is evaluating a child health promotion program, one criterion may be fewer school absence days, measured in number of days missed. Third is data collection, and fourth is analysis and interpretation of the data. Finally, the findings are presented to relevant groups or organizations for future planning decisions.

Evaluation may be formative or summative. Formative evaluation is conducted to give feedback during the development of the health program. It examines the program while it is forming, as one might wish to do with a new health education effort. Is the program process working effectively? Is the program generating the desired outcomes as it goes along? Summative evaluation is conducted after the program is complete. It is the sum of the program's final product.

Aggregate Work Compared with Small Group Work

As we have seen, aggregates, in contrast to small groups, require a different orientation and set of strategies for use by community health nurses. Despite the differences, however, there are many similarities in the approaches the nurse can apply. Let us summarize both.

Work with population groups still employs the nursing process, only its application is on a larger scale. The nurse may work alone with a small group; aggregate work involves the expertise and input of a collaborating interdisciplinary team of which the nurse is a part. With small groups, every member is expected to participate to accomplish group goals. Work with populations should also involve people in the decisions that affect them, but that involvement, of necessity, means that representatives of the group speak for the rest. We recognize that small groups have a collective identity or personality as do population groups, and we respect each group's uniqueness. Even as small groups go through stages of development, so population groups' needs change over time. Both require ongoing assessment. We employ different tools, such as epidemiological research, in working with aggregates to facilitate systematic assessment and health planning on a larger scale. Finally, external determinants of health, such as social, biologic, organizational, and environmental factors, must be considered in working with groups of any size. Their significance in the context of the total community is greater, however, when applied to work with population groups.

Summary

Groups of all sizes are an important focus for community health nursing service. A small group is two or more persons who engage in repeated, face-to-face communication, identify with each other, and are interdependent.

In preparing to work with small groups, the community health nurse must understand their different types, their essential needs, and their primary functions. There are five major types of small groups encountered by community health nurses:

1. Learning groups are those in which the primary goal is to gain an understanding in order to change behavior in some specified area.
2. Support groups aim to provide emotional reassurance and maintain healthy behaviors.
3. Socialization groups help members to learn new social roles and skills.
4. Psychotherapy groups are formed for people who need treatment of an emotional disturbance.
5. Task-oriented groups include all the groups whose primary goal is to accomplish some predetermined task.

Individuals have needs; so do groups. The small groups with which community health nurses work need clear, shared goals and an agreement about how to reach those goals. They need consistent group norms and individuals motivated to participate in the group. Finally, every group needs stable communication channels among the members. Groups have two primary types of functions — task-related functions and group maintenance functions.

Starting a small group involves determining the criteria for membership and then selecting people who are committed to the goals of the group. It is important to determine the optimal size of the group, set clear group goals, make physical arrangements for the group, and orient the members.

Every small group varies in terms of the degree of cohesiveness experienced by members. The community health nurse can build a cohesive group by assuring that its four basic needs are met and avoiding certain barriers such as open membership. Building group cohesiveness must be an ongoing process in any group.

Working with a small group is enhanced by recognizing the phases of group development: dependence, counterdependence, and interdependence. The group leader has specific functions and ways to carry out those functions. Every group also needs its members to carry out specific roles such as initiator, information seeker, informer, and clarifier. Many difficulties arise during the life of a group. In particular, the community health nurse must be alert to resolving conflicts, dealing with those who monopolize the group, and handling the nonparticipant member.

Every small group must deal with the issue of termination, the last phase in the life of a group. It is important to prepare members for termination early in the life of a group and to work through the feelings generated by termination.

Group evaluation involves assessing the ongoing group interaction as well as the final outcome. Periodic self-evaluations are useful strategies for evaluating the process of group experience. Measuring the outcomes determines to what extent the group's goals were achieved. The entire evaluation process should involve both the leader and group members.

Working with aggregates involves a different orientation and some different strategies than those employed for small group work. An aggregate, or population group, is a large, unorganized collection of people who share one or more demographic features in common, such as age, ethnic background, or vulnerability to a health problem.

Assessment strategies for working with population groups include observation, interviewing, conducting epidemiological surveys, and use of existing data. The community health nurse works collaboratively with other public health professionals to assess needs, diagnose, and plan for, implement, and evaluate interventions on behalf of population groups. Evaluation efforts address four primary types of results: outputs, outcomes, impact, and efficiency.

Work with aggregates shares similarities as well as differences with work with small groups. Community health nurses utilize the nursing process on a larger scale in work with aggregates. They work on a team. They seek input from population group representatives. They respect the group's unique features and recognize that its needs change. They employ epidemiologic research and other assessment and planning tools applicable for macro-level use. They consider the impact of external health determinants on the health of population groups.

Study Questions

1. Select a small group (not social) of which you are currently or have recently been a member. Which of the three phases of group development is it in? Would you describe this group as a healthily functioning one? Why or why not?
2. Compare and contrast a socialization group with a social group. Is socialization a health-promoting activity? What are the reasons for your answer?
3. Normally in groups we each tend to play certain typical roles. Analyze your own role behavior in groups. What roles do you commonly play as a member, and are they task or maintenance focused?
4. Imagine yourself to be the community health nurse in the case study of the Wilford County Public Health Nursing Service. You have just become a member of a planning team newly formed to assess and plan for the

needs of these adolescent girls. What are some assessment strategies you could use and suggest to the group? Discuss some specific actions you might take to begin the assessment.

References

Bennis, W. G., & Shepard, H. A. (1956). A theory of group development. *Human Relations, 9,* 415–457.

Blum, H. L. (1981). *Planning for health: Generics for the eighties* (2nd ed.). New York: Human Sciences Press.

Bradford, L., Stock, D., & Horwitz, M. (1976). How to diagnose group problems. In S. Stone, M. Berger, D. Elhart, S. Firsich, & S. Jordan (Eds.), *Management for nurses* (pp. 133–146). St. Louis: C. V. Mosby.

Churgin, S. (1981). Evaluation. In H. L. Blum (Ed.), Planning for health: Generics for the eighties (2nd ed.) (pp. 270–299). New York: Human Sciences Press.

Dever, G. E. A. (1980). *Community health analysis.* Germantown, MD: Aspen Systems.

Erikson, E. (1963). *Childhood and society* (2nd ed.). New York: W. W. Norton.

Gouldner, A., & Gouldner, H. P. (1963). *Modern sociology.* New York: Harcourt, Brace & World.

Guthrie, E., & Miller, S. (1978). *Making change: A guide to effectiveness in groups.* Minneapolis, MN: Interpersonal Communication Programs.

Hill, W. F. (1962). *Learning through discussion: Guide for leaders and members of discussion groups.* Beverly Hills, CA: Sage.

Homans, G. C. (1950). *The human group.* New York: Harcourt, Brace & World.

Konopka, G. (1954). *Group work in the institution.* New York: Whiteside.

Loomis, M. E. (1979). *Group process for nurses.* St. Louis: C. V. Mosby.

Marram, G. D. (1978). *The group approach in nursing practice* (2nd ed.). St. Louis: C. V. Mosby.

Maslow, A. (1954). *Motivation and personality.* New York: Harper & Row.

Mill, C. R., & Porter, L. C. (1976). What to observe in a group. In C. Mill & L. Porter (Eds.), *Reading book* (pp. 28–30). Washington, DC: National Training Laboratories Institute for Applied Behavioral Science.

Nutt, P. C. (1984). *Planning methods for health and related organizations.* New York: Wiley.

Pfeiffer, J., & Jones, J. E. (Eds.). (1974). *A handbook of structural experiences: Human relations training* (Vol. 1) (rev. ed.). La Jolla, CA: University Associates.

Sampson, E., & Marthas, M. (1977). *Group process for the health professions.* Somerset, NJ: Wiley.

Schutz, D. (1966). *The interpersonal underworld.* Palo Alto, CA: Science and Behavior Books.

Sweeney, B. (1975). Learning groups: Survival level, growth level. *Journal of Nursing Education, 14*(3), 20–26.

Tubbs, S. L., & Moss, S. (1974). The small group: Therapeutic communication. In S. Tubbs & S. Moss (Eds.), *Human communication: An interpersonal perspective* (pp. 231–257). New York: Random House.

Uris, A. (1964). *Techniques of leadership.* New York: McGraw-Hill.

Veninga, R. (1973). The management of conflict. *Journal of Nursing Administration, 3*(4), 12–16.

Williams, C. (1977). Community health nursing — What is it? *Nursing Outlook, 25,* 250–253.

Yalom, I. D. (1975). *The theory and practice of group psychotherapy.* New York: Basic Books.

Selected Readings

Abramson, J. H. (1974). *Survey methods in community medicine.* Edinburgh: Churchill Livingstone.

Benne, K. D. (1976). The current state of planned changing in persons, groups, communities and societies. In W. G. Bennis, K. Benne, R. Chin, & K. Corey (Eds.), *The planning of change* (3rd ed.) (pp. 68–83). New York: Holt, Rinehart and Winston.

Bennis, W. G., & Shepard, H. A. (1956). A theory of group development. *Human Relations, 9*–14, 415.

Berne, E. (1963). *The structure and dynamics of organizations and groups.* New York: Lippincott.

Blum, H. L. (1981). *Planning for health: Generics for the eighties* (2nd ed.). New York: Human Sciences Press.

Bormann, E. G., & Bormann, N. C. (1976). *Effective small group communication* (2nd ed.). Minneapolis, MN: Burgess.

Bradford, L., Stock, D., & Horwitz, M. (1976). How to diagnose group problems. In S. Stone, M. Berger, D. Elhart, S. Firsich, & S. Jordan (Eds.), *Management for nurses* (pp. 133–146). St. Louis: C. V. Mosby.

Bruhn, J. G. (1973). Planning for social change: Dilemmas for health planning. *American Journal of Public Health, 63,* 602–605.

Burnside, I. M. (1978). *Working with the elderly: Group processes and techniques.* North Scituate, MA: Duxbury Press.

Cathart, R. S., & Samovar, L. A. (Eds.). (1974). *Small group communication: A reader* (2nd ed.). Dubuque, IA: Brown.

Chopra, A. (1973). Motivation in task-oriented groups. *Journal of Nursing Administration, 3*(1), 15.

Cohen, P. (1982). Community health planning from an interorganizational perspective. *American Journal of Public Health, 72,* 717–721.

Dever, G. E. A. (1980). *Community health analysis.* Germantown, MD: Aspen Systems.

Dyer, W. G. (1973). Working with groups. In A. Reinhardt & M. Quinn (Eds.), *Family-centered community nursing: A sociocultural framework.* St. Louis: C. V. Mosby.

Green, L. (1980). *Health education planning: A diagnostic approach.* Palo Alto, CA: Mayfield Publishing.

Guthrie, E., & Miller, S. (1978). *Making change: A guide to effectiveness in groups.* Minneapolis, MN: Interpersonal Communication Programs.

Henkel, B. L. (1970). Solving health problems through small group action. In B. Henkel (Ed.), *Community health* (2nd ed.) (pp. 338–347). Boston: Allyn and Bacon.

Hill, W. F. (1962). *Learning through discussion: Guide for leaders and members of discussion groups.* Beverly Hills, CA: Sage.

Hyman, H. H. (1981). *Health planning — A systematic approach* (2nd ed.). Germantown, MD: Aspen Systems.

Kraegel, J. (Ed.). (1980). *Organization-environment relationships.* Wakefield, MA: Nursing Resources.

Larson, M., & Williams, R. (1978). How to become a better group leader? Learn to recognize the strange things that happen to some people in groups. *Nursing '78, 8*(8), 65.

Loomis, M. E. (1979). *Group process for nurses.* St. Louis: C. V. Mosby.

Marram, G. D. (1978). *The group approach in nursing practice* (2nd ed.). St. Louis: C. V. Mosby.

McLaughlin, J. (1982). Toward a theoretical model for community health programs. *Advances in Nursing Science, 5*(2), 7–28.

McLemore, M. K. M. (1980). Nurses as health planners. *Journal of Nursing Administration, 1*(9), 13–17.

Milio, N. (1975). *The care of health in communities.* New York: Macmillan.

Mill, C. R., & Porter, L. C. (1976). What to observe in a group. In C. Mill & L. Porter (Eds.), *Reading book* (pp. 28–30). Washington, DC: National Training Laboratories Institute for Applied Behavioral Science.

Neuber, K. A. (1980). *Needs assessment: A model for community planning.* Beverly Hills, CA: Sage.

Nutt, P. C. (1984). *Planning methods for health and related organizations.* New York: Wiley.

Ohlsen, M. M. (1977). *Group counseling* (2nd ed.). New York: Holt, Rinehart and Winston.

Reinhardt, A., & Chatlin, E. (1977). Assessment of health needs in a community: The basis for program planning. In A. Reinhardt & M. Quinn (Eds.), *Current practice in family-centered community nursing* (pp. 138–187). St. Louis: C. V. Mosby.

Rossi, P., & Freeman, H. (1982). *Evaluation: A systematic approach* (2nd ed.). Beverly Hills, CA: Sage.

Sampson, E., & Marthas, M. (1977). *Group process for the health professions.* Somerset, NJ: Wiley.

Shaw, M. E. (1971). *Group dynamics: The psychology of small group behavior.* New York: McGraw-Hill.

Shortell, S., & Richardson, W. (1978). *Health program evaluation.* St. Louis: C. V. Mosby.

Sweeney, B. (1975). Learning groups: Survival level, growth level. *Journal of Nursing Education, 14*(3), 20–26.

Tubbs, S. L., & Moss, S. (1974). The small group: Therapeutic communication. In S. Tubbs & S. Moss (Eds.), *Human communication: An interpersonal perspective* (pp. 231–257). New York: Random House.

Veninga, R. (1973). The management of conflict. *Journal of Nursing Administration, 3*(4), 12–16.

Veninga, R. (1982). Competency: Developing productive committees. In R. Veninga (Ed.), *The human side of health administration: A guide for hospital, nursing, and public health administrators* (pp. 153–195). Englewood Cliffs, NJ: Prentice-Hall.

Warheit, G., Bell, R., & Schwab, J. (1977). *Needs assessment approaches: Concepts and methods* (Pub. No. [ADM] 79-472). Washington, DC: National Institute of Mental Health.

Weis, C. (1972). *Evaluation research: Methods of assessing program effectiveness.* Englewood Cliffs, NJ: Prentice-Hall.

Yalom, I. D. (1975). *The theory and practice of group psychotherapy.* New York: Basic Books.

10

The Helping Relationship and Contracting

The helping relationship is a primary tool for community health nurses. It contributes to both the prevention of illness and the promotion of client health. In order to use the helping relationship skillfully in community health practice, we must understand the meaning and value of a therapeutic relationship. Unlike ordinary social relationships, it is based on mutual participation in establishing and carrying out goals. Clients and the nurse enter into a working agreement to meet specific client needs. The concept of contracting is closely tied to use of the helping relationship. This chapter examines both of these tools and discusses their integration into community health nursing practice.

The Helping Relationship: A Definition

The concept of a helping relationship has undergone a change in recent years. Traditionally, the term *helping* has implied that one individual gives help, and the other individual receives help. Viewed in this manner, the helping relationship inadvertently created a dependency relationship. Given our current consumer needs and our understanding of health care practice, this traditional model is no longer appropriate. Its weakness came from the fact that it made clients dependent on the nurse, undermined their self-confidence, and undercut their self-respect. In short, it reduced the very characteristics that the nurse hoped to foster. This traditional view of the helping relationship reduced clients' motivation to participate in the health care process and detracted from their sense of responsibility for maintaining their health.

This traditional definition has another inherent problem. It implies that the helping relationship occurs only between two individuals, the nurse and a single patient or client. Even the community health nurse working with a family, for example, may think in terms of establishing a helping relationship only with the mother or some other individual, rather than with the family as a whole. In community health nursing, the client will range from a single individual to an entire community. In the course of working, a single community health nurse might develop helping relationships with the following range of clients: (1) an elderly widower living alone in his own home, (2) an extended family of Cuban immigrants, (3) a parenting class of 15 women who have children, (4) a lumber company with 95 employees seeking to develop a wellness program, (5) a cluster of elementary schools seeking to improve nutrition among students, and (6) an entire community conducting a self-survey about health practices. Throughout this book, the term *client* refers to this broad range of individuals and groups. In order to maximize the effectiveness of the helping relationship in promoting client health, we need to redefine the meaning of this tool.

The helping relationship means *purposeful interaction between nurse and clients based on mutual participation.* This definition highlights only two basic features on the helping relationship; it has a goal and it involves both parties in setting and achieving that goal. In order to explore more fully the meaning of this relationship in the context of community health nursing, we shall examine five characteristics that distinguish it from other types of interaction, which will be referred to as simply "social relationships."

Characteristics of the Helping Relationship

EMPHASIS ON GOALS

First, the helping relationship in community health nursing is goal directed. The nurse and client recognize specific reasons why they enter into the relationship. For example, a large Thai family that recently immigrated wants to learn about nutrition; the community health nurse can provide that information. The client group and the nurse enter into the relationship with stated needs to be met and goals to accomplish. Other forms of social interaction, such as encounters between friends, often lack recognized goals.

UNILATERAL BENEFITS

Second, in community health the helping relationship is unilateral; that is, it exists for the benefit of the clients. In developing a helping relationship with the Thai immigrant family concerned about nutrition, the nurse may teach the family how to shop for food and eat in a new cultural setting. The direct benefits accrue to the family. Certainly the nurse gains satisfaction from the interaction, but the relationship is established to meet the needs of the clients. The nurse's satisfaction and growth are a side effect, not a stated objective. Many other social relationships, as among friends, business acquaintances, or professional colleagues, are bilateral. Both parties come to the relationship with an expectation of almost equivalent benefits.

EXPLICIT MUTUAL AGREEMENT

Third, in community health the helping relationship involves explicit mutual agreement. When you interact with a friend, relative, salesperson, or neighbor, the relationship operates with tacit rules; you probably do not talk about the relationship or direct your energy toward seeking an explicit consensus. The helping relationship, on the other hand, involves a reciprocal exchange in which both parties discuss what their interaction will involve. The mother, father, and grandparents in the Thai family may express their desire to provide their children with the right food. They may be concerned about loss of traditional foods and feel overwhelmed when shopping in supermarkets. They want the nurse to assist them in achieving their goals. The nurse discusses her role in giving this assistance. The relationship arises from an explicit, mutual agreement. This discussion of the goals and the nature of the relationship provides a channel within which the work of the relationship takes place.

SET RESPONSIBILITIES

Fourth, the helping relationship in community health nursing assigns set responsibilities to each party. A well-defined relationship clearly states what the client will do and what the nurse will do to accomplish the goals. The nurse, for example, might agree to take several members of the Thai family on a shopping trip, help them prepare a balanced meal, and provide reading materials on infant nutrition. The family would agree to study the materials (perhaps through an older child who can interpret for the adults), ask questions, and follow the example and instructions of the nurse. Each party to the helping relationship develops an understanding of individual responsibilities based on realistic and honest expectations. This understanding may not come with the first visit, but as the relationship develops, the nurse works toward this division of responsibilities. Together with the client, the nurse explores necessary resources, assesses the capabilities of clients, and discovers their willingness to assume tasks. This structure of recognized responsibilities is often absent in other human relationships. Two friends can enjoy long years of companionship without ever saying, "You do this and I will do these other things." A local church committee, set up to help an immigrant family, may assume all the responsibility for helping provide food for the family rather than dividing the responsibility.

SET BOUNDARIES

Fifth, the helping relationship in community health practice has set boundaries. Nearly every therapeutic relationship has a beginning and an end. A crucial part of defining the helping relationship is determining when and under what conditions to terminate it. The temporal boundaries are determined sometimes by progress toward the goal, sometimes by the number of nurse-client contacts, and often by setting a time limit. A nurse might set up eight sessions to help the Thai family with nutrition problems, or they might meet together weekly until the goal of adequate knowledge and skill was met. Other social relationships, in contrast, are generally open-ended in length. A friendship may end because of misunderstanding, or a business relationship may stop when a partner moves to another city. Table 10-1 summarizes the characteristics that distinguish the helping relationship from other social relationships.

Client Participation

This text has stressed that the helping relationship is based on mutual participation. The extent of that participation, however, varies, depending on the client's readiness and ability to participate. The level of wellness at the time of initial nurse-client encounter directly influences participation. Some people are not physically or emotionally well enough to assume an active role in the relationship. Women recently discharged from the hospital following a mastectomy, for example, have many physical and emotional adjustments with which to cope. Their families, too, must expend additional energies to provide needed support and to cope with the temporary loss of each woman's usual role in the family. They may find it difficult to engage actively in

Table 10-1
Contrast between Helping and Social Relationships

Helping Relationship	Social Relationship
Goal directed	No specific goals
Unilateral, benefits client	Bilateral, benefits both parties
Explicit mutual agreement	No consensus, casual interaction
Set responsibilities	Unstructured
Time limited, set boundaries	Open-ended in length and frequency of contacts

identifying their needs and goals at the start of the relationship. The nurse may have to take stronger initial leadership; however, the goals of a helping relationship are not abandoned. Eventually, as the women's level of wellness improves, the nurse can encourage more active participation from the clients and their families.

Sometimes clients' previous experiences with health personnel limit participation in the helping relationship. Clients from poverty areas, from different cultural backgrounds, or with little education may need extensive encouragement to participate actively in the helping relationship. Working with a Thai family, recently immigrated to the United States, will be quite different from helping a group of suburban women with infant nutrition. Clients previously regarded by health professionals as incapable of managing their own lives will also take a more passive role in the helping relationship. Even well-educated people with comfortable incomes have often learned to behave passively when dealing with physicians, nurses, or other health professionals. With all these people, unless the nurse persists in efforts to reduce the dependence of clients, the relationship can fall far short of the therapeutic goals.

The nurse's own view of the helping relationship will also influence the degree of client participation. Those nurses accustomed to relating to clients in an adult-to-child manner will restrict client involvement. If the nurse sees her position as more informed and the client's position as one of complete ignorance and need, a paternalistic relationship may develop. All clients have resources on which to build, and the community health nurse helps clients discover them.

Clients who initiate care, such as postpartum mothers who ask for home visits or families who request follow-up care after hospitalization, are frequently best able to assume an active participant role. They have already demonstrated a sense of responsibility for their health by identifying a need and asking for assistance. The nurse will still have to work carefully to build mutual participation, but its development is more likely to occur.

Skills Needed in the Helping Relationship

Communication is the lifeblood of the helping relationship. It provides the vitality and nourishment necessary to foster a healthy nurse-client relationship. For communication to take place, clients and nurses send and receive messages. As participants in the communication process, community health nurses play both roles — sender and receiver. The nurse working with an alcoholic housewife must learn to "read" the messages this woman sends. The nurse will also have to speak and act in ways that communicate effectively. Community health nursing requires two sets of communication skills — sending skills and receiving skills.

Sending Skills

Sending skills enable nurses to communicate messages effectively. Through these skills nurses convey thoughts and feelings to clients. Two important considerations will influence clarity and effectiveness of message sending. First, the extent of the nurse's self-awareness will affect the communication. Does she feel anxious, angry, impatient, or concerned? Is she tired? Do certain clients irritate her? What motives and interests does she have for wanting to communicate with these clients? Second, her awareness of the receiver will influence the sending of messages. What do these clients seem to want or need? Is the message suited to their cultural background and level of understanding? Does the message have significance for them? How do clients respond as we send the message?

Two main channels are used to send messages: nonverbal and verbal. Nonverbal messages, those conveyed without words, constitute nearly two-thirds of the messages transmitted in normal communication (Brill, 1973). We send messages nonverbally in many ways. Our personal appearance, dress, posture, and cleanliness all communicate messages about us. They may enhance or discredit what we say. Body language often speaks louder than words. Facial expressions convey acceptance or rejection, interest or boredom, and apprehension or confidence. Gestures and bodily movements such as hand clenching, finger tapping, or foot swinging all communicate strong messages to clients. Eye contact or lack of it carries additional meaning. Tone of voice and use of silence will also send nonverbal messages. Accepting food may communicate acceptance, while getting a chair for a client may say "I'm interested in your welfare."

Verbal messages communicate ideas, but they also convey attitudes and feelings. Nurses cannot assume that the intent of their words is always understood by clients. Effective sending skills depend on asking for feedback to make certain that the receiver understood the verbal message's intent. Communication can improve if speakers avoid jargon. Like all occupations, nursing has its own vocabulary. Often unfamiliar to clients, this jargon may carry different meanings or make the client feel inferior because he cannot speak that language. Mr. Jones did not know what to answer when the nurse asked if he had "voided." Mrs. Wendt felt confused when asked if she had noticed any expressions of "sibling rivalry" by her three-year-old child. When nursing jargon becomes part of everyday speech, only special effort will enable nurses to set it aside when interacting with clients. The basic rules for effective sending can be summarized in this manner: keep the message honest and uncomplicated; use as few words as possible to state it; and ask for reactions to make certain that it is understood.

Receiving Skills

Receiving skills are as important to communication as sending skills. They enable nurses to receive accurate and complete messages. Receiving skills involve not only listening to what people say but also observing their behavior. If a client says, "I haven't been feeling well," the nurse needs to discover the context of this statement. What tone of voice did the client use? What was the meaning of the client's facial expressions? What gestures accompanied the statement? When did the client mention these feelings? Effective receiving skills require training to observe these kinds of details.

The other main source of receiving is active listening, the skill of assuming responsibility for understanding the meaning of the client's message (Wismer, 1978). Instead of requiring the client to make the nurse understand, the nurse should actively work to discover what a client means. Understanding the message from the client's perspective demands carefull attention. It arises from a genuine interest in what the speaker has to say. Active listeners demonstrate their interest, perhaps by sitting forward, sustaining eye contact, nodding the head, and asking occasional questions for clarification. They concentrate in order to avoid daydreaming or the pretense of listening, both of which block communication.

Nurses can also listen actively by asking reflective questions. Such questions restate what the client has said:

Client: "Quitting smoking is impossible."
Nurse: "You feel you can't quit smoking?"

Reflective questions have a twofold purpose: to show a sincere attempt to understand accurately clients' messages, and to make clear that the messages and the clients are important to the nurse.

Active listening will communicate acceptance and increase trust, especially when a negative evaluation of the message or the way it is delivered is withheld. A critical response to the message cuts off communication. Active listening enables nurses to encourage clients to deliberate carefully and develop problem-solving skills; it avoids the pitfall of telling them what to do.

Effective communication, both sending and receiving, is strongly influenced by three factors. First, the previous experiences of both sender and receiver influence their perceptions and the meanings they attach to messages. Requests for clarification will help verify that messages are being received as intended. Second, the respective cultures of sender and receiver influence understanding and acceptance of messages. A nervous laugh, appropriate as an outlet in one culture, may appear rude and disrespectful to someone from another culture. Silence may indicate patience and thoughtfulness to one group of people but weakness or indifference to another. With many clients, the nurse will have to communicate cross-culturally, which requires patience and constant effort to ensure accurate and inoffensive messages. Third, the relationships among participants during communication can significantly influence its effectiveness. Since much of community health nursing involves families and groups, communication patterns become quite complex. When a large number of people are involved, interaction requires skill in eliciting feedback from all members and in generating a common understanding among the group.

Interpersonal Skills

In addition to effective communication, the helping relationship also requires three other interpersonal skills — showing respect, empathizing, and developing trust. Each of these skills depends on effective communication but surpasses the mere exchange of messages.

SHOWING RESPECT

Showing respect means conveying the attitude that clients have importance, dignity, and worth. Community health nurses can express respect by helping clients feel that they have valuable ideas. Nurses can let them know that they want to understand the situation from their point of view. Nurses show respect by the manner in which they address clients, for instance, by using the courtesy titles of "Mr." or "Mrs." until permission is granted to use first names. On a more subtle level, the tone of voice can either show respect or make people feel inferior and insignificant. Clients need to feel respected if they are to enter fully into the mutual exchange necessary for a true helping relationship.

EMPATHIZING

Empathizing is another important interpersonal skill. Empathy means the "ability to borrow another person's feelings . . . [and] to understand them while maintaining one's own identity" (Kalisch, 1973, p. 1548). Nurses empathize by reflecting the client's feelings, that is, by showing an attempt to understand the source and meanings of those feelings. Empathy is best expressed in the client's language. The same terms and, if possible, the same tone of voice as the clients' should be used. For example, the nurse can reflect sadness if the client seems sad. Empathy is best expressed provisionally, showing that the nurse is still attempting to ascertain the client's true feelings while allowing the client to validate each provisional expression. Empathy conveys the message, "This is the way it seems to me. Is that right?" It focuses attention on clients and their feelings. It shows that the nurse shares their concerns, and it makes clients feel important.

DEVELOPING TRUST

Developing trust is necessary for an effective helping relationship. Clients will not express their true feelings if they do not fully trust the nurse. Many

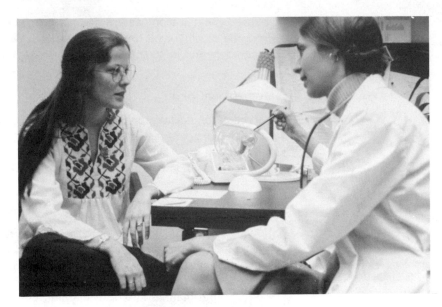

Figure 10-1
Development of trust is
crucial to an effective help-
ing relationship.

times clients will say what they think the nurse wants to hear. They may agree to a plan of action simply because they do not want to displease the nurse. They may hide true feelings because they think that the nurse is eager for a decision. Nurses develop trust by showing that they truly accept clients, that they believe in them as people. Trust generates trust; as the nurse shows confidence in clients, they will respond in kind. Treating them as fully participating partners in the relationship shows clients that they are trustworthy with responsibilities. Trust is also developed through an open, honest, and patient approach with clients. Candid discussion in a flexible time frame encourages clients to share their real feelings and to move at their own pace. As trust develops, the relationship becomes a truly helping one, focused on client needs (see Fig. 10-1).

Structure of the Helping Relationship

The skills that lead to an effective helping relationship are used within a particular structure. Awareness of this structure can greatly increase the nurse's ability to help clients. Because the relationship is bound by time, the structure involves several phases. The way nurses use their skills during the first and last phases of the helping relationship may contrast. It is useful to think of the helping relationship's following a sequential structure: (1) a beginning phase when the relationship is just being established; (2) a middle, working phase; and (3) a termination phase when the relationship ends (Brill, 1973). In the context of this process, the work of identifying and meeting client needs takes place.

The first phase is a period of establishing and defining the relationship. The nurse and clients are getting to know each other; they seek to establish communication patterns and develop trust. From these bases, they identify the clients' needs and determine the goals toward which they will work.

The middle phase occurs when nurse and clients start working together to accomplish the goals of the relationship. Their work may include assessment and planning as well as implementation and evaluation. The cycle of the nursing process will be repeated as needed during this working phase until goals are accomplished and no further goals identified.

The termination phase occurs when the need for nurse and clients to work together has ended. In many instances, clients can function on their own. When clients and nurse have grown close in the relationship, termination can be difficult. It often requires careful advance preparation to make certain that all parties understand when and why it is taking place. Termination helps to ensure a clear-cut end to the relationship. One nurse had made home visits to a refugee family for nearly a year. As the family's multiple needs declined, she decided to taper off her assistance. Two months before ending the relationship, she discussed termination with the family. At first the family members were frightened at the loss of help, but slowly they came to accept it and assumed more and more responsibility for their health needs. Had she announced the end of her visits more abruptly, the family might have easily felt confused or rejected.

The Concept of Contracting

The primary goal of community health nursing is to promote the public's health through identifying and meeting people's needs. Success demands active participation of clients. The helping relationship is "helping" only in the sense that nurses assist people in this process. Without mutual participation, clients cannot develop ability in self-care. Contracting makes the goal of self-care explicit.

The concept of self-care has a long history in community health nursing. Public health nursing, as Norris (1979) has shown, was founded on self-care concepts and originated self-care practice. More recently, self-care has come into its own through the growth of independent nursing practice. Kinlein (1977), for example, bases her independent practice squarely on this concept. She found that clients had far more capability than was believed in achieving self-care. She believes that nursing means helping clients choose the self-care practices best for them. Like the shopkeeper who expects his customers to make their own selections, the nurse treats clients as independent consumers, saying, "I believe in your ability to assume responsibility for your own health." By making self-care more explicit, contracting can become a powerful tool in community health nursing.

Contracting means negotiating a working agreement between two or more parties. They come to a shared understanding and then give consent to the purposes and terms of the transaction. Some kinds of contracts are familiar, for example, a contract connected with buying a car. Other, less obvious agreements, such as paying tuition for an education, still involve a form of contracting. As a student, you agree with an educational institution on the purposes (their financial reimbursement, your degree) and terms of the contract (regular tuition payments, regular learning opportunities), even though a formal document is not signed.

In contrast to legal contracts that are written binding agreements, the contract in a helping relationship is flexible and based on mutual understanding and trust. Sloan and Schommer (1982, p. 222) define the community nursing contract as "any working agreement, continuously renegotiable" between client and nurse. When viewed from this perspective, contracting becomes a valuable tool for community health nurses.

Features of Contracting

PARTNERSHIP

The concept of contracting as used in the helping relationship incorporates four distinctive features. The first is partnership. All aspects of contracting involve shared participation and agreement between client and nurse; they become partners in the relationship. For example, the Ericksons, an older couple who requested community health nursing visits at home, entered into a partnership with a nurse after the husband was discharged from the hospital with a colostomy. They came to an agreement on what the couple needed and what the nurse could provide. Together they developed goals, outlined methods to meet those goals, and explored resources to help achieve them. They defined the time limits for the contract as well as their separate responsibilities. The contract involved reciprocal negotiation and shared evaluation. A partnership means that both parties are responsible for setting up and carrying out the service.

COMMITMENT

Second, every contract implies a commitment. Both parties make a decision that binds them to fulfilling the purpose of the contract. In the helping relationship, contracting does not mean a binding agreement in the legal sense; rather, it is a pledge of trust and dedication. Accompanying that sense of dedication is a strong motivation to see the contract through to completion. Both parties feel responsible for keeping promises; both want to achieve the intended outcomes. When the nurse and the Ericksons identified their separate tasks, they committed themselves: "Yes, we will do thus and so. . . ."

FORMAT

Format is the third distinctive feature of the concept of contracting. Unlike many nurse-client interactions, contracting defines the terms of the relationship. Thus both client and nurse obtain a clear idea of the purpose of the relationship, of their respective responsibilities, and of the specific limits within which they will work. In other words, contracting provides a framework for the relationship. Once the terms of the contract have been spelled out, there is no question about what has to be done, who is to do it, or within what time frame it is to be accomplished. This format helps to prevent a frequently recurring problem in community health nursing — the difficulty of termination of a long-term relationship. It also helps to prevent dependency relationships from developing.

NEGOTIATION

Finally, contracting always involves negotiation. The nurse proposes to accept certain responsibilities, and then asks if the clients agree. The nurse might ask, "What do you feel you can do to achieve this goal?" A period of give and take occurs in which ideas are discussed and conclusions, which often represent compromises, are reached. A few weeks later, nurse and clients may find that terms they had agreed upon need modification. Perhaps clients have assumed more responsibility than they can realistically handle at that point in time. Perhaps the nurse does not feel comfortable teaching a complex technique and needs to utilize an outside resource. Negotiation during contracting allows for changes that facilitate the ultimate achievement of goals. It provides contracting with built-in flexibility and encourages ongoing communication between clients and nurse. Negotiation gives contracting a dynamic quality (see Fig. 10-2). It becomes a complex process that moves through eight stages, each negotiated between the nurse and clients. This process will be considered later in the chapter.

Value of Contracting

The value of contracting has been demonstrated in many settings. Contracts have been used for many years in psychiatric nursing settings to promote client self-respect, problem-solving skills, autonomy, and motivation (Davis & Woodcock, 1971; Rosen, 1978). Other disciplines, such as social work,

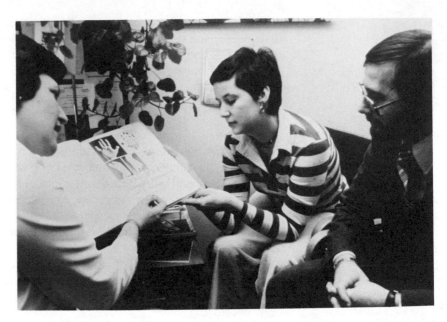

Figure 10-2
An important feature of contracting involves mutual agreement between the family and the nurse on the material they want to cover in their sessions together.

use contracting as a tool in the helping relationship to enhance realistic planning and emphasize partnership (Sauer, 1973). Educational contracts between students and instructors have proven valuable for facilitating learning (Lindberg & Simms, 1974). Community health nursing has also used the concept of contracting for many years. Without always labeling their work as such, community health nurses have contracted with clients who wanted to lose weight, mutually agreeing to certain exercise and eating patterns for clients and teaching and support responsibilities for the nurse. Often they have set a time limit, such as six months, to achieve the intended weight loss. Community health nurses have entered into contractual relationships with postpartum mothers, new diabetics, postsurgical patients, prenatal groups, and many others. In each case, a partnership developed with agreement about the purpose of the relationship and the conditions under which it would be carried out. They were, in effect, contracting.

Recognition of contracting as a tool has come more recently. Blair (1971) has described her developing awareness of the need for the nurse to encourage clients to act for themselves rather than to place them in a passive, dependent role. Using transactional analysis theory, she developed a professional treatment contract that she defined as "a mutual understanding of the reason for the service and the problems or areas that will be discussed during the [community nursing] visits" (1971, p. 588). Others have worked with the concept and refined it further. In one nursing education setting, students contracted with families and found that reaching a mutual agreement about the goals of service was beneficial to both clients and nurses (Sheridan & Smith, 1975).

278

Nurses in many settings recognize the value of the mutual participation model and use it to involve clients in the helping relationship and in use of the nursing process. Some suggest that contracting should be treated as a specific step in the helping process (Brill, 1973; Langford, 1978). As more and more nurses seek to promote client autonomy and self-care, contracting's wide applicability to nursing practice is being increasingly recognized.

Emphasis on contracting as a *method* rather than a *concept* can create problems. If one's experiences with contracts have all been business agreements, it is possible to carry the stereotype of a cold, formal arrangement into the nursing practice setting. Some nurses fear that asking clients to negotiate a contract will place clients under stress, impede the development of trust, and negatively influence the helping relationship. Others have found that some clients, who prefer to have the nurse make decisions for them, are not ready to enter into any kind of negotiation.

The concept of contracting, however, has much broader application than has simple methodology. As a concept, contracting applies basic principles of adult education — self-direction, mutual negotiation, and mutual evaluation (Gustafson, 1977). These principles become both the means and the ends of contracting. To varying degrees, all clients are able to assess, plan, implement, and evaluate in contracting, yet the concept can be applied in a variety of ways. Sloan and Schommer (1982) demonstrate that contracting can be formal or informal, written or verbal, simple or detailed, and signed or unsigned by clients and nurse. Like all nursing tools, contracting will enhance client health only if adapted to each situation.

The advantages of contracting in community health nursing can now be summarized:

1. It involves clients in their own care.
2. It motivates clients to perform necessary tasks.
3. It individualizes care by focusing on clients' unique needs, whether the client is an individual or a group.
4. It increases the possibility of achieving health goals identified by clients and nurse.
5. It develops problem-solving skills of nurse and clients.
6. It fosters client participation in the decision-making process.
7. It promotes clients' autonomy and self-esteem as they learn self-care.
8. It makes nursing service more efficient and cost-effective.

The Process of Contracting

Because contracting is rather complex, some stages will occur before others. Without some kind of sequence, negotiation of a contract can become overwhelming. Consider the fact that this working agreement depends on knowing what clients want, agreeing on goals, identifying methods to achieve these goals, knowing the resources that the nurse and clients bring to the relationship, utilizing appropriate outside resources, setting limits, deciding on responsibilities, and providing for periodic reviews. Each of these tasks requires discussion between and decision making by nurse and clients.

These tasks are incorporated into the process of contracting in a sequence that provides a guide for nurses and their clients. Sloan and Schommer (1982) describe eight phases in the process:

1. *Exploration of needs* — assessment of client's health, problems, and needs by client and nurse
2. *Establishment of goals* — discussion and agreement between client and nurse on goals and objectives
3. *Exploration of resources* — defining what client and nurse each have to offer to and expect from each other; identifying appropriate resources such as significant others, agencies, and other professionals
4. *Development of a plan* — identifying methods and activities for achieving the goals
5. *Division of responsibilities* — negotiating the activities for which client and nurse will each be responsible
6. *Agreement on time frame* — setting limits for the contract in terms of length of time or number of visits
7. *Evaluation* — periodic and final assessment of progress toward goals occurring at agreed-upon intervals
8. *Renegotiation or termination* — agreement to modify, renegotiate, or terminate the contract

As community health nurses use this process to negotiate a contract, they must adapt it to each situation. The exact sequence of phases may change and some steps may overlap. Nevertheless, the basic elements remain important considerations for successful contracting (see Fig. 10-3).

Consider the way one community health nurse used the contractual process. Eileen met the Nelsons through the agency's well-child clinic. Mrs. Nelson had been bringing 16-month-old Thor in for regular checkups and immunizations since they had moved to the city a year earlier. After becoming pregnant again, she approached Eileen about prenatal home visits to learn more about pregnancy and delivery. They made an appointment for Eileen's first visit.

Eight Phases of Contracting

EXPLORATION OF NEEDS

Eileen explained the importance of focusing the visits on Mrs. Nelson's wants. She questioned Mrs. Nelson about her previous pregnancy, concerns, and interests and suggested possible topics for discussion. In Eileen's agency,

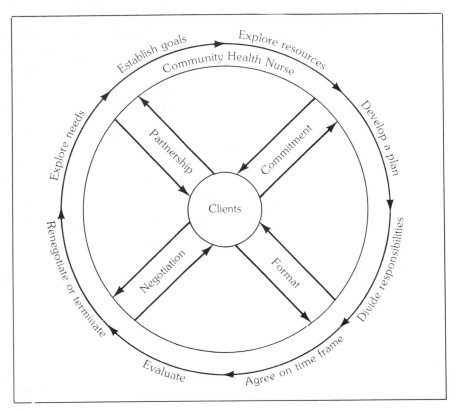

Figure 10-3
The concept and process of contracting. Contracting is based on four distinctive features shown here as spokes that support a wheel. These features form the basis for a reciprocal relationship between nurse and clients. This relationship is not static; it is a dynamic process that moves through phases, represented here as the outer rim of the wheel. The relationship moves forward, focused on meeting clients' needs, and enables the nurse to facilitate ultimate achievement of clients' goals.

the supervisor and staff had developed a prenatal catalog, a scrapbook of topics helpful to prospective mothers, which was illustrated with pictures from magazines. It was, in effect, a sales catalog that depicted many of the services the nurses could offer. Activities shown included teaching nutrition; demonstrating exercises; and discussing growth and development of the fetus, changes in the mother's body, the process of labor and delivery, postpartum developments, and care of the newborn. Eileen had found the catalog useful for helping clients to become aware of their choices and to select topics to cover in the contractual relationship. She offered to bring it on the second visit, and at that time, they would make some definite decisions about what Mrs. Nelson wanted.

ESTABLISHMENT OF GOALS

After examining and discussing the catalog items and exploring other potential health needs, Eileen and Mrs. Nelson agreed to focus on pregnancy, labor, and delivery. They agreed upon the goals of a comfortable pregnancy and a modified natural childbirth for Mrs. Nelson. To make these goals more workable, they broke them down into objectives. One, for example, was to use Lamaze breathing techniques during childbirth. Another was to eat a well-balanced diet that would make Mrs. Nelson feel energetic and still keep her weight gain under 20 pounds.

EXPLORATION OF RESOURCES

Eileen questioned further about the amount of time and energy Mrs. Nelson wanted to commit to this project. Could she spend half an hour a day, for instance, on exercises? They discussed what Mrs. Nelson was willing to do and what Eileen, given her time schedule, could realistically do. Mr. Nelson wanted to be present during teaching sessions. They also agreed that Mrs. Nelson would consult her obstetrician.

DEVELOPMENT OF A PLAN

By the end of the second visit, Eileen and Mrs. Nelson had made a list of the specific, goal-related topics to cover in each session. Beside each topic they wrote down methods and activities. For example, on the next visit, Eileen would bring teaching tools and pamphlets and explain components of a well-balanced diet during pregnancy. Mrs. Nelson, then, would prepare a sample menu for her family that included a proper balance of the foods she needed. Since Mr. Nelson was to be part of the contract, they decided to have him look over the plan, make suggestions, and meet with them on the subsequent visits. The Nelsons both agreed to be present for each appointment. They changed the visit time to late afternoon when Mr. Nelson arrived home from work.

DIVISION OF RESPONSIBILITIES

Eileen encouraged the Nelsons to take an active role in each visit. Mrs. Nelson agreed to practice the exercises half an hour daily and to keep a record of her diet. Mr. Nelson's responsibilities were to encourage his wife to stick to the diet and exercises and to practice them with her when feasible. They agreed that Eileen would be responsible for presenting new material, demonstrating exercises and other techniques, and indicating whether or not the Nelsons were performing new activities correctly.

AGREEMENT ON TIME FRAME

Their list of topics helped Eileen and the Nelsons decide on the number of visits needed. They agreed on a schedule that spread visits throughout the pregnancy and six weeks postpartum. From the start, then, all parties agreed on a tentative termination date for the relationship.

EVALUATION

A part of their plan was to do monthly evaluations to determine the satisfaction each felt with the plan and the progress being made. This built in the possibility of renegotiation; anyone could suggest needed changes at those times. At the conclusion of the contract period (six weeks postpartum), they agreed to discuss how well all the goals had been met.

RENEGOTIATION OR TERMINATION

The Nelsons and Eileen agreed to renegotiate the time frame of the contract if new needs arose. Otherwise, they would terminate the service six weeks after the baby was born.

Levels of Contracting

Community health nurses conduct the contracting process at levels that range from formal to informal. The degree of formality depends in large measure on the nurse's comfort in using this tool and clients' readiness to assume responsibility for self-care. At the most formal level, the parties usually negotiate a written contract. Drawn up by mutual agreement, each person signs it, and a third party sometimes witnesses the signing. This form of contract is sometimes used in mental health settings where the seriousness of the working agreement and the need to involve the client actively are important aspects of therapy (Davis & Woodcock, 1971). Less formal contracts, such as that with the Nelsons, are more commonly used. The nursing care plan becomes the written contract; thus no additional paper work is required. In one suburban health department, community health nurses contract with clients of a hypertension clinic. Part of their written care plan is a list of the client's goals and methods for achieving them (see Fig. 10-4). Under the column entitled "Responsibility," the nurse or client is listed as responsible for carrying out the activity.

Some situations lend themselves best to a modified use of contracting. For example, one nurse had been making regular visits to a man dying of cancer. After his death, she contracted informally with his wife to continue visits for the purpose of helping her work through the grieving process. They discussed and agreed on the goals, methods, and responsibilities each would have, but did not negotiate a formal contract. Another community mental health nurse formed a therapy group composed of her individual clients. She used modified contracting by discussing with clients the purpose of the group and the number of sessions needed, and by obtaining their agreement to attend all sessions.

Informal contracting does involve some form of verbal agreement about relatively uncomplicated tasks: "You take your pills every day as prescribed,

CLIENT-NURSE CONTRACT

Date accomplished	Goals	Date begun	Date ended	Methods	Responsibility
	1. To understand hypertension			a. Explain physiology of hypertension	N
				b. Interpret pamphlet on hypertension	C
				c. List risk factors associated with hypertension	C
	2. To decrease stress at work			a. Identify coping skills	N-C
				b. Explore possibility of job change	C
				c. List ways to relieve stress on job	N-C
				d. Design plan to relieve stress at work	C
				e. Implement plan until blood pressure is down to 115/75	C
	3. To lose 10 lb within 2 months			a. Explain nutritional factors influencing hypertension	N
				b. Design a diet plan	N-C
				c. Prepare exercise plan	C
				d. Implement plans until weight goal achieved	C

Length of contract:

Fee determination:

Signatures: Client _____ Date _____

Nurse _____ Date _____

Figure 10-4
Part of a contract developed between a client (C) and a nurse (N) in a community hypertension clinic.

and I will get a homemaker for you"; "You come to the clinic each week, and I will show you how to plan your diabetic diet." Sometimes nurses use contracting informally without realizing it. They conclude a home visit by agreeing with the family about the purpose and time of the next appointment. Conscious use of the tool, however, is a more effective way to provide structure for the relationship and foster client involvement, regardless of the level at which it is applied.

The level of contracting may also change during the development of a helping relationship. Clients often need education about their options. Initially they may have difficulty in identifying needs and making choices. The nurse can work to promote their self-confidence and help them assume increasing responsibility for their own health. Through these efforts, contracting becomes a consciously recognized part of the relationship. Clients can then become fully participating partners.

Summary

The helping relationship is a tool for promoting client health and the ability to engage in self-care. It is goal directed, unilateral in that it exists for the benefit of the client, and limited by time; it encourages mutual participation and involves clearly defined responsibilities.

Successful development of a helping relationship depends on the community health nurse's effective use of communication and interpersonal skills. To send and receive verbal or nonverbal messages well, nurses must be aware of themselves as well as of clients. It involves recognition of variables that might influence a message's interpretation. Nurses can cultivate the following skills: active listening, seeking feedback, showing respect, empathizing, and developing trust.

The helping relationship moves through three phases. During the beginning phase, the relationship is established and defined. The middle phase is a working period focused on meeting identified goals. The termination phase occurs when clients and nurse no longer need to work together.

Contracting has four distinctive features. First, it involves partnership. Contracting utilizes shared participation and two-way agreement between client and nurse. Second, it involves commitment, a promise to carry out certain responsibilities. Third, contracting's format defines goals, methods, responsibilities, and time limits. Fourth, contracting involves negotiation between clients and nurse.

The process of contracting utilizes eight phases that may sometimes vary in sequence or overlap: (1) exploration of needs, (2) establishment of goals, (3) exploration of resources, (4) development of a plan, (5) division of responsibilities, (6) agreement on time frame, (7) evaluation, and (8) renegotiation or termination.

Community health nurses practice contracting at levels ranging from formal to informal. Choice of level depends on the nurse's skill, client readiness, and demands of the situation. Clients may need assistance and instruction before they can assume the responsibilities of partners in contracting.

Study Questions

1. Describe the five characteristics of a helping relationship that distinguish it from other kinds of interactions. Discuss how you would apply these characteristics to working with a group of unwed adolescent mothers.
2. What is contracting? Discuss its four distinctive features and the advantages that contracting offers to the community health nurse.
3. Why is termination an important consideration for community health nursing practice?

References

Blair, K. K. (1971). It's the patient's problem and decision. *Nursing Outlook, 19*, 588–589.

Brill, N. I. (1973). *Working with people: The helping process.* Philadelphia: Lippincott.

Davis, R. C., & Woodcock, E. (1971). The nursing contract: An alternative in care. *Journal of Psychiatric Nursing, 9*, 26–27.

Gustafson, M. B. (1977). Let's broaden our horizons about the use of contracts. *International Nursing Review, 24*(1), 18–19.

Kalisch, B. (1973). What is empathy? *American Journal of Nursing, 73*, 1548–1552.

Kinlein, M. L. (1977). *Independent nursing practice with clients.* Philadelphia: Lippincott.

Langford, T. (1978). Establishing a nursing contract. *Nursing Outlook, 26*, 386–388.

Lindberg, J. B., & Simms, L. M. (1974). Contract grading: Incentives and rewards. *Image, 7*(1), 20–23.

Norris, C. M. (1979). Self-care. *American Journal of Nursing, 79*, 486–489.

Rosen, B. (1978). Contract therapy. *Nursing Times, 74*, 119–121.

Sauer, J. K. (1973, Summer). The process of contracting in the helping relationship. *Minnesota Welfare,* pp. 12–14, 23.

Sheridan, A., & Smith, R. (1975). Student-family contracts. *Nursing Outlook, 23*, 114–117.

Sloan, M., & Schommer, B. T. (1982). The process of contracting in community nursing. In B. W. Spradley (Ed.), *Readings in community health nursing* (2nd ed.) (pp. 197–204). Boston: Little, Brown.

Wismer, J. (1978). Communication effectiveness: Active listening and sending feeling messages. In J. W. Pfeiffer & J. Jones (Eds.), *The 1978 annual handbook for group facilitators.* La Jolla, CA: University Associates.

Selected Readings

Aiken, L., & Aiken, J. (1973). A systematic approach to the evaluation of interpersonal relationships. *American Journal of Nursing, 73,* 863–867.

Almore, M. G. (1979). Dyadic communication. *American Journal of Nursing, 79,* 1076–1078.

Avila, D., Combs, A. W., & Purskey, W. (1971). *The helping relationship sourcebook.* Boston: Allyn and Bacon.

Blair, K. K. (1971). It's the patient's problem and decision. *Nursing Outlook, 19,* 588–589.

Brammer, L. M. (1973). *The helping relationship, process and skills.* Englewood Cliffs, NJ: Prentice-Hall.

Brill, N. I. (1973). *Working with people: The helping process.* Philadelphia: Lippincott.

Combs, A. W., Avila, D., & Purkey, W. (1978). *Helping relationship — Basic concepts for the helping professions* (2nd ed.). Boston: Allyn and Bacon.

Davis, R. C., & Woodcock, E. (1971). The nursing contract: An alternative in care. *Journal of Psychiatric Nursing, 9,* 26.

Delaney, C., & Schoolcraft, V. (1977). Promoting autonomy: Clinical contracts. *Journal of Nursing Education, 16*(9), 22–28.

Gustafson, M. B. (1977). Let's broaden our horizons about the use of contracts. *International Nursing Review, 24*(1), 18–19.

Hames, C., & Joseph, D. H. (1980). *Basic concepts of helping: A holistic approach.* New York: Appleton-Century-Crofts.

Hein, E. C. (1980). *Communication in nursing practice* (2nd ed.). Boston: Little, Brown.

Kalisch, B. (1973). What is empathy? *American Journal of Nursing, 73,* 1548–1552.

Kinlein, M. L. (1977). *Independent nursing practice with clients.* Philadelphia: Lippincott.

Kron, T. T. (1972). *Communication in nursing.* Philadelphia: W. B. Saunders.

La Monica, E., & Karshmer, J. (1978). Empathy: Educating nurses in professional practice. *Journal of Nursing Education, 17*(2), 3–11.

Langford, T. (1978). Establishing a nursing contract. *Nursing Outlook, 26,* 386–388.

Levin, L. S., Katz, A., & Holst, E. (1976). *Self-care: Lay initiatives in health.* New York: Neale, Watson.

Lindberg, J. B., & Simms, L. M. (1974). Contract grading: Incentives and rewards. *Image, 7*(1), 20–23.

Loomis, M. (1979). The health care contract. In M. Loomis (Ed.), *Group process for nurses* (pp. 59–69). St. Louis: C. V. Mosby.

Milio, N. (1977). Self-care in urban settings. *Health Education Monographs, 5,* 136.

Murphy, S. (1977). Mutuality and the message: A conceptual model for nurse-client communication. *Oregon Nurse, 42,* 10.

Norris, C. M. (1979). Self-care. *American Journal of Nursing, 79,* 486–489.

O'Brien, M. (1978). *Communications and relationships in nursing.* St. Louis: C. V. Mosby.

Orlando, I. J. (1961). *The dynamic nurse-patient relationship.* New York: Putnam.

Peplau, H. E. (1952). *Interpersonal relations in nursing.* New York: Putnam.

Price, J., & Braden, C. (1978). The reality in home visits. *American Journal of Nursing, 78,* 1536–1538.

Rosen, B. (1978). Contract therapy. *Nursing Times, 74,* 119–121.

Rowan, K., & Waring, B. (1972). The teaching contract. *Nursing Outlook, 20,* 594–596.

Sauer, J. K. (1973, Summer). The process of contracting in the helping relationship. *Minnesota Welfare,* pp. 12–14.

Seeger, P. A. (1977). Self-awareness and nursing. *Journal of Psychiatric Nursing, 15*(Aug.), 24–26.

Sheridan, A., & Smith, R. (1975). Student-family contracts. *Nursing Outlook, 23,* 114–117.

Sloan, M., & Schommer, B. T. (1982). The process of contracting in community nursing. In B. W. Spradley (Ed.)., *Readings in community health nursing* 2nd ed.) (pp. 197–204). Boston: Little, Brown.

Stuart, R. B. (1971). Behavioral contracting within the families of delinquents. *Journal of Behavioral Therapy and Experimental Psychiatry, 2,* 1–11.

Ulschak, F. L. (1978). Contracting: A process and a tool. In J. W. Pfeiffer & J. Jones (Eds.), *The 1978 annual handbook for group facilitators.* La Jolla, CA: University Associates, 138–142.

Van Dersal, W. R. (1974). How to be a good communicator — And a better nurse. *Nursing '74, 4*(12), 57–64.

Wismer, J. (1978). Communication effectiveness: Active listening and sending feeling messages. In J. W. Pfeiffer & J. Jones (Eds.), *The 1978 annual handbook for group facilitators.* La Jolla, CA: University Associates, 199–222.

Zangari, M., & Duffy, P. (1980). Contracting with patients in day-to-day practice. *American Journal of Nursing, 80,* 451–455.

11

Health Teaching

Clients in community health nursing's sphere of practice have many educational needs. Families with newly diagnosed diabetic members need to understand and regulate the diabetic regimen. Young couples with their first babies want to learn aspects of infant care, such as bathing, feeding, diapering, and formula preparation. Parents of young children form a group because they want to learn about parenting. A women's self-help group seeks to develop understanding of the female role and to acquire skills in assertiveness. Senior citizens adjusting to retirement and the aging process search for increased understanding and meaningful activities. Such situations all present community health nurses with the opportunity and challenge to meet client needs through health teaching.

Teaching represents a fundamental task in the nursing profession: "All nurses function as teachers. Nurses teach patients, families, ancillary personnel, and each other. Teaching is inherent in the nurse's role whether or not the nurse consciously cultivates and exhibits teacher behaviors" (Douglass & Bevis, 1974). Education is also a basic community health nursing intervention, as we disscussed in chapter 3. Identifying a need that is best met through teaching raises a series of questions. How can nurses teach effectively? What content should they cover? What method of presentation will communicate most effectively? What pamphlets or other visual aids can nurses use as teaching devices? How do they know when the client has grasped the information or mastered the skills? In other words, what makes teaching effective, and how are teaching skills acquired? This chapter answers these questions and discusses the application of education as an intervention tool in community health nursing practice.

The Nature of Learning

The goal of all teaching is learning. Learning involves far more than the simple sharing of information. We have all been presented with information that was not interesting, relevant to our needs, or comprehensible. In such situations, we found it difficult to learn. The nurse as a teacher seeks to relate information in such a way that the learner understands and some behavior change results. Effective teaching is a cause; learning becomes the effect. Nurses cannot assume that imparting knowledge will guarantee understanding or change client health practices. To teach effectively in community health, nurses must understand the nature of learning and learning theories. We will next consider three forms of learning — cognitive, affective, and psychomotor (Bloom, 1956). Then the teaching strategies that produce these kinds of learning can be examined.

Learning Theories

What is a learning theory? A learning theory is a "systematic integrated outlook in regard to the nature of the process whereby people relate to their environments in such a way as to enhance their ability to use both themselves and their environments more effectively" (Bigge, 1982, p. 3). Since each of us, whether we know it or not, has a theory of learning and that theory, in turn, dictates the way we would teach, it is helpful to discover what ours is and how it would affect our practice as health educators.

There are many ways to view the basic nature of the learning process. Historically this perspective has changed; the major learning theories, developed over time, fall into three categories. Let us briefly examine these categories and the specific theories residing in each.

MENTAL DISCIPLINE THEORIES

Before the twentieth century, several learning theories developed that continue to influence the way many teachers teach. This category of learning theories conceives of the learner, the person, as having a substantive mind, separate from the body. Various points of view developed about the nature of the human mind. One group saw the mind of the learner as being active but innately bad and in need of correction. This group used mental discipline — drilling, testing, and more drilling — to encourage learning. Strict discipline was seen as a way to promote perseverance and willpower. This learning theory was called "theistic mental discipline."

A second group viewed the mind of the learner as active but neutral and in need of exercise to cultivate the intellect. This approach, too, used mental training and discipline as a way to develop intrinsic mental power. It became known as the "humanistic mental discipline" theory.

A third group viewed the learner's mind as both active and good and believed that the learner's mind should unfold naturally. This theory promoted a permissive style of education that centered on feelings. It was known as the "natural unfoldment " or "self-actualization" theory.

The fourth was called "apperception" learning theory. Subscribers to this theory saw the learner's mind as passive and neutral. The mind, they said, takes in ideas from the outside world and stores them in the subconscious. Learning occurs when ideas are brought to the conscious level and assimilated with other conscious ideas. As Bigge (1982, p. 35) wrote, "Apperception is a process of new ideas associating themselves with old ones."

STIMULUS-RESPONSE CONDITIONING THEORIES

This category of learning theories developed in the twentieth century and is derived from a behavioristic point of view. It says that learning is behavior change –– a response to certain stimuli. Thus the behavioristic teacher seeks to significantly change learners' behaviors through a series of selected stimuli.

Three specific theories are found in this category. The stimulus-response "bond" theory proposes that with conditioning, certain stimuli evoke certain response patterns. The causes (stimuli) are connected or "bonded" to the effects (responses). The teacher promotes acquisition of the desired stimulus-response connections so that transfer of learning can occur in another situation with the same stimulus-response elements present. Two other theories are conditioning with no reinforcement and conditioning through reinforcement. Both emphasize the promotion of desired responses but use different approaches. No-reinforcement theorists count on the learner's innate reflexive drives to accomplish the desired response after conditioning. The reinforcement theorists use successive, systematic changes in the learner's environment to enhance the probability of desired responses.

COGNITIVE THEORIES

A third category of learning theories seeks to influence learners' understanding of problems and situations, in contrast to stimulus-response conditioning, which attempts to change their behaviors. These contemporary learning theories are known as the Gestalt-field family of cognitive theories. The Gestalt-field assumption is that people are neither good nor bad — they simply interact with their environment, and their learning is related to perception. Thus, this theory defines learning as a "reorganization of the learner's perceptual or psychological world — his psychological field" (Bigge, 1982, p. 57). *Gestalt,* the German noun, in this case refers to the total configuration or pattern of related psychological theories.

The first of three theories in the Gestalt-field family is called "insight" theory. This point of view regards learning as a process in which the learner develops new insights or changes old ones. Learners sense their way intuitively but intelligently through problems. The "insight" is only useful if the learner understands its significance. A second theory, called "goal-insight," is very similar to insight theory but goes beyond intuitive hunches to tested insights. Teachers subscribing to this theory promote insightful learning but assist learners in developing higher quality insights. In the third theory, known as "cognitive-field," the learner is seen as purposive and problem centered. Teachers seek to help learners gain new insights and restructure their lives accordingly.

The progression in these three categories of learning theories reflects the trends in educational and psychological thinking. Current learning theorists generally subscribe more to the cognitive theories, but we see many evidences of the others still in practice. The way we have each been taught in our own life-learning experiences will influence the form and function of our health education. Plus, awareness of our beliefs about learning and teaching provides a base for improving our practice.

Types of Learning

COGNITIVE LEARNING

Cognitive learning involves the mind and thinking processes. It is mental knowledge. When we grasp the meaning and relationship of a series of facts, we experience cognitive learning. For example, acquisition of the following facts and relationships involves cognition: population groups have health needs; learning can meet some of those needs; community health nurses can foster learning among client populations; and effective teaching results in learning. The cognitive domain deals with "the recall or recognition of knowledge and the development of intellectual abilities and skills" (Bloom, 1956). It is useful to consider six major categories or levels in the cognitive domain (Gronlund, 1970).

Knowledge
Knowledge, the lowest level of learning, involves recall. If students can remember material previously learned, they have acquired knowledge. Nurses purposely aim for this level in teaching with some clients, particularly those who have limited ability to grasp the rationale behind prescribed health measures. For example, it is entirely appropriate to teach elderly clients the

symptoms of stroke. The nurse's goal may be for them to recall the facts about this illness rather than to understand underlying causes or treatment procedures. Clients may then remember that medication should be taken daily, that regular exercise will restore function, and that abstinence from alcohol is necessary, even though they may not grasp the reasons behind these measures.

Comprehension

The second level of cognitive learning, comprehension, combines remembering with understanding. When possible, teaching aims at instilling at least minimum understanding. Nurses want clients to grasp the meaning and to recognize the importance of suggested health behaviors. At the first level of cognitive learning, a nurse can teach a hypertensive person to take medication daily, but comprehension will occur when this individual and his family understand how his medication and life-style affect blood pressure and how control of each factor can reduce the risk of stroke. Nurses can teach pregnant women the relationship between nutrition and fetal development to help them realize the importance of a healthy diet.

Application

Application is the third level of cognitive learning. Here the learner takes understood material and applies it to new and actual situations. A more desirable level than the first two, application approaches the possibility of self-care, in which clients use their knowledge for improvement of their own health. To encourage application, the nurse can design teaching plans that show clients how to put knowledge into practice. One nurse suggested that the diabetic write down his Clinitest readings on a sheet of paper to show her at the next visit. Another, after instructing adolescents in a weight loss group about nutrition, asked each to keep a diet record for a week, draw up a diet plan, and share this plan with the group at the next meeting.

It is one thing to show a new mother how to bathe her infant; it is quite another to observe a return demonstration. The test of application is a transfer of understanding into practice. The pregnant woman who understands that her physical health and eating habits directly influence the health of her baby has not reached this level if she continues smoking and eating unbalanced foods. The diabetic who recognizes the high risk of infection has not applied this knowledge if he is careless with foot care. The construction worker who understands on-the-job hazards but seldom wears a protective hat in the work area has yet to transfer comprehension into practice.

Analysis

The fourth level of cognitive learning is analysis. At this level, the learner breaks material down into parts, distinguishes between elements, and understands the relationships among the parts. A mother, for example, analyzes when she seeks to determine the cause of an infant's crying. After viewing the total situation, she then breaks it down into variables such as hunger, pain, loneliness, type of crying, and intensity of crying. She examines these parts and draws conclusions about their relationships. Analysis precedes problem solution in the same way that diagnosis precedes treatment. The learner carefully scrutinizes all the variables or elements and their relationships to each other in order to explain the situation. Similarly, analysis precedes identification of needs because we must first study all the assessment variables before we can draw conclusions about client needs. A family that studies its own communication patterns for the purpose of identifying sources of conflict is using analysis. This level of learning becomes a preliminary step toward problem solving. In health teaching, community health nurses foster clients' analytic skills by showing them how to isolate the parts in a situation and then encouraging them to do so themselves.

Synthesis

Synthesis, a fifth level of cognitive learning, is the ability to form elements into a new whole. At this level of intellectual functioning, learners go beyond analyzing material to create something unique from it. Clients who achieve learning at this level will not only analyze their problems but also find solutions for them. For example, a nurse-teacher may assist mental health clients in a therapy group to analyze their frequent depression and then to generate their own plan for alleviating it. Synthesis combines all the earlier levels of cognitive learning to culminate in the production of a unique plan. A young couple who want to toilet train their two-year-old child learn the physiological and psychological dimensions of toilet training, analyze their own situation, and then develop strategies (their own unique plan) for training the child. Health teachers facilitate synthesis by assisting and encouraging clients to develop their own solutions with specific plans. When someone identifies a problem, they can ask clients, "What are some possible causes? Do you see anything we have overlooked about the problem?" But when the client asks for a solution after such analysis, the nurse can encourage synthesis by asking, "What are some possible solutions to this problem that you might carry out?"

Evaluation

The highest level of cognitive learning is evaluation. For the learner, to evaluate means to judge the usefulness of new material compared with a stated purpose (Gronlund, 1970). Such a judgment requires specific criteria. Clients can learn to judge, for example, the consistency of health behavior by comparing it with standards such as abstinence from smoking, maintenance of normal weight, or regular exercise. These are criteria established by others; however, clients may establish their own criteria. Parents may evaluate their parenting effectiveness when their parenting group sets up specific objectives

294

as desired outcomes. The group, for example, could design activities to enhance parent-child communication, and members could then judge their performances by using the desired outcomes as evaluation criteria. When nurse-teachers aim for this level of client learning, they have made self-care a concrete objective. Evaluation, because it goes beyond attempts at problem solving, enables the client to judge the adequacy of solutions, to critique life-style and health-related behavior, and to anticipate needed improvements.

Cognitive learning at any of the levels described can be measured easily in terms of learner behaviors. Nurses know, for instance, that clients have achieved teaching objectives for application of knowledge when their behavior demonstrates actual use of the information taught. Client roles in cognitive learning range from relatively passive (at the knowlege level) to active (at the evaluation level). Conversely, as clients become more active, the nurse-teacher role becomes less directive. Table 11-1 illustrates client and nurse behaviors for each level.

AFFECTIVE LEARNING

The second domain in which learning occurs involves emotion, feeling, or affect. This kind of learning deals with "changes in interest, attitudes, and values" (Bloom, 1956). Here teachers face the task of trying to influence what clients value and feel. Nurses want them to develop an ability to accept

Table 11-1

Cognitive Learning: Case Study in Controlling Diabetes

Level	Illustrative Client Behavior	Illustrative Nurse Behavior
Knowledge (recalls, knows)	States that insulin, if taken, will control own diabetes	Gives information
Comprehension (understands)	Describes insulin action and purpose	Explains information
Application (uses learning)	Adjusts insulin dosage daily to maintain proper blood sugar level	Suggests how to use learning
Analysis (examines, explains)	Discusses relationships between insulin, diet, activity, and diabetic control	Demonstrates and encourages analysis
Synthesis (integrates with other learning, generates new ideas)	Develops a plan, incorporating above learning, for controlling own diabetes	Promotes client formulation of own plan
Evaluation (judges according to a standard)	Compares degree of diabetic control (outcomes) with desired control (objectives)	Facilitates evaluation

ideas that promote healthier behavior patterns even though those ideas may conflict with their own values.

Attitudes and values are learned (Bigge, 1982). They develop gradually over time as the way that an individual feels and responds is molded by family, peers, experiences, and societal influences. These feelings and responses are the result of imitation and conditioning. In this way, clients acquire their health-related beliefs and practices. Because attitudes and values become part of the person, they are difficult to change unless the nurse-teacher is aware of how they develop.

Affective learning occurs on several levels as learners respond with varying degrees of involvement and commitment. At the first level, learners are simply receptive. They are willing to listen, show awareness, and be attentive. The teacher aims at acquiring and focusing learners' attention (Gronlund, 1970). This limited goal may be all clients are ready for at the early stages of the nurse-client relationship.

At the second level, learners become active participants by responding to the information in some way. At this level, clients show willingness to read educational material that nurses give them, participate in discussion, complete assignments such as keeping a diet record, or voluntarily seek out more information on their own.

At the third level, learners attach value to the information. Valuing ranges from simple acceptance through appreciation to commitment. For example, a nurse taught members of a therapy group a number of principles concerning group effectiveness. She explained the importance of a democratic group process and ways to improve group skills. Members showed acceptance when they acknowledged the importance of these ideas. They showed appreciation by starting to practice the ideas. Commitment came when they assumed responsibility for having their group function well.

The final level of affective learning occurs when learners internalize an idea or value. The value system now controls learner behavior. Consistent practice is a crucial test at this level. Clients who know and respect the value of exercise but only occasionally play tennis or do calisthenics have not internalized the value. Even several weeks of enthusiastic jogging is not evidence of an internalized value. If the jogging continues for six months, a year, and longer, learning is probably internalized.

Affective learning often remains elusive, difficult to measure. Indeed, this quality may influence community health nurses to concentrate their efforts on cognitive learning goals. Yet client attitudes and values have a major effect on the outcome of cognitive learning — desired behavior changes. For this reason, the two domains must remain linked in teaching; otherwise, results may quickly fade.

Attitudes and values can change in the same way they were first learned, that is, through imitation and conditioning (Redman, 1976). Role models, particularly those from the client's peer group, who practice the desired

Table 11-2
Affective Learning: Case Study in Family Planning

Level	Illustrative Client Behavior	Illustrative Nurse Behavior
Receptive (listens, pays attention)	Attentive to family planning instruction	Directs client's attention
Responsive (participates, reacts)	Discusses pros and cons of various methods	Encourages client involvement
Valuing (accepts, appreciates, commits)	Selects a method for use	Respects client's right to decide
Internal consistency (organizes values to fit together)	Understands and accepts responsibility for limiting number of children	Brings client into contact with role models
Adoption (incorporates new values into life-style)	Consistently practices birth control	Positively reinforces healthy behaviors

health behaviors can be a strong influence. Groups like mastectomy clubs or chemical dependency support groups can have a powerful effect. Attitudes often change when the nurse provides clients with a satisfying experience during the learning process. The nurse who recognizes client participation in a group, praises them for completing assignments, or commends them for sticking to diet plans will have more success than the nurse who only criticizes failures. Table 11-2 shows client and nurse behaviors for each level of affective learning.

To influence affective learning requires patience. Values and attitudes will seldom change overnight. Keep in mind that other forces will continue to reinforce former values. For example, a middle-aged housewife may value pursuing a career for self-fulfillment but cannot because her husband opposes an independent activity. Promoting cognitive learning by helping the client understand and try out positive health practices is also useful for influencing attitude change.

PSYCHOMOTOR LEARNING

The psychomotor domain includes visible, demonstrable performance skills that require some kind of neuromuscular coordination. Community health clients need to learn skills such as infant bathing, range-of-motion exercises, catheter irrigation, crutch-walking, breast self-examination, temperature taking, special diet preparation, and prenatal breathing exercises.

For psychomotor learning to take place, three conditions must be met. First, learners must be capable of the skill. If a nurse attempts to teach an elderly diabetic man with tremulous hands and fading vision to give his own insulin injections, it could frustrate and possibly harm him. Some other person more physically capable should probably be enlisted and taught the skill. Clients' intellectual and emotional capabilities also influence their capacity to learn motor skills. No one should expect persons of limited intelligence to learn complex skills. The degree of complexity should match the learners' level of functioning. Developmental stage is another point to consider in determining whether a skill is appropriate to teach. For example, most children can put on some article of clothing at two years of age but are not ready to learn to fasten buttons until well past their third birthday.

Learners must also have a sensory image of how to perform the skill. This is a second condition for psychomotor learning. Through sight, hearing, touch, and sometimes taste or smell, clients gain a picture of the skill. They acquire this sensory image by means of demonstration. Our first image of how to drive a car, for instance, comes from watching someone else drive. We observe their eyes, hands, and feet; the coordination between clutch and gear shift; auto speed; and road conditions. Verbal explanations enhance our understanding of the mechanics of driving. In order to teach clients motor skills effectively, the nurse has to provide them with an adequate sensory image. The nurse-teacher must demonstrate and explain slowly, one point at a time, and repeatedly if needed, until they understand the proper sequence of actions necessary to achieve the skill.

The third necessary condition for psychomotor learning is practice. After acquiring a sensory image, learners can start to perform the skill. Mastery will come over time as learners repeat the performance until it is smooth, coordinated, and unhesitating. During this process the teacher should be available to provide guidance and encouragement. In the early stages of practice the teacher may need to use hands-on guidance to give learners a sense of how the performance should feel. Similarly, a nurse demonstrates passive range-of-motion exercises on a client's wife to show her how they should feel before she learns to do them for her husband. During practice, feedback from the nurse will enable the learner to know if the skill is being performed correctly. When clients give a return demonstration, the teacher can make suggestions, give encouragement, and thereby maximize learning effectiveness.

The psychomotor domain, like the cognitive and affective domains, ranges from simple to complex levels of functioning. It is necessary to exercise judgment in assessing clients' ability to perform the skill. Even clients with limited ability can often move on to higher levels once they have mastered simple skills. Nurse behaviors that influence psychomotor learning are shown in Table 11-3.

Teaching

A sixth grade teacher recently announced to her class: "My job here is to teach; your job is to learn. I don't care whether you learn or not, but if you want to learn, that's your responsibility. I'm being paid to teach." This kind

Table 11-3
Nurse Behaviors in Psychomotor Learning

Determining Capability	Providing Sensory Image	Encouraging Practice
Nurse assesses client's physical, intellectual, and emotional ability	Nurse demonstrates and explains	Nurse uses guidance and positive reinforcement

of noncaring message only creates confusion and consternation among students. Yet, without meaning to, nurses may convey a similar message to clients. "I'm here to teach you how to get healthy and stay healthy," they say in so many words. "Whether you do or not is up to you." It is almost as though, having carried out their teaching responsibility, they can wash their hands of the whole business. How often do nurses chart, "Patient taught colostomy care," "Diabetic teaching done," "Explained medication dosage and side effects," and "Baby bath and formula preparation demonstrated" with little awareness of whether and how much learning occurred?

Teaching lies at one end of a continuum. At the other end is learning. Without learning, teaching becomes useless in much the same way that communication does not occur unless a message is both sent and received. The sixth grade teacher was trying to point this out to her students when she pushed the entire responsibility for learning on their shoulders. While we can question the effectiveness of her approach, her point remains valid. Learners must take responsibility for their own learning (Levin, 1978). Teachers obstruct that process if they assume complete responsibility for bringing about changed behavior. Clients can be led to water, but without a thirst for health information, they still will not participate in the learning process. Teaching, then, becomes a matter of facilitating both the thirst and the best conditions for satisfying it. Teaching in community health nursing means to influence, motivate, and act as catalysts in the learning process. Nurses "bring knowledge and learner together and stimulate a reaction" (Douglass & Bevis, 1974). Nurses facilitate learning when they make it as easy as possible for clients to change. To do this, the nurse-teacher needs to know basic principles underlying the teaching-learning process. Teaching also requires the use of appropriate tools to influence learning.

Teaching-Learning Principles

CLIENT READINESS

Clients' readiness to learn influences teaching effectiveness. A young primipara was not ready for prenatal teaching on fetal growth and development. She had strong fears, the nurse discovered, that "losing her figure" would make her sexually unattractive to her husband. Until these anxieties had subsided, the teaching would remain ineffective. Clients' needs, interests, and concerns determine their readiness for learning. Another factor that influences readiness is educational background. If a group of women who never completed grade school meet to learn how to care for a sick person in the home, sessions should present material simply, factually, and in terms that they understand. To discuss complex concepts of health, illness, and scientific research would be above their level of readiness.

Maturational level also affects readiness. A one-year-old child is not ready to share his toys, but a five-year-old child has reached a level that makes him ready to learn these social skills. An adolescent mother who is still working on normal developmental tasks of her age group may not be ready to learn parenting skills. Readiness of the client will determine the amount of material presented in each teaching session (Fig. 11-1). The pace or speed with which you present information must be manageable. A moderate amount of anxiety will often increase client receptivity to learning; however, high or low levels of anxiety can have the opposite effect.

Figure 11-1
The boy in this family is old enough to help measure the ingredients for the cake. His younger sister helps to stir. Their maturational levels influence their readiness to learn new tasks.

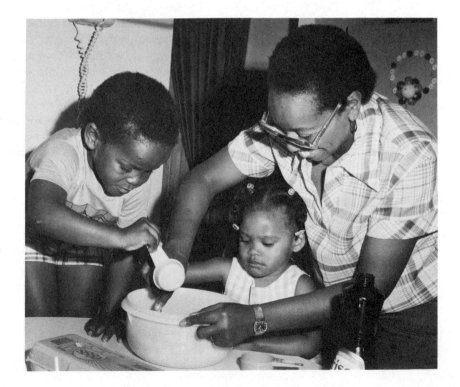

300

CLIENT PERCEPTION

Clients' perceptions affect their learning. People's perceptions, the way they see the world, act like a screening device through which all new information must pass (Marriner, 1979). Our perceptions help us to interpret and attach meaning to things. For example, one person views a piece of sculpture and exclaims over its beauty. Another person, seeing the same object, remarks on its ugliness and lack of coherence. These two people have different perceptions. In community health nursing, one client may view the experience of parenting as a positive, growth-producing relationship; another may see it as a conflict-ridden, unhappy experience to avoid. Each kind of perception has a different consequence for learning.

A wide range of variables affects human perception. These variables include values, past experiences, culture, religion, personality, developmental stage, educational and economic level, surrounding social forces, and the physical environment. Adolescent boys who have been told to stop taking drugs will resist if they perceive this instruction as an affront to their identities and independence. They want to make decisions for themselves. The nurse-teacher, recognizing the forces at work, will try to work within the boys' frame of reference by presenting information in a way that still gives them options to make their own choices. Otherwise, their perception of the situation will limit their learning.

Frequently clients use selective perception. They screen out some statements and pay attention to those that fit their values or personal desires. A nurse was teaching a client the various risk factors in coronary disease; the individual screened out smoking and obesity, paying attention only to factors that would not require a drastic change in life-style. Nurses must know their clients, understand their backgrounds and values, and learn what their perceptions are before health teaching can influence their learning potential.

CLIENT PARTICIPATION

The degree of client participation in the educational process directly influences the amount of client learning. One nurse discovered this principle when working with a group of people nearing retirement. After talking to them about the changes and needs they would face met with little response, she shifted to a different method of teaching. She distributed pamphlets and asked everyone to read each week and come prepared for discussion. Slowly the group began to participate in their own learning to a greater degree. Whenever the nurse works with clients in a learning context, one of the first questions to discuss is "What does the client want to learn?" As Carl Rogers (1969, p. 159) has said: "Learning is facilitated when the student participates responsibly in the learning process. When he chooses his own directions, helps to discover his own learning resources, formulates his own problems, decides his own course of action, lives with the consequences of each of these choices, then significant learning is maximized."

The amount of learning is directly proportional to the learners' involvement. A group of senior citizens attended a class on nutrition and aging, yet still made almost no changes in diet or eating patterns. It was not until the members became actively involved in the class, encouraged by the nurse to present problems and solutions for food purchasing and preparation on limited budgets, that any significant behavior changes occurred.

Contracting, discussed in chapter 10, can contribute to the nurse's teaching goals. It directly involves the client in a partnership to determine goals, content, and time for learning. Contracting in the context of teaching can develop a great sense of accountability in clients for their own learning.

SUBJECT'S RELEVANCE TO CLIENT

Subject matter that is relevant to the client is learned more readily and retained longer than information that is not meaningful. Learners gain the most from subject matter immediately useful to their own purposes. Consider two middle-management men taking a physical fitness course offered by their employer. One, a father of a cub scout, has agreed to co-lead his son's troop on a two-week backpacking trip in the mountains. He wants to get in shape. The second man is taking the course because it is required by the company. Its only relevance to his own purposes is that it keeps him from gaining his boss's disfavor. There can be little question about which man will learn and retain the most. The course has considerable relevance and meaning to the first man and almost none to the second.

Relevance influences the speed of learning. When a two-year-old child sees his little friend from down the street riding a tricycle, he quickly learns to peddle his own. It becomes very important to him to learn; therefore, he learns quickly. Diabetics who must give themselves daily injections of insulin learn that skill very quickly (Fig. 11-2). A housewife and mother with a broken leg rapidly learns to manage crutch-walking. Each client sees considerable relevance in the learning and thus accomplishes it with great speed. According to Rogers (1969), "There is evidence that the time for learning various subjects would be cut to a fraction of the time currently allotted if the material were perceived by the learner as related to his own purposes. Probably one-third to one-fifth of the present time allotment would be sufficient."

When subject matter is relevant to the learner, there is also greater retention of knowledge. The learner, upon seeing the usefulness of the material, develops a strong motivation to acquire and utilize it and will be less likely to forget it. Even in instances when a previously learned motor skill has not been used for many years, it is often quickly recaptured under such conditions.

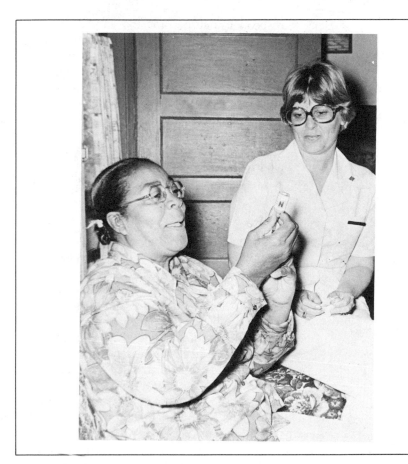

Figure 11-2
This client quickly learns to give herself daily insulin injections because she is eager to return to as normal functioning as possible.

CLIENT SATISFACTION

Clients must derive satisfaction from learning to maintain motivation and increase self-direction (Redman, 1976). Learners need to feel a sense of steady progress in the learning process. Obstacles, frustrations, and failures along the way discourage and impede learning. Many stroke patients with potential for rehabilitation give up trying to regain speech or use of paralyzed limbs because they become too frustrated and dissatisfied in the process. On the other hand, clients who experience statisfaction and progress in their speech and muscle retraining maintain their motivation and work on exercises without prompting.

Realistic goals contribute to learner satisfaction. Objectives should be set within the learner's ability, thereby avoiding the frustration that comes from a too difficult task and the loss of interest that results from one too easy. Setting objectives requires agreement on goals, periodic reviews, and revision of goals if they become too easy or too difficult. Nurses further promote clients' learning satisfaction by designing tasks with rewards. One nurse led a class for obese adolescents, and together they set the goal of a weekly three-pound weight loss. The school nurse helped the group design a plan that included counting calories and a buddy system as ways to help bring about a behavior change. If each member in the group achieved the three-pound goal, the group went on a field trip or excursion of their choice as a reward. These students found this learning experience satisfying because goals were attainable and their progress was rewarded. Instead of competing with one another, the group set out to help each member achieve the goal. As a result, most kept the weight off after the class had finished.

CLIENT APPLICATION

Learning is reinforced through application. The students in the weight loss group began immediately to count calories. They could begin to apply their knowledge. Learners need as many opportunities as possible to apply the learning in daily life. If they arise during the teaching-learning process, clients can try out new knowledge and skills under supervision. Learners are given an opportunity to start integrating the learning into their daily lives at a time when the teacher is there to help reinforce that pattern.

Take a prenatal class as an example. The learning only begins with explanations of proper diet, exercise, breathing techniques, hygiene, avoidance of alcohol and tobacco, and so on. More learning occurs as the group members discuss these issues and apply them intellectually, exploring ways they could practice them at home. Additional reinforcement comes by demonstrating how to do these activities. Sample diets, demonstrations of exercises, display of posters, pamphlets, or models may be used. The group can begin application in the classroom by making diet plans, doing exercises, role playing parenting behavior, or engaging in group problem solving. Then the members can be encouraged to apply these activities on a daily basis at home and prepare to share their results at future sessions.

Frequent use of newly acquired information fosters transfer of learning to other situations. Our major goal of prevention and health promotion depends on such a transfer. For instance, mothers who learn and practice a well-balanced diet, free of nonnutritious snacks, can be encouraged to offer more nourishing foods to their whole families. The family that practices asepsis and good hand-washing techniques when caring for a postsurgical wound can learn to transfer this same principle to prevention of infection in daily living.

Teaching Process

The process of teaching in community health nursing follows steps similar to those of the nursing process:

1. *Interaction* — establish basic communication patterns between clients and nurse.
2. *Assessment and diagnosis* — determine clients' present status and identify needs for teaching.
3. *Goal setting* — analyze needed changes and prepare objectives that describe the desired learning outcomes.
4. *Planning* — design a plan for the learning experience that meets the objectives; include the content to be covered, sequence of topics, best conditions for learning (place, kind of environment), methods, and tools (visual aids, exercises, etc.). A written plan is best; it may or may not be part of the written nursing care plan.
5. *Teaching* — implement the learning experience by carrying out the planned activities.
6. *Evaluation* — determine whether learning objectives were met and if not, why not. Evaluation measures progress toward goals and can indicate future learning needs.

Teaching occurs on many levels and incorporates various types of activities. It can be formal or informal, planned or unplanned. Formal presentations, such as lectures, are generally planned and fairly structured. Some teaching is less formal but still planned and relatively structured, as in group discussions in which questions stimulate exploration of ideas and guide thinking. Informal levels of teaching, such as counseling or anticipatory guidance, require background preparation but often no definite plan of presentation. The teaching process is guided by the client's concerns. Teaching often occurs in casual conversations, spontaneously in situations in which clients raise unexpected questions, or when a crisis arises. In these instances, nurses draw on their background of knowledge and exercise professional judgment in their teaching. Finally, nurses teach by example: actions usually speak louder than words. If a nurse teaches the importance of a healthy life-style and then lights up a cigarette, the message of her actions will carry more impact than her words. The healthy nurse who exhibits healthy practices serves as a role model as well as a health teacher.

Teaching Methods and Tools

LECTURE

There are times when the community health nurse will present information to a large group, such as a PTA meeting, a women's club luncheon, or a county board of commissioners. Under such circumstances, the lecture method, a formal kind of presentation, may be the most efficient means of communicating health information. However, lecturers tend to create a passive learning atmosphere for the audience unless accompanied by strategies devised to involve the learners. Many individuals are visual rather than auditory learners. To capture their attention, slides, overhead projections, films, or videotapes can supplement the lecture. Allowing time for questions and discussion after a lecture will also involve the learners more actively.

DISCUSSION

Two-way communication is an important feature of the learning process. Learners need an opportunity to raise questions, make comments, reason out loud, and receive feedback in order to develop understanding. Discussion, used in conjunction with other teaching methods such as demonstration, lecture, and role playing, will improve their effectiveness. In group teaching, discussion enables clients to learn from one another as well as from the nurse. One difficulty that can arise is monopolization of the discussion by one person while others seldom express themselves. The nurse-teacher must exercise leadership in controlling and guiding the dicussion so that learning opportunities are maximized. Prepared objectives and discussion organized around specific questions or topics make the discussion most fruitful.

DEMONSTRATION

The demonstration method is often used for teaching motor skills and is best accompanied by explanation and discussion. It can give clients a clear sensory image of how to perform the skill. Because a demonstration should be within easy visual and auditory range of learners, it is best to demonstrate in front of small groups. Use the same kind of equipment that clients will use in order to show exactly how the skill should be performed, and provide them with ample opportunity to practice until the skill is perfected. Again, objectives, content, and sequence of learning activities should all be planned ahead of time.

ROLE PLAYING

There are times when having clients assume and act out roles maximizes learning. A parenting group, for example, found it helpful to place themselves in the role of their children; their feelings about various ways to respond became more apparent. Reversing roles can effectively teach spouses in conflict about better ways to communicate. In order to prevent role playing from becoming a game with little learning, plan the proposed drama with clear objectives in mind. What behavioral outcomes do you hope to achieve? Define the context, the "stage," clearly so that everyone shares in the situation. Then define each role ahead of time, making sure everyone understands his performance. Emphasize that no wrong or right performance exists, merely the way people behave in everyday life. Avoid having people play themselves; it can be both embarrassing and difficult to achieve objectivity.

After the drama has concluded, elicit discussion with carefully prepared questions.

Many different tools, often used in combination, are useful during the teaching process. Visual images — pictures, slides, films, posters, chalkboards, videotapes, bulletin boards, flash cards, pamphlets, and even gestures — can enhance almost any learning. Some tools such as sound films, record players, or tape recorders provide an auditory stimulus. Other tools, for example, models or objects, allow clients both visual and tactile learning (Fig. 11-3). Still others, such as programmed instruction or games, involve learners actively through reading and activity.

Figure 11-3
Teaching methods and tools vary with clients' learning needs. On this home visit the nurse uses an egg container with labels to help an elderly woman with limited vision devise a plan for taking her medications.

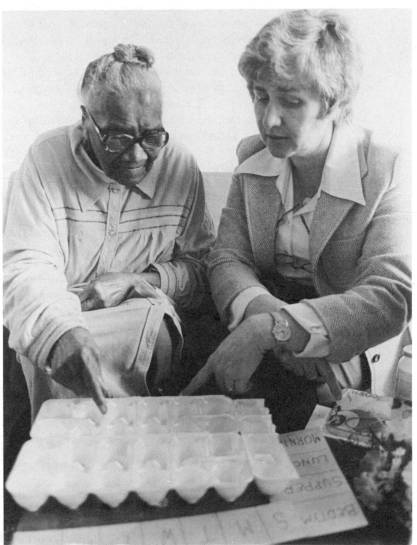

Summary

A large part of community health nursing practice involves teaching. Far more than to simply give health information to clients, the purpose of teaching is to change client behavior to healthier practices.

Understanding the nature of learning contributes to the effectiveness of teaching in community health. Learning theories include three broad categories. The first group, mental discipline theories, views learning as the promotion of mental training, ranging from strict discipline, through natural unfolding of the learner's mind, to building on the learner's store of ideas. The second category, stimulus-response conditioning, views learning as a change in behavior — responses to stimuli. Cognitive learning theories form the third category. These seek to influence learners' understanding of problems and situations through promoting their insights.

Learning occurs in three domains — cognitive, affective, and psychomotor. The cognitive domain refers to learning that takes place intellectually, through the mind. It ranges in levels of learner functioning from simple recall to complex evaluation. As learners move up the scale of cognitive learning, they become more self-directed; the nurse-teacher assumes a more facilitative role.

Affective learning means the changing of attitudes and values. Learners may experience several levels of affective involvement from simple listening to adopting the new value. Again, as the client-learner increases involvement, the nurse-teacher becomes less directive.

Psychomotor learning involves the acquisition of motor skills. Clients who learn psychomotor skills must meet three conditions: they must be capable of the skill; they must develop a sensory image of the skill; and they must practice the skill.

Teaching in community health nursing is the facilitation of learning that leads to behavior change in the client. Thus teaching is a catalytic process based on the following teaching-learning principles:

1. Client readiness for learning influences teaching effectiveness.
2. Clients' perceptions affect their learning.
3. The degree of client participation in the educational process directly influences the amount of client learning.
4. Subject matter that is relevant to the client is learned more readily and retained longer than information that is not meaningful.
5. The client must derive satisfaction from the learning to maintain motivation and increase self-direction.
6. Learning is reinforced through application.

The teaching process in community health nursing is similar to the nursing process. It includes interaction, assessment and diagnosis, goal setting, planning, teaching, and evaluation. The actual teaching may be formal or informal, planned or unplanned. Methods may range from structured lecture presentations to demonstration and role playing. Selection of a tool depends on how well it suits client-learners and helps to meet the desired objectives.

Study Questions

1. What learning theory or theories discussed in this chapter most closely reflect your own position? Discuss how you would apply it or them in your practice.
2. A children's day care center is located in your service area. What populations in this setting could be potential recipients of health teaching? How would you assess each group's learning needs?
3. Your county health board often makes decisions that appear to reflect lack of knowledge regarding health and health care. How might you "educate" them using the concepts and principles described in this chapter?
4. Discuss the differences between cognitive, affective, and psychomotor learning. Why do cognitive and affective learning need to be linked in health teaching?
5. Explore the possible use of role models as a teaching tool for community health nursing practice. What examples already exist in your community? What new ones might you develop?

References

Bigge, M. L. (1982). *Learning theories for teachers* (4th ed.). New York: Harper & Row.

Bloom, B. (Ed.) (1956). *Taxonomy of educational objectives: The classification of educational goals. Handbook I: Cognitive domain.* New York: Longman.

Douglass, L. M., & Bevis, E. O. (1974). *Nursing leadership in action-principles and application to staff situations.* St. Louis: C. V. Mosby.

Gronlund, N. E. (1970). *Stating behavioral objectives for classroom instruction.* New York: Macmillan.

Levin, L. S. (1978). Patient education and self-care: How do they differ? *Nursing Outlook, 26,* 170–175.

Marriner, A. (1979). Health teaching. In A. Marriner (Ed.), *The nursing process* (2nd ed.). St. Louis: C. V. Mosby.

Redman, B. K. (1976). *The process of patient teaching in nursing* (3rd ed.). St. Louis: C. V. Mosby.

Rogers, C. (1969). *Freedom to learn.* Columbus, OH: Merrill.

Selected Readings

Bigge, M. L. (1982). *Learning theories for teachers*. New York: Harper & Row.

Bloom, B. (Ed.). (1956). *Taxonomy of educational objectives: The classification of educational goals. Handbook I: Cognitive domain*. New York: Longman.

Borgman, M. F. (1977). Exercise and health maintenance. *Journal of Nursing Education, 16*(1), 6–10.

Bryan, N. E. (1974). Every nurse a teacher. *Australian Nurses Journal, 4*(1), 31–33.

Buford, L. M. (1975). Group education to reduce overweight: Classes for mentally handicapped children. *American Journal of Nursing, 75*, 1194–1195.

Crow, M., Bradshaw, B., & Guest, F. (1972). True to life: A relevant approach to patient education. *American Journal of Public Health, 62*, 1328–1330.

Douglass, L. M., & Bevis, E. O. (1974). *Nursing leadership in action — Principles and application to staff situations*. St. Louis: C. V. Mosby.

Flowers, L. K. (1976). The development of a program for treating obesity. *Hospital Community Psychiatry, 27*, 342–345.

Green, L. W. (1977). Evaluation and measurement: Some dilemmas for health education. *American Journal of Public Health, 67*, 155–161.

Gronlund, N. E. (1970). *Stating behavioral objectives for classroom instruction*. New York: Macmillan.

Haskin, J., Hawley, N., & Weinberger, J. (1976). Project teen concern: An educational approach to the prevention of venereal disease and premature parenthood. *Journal of School Health, 46*, 231–234.

Hein, E. C. (1978). Teaching psychosocial wellness in family and community health nursing. *Nurse Educator, 3*, 22–25.

Heit, P. (1978). Educating the nurse–community health educator to educate. *Journal of Nursing Education, 17*(1), 21–23.

Hill, W. F. (1971). *Learning — A survey of psychological interpretations*. Scranton, PA: Chandler.

Jones, P., & Oertel, W. (1977). Developing patient teaching objectives + techniques: A self-instructional program. *Nurse Educator, 2*(5), 3–18.

Knowles, M. (1970). *The modern practice of adult education*. New York: Associated Press.

Knowles, M. (1975). *Self-directed learning: A guide for learners and teachers*. New York: Associated Press.

Kopelke, C. E. (1975). Group education to reduce overweight . . . in a blue-collar community. *American Journal of Nursing, 75*, 1993–1995.

Kyle, J. R., & Savino, A. B. (1973). Teaching parents behavior modification. *Nursing Outlook, 21*, 717–720.

Leahy, K. M., & Bell, A. T. (1952). *Teaching methods in public health nursing*. Philadelphia: W. B. Saunders.

Levin, L. S. (1978). Patient education and self-care: How do they differ? *Nursing Outlook, 26,* 170–175.

Marriner, A. (1971). The role of the school nurse in health education. *American Journal of Public Health, 61,* 2155–2157.

Marriner, A. (1979). Health teaching. In A. Marriner (Ed.), *The nursing process* (2nd ed.). St. Louis: C. V. Mosby.

Milio, N. (1976). A broad perspective on health: A teaching-learning tool. *Nursing Outlook, 24,* 160–163.

Milio, N. (1976). A framework for prevention: Changing health-damaging to health-generating life patterns. *American Journal of Public Health, 66,*435–439.

Mohammed, M. F. (1964). Patients' understanding of written health information. *Nursing Research, 13,* 100–108.

Murray, R., & Zentner, J. (1976). Guidelines for more effective health teaching. *Nursing '76, 6*(2), 44–53.

Narrow, B. (1979). *Patient teaching in nursing practice: A patient and family-centered approach.* Somerset, NJ: Wiley.

Neeman, R. L., & Neeman, M. (1975). Complexities of smoking education. *Journal of School Health, 45*(1), 17–23.

Pohl, M. (1973). *The teaching function of the nursing practitioner* (2nd ed.). Dubuque, IA: Brown.

Redman, B. K. (1980). *The process of patient teaching in nursing* (4th ed.). St. Louis: C. V. Mosby.

Reilly, D. E. (Ed.). (1978). *Teaching and evaluating the affective domain in nursing programs.* Thorofare, NJ: Charles B. Slack.

Richie, N. D. (1976). Some guidelines for conducting a health fair. *Public Health Reports, 91,* 261–264.

Robinson, G., & Filkins, M. (1964). Group teaching with outpatients. *American Journal of Nursing, 64,* 110–112.

Rogers, C. R. (1969). *Freedom to learn.* Columbus, OH: Merrill.

Schweer, J. E., & Gebbie, K. M. (1976). *Creative teaching in clinical nursing.* St. Louis: C. V. Mosby.

Simmons, J. (Ed.). (1975). Making health education work. *American Journal of Public Health, 65*(Oct. Suppl.), 1–49.

Stewart, R. F. (1974). Education for health maintenance. *Occupational Health Nursing, 22*(6), 14–17.

Thompson, W. (1978). Health education: II. How do we communicate? *Nursing Times, 74,* 1561–1562.

Tinch, J. (1975). For sickness or for health? *Nursing Mirror, 140*(17), 71–72.

Valadez, A. M., & Heusinkveld, K. B. (1977). Teaching nursing students to teach patients. *Journal of Nursing Education, 16*(4), 10–14.

Veninga, K. A. (1983). How to establish a nutrition education program. *Occupational Health Nursing, 12,* 34–38.

12

Community Crisis Prevention and Intervention

All human beings, individually and collectively, experience periods of upset, trouble, even danger. A teenager discovers she is pregnant. The father and breadwinner in a family loses his job. A beloved leader dies. A man faces retirement. An accident at a nuclear power plant threatens a community. A woman has her first baby. These life experiences can produce stress and anxiety. Each event can cause changes in peoples' behavior; each can require days, weeks, even months of adjustment and coping. When that happens they may become times of crisis.

People respond differently to a potential crisis. Some see the event as a challenge; others see it as adversity. What one person experiences as crisis, another treats as a normal occurrence. Some seek out the help they need and come through the experience unscathed, perhaps even stronger than before. Others, unable to cope, incur severe, sometimes permanent, damage.

Regardless of their responses, people in a crisis-producing situation need help. Equally important, they are receptive to help. Community health practitioners have a unique opportunity to provide that assistance because they can see clients frequently and in a broad environmental context. Not only can they give assistance during a time of crisis, but, more important, they can help people equip themselves with the tools needed for crisis management and prevention. In particular, community health practitioners are concerned about crises or potential crises at the aggregate level. When the Three Mile Island nuclear power plant accident occurred, for example, it created a crisis

312

for families, groups, communities, and, indeed, our whole society. Major professional challenges in community health are to prevent crises and to help people in crisis. This chapter examines how nurses can sharpen their knowledge and skills in the practice of crisis prevention and intervention for community health.

Crisis Theory

Our understanding about crises has grown considerably. At one time, we equated crisis only with disaster; it might have been natural (a hurricane), economic (a stock market crash), political (a presidential assassination), environmental (water polluted with chemicals), personal (death of a loved one), or another form of disaster. Researchers have studied the nature of crisis and have now developed a body of knowledge called *crisis theory*. Initially limited to the field of mental health, crisis theory now influences every field of health care. We know, for example, that a crisis is not an event per se, but rather people's perception of the event. We know that different kinds of crises occur; we can explain why people respond the way they do in a crisis; we can predict the phases that people go through in a crisis of any kind. These are important aspects to understand before attempting to prevent, manage, or intervene in crises.

Dynamics of Crisis

How does a crisis occur? People as living systems behave in certain ways, which are generally unconscious, in order to maintain relative equilibrium within themselves and in their relations with others. When some internal or external force disrupts the system's balance and alters its functioning, loss of homeostasis occurs. To restore equilibrium, people attempt to cope. They develop problem-solving behaviors that become habitual through repeated, although not always successful, use. Caplan (1964) points out that during the brief period before a problem is resolved, people experience tension. But the tension is manageable because they know from previous problem-solving successes that the outcomes will be positive. They have also learned techniques for handling the tension. For example, Sharon has a flat tire while driving her car. This event creats a brief period of tension. But as Sharon locates the spare and begins to jack up the car, her anxiety subsides. She uses her knowledge to solve the problem.

In a crisis, the dynamics change. The problem is unfamiliar and greater than usual. It calls for a dramatic alteration of people's accustomed role, responsibilities, or both. Tension develops. They try their customary problem-solving responses only to find them inadequate. It becomes impossible to restore equilibrium; anxiety mounts. If, instead of having a flat tire, Sharon is caught in a blizzard with blinding snow and driving winds obliterating her vision and making temperatures drop to levels that threaten her survival, she cannot use her past experience to solve the problem. Her anxiety may rise and a crisis ensue.

The problem persists and tension grows more apparent. People continue to apply their usual problem-solving techniques or direct their efforts toward handling the tension. Sharon, for example, may think about walking to the nearest farmhouse or tell herself, "No, I should stay with the car and try to keep warm until help comes." If these efforts fail to solve the problem, the feelings of anxiety and inadequacy will increase: "A person in this situation feels helpless — he is caught in a state of great emotional upset and feels unable to take action *on his own* to solve the problem" (Aguilera & Messick, 1978, p. 1).

Increased stress caused by a further rise in tension and anxiety serves as a catalyst for some people to resolve the problem. Realizing that they cannot solve it on their own with their usual coping mechanisms, they mobilize new internal resources, seek outside help, or both, or they define the problem in a new way that makes it manageable. Community residents in a Midwestern town following a sudden spring storm faced a rapidly rising river and the threat of flood. After the initial shock and disorientation, they mobilized to form teams — one for rescue and first aid, one for sandbagging the river banks, and one to evacuate low-level area homes. As a result no lives were lost and minimal property damage occurred. Their efforts were successful.

For others, the problem remains. Stimulated by the same tension, they may seek inappropriate solutions without success. The help they receive may not redefine their problem in a realistic and workable manner. They may choose to avoid the problem by resigning themselves to it or minimizing its importance. Tension and anxiety mount rapidly or gradually, but ultimately people reach a point beyond which they can no longer function. Drastic results can follow, such as suicide, mass hysteria, heart attacks, psychotic breaks, and family or group disintegration.

Caplan (1964) has summarized in four stages the effect of rising tension on the functioning of people in crisis:

1. Tension develops (as a result of precipitating event)	People use customary problem-solving responses in order to restore equilibrium.
2. Tension increases	Failure to cope leads to feeling upset and ineffectual.
3. Tension rises further	Increased tension acts as a stimulus to mobilize internal and external resources. People try to redefine the situation and may solve the problem, in which case tension abates.

4. Tension reaches threshold

If problem continues unsolved (or avoided), the breaking point is reached, causing major disorganization both socially and individually.

Thus, in a crisis, a certain amount of tension or stress may promote problem resolution and restoration of equilibrium. However, stress that becomes too intense and is unrelieved will ultimately lead to system breakdown (Veninga & Spradley, 1981, p. 35).

Definition of Crisis

Crisis is a temporary state of severe disequilibrium for persons who face a situation they find threatening that they can neither escape nor solve with their usual coping abilities (Caplan, 1964; Fink, 1967).

Let us look at several key characteristics of this definition in the context of a family in which the father is killed unexpectedly in a plane crash (Caplan, 1964). Crisis begins with a sense that things are *out of balance*. It causes the awareness of being upset, a state of considerable disequilibrium with resulting tension. Crises create "sudden discontinuities in the functioning pattern" (Caplan, 1964, p. 39). The man's wife and three children feel shattered by the news. The rhythm of their family life comes to a halt. Bills go unpaid; someone else must prepare meals. The family has been pushed out of balance.

Crisis is a *temporary condition*. A system's strong need to regain homeostasis means that the disequilibrium of a crisis does not go on indefinitely. Most crises last from four to six weeks (Aguilera, 1978). In this family, as shocking as the loss might seen, life begins to return to a more regular pattern in a few weeks. Although the members will feel the loss of husband and father for years, the crisis will soon disappear.

A crisis involves *cognitive uncertainty*. Much stress comes from not understanding the situation and not knowing its outcome. Immediate questions about notifying friends and planning the funeral raise uncertainty for the family that has lost a father. Long-range questions can plague every family member.

A crisis situation is *hazardous*. For the persons involved, crisis represents an actual loss (the death of a loved one), the threat of a loss (terminal illness), or an overwhelming challenge (the offer of an important job). With her husband dead, the wife faces sudden financial insecurity. She may have also lost her major source of emotional support.

Crisis brings on *psychophysiological symptoms*. People react somatically to the stress. They may experience appetite fluctuations, sleeplessness, body aches, nausea, muscle tension, perspiration, rapid pulse, and other signs of anxiety, as well as fear, shame, guilt, or excitement. The specific reaction depends on the nature of the situation, how it is perceived, and inherited tendencies. The children who have lost their father become irritable, cry, and may feel sick. The wife and mother may experience shortness of breath and exhaustion.

A crisis situation is *inescapable*. People face an unavoidable demand for change. The experience cannot be reversed or ignored. It requires some kind of action or response. When the head of a household dies suddenly, the other family members cannot escape the loss. Death brings inevitable changes for each of the remaining individuals.

Crisis often reveals *inadequate coping skills*. Habitual problem-solving resources do not work in this situation. The children have all known times when their father was absent from the family and have developed ways to cope with such temporary loss. But in this crisis situation, their father's death means permanent loss. They cannot deal with it in the same way.

Crisis creates a feeling of *helplessness*. The person feels overwhelmed, paralyzed, and unable to think or take action on his or her own. It is a time when the family members may ask others what to do. Sometimes helplessness takes the form of immobility; the wife may be unable to make even the simplest decisions.

Crisis elicits *exaggerated defense mechanisms*. Behaviors such as rationalizing excessively, compensating for losses, and blaming others are often evident. The wife may blame her husband's boss for overworking him and making him take the business trip that ended fatally.

Each crisis presents a unique problem, one too difficult for the person to solve alone with his normal coping mechanisms yet one too important to ignore. The problem represents a threat to the satisfaction of some basic need. An imbalance exists between supply and demand: the resources of the person are insufficient under the circumstances.

Every crisis constitutes a turning point. It presents people with an opportunity for growth toward a healthier state; it also brings the danger of increased vulnerability to illness. Growth occurs when we mature in the crisis and develop more effective problem-solving skills. Some persons, drawing on new resources, redefine the crisis of divorce, for instance, as a challenge to make a new life, to discover themselves and their potential, and to learn to establish healthier relationships with others. Those who engage in healthy adaptation during a crisis will emerge unharmed, even strengthened. They have become prepared to cope with similar events in the future.

Crises, however, present dangers as well as provide opportunities. The loss of homeostasis increases people's vulnerability to illness, mental or physical, and regression (Murray & Zentner, 1975). Some divorced persons, for instance, may not handle the crisis well; they may not accept or receive adequate help from others and become bitter, withdrawn, and resentful. These individuals have moved toward an unhealthy outcome as a result of maladaptive behavior. Ways in which the nurse can help the person or group handle crisis adaptively will be examined later.

Kinds of Crises

When the disease acquired immune deficiency syndrome (AIDS) struck the city of San Francisco a few years ago, panic and fear spread quickly. Who would contract the rapidly developing symptoms next and perhaps die? The situation threatened the very lives of the community. An overwhelming feeling of helplessness arose as public health authorities and city officials struggled to control the disease and identify its cause. For many people it was clearly a crisis.

Other less dramatic and less threatening events can still create anxiety and stress. They also require coping skills beyond those regularly practiced by the persons involved. A young couple is overwhelmed at the responsibility of becoming parents. An elderly woman panics at the thought of moving to a nursing home. A deteriorating neighborhood is threatened by a rise in crime. Like the AIDS disease outbreak, these too are crises, but of a different magnitude.

There are two kinds of crises. The AIDS disease event exemplifies a situational (or accidental) crisis. The other kind is a maturational (or developmental) crisis.

Maturational Crises

Maturational crises are periods of disruption that occur at transition points in normal growth and development. The people involved feel threatened by the demands placed on them. They have difficulty making the changes necessary to fit the new stage of development.

During the process of normal biopsychosocial growth, we go through a succession of life cycle stages. These begin with birth and continue through old age, each stage quite different from the previous one. As we leave one stage and enter a new one, we experience a transitional period characterized by changes in role expectations and behavior. It is a period of upset and disequilibrium. In recent years popular writers like Sheehy (1976), Levinson (1978), and Goodman (1979) have called these periods "passages," "transitions," and "turning points." They are the times when maturational crises occur (Fig. 12-1).

Groups and communities, too, develop through successive stages that frequently parallel the birth–to–old age pattern. Theorists have variously described the stages of group growth (Sampson & Marthas, 1977), which chapter 9 summarizes as dependence, counterdependence, and interdependence. Community development may be less easily distinguished. None-

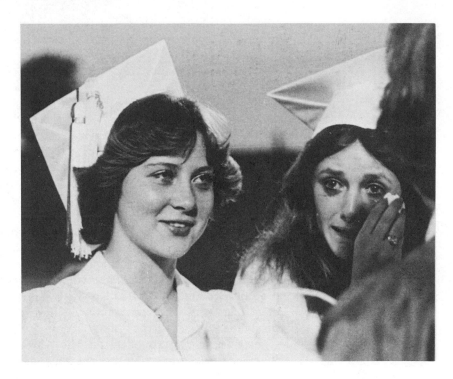

Figure 12-1
Graduation, like any maturational transition, is a time of mixed feelings. Some individuals can take it in stride. For others, it may become a time of crisis.

theless, anthropologists, sociologists, philosophers, historians, and other social scientists down through the years have observed and recorded the birth, rise, decline, and sometimes renewal (Gardner, 1981) of societies, communities, and other aggregates of people. Groups and communities, like most living systems, encounter stages of growth with accompanying transitions that require adaptation and lead to what can be described as "maturational" crises. For example, a new community may find that its growing population of young children lacks adequate playgrounds and recreational activities. The community is experiencing a maturational transition that requires adaptation.

Most maturational crises begin with a gradual onset. The change is evolutionary rather than revolutionary. We can anticipate and even prepare to start school, enter adolescence, leave home, get married, have a baby, retire, or die. People move into and through each transitional period knowing in advance that some kind of change will be required. So, too, with communities. A new town needs to develop its schools, businesses, city ordinances, recreational areas, hospitals, law enforcement, and churches. As it grows, the needs change to maintenance and controlled expansion. In many instances, we have already seen other people or communities of people experience these transitions. As a result, maturational crises have a degree of predictability. They offer the possibility of a period of time for anticipation and adjustment.

318

Maturational crises arise from both physical and social changes. Each new life stage confronts us with changed relationships, responsibilities, and roles. Consider the transition to parenthood, for example. It demands a change in role from caring for oneself and one's mate to include nurturing, caring for, and protecting a completely helpless child. Relationships with other adults, other children, and even one's own parents also change. Parenthood becomes an entrance into a previously unexperienced part of the adult world. New parents may fear the unknown. Will this infant develop normally? Can I give adequate care? Parents often feel anxiety over the responsibility of shaping this new person's life and satisfying society's expectations for their child's proper education and training. They may worry about the increased financial burden and struggle with mixed feelings about giving up a large measure of freedom. A community may find it lacks adequate resources to cope with increasing law enforcement demands, or a small town may struggle with its identity as it increases in size and loses its unique intimacy. These transitions place on people considerable stress, which contributes to tension build-up, feelings of helplessness, and resultant crisis. Some people adapt quickly; others cannot cope, probably because earlier maturational crises went unresolved. If people lack a repertoire of adaptive skills, a crisis can become major and disastrous. We can easily see how abused children become abusive parents when most, if not all, of their maturational crises have been detrimental rather than healthy.

CASE EXAMPLE

> Marcia Sand is 39 years old. Married for 22 years, she has been a capable homemaker and mother of 4 children. Her husband, Lou, a construction worker for the past 20 years, thinks Marcia does a "super job at home." In the past, Marcia's time was filled with cooking, laundry, cleaning, shopping, and meeting the endless demands of the family. Their limited income prompted her to adopt many money-saving strategies. She made most of her own and the children's clothes, did all her own baking, and raised vegetables in her backyard garden. Now the youngest of the children, Tommy, has just left home to join the Navy. Her husband spends much of his spare time at the local bar with his friends, leaving Marcia alone. With a nearly empty house and little need for cooking, baking, and sewing, Marcia has lost her sense of usefulness. She thinks of taking a job, but knows her choices are limited because she has only a high school education. Marcia has not slept well in weeks; she wakes up tired and drags through the day barely able to manage the simplest task. She cries frequently but does not know why. Her hair, always neat and attractive in the past, looks bedraggled, and her shoulders slump. "I just can't seem to get on top of things anymore," she complains.

Marcia has entered a maturational crisis that is sometimes called the "empty nest syndrome." She faces a turning point in her life, a time when parenting has ended. Leaving her satisfying homemaker role, she faces a new life stage filled with unknowns, changes, and a seeming lack of purpose. The

319

transition came about gradually, almost imperceptibly, but now she must deal with it. Yet she feels unable to cope and wishes to turn to someone who would understand and lend her strength. She can be helped, but her crisis could also have been prevented.

Situational Crises

A situational crisis is an acute state of disequilibrium precipitated by an unexpected external event perceived as hazardous. It requires behavioral changes and coping mechanisms beyond the abilities of the people involved.

Sudden events over which we have little or no control come in many forms (Fig. 12-2). A flood destroys a family's home and all their possessions.

Figure 12-2
This flood in Wilkes-Barre, PA, July 1972 created a situational crisis for that community. Here, Red Cross disaster workers search for victims in the flood-inundated downtown area.

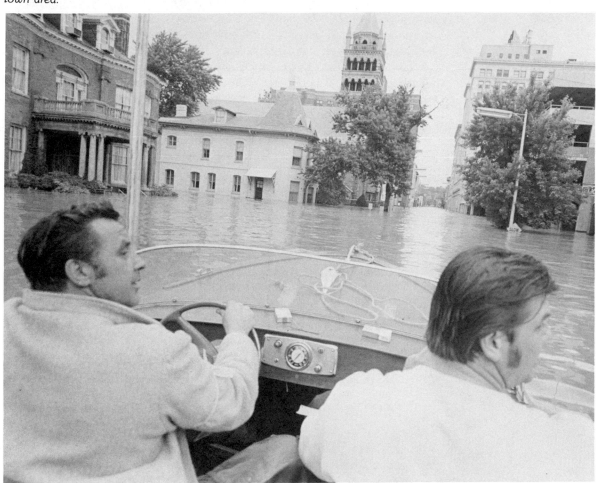

Another family loses its young mother through cancer. A group of workers lose their jobs. After 25 years of marriage, a couple gets divorced. An epidemic of serious influenza strikes a city. These kinds of events, which involve loss or the threat of loss, represent life hazards to those affected. Some crisis-precipitating events can be positive, such as a significant job promotion or news of a large inheritance; however, they still make increased demands on individuals (Caplan, 1964). Integrity is threatened and equilibrium disrupted during these situational or accidental crises.

Situational crises arise from external sources, that is, events or conditions generally outside of people's normal life processes. They are extraordinary experiences. They create life changes and disrupt equilibrium by imposing stresses that are usually foreign to ordinary living. The result is overwhelming tension and incapacitation. Natural disasters, for example, are clearly an external cause of a situational crisis. Said one client, "I shall never forget my feelings when one of my high school classmates was killed instantly by lightning. Mel was a popular boy, and his death threw us all into crisis."

Community health nurses see an almost infinite variety of situational crises; included are debilitating disease, economic misfortune, unemployment, physical abuse, divorce, unwanted pregnancy, chemical abuse, sudden death of a loved one, tragic accidents like a mine explosion, and many others. In each situation, people feel overwhelmed and need help to cope. Skilled intervention can make the difference between a healthy or unhealthy outcome.

CASE EXAMPLE

The Cooper family eagerly anticipated the birth of their first child. When they first learned that Danny had a harelip and cleft palate, Jan and Frank were numb. They were immediately overwhelmed by the shock of seeing their disfigured baby and worried about the possibility of other defects. Then came the first painful days adjusting to Danny's appearance and trying to feed and care for him. Jan and Frank alternated between feelings of guilt ("Perhaps we didn't do something right during pregnancy!") and resentment ("Why did this have to happen to us?"). Added to these anxieties was the specter of several corrective surgeries. Each operation threatened them with the risk to Danny, the stress of hospitalization, the struggle to stay with Danny while juggling jobs, the consequences to home life, and the impossible financial costs. How could they handle it all? They felt unable to cope.

As with most situational crises, this one took the Coopers completely by surprise. It upset their normal pattern of living and disrupted their equilibrium. The onset was sudden, precipitated by an event that they perceived as threatening to their well-being. Unlike maturational crises that are brought on by normal demands of growth, their child's congenital defect was externally imposed. And it required behavior changes and adjustments that the Coopers' usual coping abilities were not equipped to handle. These abilities needed help too.

Maturational and situational crises share the characteristics of crises in general described earlier. Their major differences are summarized in Table

Table 12-1
Major Differences between Types of Crises

Maturational Crisis	Situational Crisis
Part of normal growth and development	Unexpected period of upset in normalcy
Precipitated by a life transition point	Precipitated by a hazardous event
Gradual onset	Sudden onset
Response to maturational demands and society's expectations	Externally imposed "accident"

12-1. These two kinds of crises can overlap in actual experience. The Coopers, for example, experienced a maturational crisis (birth) and a situational crisis (birth defect) simultaneously; thus their stress was compounded. A maturational crisis of midlife may become complicated by situational crises such as divorce and job change occurring at the same time. The transition a child faces entering school may occur at the same time the family moves to a new neighborhood and a new infant joins the family. The child must share his parents' attention and affection with a new sibling at a time when all the resources the child can muster are needed. Overlapping crises are not uncommon, and they compound the stress felt by the persons involved. A team of football players, for example, experiencing the shock of an unexpected and embarrassing defeat is composed of individuals who may also be undergoing separate maturational or situational crises of their own. Research has shown that these accumulated stresses can lead to ill health (Holmes & Rahe, 1967). Those who might normally work through one crisis in a healthy way may find that compound events overwhelm them and cause disaster.

Crisis Prevention

Many people go through crises unnecessarily, ones that might have been prevented. Other crises could be shortened in length or diminished in intensity through preventive measures. Because of the nature and philosophy of community health practice, nurses should place a high priority on crisis prevention. Community health nurses are in a unique position to prevent or detect crises early. They encounter clients or would-be clients in their natural settings where direct observation and discussion can occur. Also, through their participation in communities' communication networks, they can learn about potential family and community problems.

Primary Prevention

We shall consider crisis prevention in terms of its three levels — primary, secondary, and tertiary. Primary crisis prevention means keeping the crisis from ever happening; action completely obstructs its occurrence. Both maturational and situational crises can, in many cases, be prevented. Let us examine what this prevention involves.

A primary crisis prevention program in community health has two major goals (Caplan, 1964). The first objective is to make certain that people have adequate provision for basic needs. For the community health nurse, this goal involves health promotion. Any activity that fosters healthful practices and counteracts influences detrimental to healthy living can help prevent a crisis. For instance, nurses teach and encourage safety practices in the home and workplace. They work for stronger legislation and enforcement to keep drunk drivers off the roads. They promote improved nutrition for adolescents. Healthy people will have less trouble coping with crises that occur than those in poor health. Health promotion should deal with physical, psychological, sociocultural, and spiritual needs. Like purchasing insurance or depositing money in an account, storing up reserves in these areas safeguards clients against stressful times.

The second goal of primary crisis prevention is anticipatory action. Because maturational crises are often predictable, community nurses can help clients prepare for them. Clients can discuss with the nurse the kinds of adjustments and role changes the next transition period will require. Marcia Sand could have avoided an empty nest midlife crisis through anticipatory planning. Knowing that the children would inevitably leave home and that they contributed to her primary satisfactions in life, Marcia could have made plans to start developing new relationships and new work outlets. Placing an aging parent in a nursing home is often very stressful for the entire family, an event that anticipatory planning can make less intense, averting a crisis. Even situational crises, like many "accidents," are often predictable. There may be a family history of myocardial infarctions, for example, but family members can change lifestyles to prevent heart attacks in the living generations. Making changes in diet, exercise patterns, and job choices as well as learning stress-coping skills may greatly reduce the risks.

Anticipatory work means experiencing some of the feelings of loss, tension, or anxiety before the crisis-precipitating event occurs. It is much easier to do this at a time when energy and intellectual processes are at a high level of functioning. Anticipatory work dissipates the impact of the crisis event. Grief work, for example, can begin before the terminally ill family member actually dies. If such preparations are made, a crisis of large proportions can thus be prevented.

Secondary Prevention

Secondary crisis prevention focuses on early detection and treatment. It seeks to reduce the intensity and duration of a crisis and to promote adaptive behavior. Community health nurses often encounter clients in the early stages of a crisis. A mobile home community, devastated by a tornado, can be assisted with the help of other professionals to find emergency assistance to prevent group disintegration and mental health problems.

During the course of normal practice, community health nurses can watch for signs that people may be entering a crisis. By considering suspect any event that might potentially provoke crisis, the nurse can monitor clients' responses. Several simultaneous or rapidly succeeding stress events may forecast impending crisis. One family appeared to handle a job loss well; family members coped adequately with the death of a grandparent a few weeks later. However, their crisis became full-blown when the mother of the family learned she must have surgery. Nursing intervention at an early stage could have prevented the crisis from reaching major proportions and enabled the family to regain equilibrium sooner.

Tertiary Prevention

Tertiary crisis prevention involves reducing the amount and degree of disability or damage resulting from crisis. Although it involves rehabilitative work, it can help clients' recovery and reduce the risk of future crises. In this sense, it is a preventive measure. Clients can easily become caught in a web of maladaptive responses. For instance, workers laid off from their jobs do not recover from the experience, remain bitter and hostile, and reinforce one another's heavy drinking. A grieving widower continues for months or years to deny his wife's death, withdraws socially, and develops chronic physical problems. A person in the crisis of old age cannot accept her aging and adopts bizarre and offensive dress and mannerisms. Tertiary crisis prevention involves helping these clients to face the reality of their present stiuation and to develop improved coping skills. Working with individuals in groups is a particularly effective means of providing support, reality orientation, and the prevention of further disability.

Phases of a Crisis

Regardless of the kind of crisis — situational or maturational — people follow a fairly predictable pattern when they respond to the event and seek to regain equilibrium. This pattern progresses in four phases — shock, withdrawal, acknowledgment, and resolution (Caplan, 1964,; Fink, 1967; Murray & Zentner, 1975) (see Table 12-2).

efforts to resolve the crisis. The people who have lost jobs, for example, can no longer deny that it has happened. There is recognition and gradual, albeit painful, acceptance of the loss. Assessing the situation's significance and planning for its management can now begin.

However, the harshness of reality frequently leads to depression expressed in apathy, agitation, remorse, or bitterness. Divorced persons may feel at fault or, conversely, that they have been treated unfairly. The pain of rejection, loss of relationships, and anxiety about how to cope with the present and future can all combine to create severe depression. The acknowledgment phase is a time of mourning, self-depreciation, and emotional decline. From these feelings, however, and with outside help, a restructuring of coping abilities begins. People move from disorganized thinking to redefining and attempting to solve the problem. Their behavior becomes more purposeful, planning more realistic. Tension, though still felt, is converted into a constructive energy force.

Again, maladaptive responses can occur when people retreat from this phase and continue to deny the problem. Some choose long-term nonreality or the more drastic escape of suicide. Most people, however, discover that the acknowledgment phase is often completed within a few weeks.

Adaptation

The final phase of crisis occurs as people engage in successful problem resolution and adaptation to a new life. They not only face reality but test it by restructuring their lives to make them workable. The adaptation phase is marked by feelings of hope and a positive approach to problem solving. The level of anxiety diminishes as people gain a new sense of identity and self-worth. They can talk about the situation openly. They reorganize their thinking toward effective reconstruction, making the best use of their own and other available resources. Their behavior is directed toward mastering the situation and stabilizing the change. People who successfully complete the adaptation phase, which may last for weeks or months, have developed new coping abilities. They have grown stronger, more mature, and better equipped to deal with future crises.

It is helpful for the nurse to recognize the pattern that emotions follow throughout the crisis sequence. Emotions are initially high, then begin to decline rapidly during the shock phase as people feel overwhelmed and increasingly anxious. If it is a crisis for a group, anxiety seems to spread from one person to another. Emotional decline's lowest point occurs at the end of the defensive retreat phase, resulting in depression and exhaustion. In the acknowledgment phase, the emotional level begins to climb as people start to face and cope with reality. Finally, emotions are back to a normal level of functioning by the end of the adaptation phase (Hirschowitz, 1966).

In the crisis sequence, each succeeding phase lasts longer than the previous

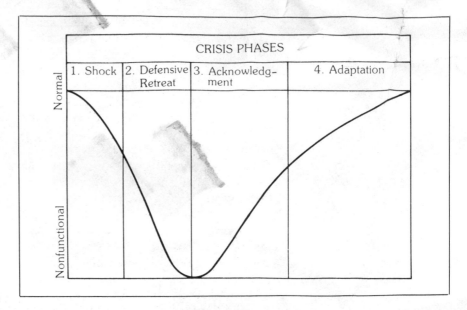

Figure 12-4
Varying emotional levels
during crisis.

one; thus, an increasing amount of adaptive energy is required. Effective
professional intervention may significantly reduce the length of time spent
in each phase. Figure 12-4 depicts the emotional curve in relation to the
varying lengths of each phase. These phases parallel the Kübler-Ross (1969)
stages of dying — shock, denial, anger, bargaining, depression, and acceptance.
They have also been expressed as (1) Who, me?; (2) Not me!; (3) Why
me?; and (4) Yes, me. The latter sequence provides a colloquial but useful
description of the crisis stages.

Crisis Intervention

People in crisis need help. They often desperately want help. The crisis and
its associated disequilibrium has a two-fold effect on the individuals involved.
It renders them temporarily helpless, unable to cope on their own, and thus
makes them especially receptive to outside influence. Also, this very desire
for assistance triggers a helping response from the people nearby. Caplan
(1964, p. 48) explains that "in crisis . . . , as the individual's tension rises
to a climax, he begins not only to mobilize his own resources, but also to
solicit help from others. The signs of his increasing tension appear to have
a significant effect on others, so that they are stimulated to come to his
assistance. This reciprocal pattern of seeking and offering help appears to
have primitive biosocial roots; similar phenomena can be found in many
social animals."

The significance of this phenomenon cannot be overemphasized. People in crisis will seek and generally receive some kind of help, but the nature of that help can rule in favor of or against a healthy outcome. Clients' desires for assistance give the helping professional a prime opportunity to intervene; this opportunity also presents a challenge to make that intervention as effective as possible.

Goal

The primary goal of crisis intervention is to reestablish equilibrium. Minimally that goal involves resolving the immediate crisis and restoring clients to their precrisis level of functioning. Ultimately, however, intervention seeks to raise that functioning to a healthier, more mature level that will enable them to cope with and prevent future crises. As we discussed earlier, crises tend to be self-limiting, which causes intervention time to last from four to six weeks (Aguilera & Messick, 1978). The urgency of the situation and its time limitations require the prompt, focused attention of clients and nurse working together to achieve intervention goals.

Methods

Crisis intervention in community health may utilize one or both of two approaches, generic and individual. For the majority of crisis encounters, the generic approach is more appropriate.

GENERIC APPROACH

The generic approach designs intervention to fit a particular type of crisis. That is, treatment focuses on the nature and course of the crisis, rather than on the psychodynamics of each client (Aguilera & Messick, 1978). Crisis intervention using the generic approach is tailored to a specific kind of crisis, situational or maturational, and includes four important elements: (1) direct encouragement of adaptive behavior, (2) general support, (3) environmental manipulation, and (4) anticipatory guidance (Jacobson, Strickler, & Morely, 1968). For example, the generic approach used with mastectomy clients encourages discussion and analysis of feelings, uses exercises to regain physical functioning, and creates a supportive, caring atmosphere. The nurse helps in fitting and use of prostheses, rebuilding of self-image, and strengthening of self-esteem through positive interpersonal relationships. The community nurse also prepares clients to handle future feelings of depression and anxiety related to bodily disfigurement and the possibility of metastasis.

The generic approach does not require advanced professional psychotherapy skills. More important for community health practice, it works well with families, groups, and even communities caught in crisis. The community health nurse may lead a group of cancer patients; grieving spouses; adolescents struggling with developmental crisis; or an entire community recovering from flood, tornado, or some other disaster. The generic approach allows the nurse to intervene with any group of people who have a crisis in common. It offers a broad base of support, since such a group can offer resources for the members beyond those brought by the nurse. Whether a family or a group of divorcées, new ostomy patients, or new retirement home residents, clients can benefit from the generic approach in a time of crisis.

INDIVIDUAL APPROACH

The individual approach is used when clients do not respond to the generic approach or need special therapy. Individual crisis intervention should not be confused with individual psychotherapy. The latter tends to focus on clients' developmental past, although the extent of that focus depends on the type of psychotherapy. Crisis intervention, on the other hand, directs treatment toward the immediate state of disequilibrium, identifying its causes and developing coping mehcanisms. Family members or significant others are included during the process of crisis resolution. An entire group may need this type of intervention. When this approach is needed, clients are usually referred to a professional with specialized training.

Steps for Intervention

Crisis intervention in community health assumes that clients have resources (Fig. 12-5). If their potential for managing stress events can be tapped, people in crisis will need minimal direct assistance. In accordance with the self-care concept, crisis intervention seeks to identify and build on client strengths. Aguilera and Messick (1978) outline a series of four steps for intervention during crisis.

ASSESSMENT

Initially, the nurse must assess the nature of the crisis and the clients' response to it. How severe is the problem, and what risks do the clients face? Are other people also at risk? Assessment must be rapid but thorough, focusing on some specific areas.

First, concentrate on the immediate problem in order to make an accurate diagnosis. Why have they asked for help right now? How do they define the problem? What happened to precipitate the crisis? When did it occur? Was it a sudden accidental event or a slower developmental one?

Next, focus on the clients' perception of the event. What does the crisis mean to them, and how do they think it will affect their future? Are they viewing the situation realistically? When crisis occurs to a family or group,

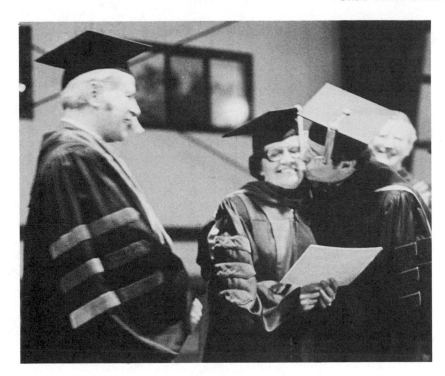

Figure 12-5
Many women avert midlife crisis by returning to school and starting a new career after raising their children.

some members see the situation differently from others. During intervention, all should be encouraged to express themselves, to talk about the crisis, and to share their feelings about its meaning. Acceptance of the range of feelings is important.

Determine what persons are available for support. Consider family, friends, clergy, other professionals, community members, and agencies. To whom are clients close and whom do they trust? One advantage of group intervention is that the members provide some of this support for each other. In subsequent sessions, the *quality* of support should be evaluated. Sometimes a well-meaning individual may worsen the situation or deter clients from facing and coping with reality.

Next, assess the clients' coping abilities. Have they had similar kinds of experiences in the past? What techniques have they previously used to relieve tension and anxiety? Which ones have they tried in this situation, and if they have not worked, why not? Clients should be encouraged to think of other stress-relieving techniques, perhaps ones used formerly, and to try them.

Finally, and of crucial importance, find out if there is a possibility of suicide or homicide. Ask directly and specifically about any plans or hints of anyone to kill himself or anyone else. If plans are specific and the threat appears real, psychiatric referral is indicated. Do not discount threats as idle talk.

PLANNING THERAPEUTIC INTERVENTION

Several factors influence the extent of the clients' disequilibrium; try to determine them before making intervention plans. The major balancing factors — clients' perception of the event, situational supports, human resources, and clients' coping skills — have been assessed in the first step (Aguilera & Messick, 1978). While continuing to explore these, the nurse now also considers clients' general health status, age, past experiences with similar types of situations, sociocultural and religious influences, and the actual assets and liabilities of the situation. This additional assessment helps to clarify the situation and gives the nurse the opportunity to encourage further clients' participation in the resolution process. If clients remain in the defensive retreat phase of crisis, they can complete only simple tasks until they face reality and begin problem solving.

The plan is based on the kind of crisis (situational or maturational, acute or chronically recurring), the crisis's effects on the clients (can they still work, go to school, keep house?), the phase of crisis the clients are in, the ways significant others are affected and respond, and the clients' strengths and available resources.

Using the problem-solving process, nurse and clients develop the plan. They review the event that precipitated the crisis, obvious symptoms, and the disruption in the clients' lives. The plan may focus on one or several areas. For instance, clients may need to grasp intellectually the meaning of the crisis, to engage in greater expression of feelings, or both. Part of the plan may be directed toward finding appropriate replacement, such as temporary housing, emergency financial aid, or physical care, for material losses. Another part may focus on helping clients to identify and use more effective coping techdniques or locate supportive agencies and resource persons. The plan will also include the development of realistic goals for the future.

INTERVENTION

During intervention it is important for nurse and clients to continue to communicate. They should discuss what is happening, review the plan and the rationale behind its elements, and make appropriate changes in the plan when indicated. It is helpful to assign definite activities at the end of each session so that clients can try out different solutions and evaluate various coping behaviors.

The intervention step is enhanced by use of the guidelines below (Cadden, 1964; Morely, Messick & Aguilera, 1967; Murray & Zentner, 1975).

Demonstrate Acceptance of Clients

A crisis will often shatter the ego. Clients need to feel the support of a positive, caring person who does not judge their feelings or behavior. Some negative expressions such as anger, withdrawal, and denial are normal aspects of the early phases of crisis. Accept them as normal.

Help Clients Confront Crisis

Clients need to face and discuss the situation. Expressing their feelings reduces tension and improves reality perception. Recounting what has actually occurred may be painful, but it helps clients confront the crisis. Do not assume that once clients have told about the event, no further recounting is necessary. Each time the story is told, they come closer to dealing realistically with the crisis.

Help Clients Find Facts

Distorted ideas and unknown factors of the situation create additional tension and may lead to maladaptive responses. For instance, it would help the Coopers to know that their son's cleft palate was unpreventable. Facts about surgical treatment and speech training would also be important for them to know.

Help Clients Express Feelings Openly

Suppressed feelings can be harmful. For instance, a widow may feel guilty that she is glad her husband is gone. Expression of these feelings helps reduce tension and gives clients an opportunity to deal with them.

Do Not Offer False Reassurance

Clients need to face reality, not avoid it. A statement such as "Don't worry, it will all work out" is demeaning and meaningless. Rather, make positive statements about faith in their ability to cope: "It is a very difficult situation, but I believe you will be able to deal with it."

Discourage Clients from Blaming Others

Clients often blame others as a way to avoid reality and the responsibility for problem solving. Withhold judgment when they blame others, but point out other causal factors and avenues for dealing with the situation.

Help Clients Seek Out Coping Mechanisms

Explore and test old and new techniques to reduce stress and anxiety. Ask questions. What are all the things clients and nurse might do together to resolve the problem? What are the things that need to be done? What do clients think they can do? This assistance gives clients more adaptive energy to work toward resolution.

Encourage Clients to Accept Help

Denial in the early phases of crisis cuts off help. Encouraging clients to acknowledge the problem is a first step toward acceptance of help. Often, however, clients fear the loss of their independence and the invasion of their privacy. They may state, "We ought to be able to handle this problem." At this point, the community nurse can assure clients that people in a crisis of this sort almost always need help. Preparing people to accept help will enable them to make the best use of what others have to offer.

Promote Development of New Positive Relationships

Clients who have lost significant persons through death or divorce should be encouraged to find new people to fill the void and provide needed supports and satisfactions.

RESOLUTION AND ANTICIPATORY PLANNING

In the final step, clients and nurse evaluate, stabilize, and plan for the future. First, evaluate the outcome of the intervention. Are clients using effective coping skills and exhibiting appropriate behavior? Are adequate resources and support persons available? Is the diagnosed problem solved, and have the desired results been accomplished? Analysis of these outcomes gives a greater understanding for coping with future crises.

To stabilize the change, identify and reinforce all the positive coping mechanisms and behaviors. Discuss why they are effective and how to use them in future stress situations. Summarize the crisis experience, emphasizing the clients' successes with coping in order to reconfirm progress and reinforce self-confidence. Point to evidence that they have reached their precrisis, or an even higher, level of functioning.

Clients' plans for the future should include setting realistic goals and means for implementing them. Review with clients how their handling of the present crisis can help them cope with, minimize, or preferably prevent future crises.

Summary

Crisis is a temporary state of severe disequilibrium for persons who face a threatening situation. It is a state that they can neither avoid nor solve with their usual coping abilities. A crisis occurs when some force disrupts normal functioning and thus causes a loss of homeostasis. A crisis creates tension; subsequently, efforts are made to solve the problem and reduce the tension. When such efforts meet with failure, people feel upset, redefine the situation, try other solutions, and, if failure continues, eventually reach the breaking point.

There are two kinds of crises, situational and maturational. Maturational crises are disruptions that occur during transitional periods in normal growth and development. They usually have a gradual onset and are often predictable. Situational crises, on the other hand, are precipitated by an unexpected external event. They have a sudden onset.

Crises can be prevented or their frequency and intensity can be diminished. Primary crisis prevention seeks to obstruct occurrence of crisis through promoting a high level of wellness and teaching people to anticipate and thus avoid possible crises. Secondary crisis prevention focuses on early detection and treatment. Tertiary crisis prevention seeks to reduce the degree of disability resulting from crisis.

Crises tend to progress through four stages — shock, defensive retreat, acknowledgment, and adaptation. People's perception of the crisis changes through these four stages, as do emotional response, cognitive ability, and behavior.

People in crisis both need and seek help. Crisis intervention builds on these two phenomena to achieve its primary goal — reestablishment of equilibrium. The two major methods for crisis intervention are the generic and individual approaches. The generic approach deals with a single type of crisis, such as rape, and often works with groups of people caught in the same crisis. The individual approach is used when clients do not respond to the generic approach or need additional therapy. Crisis intervention begins with assessment of the situation; then a therapeutic intervention is planned. Next, the nurse carries out the intervention, building on the strengths and self-care ability of clients. Finally, resolution and anticipatory planning to avert possible future crises occur.

Study Questions

1. What are the major differences between a maturational and a situational crisis? Give an example of each from your own experience.
2. Describe a maturational crisis experienced by a community known to you. What was this community's response? Describe some actions a community health nurse might have taken (alone or with a team) to help this community cope with the crisis.
3. Mobile home communities are frequent victims of tornadoes. What preventive actions could the community health nurse take? Design actions at each level of prevention.

References

Aguilera, D. C., & Messick, J. M. (1978). *Crisis intervention: Theory and methodology* (3rd ed.). St. Louis: C. V. Mosby.

Cadden, V. (1964). Crisis in the family. In G. Caplan, *Principles of preventive psychiatry* (pp. 288–296). New York: Basic Books.

Caplan, G. (1964). *Principles of preventive psychiatry*. New York: Basic Books.

Fink, S. L. (1967). Crisis and motivation: A theoretical model. *Archives of Physical and Medical Rehabilitation, 48,* 592.

Gardner, J. (1981). *Self-renewal: The individual and the innovative society* (rev. ed.). New York: Norton.

Goodman, E. (1979). *Turning points.* New York: Doubleday.

Hirschowitz, R. G. (1966). Crisis/transition sequence. In *Levinson Letter.* Cambridge, MA: Levinson Institute.

Holmes, T., & Rahe, R. (1967). The social readjustment rating scale. *Journal of Psychosomatic Research, 11,* 213–217.

Jacobson, G., Strickler, M., & Morely, W. (1968). Generic and individual approaches to crisis intervention. *American Journal of Public Health, 58,* 339–341.

Kübler-Ross, E. (1969). *On death and dying.* New York: Macmillan.

Levinson, D. J. (1978). *The seasons of a man's life.* New York: Knopf.

Morely, W. E., Messick, J. M., & Aguilera, D. C. (1967): Paradigms of intervention. *Journal of Psychiatric Nursing, 5,* 537–540.

Murray, R., & Zentner, J. (1975). *Nursing concepts for health promotion.* Englewood Cliffs, NJ: Prentice-Hall.

Sampson, E., & Marthas, M. (1977). Theories of group development. In E. Sampson & M. Marthas (Eds.), *Group process for the health professions.* New York: Wiley.

Sheehy, G. (1976). *Passages: Predictable crises of adult life.* New York: Dutton.

Veninga, R., & Spradley, J. (1981). *The work stress connection.* Boston: Little, Brown.

Selected Readings

Aguilera, D. C., & Messick, J. M. (1978). *Crisis intervention: Theory and methodology* (3rd ed.). St. Louis: C. V. Mosby.

Brandon, S. (1970). Crisis theory and possibilities of therapeutic intervention. *British Journal of Psychiatry, 117,* 541–545.

Brose, C. (1973). Theories of family crisis. In D. Hymovich & M. Barnard (Eds.), *Family health care* (pp. 271–283). New York: McGraw-Hill.

Cadden, V. (1964). Crisis in the family. In G. Caplan *Principles of preventive psychiatry* (pp. 288–296). New York: Basic Books.

Caplan, G. (1964). *Principles of preventive psychiatry.* New York: Basic Books.

Chandler, H. M. (1972). Family crisis intervention: Point and counterpoint in the psychosocial revolution. *Journal of the American Medical Association, 64,* 211–215.

Christ, J. (1972). The adolescent crisis syndrome: Its clinical significance in the outpatient service. *Psychiatric Forum, 3*(1), 25–32.

Clark, T. (1976). Counseling victims of rape. *American Journal of Nursing, 76,* 1964–1966.

Clark, T., & Jaffe, D. T. (1972). Change within youth crisis centers. *American Journal of Orthopsychiatry, 42,* 675–679.

Collins, M. (1977). *Communication in health care: Understanding and implementing effective human relations.* St. Louis: C. V. Mosby.

Comstock, B., & McDermott, M. (1975). Group therapy for patients who attempt suicide. *International Journal of Group Psychotherapy, 25*(1), 44–47.

Donner, G. J. (1972). Parenthood as a crisis. *Perspectives in Psychiatric Care 10*(2), 84–87.

Dzik, R. S. (1976). Transactional analysis in crisis intervention. *Journal of Gynecological Nursing, 5*(1), 31–36.

Ebersole, P. P. (1976). Crisis intervention with the aged. In I. M. Burnside (Ed.), *Nursing and the aged.* New York: McGraw-Hill.

Eisler, R., & Hersen, M. (1973). Behavioral techniques in family-oriented crisis intervention. *Archives of General Psychiatry, 28*(1), 111–116.

Fallom, C. W. (1973). Providing relevant brief services to couples in marital crises. *American Journal of Orthopsychiatry, 43,* 235–237.

Fink, S. L. (1967). Crisis and motivation: A theoretical model. *Archives of Physical Medicine and Rehabilitation, 48,* 592–597.

Foreman, N. J., & Zerwekh, J. V. (1971). Drug crisis intervention. *American Journal of Nursing, 71,* 1736–1738.

Freudenberger, H. J. (1974). Crisis intervention, individual and group counseling, and the psychology of the counseling staff of a free clinic. *Journal of Social Issues, 30*(1), 77–81.

Golan, N. (1969). When is a client in crisis? *Social Casework, 50,* 389–391.

Goldstein, S., & Giddings, J. (1973). Multiple impact therapy: An approach to crisis intervention with families. In G. Specter (Ed.), *Crisis intervention* (Behavioral Publications No. 210) (pp. 193–204). New York: Behavioral Publications.

Hall, J. E., & Weaver, B. (Eds.). (1974). *Nursing of families in crisis.* Philadelphia: Lippincott.

Hitchcock, J. M. (1973). Crisis intervention — The pebble in the pool. *American Journal of Nursing, 73,* 1388–1390.

Hoff, L. (1978). *People in crisis: Understanding and helping.* New York: Addison-Wesley.

Holstrom, L., & Burgess, A. (1975). Assessing trauma in the rape victim. *American Journal of Nursing, 75*(8), 1288–1290.

Hott, J. R. (1976). The crisis of expectant fatherhood. *American Journal of Nursing, 76,* 1436–1440.

Hott, J. R. (1977). Mobilizing family strengths in health maintenance and coping with illness. In A. Reinhardt & M. Quinn (Eds.), *Current prac-*

tice in family-centered community nursing. St. Louis: C. V. Mosby.

Jacobson, G. (1974). Emergency services in community mental health: Problems and promise. *American Journal of Public Health, 64,* 124–127.

Jacobson, G., Strickler, M., & Morely, W. (1968). Generic and individual approaches to crisis intervention. *American Journal of Public Health, 58,* 339–341.

Kübler-Ross, E. (1969). *On death and dying.* New York: Macmillan.

Lavietes, R. L. (1974). Crisis intervention with ghetto children: Mythology and reality. *American Journal of Orthopsychiatry, 44,* 241–245.

Marks, M. J. (1976). The grieving patient and family. *American Journal of Nursing, 76,* 1488–1491.

Marmer, J. (1972). The crisis of middle age. In L. H. Schwartz & J. L. Schwartz (Eds.), *The psychodynamics of patient care.* Englewood Cliffs, NJ: Prentice-Hall.

McClellan, M. S. (1972). Crisis groups in special care areas. *Nursing Clinics of North America, 7,* 363–371.

Messick, J. M. (1972). Crisis intervention concepts: Implications for nursing practices. *Journal of Psychiatric Nursing, 10*(5), 3–7.

Morely, W. E., Messick, J. M., & Aguilera, D. C. (1967). Crisis: Paradigms of intervention. *Journal of Psychiatric Nursing, 5,* 537–540.

Nakushian, J. (1976). Restoring parents' equilibrium after sudden infant death. *American Journal of Nursing, 76,* 1600–1604.

O'Brien, M. J. (1978). *Communication and relationship in nursing* (2nd ed.). St. Louis: C. V. Mosby.

Parad, H. J. (Ed.). (1965). *Crisis intervention.* New York: Family Service Association of America.

Price, J. L., & Braden, C. (1978). The reality in home visits. *American Journal of Nursing, 78,* 1536–1538.

Rapoport, R. (1963). Normal crises, family structure, and mental health. *Family Process, 2,* 68–76.

Selkin, J. (1975, January). Rape. *Psychology Today,* pp. 71–76.

Specter, G. (1973). *Crisis intervention* (Behavioral Publications No. 210). New York: Behavioral Publications.

Strickler, M., & LaSor, B. (1970). The concept of loss in crisis intervention. *Mental Hygiene, 54,* 301–303.

Van Antwerp, M. (1970). Primary prevention: A challenge to mental health associations. *Mental Hygiene, 54,* 453–457.

Williams, F. (1971). Intervention in maturational crises. *Perspectives in Psychiatric Care, 9,* 240–242.

Woehning, M., & Martinson, I. (1975). Family nursing during death and dying. In B. W. Spradley (Ed.), *Contemporary community nursing* (pp. 405–411). Boston: Little, Brown.

Zelbach, J. Z. (1971). Crisis in chronic problem families: Psychiatric care of the underprivileged. *International Psychiatry Clinics, 8*(2), 101–105.

three

Care of Communities

13

The Community:
Assessment and Planning

A central theme of this book has been community health nursing's involvement in promoting the health of aggregates of people. This idea has been emphasized because, in both subtle and direct ways, our culture works against it. The value of individualism is one of the greatest barriers to carrying out the mission of community health nursing.

Individualism and Community Health

Every society has a small number of core values that give meaning to life. In the United States, for example, we value success and material rewards. Such values provide motivation for millions of people. They uphold the work ethic; they become the measures by which we elevate successful and wealthy people to the status of popular heroes. The very existence of our society and its way of life depends on a deep commitment to such values. We learn them early in life and come to take them for granted as the way things ought to be. One value that most Americans hold as God-given, a value that profoundly influences the entire practice of nursing, is individualism.

Nearly every social observer who has written about American society has identified this value. A cornerstone of our civilization, this basic premise underlies most of our institutions. "Protect the rights of the individual"; "Equal justice for all under the law"; "Life, liberty, and the pursuit of happiness for all individuals'' are familiar cries. More than 40 years ago, the sociologist Robert Lynd described this value: "Individualism, 'the survival of the fittest,' is the law of nature and the secret of America's greatness; and restrictions on individual freedom are un-American and kill initiative'' (Lynd, 1939, p. 60).

We reward individual effort in the school and in the workplace. Our criminal justice system punishes individual crimes far more harshly than corporate crimes. A woman who steals five dollars in a southern state serves several years in prison; a large oil company that steals millions by overcharging customers pays a relatively small fine or suffers no punishment at all. Health care in our society is dominated by a commitment to the treatment of individuals. The vast majority of our research, personnel, and health care institutions engage in the care of individual illness rather than promote community health.

How does this value of individualism affect community health nursing? All nurses are first educated and trained in the individualistic perspective of clinical nursing. The individual patient is the focus of nursing service. Moreover, this early education is supported by powerful cultural premises; together, they create a mind-set that nurses bring into community health nursing. Unless nurses become aware of this mind-set and consciously set it aside, clients will remain individuals instead of families, groups, organizations, populations, and communities (*Redesigning Nursing Education*, 1973).

This mind-set is influenced by three pervasive myths, all touched on in earlier chapters.

The Location Myth

Community health nursing is only clinical nursing outside the hospital setting. This myth silently influences nurses to think of their task as simply nursing *in* the community. Community health nursing, from this perspective, seems to have the merit of reducing hospital costs. It is easy to think that patients do not have to spend so much time in the hospital; health professionals can treat them and care for them in their homes. Instead, community health nursing is practice *to* and *with* the community. It may include the hospital.

The Skills Myth

Community health nursing employs only the skills of clinical nursing when working with community clients. This myth leads many nurses to assume their clinical skills are completely adequate for community nursing. It can lead them to overlook a large and sophisticated body of knowledge required for effective community health nursing. When unquestioningly accepted, this myth causes nurses to discount key concepts such as health, culture, family dynamics, and group process, or an essential epidemiological approach.

342

The Client Myth

Community health nursing involves working with communities, but the individual in a family context is the primary client. This myth prevents us from taking a wide perspective, one that sees the health of families, groups, subpopulations, communities, and populations as central to community health nursing practice.

In order to escape the constricting influence of this final myth, it is useful to think of six different levels on the community health nursing scope of practice continuum, ranging from individuals to aggregates. On a typical day, a community health nurse might well work at all six levels. In a city such as Atlanta, Georgia, as a community health nurse, you might leave an agency to visit an unmarried adolescent in the last trimester of her pregnancy. As you offer service to this individual, you will also assess her family as a group and seek to promote the health of that family. You might invite this young woman to a group of expectant mothers with whom you will meet that evening. Before noon, let us say that you stop by The Family Tree on Selby Avenue to meet with the staff for a discussion of how to reach the subpopulation of teenage girls in the neighborhood. In the early afternoon you meet with other staff at your agency to discuss assessing the population of unmarried, pregnant adolescents in the city of Atlanta. Before you finish your day's work, you might stop by the city council hearing room to participate in a hearing on a local ordinance regarding abortion, or you might visit the Georgia state legislature for a committee hearing on the use of state funds for abortion by women on welfare. These last two activities involve nursing practice at the community level.

Table 13-1 summarizes some of the major differences among the various levels of nursing practice. Chapters 15 and 16 describe the family as client, the characteristics of a healthy family, and ways to provide nursing service to families. We have examined the nature of groups, what causes groups to function effectively, and how community health nurses can work with groups. In chapter 9, we also discussed working with populations and subpopulations. Now we will shift our attention to the community as an aggregate.

Although community health nurses work at all six levels of practice, working with communities is of considerable significance for two important reasons. First, the community, geographically defined, directly influences the health of individuals, families, groups, subpopulations, and populations. When the city of Los Angeles failed to take aggressive action to stop air pollution, this failure affected the health of millions of people. Similarly, when a community improves its water supply, this action affects the health of families, groups, and people at all the other levels. Second, working with communities is important because it is at this level that most health service provision occurs. Health information is developed by community agencies, as are the services required by families and groups.

Table 13-1
Variations in Scope of Community Health Nursing Practice

	Client	Example	Characteristics	Health Assessment	Nursing Involvement
Individual	Individual	Kim Murphy	One person with various needs	Individual health assessment	A dyad; interaction with the individual
	Family	Murphy family, seven members	A small group based on kin ties; specific roles	Family health assessment	Family visits; interaction with members as a group
	Group	Parenting group; Alanon club	Two or more people; face-to-face communication; interdependency	Assessment of group effectiveness in fulfilling its functions	Group participation; having a role in meetings
Aggregate	Subpopulation	Unmarried pregnant adolescents in a school district	Large group; shared characteristics (subset of a larger group)	Assessment of collective health problems and needs	Study of and planning for meeting specific health needs
	Community	St. Paul, MN, Macalester neighborhood	An aggregate of people in a specific location organized in a social system	Survey of community characteristics, such as vital statistics and competence	Membership in organizations such as a health planning council
	Population	U.S. elderly; all diabetics in one state	A large, unorganized aggregate based on some demographic feature	Survey of health needs and vital statistics	Researching the population; planning and setting up services

The community health nurse, then, must deal with the community as the client. Understanding the community is a prerequisite for effective service at every level of community nursing practice.

The Community as Client

Community is a term that we use in many different ways. Some people talk about the "community of professional nurses," those nurses who are trained and work in the field. On a small college campus in the south, students and faculty talk about the "college community." You probably think of your hometown or city as a "community." On occasion, the president of the United States will refer to the "American community." In England and France, people talk about the "European Economic Community," and spokespeople for the United Nations refer to the "world community."

In chapter 1, we defined a community as having three features: (1) a location, (2) a population, and (3) a social system (Lynd, 1939). This three-dimensional view, represented in Figure 13-1, especially suits our idea of a local community. The size of a local community can vary by expanding or constricting the geographic boundary. The community of Seattle, for example, may refer to the city as defined by all the people within the city limits. But we also speak of "greater Seattle," a community composed of the city, its suburbs, and many other small towns located near Seattle. A community health nurse might want to restrict the size of the community within Seattle to the Wallingford district. If you worked in the Washington State Health Department in Olympia, you would probably think of your community as the entire state. However, all these communities still share the three common denominators of a single location, population, and social system.

Think of these three dimensions of every community as a rough map you can follow whether you are working in a rural town of 250 people or in the city of Chicago. This concept of community is a useful tool for assessing

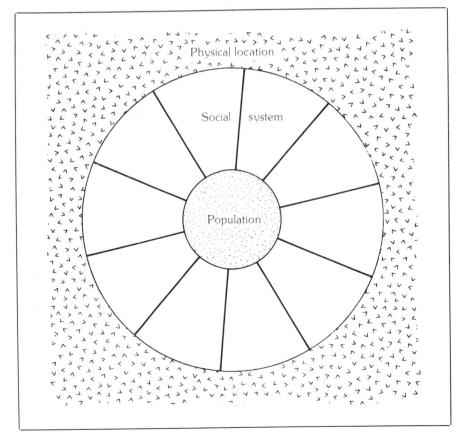

Figure 13-1
A community has (1) a physical location, represented here by the square boundary; (2) a population, shown here by the central circle; and (3) a social system, divided here into subsystems.

needs or planning for service provision, whether the particular community is a refugee camp in Cambodia or the state of New Hampshire. As we consider each dimension, we will pay particular attention to the questions that must be asked to assess the health of a community.

Location

Every community carries out its daily existence in a specific geographic location. The health of a community is affected by this location, by the location of health services, the geographic features, climate, plants, animals, and the human-made environment. The community health nurse will want to become aware of all these location variables and their implications for community health.

The location of a community places it in an environment that offers resources and also poses threats. The healthy community is one that makes wise use of its resources and is prepared to meet threats and dangers. In assessing the health of any community, it is necessary to collect information not only about these location variables, but also about how the community relates to them. Do groups cooperate to identify threats? Do health agencies cooperate to prepare for an emergency such as flood or earthquake? Does the community communicate information about resources and dangers to its members?

Guiding the nurse in assessing the health of any community is a Community Profile Inventory (Tables 13-2 to 13-4). It is divided into three parts — location, population, and social system — in order to conform to our definition of a community. Although not exhaustive, it suggests the implications for community health of each variable, provides a set of community assessment questions, and some information sources. Let us consider the six location variables that define, in part, every human community.

BOUNDARY OF COMMUNITY

In order to talk about the community in any sense, one must first discover its boundary. All measurements of wellness and illness within the community depend on knowing the unit under consideration. However, all communities are also related to other communities, and it is important to know about such locations. If nurses are working in a small community of 5,000 persons, they need to know whether it is part of a huge metropolis or an isolated rural town.

LOCATION OF HEALTH SERVICES

If the members of a town must travel 300 miles to the nearest clinic or dental office, the health of the community will be affected. When assessing

346

Table 13-2
Community Profile Inventory: Location Perspective

Location Variables	Community Health Implications	Community Assessment Questions	Information Sources
Boundary of community	Basis for measuring incidence of wellness and illness Basis for determining spread of disease	Where is community located? What is its boundary? It is a part of a larger community? What smaller communities does it include?	Atlas State maps County maps City maps Telephone book City directory Public library
Location of health services	Use of health services depends on availability and accessibility	Where are major health institutions located? What necessary health institutions are outside the community? Where?	Telephone book Chamber of commerce State health department County or local health departments Maps Public library
Geographic features	Injury, death, and destruction from floods, earthquakes, volcanoes Recreation opportunities at lakes, seashore, mountains	What major land forms are in or near the community? What geographic features pose possible threat? What geographic features offer opportunities for healthful activities?	Atlas Chamber of commerce Maps State health department Public library
Climate	Extremes of heat and cold affect health and illness Extremes of temperature and precipitation may tax community's coping ability	What is average temperature and precipitation? What are extremes? What climatic features affect health and illness? Is community prepared to cope with emergencies?	Weather atlas Chamber of commerce State health department Maps Local government Weather bureau Public library
Flora and fauna	Poisonous plants and disease-carrying animals can affect community health Plants and animals offer resources as well as dangers	What plants and animals pose a possible threat to health?	State health department Poison control center Police department Emergency rooms Encyclopedia Public library
Human-made environment	All human influences on environment (housing, dams, farming, type of industry, chemical waste, air pollution, etc.) can influence levels of community wellness	What are major industries? How has air, land, and water been affected by humans? What is quality of housing? Do highways allow access to health institutions?	Chamber of commerce Local government City directory State health department University research reports Public library

Table 13-3
Community Profile Inventory: Population Perspective

Population Variables	Community Health Implications	Community Assessment Questions	Information Sources
Size	The number of people influences number and size of health care institutions Size affects homogeneity of the population and its needs	What is the population of the community? Is it an urban, suburban, or rural community?	State health department Census data Maps City or town officials Chamber of commerce
Density	Increased density may increase stress High and low density often affect the availability of health services	What is the density of the population per square mile?	Census data State health department
Composition	Composition of the population often determines the types of health needs	What is the age composition of the community? What is the sex composition of the community? What is the marital status of community members? What occupations are represented and in what percentages?	Census data State health department Chamber of commerce U.S. Department of Labor Statistics
Rate of growth or decline	Rapidly growing communities may place excess demands on health services Marked decline in population may signal a poorly functioning community	How has population size changed over the past two decades? What are the health implications of this change?	Census data State health department
Cultural differences	Health needs vary among subcultural and ethnic populations Utilization of health services vary with culture Health practices and extent of knowledge affected by culture	What is the ethnic breakdown of the population? What racial groups are represented? What subcultural populations exist in the community? Do any of the subcultural groups have unique health needs and practices? Are different ethnic and cultural groups included in health planning?	Census data State health department Social and cultural research reports Human rights commission City government Health planning boards
Social class	Class differences influence the utilization of health services Class composition influences cost of public health services	What percentage of the population falls into each social class? What do class differences suggest for health needs and services?	State health department Census data Sociological reports

Table 13-3 Continued

Population Variables	Community Health Implications	Community Assessment Questions	Information Sources
Mobility	Mobility of the population affects continuity of care Mobility affects availability of service to highly mobile population	How frequently do members move into and out of the community? How frequently do members move within the community? Are there any specific populations, such as migrant workers, that are highly mobile? How does the pattern of mobility affect the health of the community? Is the community organized to meet the health needs of mobile groups?	State health department Census data Health agencies serving migrant workers Farm labor offices

Table 13-4
Community Profile Inventory: Social System Perspective

Social System Variables	Community Health Implications	Community Assessment Questions	Information Sources
Health system Family system Economic system Educational system Religious system Welfare system Political system Recreation system Legal system Communication system	Each system must fulfill its functions for a healthy community Collaboration among the systems to identify goals and problems affects health of community Undue influence of one system on another may lower the health of the community Agreement on the means to achieve community goals affects community health Communication among organizations in each system affects community health	What are the functions of each major system? What are the major subsystems of each system? What are the major organizations in each subsystem? How well do the various organizations function? Are the subsystems in each major system in conflict? Is there adequate communication among the major systems? Is there agreement on community goals? Are there mechanisms for resolving conflict? Do any parts of the total system dominate the others? What community needs are not being met?	Chamber of commerce Telephone book City directory Organizational literature Officials in organizations Community self-study Community survey Local library Key informants

a community, the community health nurse will want to identify the major health institutions and where they are located. In one city, for example, the alcoholism treatment center for skid row alcoholics was located 30 miles outside of the city. This location profoundly affected who volunteered for treatment and how long they remained at the center. The location of services may be restricted from some members who have transportation problems. If a well-baby clinic is located on the edge of a high-crime district, parents may be discouraged from using it. It is often enlightening to place the major health institutions, both inside and outside the community, on a map that shows their proximity and relation to the community.

GEOGRAPHIC FEATURES

Communities have been constructed in every conceivable physical environment. Mountain communities face problems that are foreign to a desert town. A healthy community takes into consideration the geography of its location, identifies the possible problems and likely resources, and responds in an adaptive fashion.

In Anchorage, Alaska, the community is set in the midst of mountains and almost on top of a geologic fault line. The same is true for San Francisco, where in 1906, a massive earthquake destroyed many buildings and fire swept through the city. Seven hundred persons died. In such places, the health of the community would be partly determined by its preparedness for an earthquake and its ability to cope when such a crisis occurred.

A geographic feature such as a lake offers food supplies for community members. A healthy community uses such a local resource in many ways, for instance, as a source of food, recreation, or water supply. The same resource, however, can also present a public health danger if drownings or contamination of fish occur. Sometimes the contamination comes from far distant communities. In Ontario, Canada, a series of lakes called the Lac la Croix is a valuable resource for the Ojibway Indian communities. They depend on fish from the lakes for their livelihood. However, in recent years, acid rain has begun to affect the lakes and the fish. Coal-burning power plants in the United States and Canada emit large amounts of sulfur dioxide that rise high in the air and are then blown by strong winds over the Lac la Croix chain of lakes. In the atmosphere, the sulfur dioxide reacts with water vapor to form sulfuric acid, which then falls to earth in the rain and snow, eventually finding its way into the lakes. As the acidity of lakes rises, the egg-producing ability of the fish drops. More immediately, the acid in the water changes mercury in the lake sediment into methyl mercury, which is easily absorbed by the fish. A major food supply has thus become contaminated for the Ojibway Indian communities.

350

CLIMATE

The climate also has a direct influence on the health of a community. When Buffalo, New York, is blanketed with deep winter snows, members of this community are sometimes immobilized for days. Deaths from coronary occlusions increase as people attempt to shovel their walks and uncover their cars. The intense summer heat of another location, such as Phoenix, Arizona, can create other health problems. Skin cancer, for example, is highest in states that constitute the Sunbelt. A healthy community will encourage physical activity among its members, but the climate, in turn, affects this activity. Although long cold winters can restrict activity, one community, St. Paul, Minnesota, holds an annual Winter Carnival, which includes sporting events. Parades, ice sailing, dogsledding, a treasure hunt, and hot air balloon races bring thousands of people out-of-doors at a time when they might otherwise be confined by the weather.

FLORA AND FAUNA

Plant and animal populations in a community are often determined by location. The way a community responds to these populations, whether wild or domestic, can affect the health of the community. In Covina, California, black widow spiders make up part of the local insect population. The poison from a single bite may cause injury and death. In Seattle, Washington, a bushy, attractive plant, known as Deadly Nightshade, grows in yards and vacant lots. It has an appealing black berry that appears edible. However, it contains the drug belladonna, and people have died from ingesting the berries. The community health nurse will want to know about the major sources of danger from plants and animals in the community. Are there community agencies that provide educational information about these dangers? Does the populace understand their significance? Are emergency services, such as a poison control center, available to community members?

HUMAN-MADE ENVIRONMENT

Every community is located in the midst of an environment created and transformed by human ingenuity. We build houses and other buildings; we dump wastes into streams or vacant lots; we fill the air with gasses; we build dams to control streams. All these human alterations of the environment have important implications for community health.

A community health nurse might improve the health of a community by working for legislation to prevent disposing of waste chemicals into water or landfills. Had such legislation been passed years ago, the disaster at New York's Love Canal, where toxic wastes are still seeping into the homes and yards of victimized citizens, might have been prevented.

One way in which we alter the environment is through agricultural activity. Southern Wisconsin is in the heart of midwest farmland. The rich harvests attract thousands of seasonal workers, farm migrants, every year. Because of their nomadic life-style and their rural location, the health of migrants suffers. Community assessment in this area would include a careful examination of the migrant population, the health services available to them, their housing accommodations, and the community's economic resources.

Every community exists in some physical location. This fact has important implications for the community's health and any plans to assess or improve it. Table 13-2 shows the first part of a provisional assessment tool, the Community Profile Inventory. It will help the nurse sense the health implications of geographic location as well as give some direction for assessing any community.

Population

When we consider the community as the client, the second dimension to examine is the population of the total community. As discussed in chapter nine, one level of practice in community health nursing is working with special population groups. These population groups may be within a community or cut across many communities. For example, health care for the elderly population may be carried out in a city such as Des Moines, Iowa, or in the entire state of Iowa. However, from the perspective of the community itself, the population consists not of a specialized aggregate, but of all the diverse people who live within the boundaries of the community. As Sanders and Brownlee (1979, p. 413) have said, "A community can be viewed as a population, as a collection of people. Health authorities conduct demographic analyses in order to determine the extent of maternity, morbidity, and mortality within a community."

The health of any community is greatly influenced by the population that lives in it. Different features of the population suggest health needs and provide a basis for health planning. A healthy community has leaders who are aware of the population's characteristics, know its different needs, and respond to those needs. Community health nurses can better understand any community by knowing about population size, density, composition, rate of growth or decline, cultural differences, social class, and mobility (Figs. 13-2 and 13-3). Let us consider each of these population variables briefly.

SIZE

The town of Dover, Delaware, with less than 10,000 people, and the city of Los Angeles, California, have radically different health problems. If a single hepatitis case occurred in Dover, health officials would likely learn of it. It would be relatively easy to trace the course, check the few restaurants

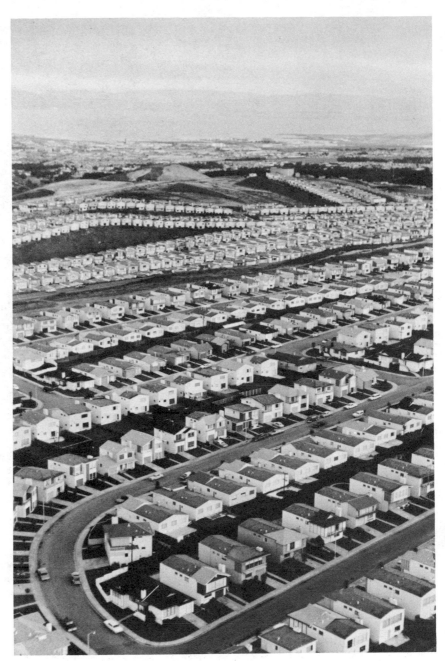

Figure 13-2
Many factors affect a community's health. Urban sprawl, shown here in this San Francisco suburb, influences commuting distance to work, pressures to conform to neighborhood standards, and many other variables affecting life-style and health.

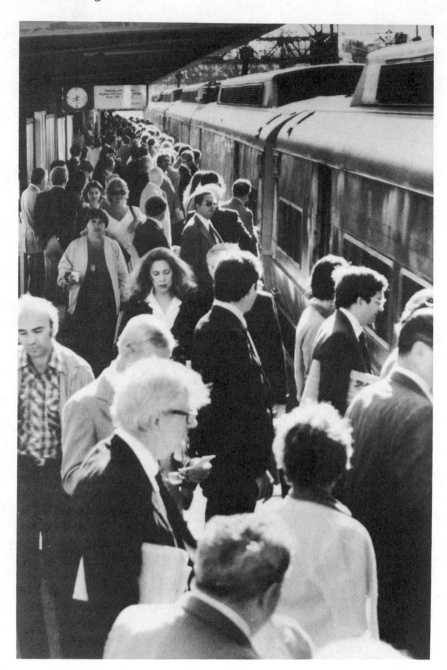

Figure 13-3
A community's resources,
including its public transportation system, pro-
foundly affect its health.
Here white-collar workers
crowd together to catch
their commuter train.

in town, and interview people about sanitation practices. However, many cases might occur in Los Angeles without the health department's knowledge. Moreover, if these cases were discovered, tracing the source of contamination might involve a long and complicated search. This is only one small way in which population size might affect the health of a community, but it also would influence the presence of slums, heterogeneity of the population, and almost every conceivable area of health need and service. One of the first things community health nurses need to know about a community is its size.

DENSITY

In some communities, thousands of people are crowded into high-rise housing. In others, such as farm communities, people live at great distances from one another. We do not yet know the full impact of living in high-density communities, but some research has already shown that crowding affects individual and community health. A study of Ohio farmers, living in low-density communities, suggests that the absence of stress from crowding may contribute to their reduced rate of coronary artery disease (Nagi, 1959).

A low-density community may have other problems. When people are spread out, health care provision may become difficult. There may not be enough resources in the form of taxes to support public health services. Rural communities often suffer from inadequate supply of health care personnel, ranging from private physicians to community health nurses. A healthy community will take into consideration the density of its population. It will organize in ways to meet the differing needs created by its density levels; for example, it will recognize differences in density between the inner city and the suburbs and allocate services accordingly.

COMPOSITION

Communities differ in the types of people who live within their boundaries. A retirement community in Florida whose majority of members are over 65 years of age has one set of problems. A city with a higher number of women in the childbearing years will have another set of problems. A healthy community is one that takes full account of differences in age, sex, educational level, and occupation of its members.

Occupations may be diversified among many industries or concentrated in a single field. In a town where 75 percent of the workers are employed by a textile mill, the community lives under the threat of cotton dust, the cause of brown lung disease. Some textile mill communities ignore this danger, do nothing to inform workers of the dangers they face, and provide little help for older workers who are laid off as a result of contracting this disease. A community nurse working to improve the health of this type of community would need to visit the textile mill, check on safety precautions such as face masks, and work to instigate regular lung examinations for all workers. Community leaders would have to become aware of the problem. Such a nurse might find it necessary to become an advocate for workers and organize them to negotiate with the textile mill managers for improving conditions in the mill. Understanding a community's composition is the first step in determining its level of health.

RATE OF GROWTH OR DECLINE

Community populations change over time. Some grow rapidly, thus putting extreme demands on the provision of health services. Others, because of economic change, may decline. Any fluctuation in population size can affect the health of the community. As population declines, community leadership may also decline. Even a stable community can have problems; for instance, members may resist needed change because they see little fluctuation in their population.

CULTURAL DIFFERENCES

A community may be composed of a single cultural group. A Pennsylvania farming town may share a common commitment to traditional Pennsylvania Dutch heritage. An Indian reserve in Washington state may reflect a single cultural tradition of Snohomish Indians. In many communities, however, several cultures or subcultures may be present. If a city has a large Hispanic population, a cluster of Native Americans who live in the inner city, and a scattering of Vietnamese refugees, the cultural differences among these members will influence the health of the community. A university town in a southern state had a large influx of students from Iran, Iraq, Greece, Turkey, Saudi Arabia, and other Middle Eastern countries. When Iranian militants in Teheran held American citizens hostage, their action had a direct effect on the university town. A healthy community is aware of such cultural differences and moves quickly to promote understanding between subcultural groups.

SOCIAL CLASS

Social class refers to the ranking of groups within society by income, education, occupation, prestige, or a combination of these indexes (Goode, 1977). Upper-class people are generally rich, educated, and in the most powerful positions. Lower-class people tend to be uneducated, poor, held in low esteem, living on subsistence incomes or less, and powerless. In between is the group that makes up the majority of the population — the middle class. Professionals and white-collar workers form a large portion of this

356

group. Further class distinctions are used to designate people who fall along the wide range within the middle-class category. For instance, "lower-middle" describes people with less prestigious occupations who are less affluent and sometimes less educated than most middle class people but not truly "poor." There is no absolute agreement on the income amounts used to designate each category other than the government formula used to compute poverty level. Nor is there agreement on other indexes; consequently, the labeling tends to be very subjective. Although class distinctions are arbitrary, class rankings by such indexes as occupation or wealth (income plus assets) correlate with many different social patterns and are used frequently as research measures. Occupational level, in particular, has proven a reliable measure with extraordinarily similar rankings among all societies for which there are data. The reason for this, Goode (1977, p. 272) points out, is that "people at higher occupational levels enjoy higher incomes; typically they have more education; they have more political influence; and they receive more esteem from others."

Some communities appear to be primarily middle class; others have large numbers of lower-class members. Still other communities may have a sprinkling of each social class. We know that social classes have different health problems, resources for coping with illness, and ways of using health services (Freeman, Levine, & Reeder, 1979). A healthy community recognizes these differences and creates health care services to meet these varied needs.

MOBILITY

American people are a mobile population. We move to go to college, take a new job, or seek new climates upon retirement. This mobility has a direct effect on the health of communities. If the population turnover is extensive, continuity of care may suffer. Leadership for improving the health of the community may change so frequently that concerted action becomes difficult. High turnover may require special attention to health education about local conditions.

Population groups may arrive and depart in seasonal swings; migrant farm workers and college students can both affect a community. The community health nurse will want to identify those populations that are seasonally mobile. They not only present special health needs, but may place an added burden on a community. If a town of 3,000 people has an annual influx of 10,000 students who disappear in the summer, members must prepare to meet this population change. A healthy community neither ignores nor overreacts to this kind of mobility. Rather, it identifies the nature of population change, determines the needs created by such change, and organizes to meet those needs.

As community nurses consider the population dimensions of the community, they will take a long step toward uncovering the true character of the community. Each of the variables related to population will suggest clues to the relative health of the community itself. Table 13-3 presents the second part of the Community Profile Inventory. It identifies the seven population variables, suggests some implications for community health, and provides several community assessment questions as well as possible sources of information.

Social System

Every community has a third dimension, a social system. A social system consists of parts, such as the local government, churches, families, and hospitals, that are linked together. The parts interact with and influence each other. Whether assessing a community's health, developing new services for the elderly within the community, or promoting the health of several familes, the community nurse needs to understand the community as a social system. A community health nurse working in a tiny village in Alaska needs to grasp the social system of that village no less than a nurse working in Washington, D.C., needs to understand the social system of our country's capital.

THE WHOLE COMMUNITY: CASE STUDY

A social system is an abstraction. For this reason, it can be elusive and difficult to grasp. Let us start with a specific example of a community of 20,000 people, which we will call Centerville. If you visited Centerville, you would not see the social system. It does not exist as a concrete reality, something that you can see, touch, or smell. What you would observe in Centerville is people. They would be walking, talking, playing, paying bills, performing surgery, saying prayers, water skiing, voting, and doing all the other things common in a community. Where, then, is the social system of Centerville? We can see how social scientists conceive of a community's social system by focusing briefly on a single individual.

Consider Marian Branch, mother of four children, director of the Centerville Public Health Nursing Agency. If you followed Marian Branch around for a few days, you would notice that she repeats certain activities. She prepares breakfast for her family each morning; she meets with her staff each day at the agency; she shops for food and clothes. If you expanded your observation to several weeks or months, other patterns of behavior, such as church attendance, participation in a subcommittee of the Centerville City Council, and theater patronage, would appear.

From a social system perspective, these patterns of activities make up the roles that Marian Branch enacts in the course of her daily life. She acts in the capacity of mother, agency director, store customer, church member, and Centerville City Council subcommittee member. When we take specific actions of a person and group them into patterns, we have identified social roles. Keep in mind, however, that these roles are only abstractions from observable concrete actions.

We can also look for patterns among roles, such as those enacted by Marian and the people whom she encounters. In doing so, we quickly discover that certain roles are closely connected: interaction occurs between mother and daughter, nursing supervisor and staff nurse, customer and sales clerk, and church member and clergyman. These new patterns that emerge among roles form the basis of *organizations*. Some organizations, such as the Branch family, are informal; others, such as the Centerville City Council subcommittee, are formal. However, all organizations are constructed from roles that are enacted by individual citizens. You can see that by discussing organizations we have moved another rung up the ladder of abstraction.

Patterns of similarity can also be found among organizations. As people move in and out of organizations, playing out their roles, they connect with people from other organizations. When a group of organizations are thus linked and when they have similar functions, we can begin to refer to systems and subsystems. For example, as a patron of the theater in Centerville, Marian Branch participates in the recreation system of the community. The Centerville Public Health Nursing Agency is linked to the Centerville Health Department, Centerville Hospital, Centerville Nursing Home, and other organizations that make up the health system of this community. The city council is part of the political system; Marian's church is part of the religious system. These systems all interact because people, in their various roles, move in and out of organizations, connecting with other people from still other organizations.

As a rough map of a community's social system, Figure 13-4 shows the ten major systems common to all communities. The people (or population) are represented by the circle at the center. They become part of the social system by virtue of the roles they enact, roles that form organizations and ultimately one or another major community system.

You may ask why it is important to understand Centerville, or any other community, as a social system. Perhaps you consider a social system as merely an abstract idea about a community. It may be abstract, but it reflects an important reality: the various community systems have a profound influence on one another. Because this interaction among parts determines the health of the whole, it is the total system that concerns community health nurses.

Let us consider one aspect of the health of Centerville. The city's department of health reported more than 75 pregnancies among teenage girls, a large number for the size of this community. This situation has placed a marked strain on the families of these girls as well as caused increased demands for services from the health system. Because the vast majority of these pregnancies are unwanted, they present a problem for the unwed teenage parents, their families, and eventually, the community. What will happen to the babies of these girls? Evidence from research suggests that, in the future, the girls are

359

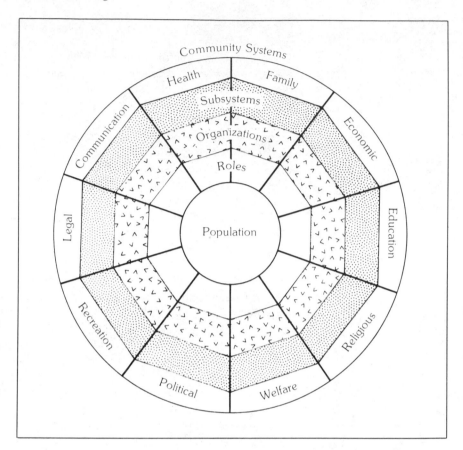

Figure 13-4
The community as a social system. Each of the ten major systems of a community includes a number of subsystems that are made up of organizations. Members of the community occupy roles in these organizations.

likely to have larger families, depend more frequently on the welfare system, and have a higher number of health problems than women who were not teenage mothers. How is the community responding to this situation? Its response gives us clues to the overall health of Centerville.

For one thing, the problem has been ignored, a sign of defense rather than adaptation. When it does come to public attention, it divides various groups. Families blame the schools; school officials in turn blame the changing sexual mores represented in motion pictures. Some members of the health system asked Planned Parenthood to set up an office and clinic in Centerville in an effort to resolve the problem. Almost immediately, however, the religious system entered the picture with groups forming to picket Planned Parenthood facilities because of the association's stand on abortion. Planned Parenthood set up its office in an old restaurant on the edge of one business district in Centerville. Individuals from the religious and economic system (local businessmen) joined to file suit to prevent Planned Parenthood from occupying the old building. Within months, every major system of this community was involved in the problem, yet it was as far from solution as ever. Indeed, the original problem had almost fallen by the wayside as community members fought over the issues of abortion and the Planned Parenthood headquarters. Vandals set several fires that destroyed part of the building. Pickets daily called attention to this unwanted health agency. Moreover, in the midst of the trouble, more teenagers, some with parents who were deeply involved in the conflict, became pregnant.

Community health nurses work in such community situations. Their goal is to assess the community's level of health, identify needs, set priorities, and then work with community members to raise the level of health. It is a complex yet challenging task. All the ways to assess the community as a social system cannot be described within the scope of this chapter, but the last part of the Community Profile Inventory (Table 13-4) suggests some of the health implications for the major systems. It also offers some suggestions for making an assessment of each system.

A PART: THE HEALTH SYSTEM

Although community health nurses must have some understanding of all the systems in a community and how they interact, the health system is of particular importance. Let us compare community assessment, for a moment, with individual health assessment. Then we can examine the health system in greater depth, as an example of how a community health nurse might conduct a more detailed study of a community.

Initial assessment of individuals begins with a survey of major systems. One does not begin by minutely examining the health of each cell, but concentrates instead on the overall condition of the individual. This survey usually involves a head-to-toe examination during which one looks for indications of wellness and illness in the respiratory, musculoskeletal, glandular, skin, and circulatory systems, among others.

Initial assessment of a community also begins with a survey of major systems. Instead of asking, "Is the traffic policeman doing his job?" or "Is the mayor an effective leader?" one would inquire about the political system as a whole. What are its constituent parts? Are there any signs of health or illness?

When beginning an examination of a single person, the nurse asks whether the major body systems are functioning well or poorly. Pulse rate and blood pressure checks provide information about the level of functioning in the circulatory system. In order to answer questions about a system's level of functioning, one must first know its function, that is, the job it has to do as part of the larger system, the body.

The same holds true for community assessment. The nurse might ask, for example, "How well does the communication system keep citizens informed about important matters?'' This question implies that this system has a basic function, information dissemination. The nurse might also ask, ''Does the educational system offer equal education to all children of the community?,'' which implies that this system's function is to offer learning opportunities to everyone in a particular age group.

Each of the major systems in Figure 13-4 has developed over time in a community to meet the needs of its members. The major function of the health system is to promote the health of the community. Community assessment does not merely ask if, but also how well the system is functioning. What is the level of health promotion as carried out by the health system of a community? In order to answer this question, which can be applied to any system, one needs a clear notion about the subsystems, organizations, and roles that make up the system.

Let us say that in examining an individual patient, you have surveyed all the general systems of the body and discovered that the person has an elevated blood pressure. You will now want to move from your initial survey to a more detailed examination of the circulatory system or other parts of the body. Any evidence of inadequate functioning becomes a warning signal for more careful assessment.

The same rule should be followed in community assessment. The rate of teenage pregnancies in Centerville signals inadequate functioning of some systems; perhaps the family, educational, religious, health, or all these systems need improvement. Thus, you want to take a closer look. What community values influence sexual behavior among adolescents? What sex education programs are available to this population? Does the health system provide information and counseling? Like high blood pressure in a single person, this sign in Centerville may quickly lead to discovery of many other underlying problems. They might require care as simple as regular exercise or as complicated as major surgery, each solution translated into community terms.

What are the components of the health system? Figure 13-5 abstracts one segment from our illustration of the community social system — the health system. It is composed of eight major subsystems, each with one or more organizations. Although the community health nurse must be aware of all the systems in a community, the health system is of central importance. Figure 13-5 shows some representative types of organizations for each of the major subsystems. Keep in mind that each of these organizations also has members with many different roles, and the health of the entire system depends, in part, on how well these roles are carried out.

Community Dynamics

Our discussion to this point may have suggested that the community is a rigid structure composed of a geographic location, a population, and a social system. Yet every community has a dynamic quality. Think of the diagram

362

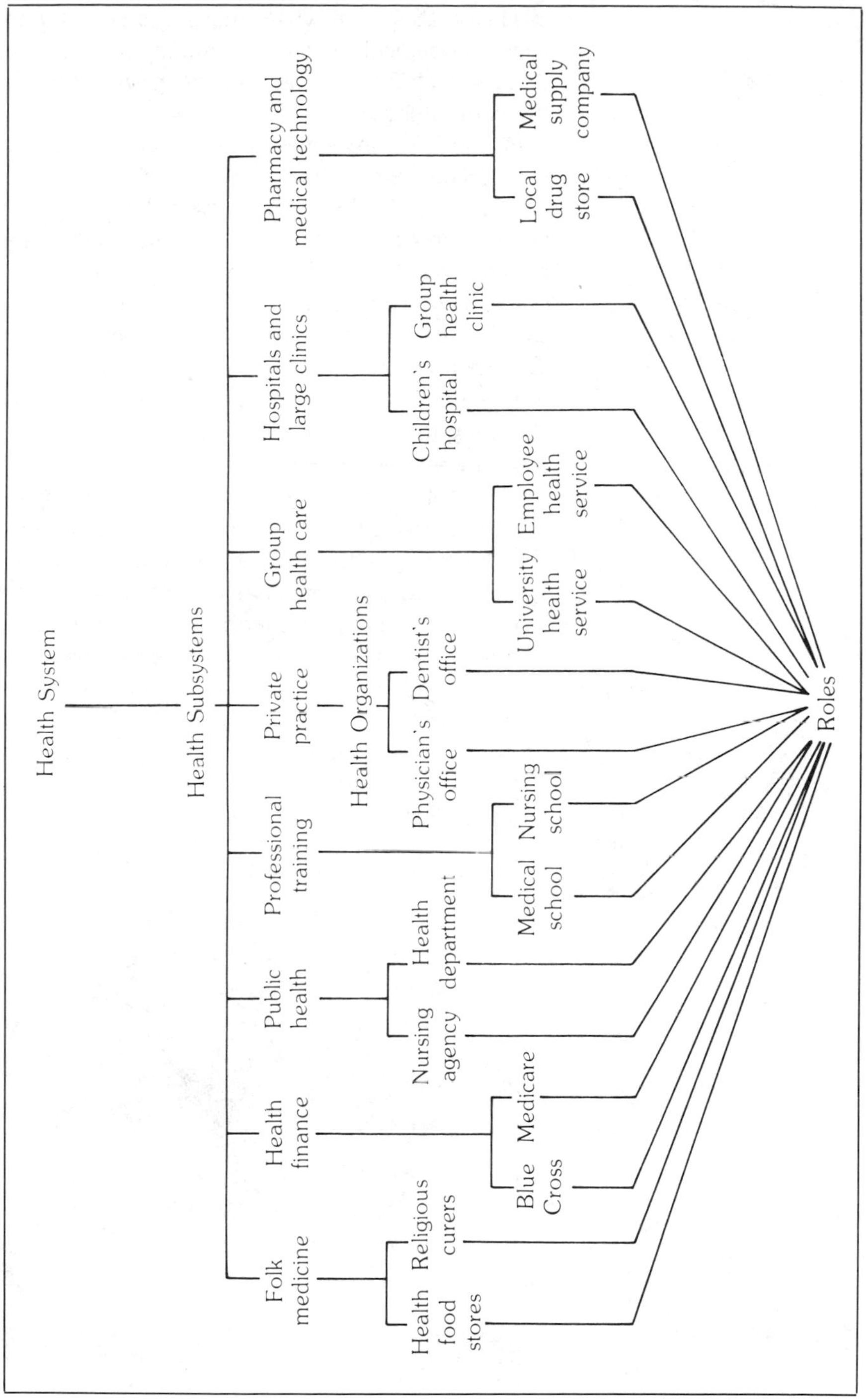

Figure 13-5
Components of the health
system. (For a detailed discussion of the health system with slightly different
categories of subsystems,
see I. T. Sanders and
A. Brownlee [1979, p.
411]).

363

in Figure 13-4 as a wheel that turns rather than as a static structure. Two factors in particular affect community dynamics: citizen participation in community health programs and the power and decision-making structure of the community (Lynd, 1939).

In some communities, citizens show little concern about public health issues. They expect health officials to take entire responsibility: "That's what we pay them to do." When apathy abounds, community health nurses will probably have to work on community education and awareness. In other communities, participation may be widespread but either uninformed or obstructive. The example of the Planned Parenthood Clinic in Centerville suggests that citizens can block the development of some programs or at least hamper them. It is much more difficult to work in a community where groups have become polarized by issues such as abortion and fluoridation. Assessing the type and extent of citizen participation will be a necessary first step in community work.

The goal of encouraging responsible participation touches on the concept of self-care discussed in earlier chapters. One goal of community nurses when working with families or groups is to encourage people to take responsibility for their own health care. They have the right to make decisions, to have adequate information, and to consult widely about their own health. The nurse's role is to encourage the full development of a self-care attitude. On a community level, self-care occurs when citizens become committed to the goal of a healthy community (Fig. 13-6). Such a commitment includes responsible involvement in assessing, planning, and carrying out programs to meet community needs (Kinlein, 1978). Community self-care is community health nursing's goal.

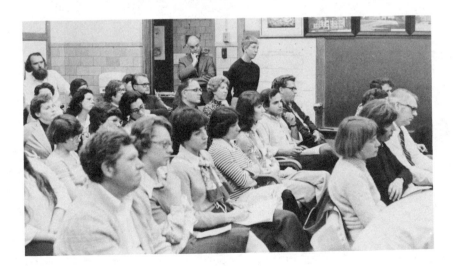

Figure 13-6
A healthy community encourages its citizens to participate in decision making. Here citizens are involved in a town meeting discussion.

364

The second factor, the power and decision-making structure, is a central concern to anyone wishing to bring about change. The description of the community as a social system may suggest that power and decision making reside primarily in the political system, but that is not the case. Sanders and Brownlee (1979, p. 421) have argued against oversimplifying the decision-making process: "In its naivest, simplest terms this [oversimplification] blandly states that (1) *every* community has an identifiable power clique and (2) that if you get the members on your side, all of your problems will be solved."

Decision making in any community is much more complex than this description. Sanders and Brownlee (1979) suggest that power is distributed unevenly among members of organizations in various community systems. A *key leader* may have influence in more than one system, but that power will be diffuse. Seldom does a public health official have power in the religious system or a clergyman in the legal system. A *dominant leader* is one who has specific power, but only within a single community system. An *organizational leader* will have power, but only within a single organization, not in the entire system. Sanders and Brownlee also say that key and dominant leaders will often work through other, less powerful leaders, which they call *functionaries, issue leaders,* and *spokesmen.* We will return to the problem of leadership and the types of leaders in chapter 20.

Although power and decision making in any community are complex, Sanders and Brownlee (1979) do suggest several propositions to use as general guidelines for understanding this aspect of a community's dynamics.

1. Because communities differ widely in their power structures, do not assume that what you know about one community will be true of another.
2. The leaders within the health system have different degrees of power and varying spheres of influence; a knowledge of these differences is prerequisite to effective community work.
3. Those leaders whose power is limited to the health system or organizations often have a network of contacts with similar leaders in other systems. Many of the decisions are made informally through this network.
4. Power does not automatically flow through the established bureaucratic channels. Locate the informal patterns of power and decision making.
5. Beware of leaders who speak authoritatively on issues outside their sphere of power. Their power may be more apparent than real.
6. Leaders from the health system may become key leaders with power that extends far beyond the health system.
7. Learn to distinguish between political, economic, and social power; then use the appropriate combination needed to promote community health issues.

8. Do not overestimate the support of key leaders or power cliques; their support may be helpful but still leave much organizational work to be done.
9. Try to encourage participation in the decision-making process at every level, from average citizen to key leader.
10. You can assume that leaders in one part of a community are ignorant of needs and problems in other parts of the system. When you contact such leaders, recognize that you will have to educate them in community health issues.

Types of Community Assessment

When dealing with an individual patient, it is important to know whether to record temperature and check all vital signs or recommend a complete physical examination with thorough laboratory analysis. The same is true for community assessment. In some situations, an extensive community study becomes the first priority. In others, all that is needed is a study of one system or even one organization. At other times community health nurses may need to familiarize themselves with an entire community without going into any depth, in other words, to perform a cursory examination. The type of assessment will depend on variables such as the needs that exist, the goals to be achieved, and the resources available for carrying out the study. Although it is impossible to make such a decision ahead of time, it will be much easier if the nurse beginning a study understands the several different types of community assessment.

Comprehensive Assessment

The comprehensive assessment seeks to discover all the relevant community health information. It begins with a review of existing studies and all the data presently available on the community. A survey would compile all the demographic information on the population, such as its size, density, and composition. Key informants would be interviewed in every major system — education, health, religious, economic, and others (Neuber, Atkins, Jacobson, Reuterman, 1980). Then more detailed surveys and intensive interviews would yield information on organizations and the various roles in each organization. A comprehensive assessment would not only describe the systems of a community but also how power was distributed throughout the system, how decisions were made, and how change occurred.

Because comprehensive assessment is an expensive, time-consuming process, it is seldom performed. Indeed, in many cases such a thorough research plan might be a waste of resources and repeat, in part, many other studies.

Performing a more focused study based on prior knowledge of needs is often a better strategy. Yet knowing how to conduct a comprehensive assessment has an important influence over the approach to a more focused study.

Familiarization

The second kind of community assessment is also the most necessary. Familiarization involves studying data already available on a community, and perhaps gathering a limited amount of firsthand data, in order to gain a working knowledge of the community. Such an approach has been used in nursing students' community survey courses (Flynn, Gottschalk, Ray, & Selmanoff, 1978; Ruybal, Bauwens, & Fasla, 1975). This type of assessment is needed whenever the community health nurse works with families, groups, organizations, or populations. It provides a knowledge of the context in which these other aggregates exist.

Consider use of community familiarization when the main concern is a single family. Let us say that you, as the community health nurse, visit the Angelo family on the edge of Philadelphia. During your first few visits, you gather information, learning that the family is Italian-American and that there are four children. The father has been out of work for six months; the oldest boy has been in trouble with the juvenile authorities; a younger child is deaf; their house appears run-down to you. You assess this family, trying to determine its coping ability, its level of health.

However, even this task is almost impossible without some knowledge of the community. Is theirs an Italian-American neighborhood? What is the extent of unemployment in this city? What are the services for the deaf? Are all the houses in this part of town old and in need of repair? Once you begin working with the family, familiarity with the community becomes even more imperative. You discover that as a result of the Angelos' low income, family conflicts are intense. The family members seldom get out; they make almost no use of the community's recreational system. Before you can help them make use of it, however, you must find out what resources are available. As you familiarize yourself with the community, you discover a group called "Friends of the Deaf," which sponsors a group for parents of deaf children. You can now help Mr. and Mrs. Angelo become part of that group. A quick survey of the religious system in the community reveals two job transition support groups, one of which will welcome Mr. Angelo. In the meantime, you will want to find out about the welfare system and how this family can benefit from its services. Even your own attitude toward the family will change as you study the community. For instance, if you discover that a strike closed down the plant where Mr. Angelo worked for 20 years, you can then view his unemployment from a broader perspective.

However, familiarization will go beyond connecting the family to the community and its resources. Whatever role nurses play in a community, they will want to be making a continuous study, an ongoing assessment. Whether nurses become client advocates, working with the local government, or operate from a nursing agency serving the elderly, this kind of assessment is a prerequisite for their work.

Problem-oriented Assessment

The third kind of assessment begins with a single problem and then assesses the community in terms of that problem. Assume that when you check around for services available for the Angelos' deaf child, you discover that there are none. Confronted with this problem, one family with one deaf child, you could make a problem-oriented community assessment. Your first step would be to seek to discover the incidence of childhood deafness, both in the community and in the state. Second, you might begin interviewing officials in the schools and health institutions to find out what has been done in the past with such problems. You could check the local library to find out what resources are available on the subject of deafness. Do they subscribe to *The Deaf American*? Are there interpreters available for adults who use sign language? How do hospitals and courts approach deafness? Are there any clubs or other organizations for deaf adults? Is there a state school for the deaf and where is it located?

The problem-oriented assessment is commonly used when familiarization is not sufficient and a comprehensive assessment is too expensive. It is the type of assessment that responds to a particular need. The data you collected will be useful in any kind of planning for a community response to the problem.

Community Subsystem Assessment

In the community subsystem assessment, the community health nurse focuses on a single dimension of community life. For example, the nurse might decide to survey churches and religious organizations to discover their role in the community. What kinds of needs do the leaders in these organizations believe exist? What services do these organizations offer? To what extent are services coordinated within the religious system and between it and other systems in the community?

The community subsystem assessment can be a useful way for a team to conduct a more thorough community assessment. If five members of a nursing agency divided up the ten systems in the community, and each person did an assessment of two systems, they could then share their findings and create a more comprehensive picture of the community and its needs.

Community Assessment Methods

Community health needs may be assessed through a variety of methods. We will discuss two. Surveys, among the most commonly used, provide a broad range of data and are helpful when other sources are not available. According to Dever (1980, p. 147), "The basic objective of planning and conducting community health surveys is to determine the occurrence and distribution of selected environmental, socioeconomic, and behavioral conditions important to disease control and wellness promotion." Thus, the nurse may choose to conduct a survey to determine health care utilization patterns, immunization levels, demographic characteristics, or health beliefs and practices. The survey method involves nine steps needed to ensure an adequate design and appropriate collection of data (Dever, 1980, p. 147):

1. Determine the objectives.
   — what information is needed?
   — why is it needed?
   — how accurate does it need to be?
2. Define the study population.
   — what groups will be studied?
   — what are their distinguishing characteristics? (i.e., age, occupation, location)
3. Determine data to be collected.
   — what specific data will be collected? (i.e., behavior, opinions, beliefs)
   — what sources will provide this data? (i.e., records, people)
   — how will you measure this data?
4. Select sampling unit.
   — will it be an individual, a household, a city block?
   — what sample size is needed?
   — what sampling method is most appropriate and feasible?
5. Select contact method.
   — what will the data gathering method/instrument be ? (i.e., interviews, telephone calls, questionnaires)
   — will you exclude any types of organizations or facilities? (i.e., omit interviews in businesses)
6. Develop the method.
   — (i.e., construct questionnaire or interview guide)
7. Organize and conduct the survey
   — identify and train data collectors (i.e., interviewers)
   — pretest and adjust instrument
   — supervise actual collection
   — plan for nonresponses or refusals
8. Process and analyze data.
   — code, keypunch, tabulate?

— apply appropriate statistical methods, as indicated
— determine relationships and significance
9. Report the results.
— include implications and recommendations.

A descriptive epidemiological study is another important methodology applied particularly to problem-oriented needs assessment. Its design and use are detailed in chapter 8. Choice of assessment method varies depending upon the reasons for data collection, goals and objectives of the study, and available resources.

The Healthy Community

Throughout this chapter, it has been emphasized that community health nursing's role is to promote the health of the entire community. Included in our discussion were suggestions about the characteristics of a healthy community. However, what is a healthy community? If health practitioners are going to assess a community, set goals for community health, plan to improve the health of a community, and work toward goals, they require some criteria of wellness, health, and competence.

To begin, there is no such thing as the perfectly healthy community. All aggregates exist in a relative state of health. New needs emerge every day; the system is threatened or weakened and must respond to maintain homeostasis. Thus, whatever the concept of a healthy community is, it will be a relative idea.

Because of their complexity, criteria for healthy communities must be discussed cautiously. At present, there is not wide agreement on such criteria. We can begin with a classic article, "The Competent Community," by Leonard Cottrell, Jr. (1976). His concept of competence is close to current ideas of wellness expressed in this text. It is important to keep in mind that this discussion of community competence refers to the collective functioning of the total community unit, not to its various parts, like single agencies, families, or individuals (Goeppinger, Lassiter, & Wilcox, 1982). Cottrell argues that a competent community is one whose various systems have four important characteristics (pp. 195–209):

1. They can collaborate effectively in identifying community needs and problems.
2. They can achieve a working consensus on goals and priorities.
3. They can agree on ways and means to implement the agreed-upon goals.
4. They can collaborate effectively in the required actions.

370

These general requirements take us closer to an understanding of a healthy community. However, we must still determine the factors that enable a community's systems to work together in these ways. Cottrell (1976) suggests several essential conditions for community competence: (1) commitment of members, (2) self-awareness and awareness of others among groups, (3) clarity of situational (positional) definitions, (4) articulateness of various subgroups, (5) effective communication, (6) conflict containment and accommodation, (7) participation (community involvement), (8) management of relations with the larger society, and (9) machinery for effective decision making. Drawing from this list and other sources, we can use the following adaptation as a guide for assessing a healthy community:

1. A healthy community is one in which members have a high degree of awareness that "we are a community."
2. A healthy community uses its natural resources while taking steps to conserve them for future generations.
3. A healthy community openly recognizes the existence of subgroups and welcomes their participation in community affairs.
4. A healthy community is prepared to meet crises.
5. A healthy community is a problem-solving community; it identifies, analyzes, and organizes to meet its own needs.
6. A healthy community has open channels of communication that allow information to flow among all subgroups of citizens in all directions.
7. A healthy community seeks to make each of its systems' resources available to all members of the community.
8. A healthy community has legitimate and effective ways to settle disputes that arise within the community.
9. A healthy community encourages maximum citizen participation in decision making.
10. A healthy community promotes a high level of wellness among all its members.

Planning for the Health of a Community

Planning for community health is based on assessment of the community. Once community health nurses have this essential information, they can determine needs, rank them, establish goals and objectives, and develop a plan of action. The nursing process, detailed in chapter 7, again becomes an important tool to facilitate nursing practice, this time with the community as the client. Throughout this chapter, we have discussed elements to consider in planning for community health. We have examined characteristics of a healthy community (one is illustrated in Figure 13-7) as a guide to assessing the health of the community that community health nurses seek to serve. Nurses also need to understand what a healthy community is in order to establish planning objectives; in other words, they need to know what to aim for. A health subsystem with deficient communication patterns, for instance, will require intervention if health care services in the community are to function effectively.

Aggregate-level nursing practice requires teamwork. The job of planning for the health of an entire community or a community subsystem of necessity means that the nurse will be collaborating with other professionals. Working with a health board task force to recommend methods for improved communication between health care agencies is one way the nurse works as a team member in serving the community as the client. All sound public health practice depends on pooling resources, including people, in ways that will best serve the public. Whether health service is aimed at the individual, family, group, subpopulation, population, or community, the consumer of that service is an equally important member of the team. In planning for a community's health, the community (represented by appropriate individuals and agencies) must be involved. Community health nurses cannot lose sight of the need for client involvement at all levels and in all stages of community health practice.

Figure 13-7
Healthy communities pro-
vide needed resources for
all their citizens. This city
park in Boston offers
scenic beauty as well as
play equipment for active
children.

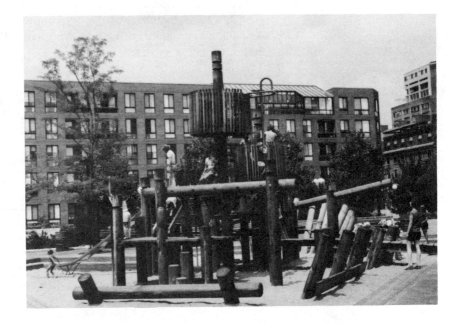

Summary

A major mission of community health nursing practice is to promote the health of aggregates of people. A strong value of individualism in the United States distracts nurses from a broad focus. It has led to three pervading myths: (1) community health nursing is only clinical nursing outside the hospital setting; (2) community health nursing employs only the skills of basic nursing when working with community clients; and (3) the primary client in community health nursing is the individual in a family context. Rather, community health nursing is practice with and to the community. It employs basic nursing expertise but adds many important concepts and skills from public health. Moreover, its practice ranges along the community health nursing scope of practice continuum from individuals to aggregates.

Any geographic community has three important dimensions to consider when assessing its health needs: location, population, and social system. The effect of a community's location may be further analyzed by considering such variables as its boundary, location of health service, geographic features, climate, flora and fauna, and human-made environment. The health of a community is also influenced by its population. Knowledge of features, such as the population size, density, composition, rate of growth or decline, cultural differences, social class, and mobility, helps the community health nurse to better understand the community. The third dimension of a community, its social system, includes ten major systems (including the health system) and many subsystems. Each subsystem is composed of organizations whose members assume various roles. A Community Profile Inventory details the community health implications of each dimension, poses assessment questions for the nurse to ask, and suggests sources of information.

Initial assessment of a community begins with a survey of the major systems to determine how well they are functioning. Evidence of malfunctioning in any part becomes a stimulus for further and more detailed analysis.

Community dynamics, the driving forces that govern a community's functioning, must also be considered when assessing community health. Two factors, in particular, affect community dynamics: citizen participation in community health programs and the power and decision-making structure. Community health nurses need to encourage community self-care by promoting community-level involvement in, commitment to, and responsibility for, its own health. Nurses also need to recognize the sources of community influence in order to use the system effectively to promote community health.

There are different types of community assessment. A comprehensive assessment surveys the entire community in depth, gathering thorough original data. A familiarization assessment studies available data, perhaps adding some firsthand data, to gain a general understanding of the community. Problem-oriented assessment focuses on a single problem and studies the community in terms of that problem. Community subsystem assessment examines a single facet of community life. There are many methods for assessing a community's health. Two important ones are surveys and descriptive epidemiological studies.

A healthy community has a number of characteristics that health practitioners look for when assessing its health. Among them are a sense of unity, ability to collaborate and communicate effectively, a problem-solving orientation, ability to utilize yet conserve resources, and ability to handle crises and conflict.

Planning for community health draws on a thorough assessment and utilizes the nursing process. It involves a team effort by professionals and community personnel.

Study Questions

1. Why is it important to understand and work with the community as a total entity?
2. How does defining the total community as the client change the community health nurse's practice? List some specific examples of how this concept might be applied.
3. If you were part of a health planning team concerned about the health needs of the elderly in your community, what are some location, population, and social system variables you would want to assess? Name some of the sources from which you might collect the data.
4. Under what circumstances might you choose to conduct a problem-oriented community health assessment? What method would you consider using to conduct this assessment, and how would you carry it out?

References

Cottrell, L. S., Jr. (1976). The competent community. In B. H. Kaplan, R. N. Wilson, & A. H. Leighton (Eds.), *Further explorations in social psychiatry* (pp. 195–209). New York: Basic Books.

Dever, G. E. A. (1980). *Community health analysis: A holistic approach.* Germantown, MD: Aspen Systems.

Flynn, B., Gottschalk, J., Ray, D., & Selmanoff, E. (1978). One master's curriculum in community health nursing. *Nursing Outlook, 26,* 633–637.

Freeman, H. E., Levine, S., & Reeder, L. G. (Eds.). (1979). *Handbook of medical sociology* (3rd ed.). Englewood Cliffs, NJ: Prentice-Hall.

Goeppinger, J., Lassiter, P., & Wilcox, B. (1982). Community health is community competence. *Nursing Outlook, 30,* 464–467.

Goode, W. J. (1977). *Principles of sociology.* New York: McGraw-Hill.

Kinlein, L. (1978). Nursing and family and community health. *Family and Community Health, 1*(1), 57–68.

Lynd, R. (1939). *Knowledge for what? The place of social science in American culture.* Princeton: Princeton University Press.

Nagi, S. Z. (1959, October). Factors related to heart disease among Ohio farmers. *Ohio Agricultural Experiment Station Research Bulletin,* p. 842.

Neuber, K. A., Atkins, W. T., Jacobson, J. A., and Reuterman, N. A. (1980). *Needs assessment: A model for community planning.* Beverly Hills, CA: Sage.

Redesigning nursing education for public health: Report of the conference (Pub. No. 75-75). (1973). Bethesda, MD: U.S. Department of Health, Education and Welfare.

Ruybal, S. E., Bauwens, E., & Fasla, M. (1975). Community assessment: An epidemiological approach. *Nursing Outlook, 23,* 365–368.

Sanders, I. T., & Brownlee, A. (1979). Health in the community. In H. E. Freeman, S. Levine, & L. G. Reeder (Eds.). *Handbook of medical sociology* (3rd ed.) (pp. 412–433). Englewood Cliffs, NJ: Prentice-Hall.

Selected Readings

Aneshensel, C., Frerichs, R., Clark, V., and Yokopenic, P. (1982). Telephone versus in-person surveys of community health status. *American Journal of Public Health, 72,* 1017–1021.

Blum, H. L. (1981). *Planning for health: Generics for the eighties* (2nd ed.). New York: Behavioral Publications.

Boyle, J. S. (1973). Community assessment. In A. Reinhardt & M. Quinn (Eds.), *Family-centered community nursing.* St. Louis: C. V. Mosby.

Brill, N. (1976). *Teamwork: Working together in the human services.* Philadelphia: Lippincott.

Burke, E. M. (1979). *A participatory approach to urban planning.* New York: Human Sciences Press.

Carter, D., & Lee, P. (Eds.). (1972). *Politics of health.* New York: Medcom.

Cottrell, L. S., Jr. (1976). The competent community. In B. H. Kaplan, R. N. Wilson, & A. H. Leighton (Eds.), *Further explorations in social psychiatry* (pp. 195–209). New York: Basic Books.

Dever, G. E. A. (1980). *Community health analysis: A holistic approach.* Germantown, MD: Aspen Systems.

Ellig, R. H., & Lee, O. J. (1972). Formal connections of community leadership to the health system. In E. G. Jaco (Ed.), *Patients, physicians, and illness: A sourcebook in behavioral science and health* (2nd ed.). New York: Free Press.

Flynn, B., Gottschalk, J., Ray, D., & Selmanoff, E. (1978). One master's curriculum in community health nursing. *Nursing Outlook, 26,* 633–637.

Frankle, R. T., & Owen, A. Y. (1978). *Nutrition in the community: The art of delivering services.* St. Louis: C. V. Mosby.

Freeman, H. E., Levine, S., & Reeder, L. G. (Eds.). (1979). *Handbook of medical sociology* (3rd ed.). Englewood Cliffs, NJ: Prentice-Hall.

Goeppinger, J., Lassiter, P., & Wilcox, B. (1982). Community health is community competence. *Nursing Outlook, 30,* 464–467.

Hanchett, E. (1979). *Community health assessment: A conceptual tool kit.* New York: Wiley.

Hays, B., & Mockelstrom, N. R. (1977). Consumer survey: An approach to teaching consumer participation in community health. *Journal of Nursing Education, 16,* 30–33.

Klein, D. C. (1968). *Community dynamics and mental health.* New York: Wiley.

Knight, J. H. (1974). Applying nursing process in the community. *Nursing Outlook, 22,* 708–710.

Kramer, R. M., & Specht, H. (Eds.). (1975). *Readings in community organization practice.* Englewood Cliffs, NJ: Prentice-Hall.

Logan, R. (1964). Assessment of sickness and health in the community — Needs and methods. *Medical Care, 2,* 173–175.

MacStravic, R. (1978). *Determining health needs.* Ann Arbor, MI: Health Administration Press.

Milio, N. (1975). *The care of health in communities: Access for outcasts.* New York: Macmillan.

Miller, M., & Stokes, C. (1978). Health status, health resources, and consolidated structural parameters: Implications for public health care policy. *Journal of Health and Social Behavior, 19,* 263–279.

Moe, E. V. (1977). Nature of today's community. In A. Reinhardt & M. Quinn (Eds.), *Current practice in family-centered community nursing.* St. Louis: C. V. Mosby.

Mullane, M. K. (1975). Nursing care and the political arena. *Nursing Outlook, 23,* 699–701.

National Commission on Community Health Services. (1967). *Health is a community affair.* Cambridge, MA: Harvard University Press.

Neuber, K., Atkins, W. T., Jacobson, J. A., and Reuterman, N. A. (1980). *Needs assessment: A model for community planning.* Beverly Hills, CA: Sage.

Perlman, R., & Gurin, A. (1972). *Community organization and social planning.* New York: Wiley.

Redesigning nursing education for public health: Report of the conference (Pub. No. 75-75). (1973). Bethesda, MD: U.S. Department of Health, Education and Welfare.

Ruybal, S. E. (1978). Community health planning. *Family and Community Health, 1*(1), 9–18.

Ruybal, S. E., Bauwens, E., & Fasla, M. (1975). Community assessment: An epidemiological approach. *Nursing Outlook, 23,* 365–368.

Sanders, I. T. (1963). The commuinity: Structure and function. *Nursing Outlook, 11,* 642–646.

Sanders, I. T., & Brownlee, A. (1979). Health in the community. In H. E. Freeman, S. Levine, & L. G. Reeder (Eds.), *Handbook of medical sociology* (3rd ed.) (pp. 412–433). Englewood Cliffs, NJ: Prentice-Hall.

Shamansky, S., & Pesznecker, B. (1981). A community is. . . . *Nursing Outlook, 29,* 182–185.

Simmons, H. J. (1974). Community health planning — With or without nursing. *Nursing Outlook, 22,* 260–264.

Stokinger, M., & Wallinder, J. (1979). A graduate practicum in health planning. *Nursing Outlook, 27,* 202–205.

Storck, J. (1968). Assessing the community's health in times of change. *Public Health Reports, 81,* 821–830.

Weeks, M., Kulka, R., Lessler, J., & Whitmore, R. (1983). Personal versus telephone surveys for collecting household health data at the local level. *American Journal of Public Health, 73,* 1389–1394.

14

Preschool and School-age Populations

Healthy children are a vital resource to ensure the future well-being of the nation. They are the parents, workers, leaders, and decision makers of tomorrow, yet their health and safety depends on today's decisions and actions. Their future lies in our hands.

Children are an important population group of concern to community health nursing. To understand the nurse's role in serving this population, we must first ask some questions. What are the health needs of children as an aggregate? What infant, preschool, school-age, and adolescent populations are at greatest risk of poor health? What health programs are available to serve these groups and what others are needed? This chapter addresses these questions by summarizing the state of children's health. The subject is treated extensively in many excellent sources; a number are listed at the conclusion of the chapter. You are encouraged to explore them for greater depth and breadth of understanding. For our purposes here, we examine the subject in order to obtain a clearer conception of specific populations at risk and a better grasp of the community health nurse's contribution to those groups.

Children's Health Needs

Child welfare has been a subject of great concern in this country for many years. As a nation, we have emphasized its importance through development of numerous laws and services, yet the needs of millions of children continue to go unmet. Consider the following facts about children in the United States (Children's Defense Fund, 1979):

One in seven children has no regular source of health care.

Eighteen million children, or one in three, have never been to a dentist.

More than 10 million children — one child in six — lives in poverty (this makes children the poorest group in America).

Minority children are disproportionately poor (one in four Hispanic children and two in five black children live in poverty).

Over half the children from families headed by a woman lived in poverty in 1978. Fifty percent of families headed by black females are on welfare.

These facts clearly indicate the need for improvement in our efforts to prepare children adequately for the future.

Childhood Mortality

Specifically, what are children's health needs? The health of children generally has improved a great deal since the early 1900s. Childhood mortality rates have dropped dramatically. We have seen the threat of major child-killing infectious diseases, such as diphtheria, pneumonia, and tuberculosis, significantly reduced. Now, according to the National Center for Health Statistics (Public Health Service, 1979, p. 33), the major cause of death among children in the United States over the age of one year is accidents, causing 45 percent of total childhood mortality. Motor vehicle accidents are the largest killer, responsible for 20 percent of childhood deaths. Infants under one year are at greatest risk as motor vehicle passengers, preschoolers as pedestrians, school-age children as cyclists, and adolescents as drivers and riders of automobiles and motorcycles (Bell, Ternberg, & Bower, 1980). Use of appropriate restraints in motor vehicles (see Figure 14-1) has proved effective in reducing child deaths and injuries (Avery, 1980).

All other accidents account for the second leading cause of death among children aged five to 14 years and are the first cause of death (above motor vehicle accidents) for children aged one to four years. Falls, drownings, burns, and poisonings lead the list of threats in this category (Tyrell, 1981). In the "other accidents" category, deaths from falls rank highest. Drownings are next and account for 8 percent of childhood deaths; fires, for 6 percent. Poisonings, particularly from toxic substances in the home, such as cleaning

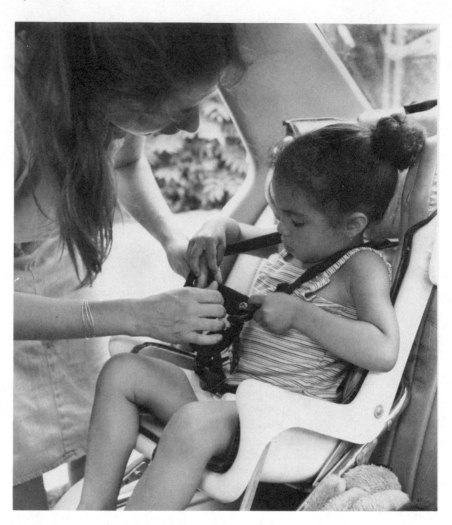

Figure 14-1
Appropriate use of re-
straints in motor vehicles
can prevent many child-
hood injuries and deaths.

compounds, drugs, and pesticides, pose a special hazard for young children. For inner-city children, lead poisoning (from ingested paint chips) and automobile exhaust are additional threats.

Among older children most accidents are associated with recreational activities and equipment (Public Health Service, 1979, p. 39). Football, basketball, and bicycle riding account for the leading causes of emergency room visits among 12- to 17-year-olds. Bicycle, swing, and skateboard accidents lead the causes of emergency room visits in the six to 11 age group.

The loss of children's lives resulting from all accidents combined suggests a staggering number of years of productive life lost to society. Congenital anomalies and homicides are two other major causes of death among children.

Homicides have risen at a frightening rate since 1925, showing a sixfold increase for one- to four-year-old children and a twofold increase for the five to 14 age group. Child homicides occurring to children under the age of three most often result from family violence, but homicides involving children over the age of 12 generally involve violence outside of the home ("Child Homicide," 1982).

Childhood Morbidity

Although childhood mortality rates have markedly decreased, morbidity rates are high. The most common types of acute conditions are respiratory illnesses (which account for the largest group), injuries, infectious and parasitic diseases, and digestive diseases (Hanlon & Pickett, 1984, p. 419). During the preschool and school-age years, children undergo significant physical and emotional changes, increase their contact with other people, and experience many new life events. All these factors serve to increase their vulnerability to injury and disease.

Other child health problems, less easy to detect and measure but often as debilitating, are those of emotional, behavioral, and intellectual development. These include learning disabilities, behavior disorders, developmental disabilities, speech and vision problems, and neuroses and psychoses. They have been called the "new morbidity" (Public Health Service, 1979, p. 36). Although these problems are not new, awareness and concern for them has increased as other life-threatening childhood diseases have diminished.

There is no precise etiology for these childhood developmental problems. Usually multiple causes, such as genetic, emotional, environmental, and cultural influences are involved for children with learning disorders and behavior problems. A deprived environment and poor nutrition have been associated with mental retardation (Public Health Service, 1979, p. 37). Increased aggressive behavior among children has been attributed to violence on television (Comstock, 1981).

Child abuse and neglect form a serious threat to children's health, both physical and emotional: "Abuse and neglect . . . account not only for many injuries, burns and other seeming accidents in children but also for brain damage, emotional scars, and even deaths. There are also children who are victims of sexual abuse, incest, and rape" (Public Health Service, 1979, p. 37). The problem is difficult to detect and often underreported; estimates range from 200,000 to four million cases a year (Public Health Service, 1979, p. 38).

Causes of this behavior generally derive from unstable family situations where immaturity, stress, poverty, or alcoholism may be present, singly or in combination. Abusive adults have often been abused children themselves, carry low self-images into their adult lives, and are unable to cope with the demands of parenting or parent-substitute roles: "Abusing parents are often immature, dependent, unable to handle responsibility. They have low self-esteem, strong beliefs about the value of physical punishment, and misconceptions about children's competence to understand and perform according to their expectations. They frequently make unreasonable demands and, during time of crisis, may direct their anger and frustration at a child. They often are isolated socially and have difficulty seeking help" (Public Health Service, 1979, p. 38).

Families at high risk for child abuse may be those chronically troubled or temporarily stressed. Teenage mothers and families with closely spaced children may also be more likely to engage in abusive behavior. Although poverty and lack of education are often linked with child abuse, no socioeconomic level is immune.

A greater incidence of child abuse outside the home is coming to public attention. Physical and emotional maltreatment of children in institutions, such as day care centers, nursery schools, and children's theater should alert the community health nurse to watch for this problem on a broader scale than only within the family.

Infant Health Problems

The past 50 years marks a steady decline in infant mortality that has resulted mostly from improved health care and general living standards. The infant mortality rate for 1982 was 11.2 per 1,000 live births (National Center for Health Statistics, 1983) as compared with 28 in 1949 and 100 in 1915. However, in the United States we still lose 45,000 infants each year (Hanlon & Pickett, 1984, p. 404), and the first year of life continues to be the most hazardous until age 65. Infant deaths are most commonly owed to congenital anomalies, respiratory distress, sudden infant death syndrome, and premature delivery. Twice as many black infants die as white infants, although race is less the determinant than is socioeconomic status and lower education.

Several important variables influence which groups of infants are most at risk. The two greatest threats to infant survival and health are low birth weight and congenital anomalies (Public Health Service, 1979). Low birth weight (under 2,500 gm) is directly related to higher infant mortality and morbidity rates. The surgeon general's report on health promotion and disease prevention describes low birth weight as "the greatest single hazard for infants, increasing vulnerability to developmental problems — and to death" (Public Health Service, 1979, p. 21). The most important cause of low birth weight is inadequate prenatal care, accompanied by poor maternal nutrition plus smoking and alcohol and drug abuse during pregnancy. Other factors associated with low birth weight are race — 13 percent of babies with low birth weights are born to blacks, 6.2 percent to whites (Kleinman, 1981) — lower socioeconomic status, fewer years of education, and youth and unmarried status of the mother.

382

Congenital anomalies stem partly from genetic and environmental causes and partly from interactions between the two. Though many birth defects cannot be prevented, others can. Exposure of the fetus to toxic or infectious agents during pregnancy, such as rubella during the first trimester, radiation, drugs such as thalidomide and diethylstilbestrol, alcohol, and cigarette smoking, has clearly been associated with high levels of fetal abnormalities.

Other infant health problems that signal groups at risk include premature birth, injuries at birth, respiratory difficulties, sudden infant death syndrome, accidents, infant abuse, malignancies, poor infant nutrition, and parental inadequacy.

Preschool Health Problems

The preschool population, ages one through four, has a low mortality rate that is becoming lower every year. Currently it is 0.66 deaths per 1,000 live births, compared with 20 per 1,000 at the beginning of the century (Hanlon & Pickett, 1984, p. 406). We can credit this dramatic change to the prevention and control of the acute childhood communicable diseases. The major cause of death is accidents (falls, drownings, burns, poisonings) followed by motor vehicle accidents, congenital anomalies, and malignant neoplasms.

As pointed out earlier, however, morbidity rates in this group are exceptionally high. Preschool children experience a high frequency of acute illnesses, the total number of which exceeds that of any other age. These account for a large number of days of restricted activity and disability requiring bed rest. Respiratory illness makes up 80 percent of these acute conditions (Pilliteri, 1981, p. 241). Preschoolers are vulnerable to many types of accidents. Their nutritional and dental health needs are great during this rapid growth period, and their future mental health as adults will be influenced by how well their emotional needs are met during this phase.

School-age Health Problems

As with preschool children, the mortality rates of schoolchildren are low and decreasing; they have dropped from 4 per 1,000 in 1900 to 0.6 per 1,000 currently. Again, we can credit this reduction to effective prevention and control of the acute infectious diseases of childhood. In 1900 the leading causes of death among this group were diphtheria, accidents (but not motor vehicle accidents), pneumonia and influenza, tuberculosis, and heart disease. Today motor vehicle accidents lead the list of causes of death for children ages 5 to 14 followed by all other accidents, congenital malformations, and homicide.

Morbidity in schoolchildren, however, is high. Children of this age group are most often affected by respiratory illness, followed by injuries, infectious and parasitic diseases, and digestive conditions. Among school children, the incidence of measles, rubella (German measles), pertussis (whooping cough), and infectious parotitis (mumps) has dropped considerably because of widespread immunization efforts. Yet more cases than should still occur, some with potentially serious complications, for example, birth defects from rubella and nerve deafness from mumps. Chicken pox, because no immunization for it is yet widely accepted and used, continues to be a frequent childhood illness.

Behavioral disorders and developmental disabilities are problems of this age group, often because they become exacerbated when the child enters school. The prevalence of these problems is difficult to measure epidemiologically, but one estimate places "clinical maladjustment" rates for schoolchildren at 11 percent (Hanlon & Pickett, 1984, p. 419).

Handicapped schoolchildren, those with one or more chronic disabilities that limit activities, make up 3.9 percent of the school-age population and this figure is rising (Newacheck, Budetti, & McManus, 1984). Handicaps include speech (15.2 per 1,000), hearing (14.3 per 1,000), and visual (11.3 per 1,000) defects, and partial or complete paralysis (2 per 1,000) (Hanlon & Pickett, 1984, p. 419).

Other health problems found in this age group are nutritional problems — primarily overeating and inappropriate food choices — and poor dental health. Obesity often begins in childhood and becomes a risk factor for heart disease, hypertension, and diabetes. Obese children are three times more likely to become obese adults (Jonides, 1982). Schoolchildren's diets, many unreasonably high in sugar and fat, are increasing the incidence of coronary arteriosclerosis and dental caries in this population group. The average American child, by age 11, has three decayed permanent teeth. When that child reaches 17, eight or nine permanent teeth are filled, decayed, or missing (Public Health Service, 1979, p. 41).

Adolescent Health Problems

Adolescents, during the period roughly encompassing the teen years, encounter many complex changes, physically, emotionally, cognitively, and socially. Rapid and major developmental adjustments create a variety of stresses, with concomitant problems, that have an impact on their health.

Mortality and morbidity rates for adolescence are low overall and demonstrate considerable improvement over the early 1900s. However, people in this age group die 2.5 times more often than younger children, and since 1960 the adolescent death rate has been gradually increasing (Public Health Service, 1979, p. 43).

What are the health problems of adolescents? Violent death and injury head the list of major threats to life and health. For whites (male and female), motor vehicle accidents cause the greatest number of deaths, followed by all other accidents, suicide, and homicide. For nonwhites (male and female), homicides are the leading cause of death, with motor vehicle accidents second and all other accidents third. Suicides are fourth for nonwhite males and sixth for nonwhite females (after malignant neoplasms and heart disease) (Hanlon & Pickett, 1984, p. 421). Adolescent males are at greatest risk in this population group, having a death rate nearly three times higher than that of females. When combined, accidents, homicides, and suicides cause nearly three-fourths of all adolescent deaths. Responsibility for these has been attributed "to behavior patterns characterized by judgmental errors, aggressiveness, and, in some cases, ambivalence about wanting to live or die. Certainly, greater risk-taking occurs in this period of life" (Public Health Service, 1979, p. 43).

Another set of health problems for adolescents relates to life-style and behavior patterns. They include alcohol and drug abuse, unwanted pregnancies, sexually transmitted diseases (STDs), and poor nutrition. For adolescents, alcohol is the most serious drug abuse problem. In 1980, 19 percent, or 3.3 million young people of those aged 14 to 17, were problem drinkers (Alcohol, Drug Abuse and Mental Health Administration, 1980). This age group tends to consume alcohol less frequently (an average of once monthly) than adults do, but when adolescents do drink they drink large quantities and they experience more frequent episodes of intoxication than adults, thus increasing the chances of violent behavior and motor vehicle accidents. Cigarette smoking continues to be "the most significant preventable health problem of adolescents" (Hanlon & Pickett, 1984, p. 422). It is decreasing among males and increasing among females but less overall since 1974. An increasing number of adolescents smoke marijuana and take stimulants — amphetamines — frequently. Illegal use of substances such as cocaine, hallucinogens, and prescription medications tends to be more common with older adolescents and young adults (18 to 25 years of age) than with younger adolescents. Drug abuse among young people was almost unknown before 1950 and rare before 1962. Now, adolescent drug experimentation and use pose serious physical and psychological threats.

Increasing sexual activity among adolescents creates two other significant health problems for this age group. According to the Surgeon General's Report (Public Health Service, 1979, p. 48), "One-fourth of American teenage girls have had at least one pregnancy by age 19." Each year 10 percent of all teenage girls become pregnant (two-thirds of those are unmarried), and at least a third terminate their pregnancies. Young mothers are at high risk of bearing infants with low birth weight, less because of their biologic age (except for preteen mothers whose youth increases their risk) than because of other associated factors, such as smoking and alcohol consumption (Merritt, Laurence, & Naeye, 1980). They are also at risk for a greater number of physical, psychological, and social problems, including disrupted schooling, as a result of pregnancy (President's Commission, 1981). Those who choose to end their pregnancies with abortion encounter other physical and psychosocial complications, including emotionally wrenching ethical dilemmas. STDs, particularly gonorrhea and syphilis, pose another threat to adolescent health and are increasing in this age group despite improved treatment and reporting. Other STDs, notably genital herpes and nonspecific urethritis, have become major public health problems. Combined with gonorrhea and syphilis, they strike approximately 8 million to 12 million young people a year (Public Health Service, 1979, p. 49). Serious complications can result from these diseases, including sterility in young women who have pelvic inflammatory disease.

Poor nutrition and obesity are common among adolescents, whose eating habits often consist of nonnourishing snacks (Figure 14-2) and unhealthy diets (Langford, 1981). Among adolescent girls, two problems of mounting incidence and gravity are anorexia nervosa and bulimia. While creating nutritional problems in that they starve their victims, these diseases have emotional etiologies that pose a complex challenge to treatment.

Figure 14-2
Fast foods are popular with young people whose frequently poor eating habits can lead to health problems.

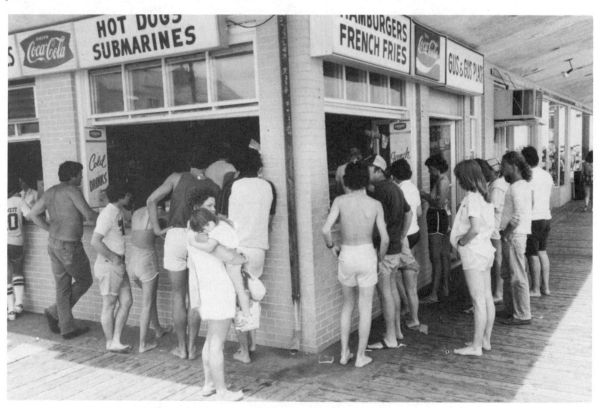

Health Services for Children and the Nurse's Role

What is being done to meet children's health needs? In response to the nation's inadequate services for children, the Select Panel for the Promotion of Children's Health, established in 1978, developed health goals for children and expectant mothers in the United States and designed a plan to achieve the goals (Hanlon & Pickett, 1984, p. 400). The panel, in 1981, found that the current health care system had not kept up with children's changing health needs, with advanced technology, or with epidemiological research. The panel emphasized a need for more disease and injury prevention through programs addressing environmental concerns. It recommended that health services focus on the relationship between health and behavior, and it urged improved nutrition. Members recommended a reconstitution of the former Children's Bureau into a new Maternal and Child Health Administration, to be housed in the Public Health Service, and the consolidation of maternal-child functions at the state level into a single agency. These recommendations are being carried out in many areas.

A variety of programs now exist that directly or indirectly serve the health needs of children. Community health nurses play a major and vital role in delivering these services. In community health, they fall into three categories approximating the three practice priorities of community health nursing practice — preventive health programs, health protection, and health promotion.

Preventive Health Programs for Children

Proper *prenatal care* makes a significant difference in maternal health and the subsequent health of the infant. More community health programs seek out high-risk mothers, those least likely to obtain regular care during pregnancy, and emphasize maternal nutrition, particularly adequate protein and caloric intake, smoking cessation, reduction of alcohol consumption, and social and family support. The WIC (Women, Infants, and Children) program has been particularly successful in reducing the number of low birth weight infants. Community health nurses play a vital role in teaching good health habits during pregnancy, especially with unwed mothers, and preparing the mother for care of the baby.

Health departments and private services continue to offer *immunization* against each of the seven major childhood infectious diseases — measles, mumps, polio, rubella, diphtheria, pertussis, and tetanus — any of which can cause permanent disability and some even death. Although their threat has been substantially reduced, vigilance cannot be relaxed. Low immunization levels in many areas, particularly among the poor, plus disease increases signal the need for constant surveillance, outreach programs, and educational efforts. Community health nurses are deeply involved in each of these preventive activities. Health departments and schools often work collaboratively to provide immunization services (Table 14-1). A compulsory immunization law, varying in its application from state to state, has enabled public health personnel to carry out these preventive services.

Parental support services, available through many public and private agencies including churches, have a long-range effect on children's health. Emotionally healthy parents and stable families offer a healthful environment and support system for growing children. Community health nurses provide teaching and counseling services to parents in their homes and in groups. Discussing parenting concerns and increasing parents' understanding of normal child growth and development allay fears and prevent problems. Through such efforts, family violence and abuse can be averted.

Family planning programs, often stationed strategically near schools and in inner cities, provide birth control information and counseling to young people. Community health nurses, in collaboration with an interdisciplinary team, are usually the primary care providers in these programs. Their major goals are to prevent teenage pregnancy, educate teenagers about reproduction and contraception, and encourage responsible sexual behavior.

Providing *STD services* has been more difficult. Young people affected with one of these diseases are often afraid or embarrassed to seek help. Furthermore, community health professionals receive very little training in this area and may be uncomfortable and judgmental in their approach. Vulnerable groups, particularly young minorities, inner city residents, and homosexuals, are being reached, however. Quality services and nonjudgmental

Table 14-1
Childhood Immunization Schedule

Age*	Diphtheria Pertussis Tetanus	Polio	Measles	Rubella	Mumps
2 months	x	x			
4 months	x	x			
6 months	x	x(optional)			
15 months**			x	x	x
18 months	x	x			
4–6 years	x	x			
14–16 years***	x				

*It is recommended that immunizations begin in early infancy but can be initiated later under physician direction.
**Measles, rubella and mumps vaccines may be combined in a single injection and given about 15 months of age.
***A sixth tetanus-diphtheria booster should be given at 14–16 years, then every 10 years.
Source: Parents' Guide to Childhood Immunization, (1979) USDHEW, Center for Disease Control. Atlanta, GA: U.S. Government Printing Office.

attitudes attract young people who need help and are being offered through STD clinics, family planning clinics, private physicans, schools, and employers. Community heatlh nurses, stationed in most of these settings, are generally the professionals who deal most directly with these clients. Improved public awareness and education, screening of high-risk groups, appropriate antibiotic treatment of infected individuals, and identification and treatment of sexual contacts have all served to reduce the threat of STDs.

Treatment and prevention of alcohol and drug abuse is another difficult task. Many social and economic influences promote chemical abuse and dependency, complicating the reversal of these effects. Recommended strategies and areas in which community health nurses working with aggregates can be more involved include (Public Health Service, 1979, p. 127):

1. Prevention through early and ongoing education,
2. Working to make the social climate less accepting of these behaviors,
3. Reducing stress factors contributing to chemical abuse, and
4. Law enforcement.

Educational efforts to discourage alcohol and drug use have often been ineffective, some even creating an incentive to experiment with them. Educational strategies that have been most successful have focused on the young person's individual responsibility for daily decisions affecting his or her health (Public Health Services, 1979, p. 127). Thus, programs such as youth service clubs and community activities that encourage children and adolescents to be responsible and to make wise choices affecting their well-being and that promote self-worth can serve as useful preventive measures.

Health Protection Programs for Children

Accidents and injury control programs serve a critical role in protecting the lives of children. Efforts to prevent motor vehicle accidents, a major killer, include driver education programs, better highway construction (reducing sharp curves and improving signs), and continuing research into the causes of various types of crashes. Injury prevention and reduction has been addressed through strategies such as use of safety restraints (particularly specially designed ones for infants and small children), air bags, substituting other modes of travel (air, rail, or bus), lower speed limits, stricter enforcement of and penalties associated with drunk driving laws, safer automobile design, and helmets for motorcyclists.

Falls, the major killer of preschool children and the cause of deaths and injuries for millions of other children each year, occur mostly in the home. Here the community health nurse plays a major role in observing potential hazards, teaching safety measures, and reinforcing positive practices. Preventive and protective measures may be achieved through simple and inexpensive changes in the home and furniture design. They include guards on windows and across stairways, safer walking surfaces, elimination of sharp objects or modification of surfaces that a child might fall against, and closer supervision of young children.

Child deaths and injuries from burns result primarily from house fires, but also from electrical burns and scalds. Many local fire departments and public health programs offer safety education in this area, emphasizing the use of heat- and smoke-detecting systems, fire drills, and home evacuation plans; less flammable structural materials, furnishings, and clothing; and careful smoking. Scalds occur in kitchens and bathrooms most often. Children can be protected by keeping pot handles turned toward the center of the stove and by modifying water temperatures in water heaters.

Safety programs also seek to protect children against the hazards of poisonings, ingestion of prescription and over-the-counter drugs, product-related accidents (unsafe toys, bicycles, skateboards, playground equipment, and furniture), and recreational accidents, including drownings and sport injuries. Safety services assume various forms. Poison control centers in many localities offer information and emergency assistance. Toxic household substances, such as cleaning supplies, must be clearly labeled, and harmful drugs packaged with special seals and safety caps. Product safety is monitored by the Federal Consumer Product Safety Commission. Greater efforts are being made to reduce recreational injuries through improved boating and swimming regulations, water safety measures, team sports safety measures, and better protective equipment and playfields for sports participants, including football helmets that don't injure other players and obstacle-free zones around playing fields. Generally, the community health nurse can educate families to recognize potentially hazardous situations and encourage efforts to eliminate them.

Programs to reduce environmental hazards begin at the federal level with the government setting and enforcing pollution standards and dealing with environmental contamination that poses health risks. At the state and municipal government levels, measures include monitoring air and drinking water safety, providing proper sewage disposal, controlling ionizing radiation, enforcing auto safety and emission standards, and regulating agricultural chemicals and pesticides. Locally, protective measures include educational programs warning against toxic agents in the environment, community surveillance, and enforcement of environmental health standards. At all levels, epidemiologic research probes the causes and seeks answers to provide better protection for the public. Community health nurses need to be alert to environmental hazards and work collaboratively with other members of the public health team to report problems and educate clients. Improved environmental control protects today's children against disease and disability and tomorrow's children against birth defects and the long-range hazards of environmental contamination (Figure 14-3).

We have learned in community health that infectious diseases can be

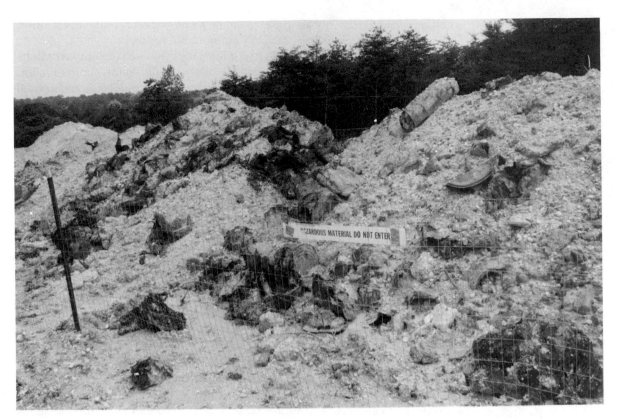

HAZARDOUS MATERIAL DO NOT ENTER

Figure 14-3
Toxic materials in the environment pose a serious threat to children's health — immediately and long range.

controlled and in some cases eliminated. Witness the successful worldwide eradication of smallpox, the dramatic decline in paralytic polio, and the decreasing incidence of the other communicable diseases of childhood. *Control of infectious diseases* comes largely through a two-pronged effort. One is wide-scale, persistent immunization programs, discussed earlier. The second is rigorous monitoring and surveillance of communicable disease incidence. Such surveillance is done continuously in the United States through the efforts of the federal Center for Disease Control in collaboration with state and local health departments. Surveillance involves four basic activities (Public Health Service, 1979, p. 117):

1. Case finding — of disease or exposure to disease, done by community health professionals.
2. Case reporting — to public health officials, by health care providers, schools, industries.
3. Analysis and interpretation — of communicable disease data to determine implications.
4. Appropriate response — with control measures.

Community health nurses do case finding and reporting and assist other health team members with carrying out control measures.

Programs protecting children against infectious diseases encompass efforts such as closing swimming pools with unsafe bacteria counts, immunization campaigns in conjunction with influenza outbreaks, or surveillance and control efforts in hospital pediatric units to reduce the incidence and threat of iatrogenic disease.

Services to protect children from abuse are much less developed or effective. A variety of factors account for this. Most child abuse occurs in the home; thus, only the most blatant situations become evident to outsiders (Figure 14-4). Community health nurses and physicians who see injured children may find parents' explanations plausible and not suspect or want to believe that foul play might be responsible. Avoidance of legal involvement keeps others from reporting suspected cases. A model law passed in 1963 (Children's Bureau, 1963) required mandatory reporting of suspicious cases of child abuse. In 1966, the American Academy of Pediatrics developed recommendations for an improved reporting, record keeping, and intervention system that would provide legal immunity to the reporting professional ("Maltreatment of Children," 1966). Currently, all the states have developed adaptations of the model law, professionals and the public are more aware of the problem, and there is an increase in reporting. Nonetheless, it is estimated that only 1 percent of battered child cases are actually reported (Hanlon & Pickett, 1984, p. 522). In 1974, the National Center for Child Abuse and Neglect was established as a result of the Child Abuse Prevention and Treatment Act. The center collects and analyzes information on child abuse and neglect, serves as an information clearinghouse, publishes educational materials on the subject, offers technical assistance, and conducts research into the problem. The surgeon general's report on health promotion and disease prevention suggests a multifaceted approach to dealing with child abuse and neglect. It recommends "parent education, enhancement of community and social support systems, assistance to abusing parents through collaborative efforts of public and private sector, and projects designed to create an integrated health and social service delivery system" (Public Health Services, 1979, p. 38). The effectiveness of local programs depends, in large measure, on the willingness of community health professionals to work as a team to detect, report, and develop interventions for abusers and abused children (Hanlon & Pickett, 1984, p. 523). The community health nurse is in a unique position to detect early signs of neglect and abuse, establish rapport with abusing parents, family members, or others, and assist with appropriate interventions and referrals.

Fluoridation of community water supplies is the most effective, safe, and low-cost means of *protecting children's dental health*. Fluoride makes teeth less susceptible to decay by increasing resistance to the bacteria-produced acid in the mouth. Presently only about one-half of the U.S. population has

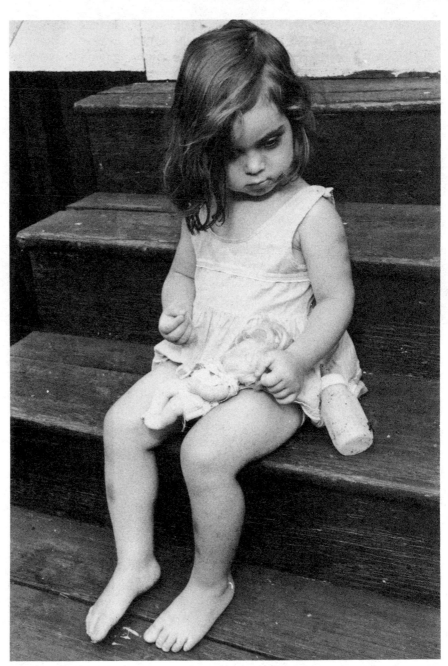

Figure 14-4
The abused child's experience will strongly influence her future perceptions of the parenting role.

access to fluoridated water. Fluoride rinses, dietary supplements, and direct applications are other methods used to protect children's teeth but with less success. Public acceptance of community water fluoridation has been slow, despite 35 years of research demonstrating its unquestioned safety and effectiveness. In addition to regular dental care, good nutrition, and proper oral hygiene, community health nurses can safely promote public water fluoridation as an important program for protecting children's dental health.

Health Promotion Programs for Children

Early childhood development programs serve an increasingly important function for the escalating number of children enrolling in day care centers and preschools. At least half of all children today have mothers who work, and that figure is rising. Economic pressures eat into family time together and often diminish the quality of children's physical and psychosocial nourishment. Childhood development programs, like Head Start, provide physical, emotional, intellectual, and social stimulation during a critical period of children's growth when impressions are being made and patterns formed that will influence what kind of adults these children will be in the future. Comprehensive preschool programs promote good physical health, proper nutrition, a positive self-concept, and cognitive and social skill development. Many such programs exist, but more are needed. The quality of day care and preschool programs varies considerably. Licensing laws can only regulate minimum safety and health standards. In addition, numerous child care operations are too small to require licensing, leaving their quality open to individual discretion. Community health nurses can influence the quality of day care and preschool programs through active educational efforts and through monitoring of health and safety standards.

Nutrition and weight control programs form another important set of health promotion services. Children need to learn sound dietary habits early in life to establish healthy lifelong patterns. Some preschool and school programs teach, as well as provide, good nutrition and encourage the kinds of eating patterns that prevent obesity. For overweight children and adolescents, there are a number of weight control programs available through schools, health departments, community health centers, health maintenance organizations, and private groups. Adolescents are particularly vulnerable to media and peer pressures for nonnutritive snacks, including diet sodas, based on a desire to be accepted and to acquire a trim figure. Fad diets can also be harmful if not nutritionally balanced. Programs aimed at nutritionally sounder advertising are having a positive effect. Parents and children are becoming more aware of harmful foods, such as cholesterol from animal fats, the need to eat less sugar and salt, and the need to eat right to feel and look good. The nurse, through nutrition education and reinforcement of positive practices, plays a significant role in promoting the health of these children.

394

The value of *exercise and physical fitness programs* for young people has been recognized for some time. Organized groups, such as the YMCA, YWCA, Boy and Girl Scouts, and Campfire Girls, have offered sports and character development programs for many years. Good preschool programs provide equipment and opportunities for large-muscle activity as well as fine motor development. Schools, parks, and recreation centers encourage exercise through use of playground equipment and organized sports activities. Despite these opportunities, many young people do not exercise often enough or vigorously enough. And minorities, females, and inner-city residents exercise less than white, suburban males (Public Health Service, 1979, p. 134). Even team sports keep players inactive much of the time and are not activities that young people continue in their adult lives. More comprehensive physical education programs that encourage vigorous exercise and self-discipline as lifetime habits would better serve the health needs of this population group. Community health nurses can promote such programs through the schools as well as encourage these activities in their contacts with students of all ages (Figure 14-5).

The demonstrated hazards of cigarette smoking, alcohol, and drug abuse have prompted the development of *substance abuse programs* particularly targeting children and adolescents. School health educational efforts, involving school nurses, have been a major source of influence encouraging students to make responsible decisions about smoking, drinking, and other behaviors affecting their health. Health departments, community health nursing agencies, and private groups, such as the American Cancer Society and the National Lung Association, also provide educational materials and promote antismoking and drug use prevention campaigns. The more successful programs emphasize how the human body works and how behavior affects it. They also help young people resist social pressures to smoke and take drugs by pointing out that those who do are in the minority and by showing the deleterious effects of these practices. Using students themselves as health educators is a positive use of peer pressure and has proved to be a successful means of influencing attitudes (Public Health Service, 1979, p. 124). Other groups, like 4-H clubs, churches, the Catholic Youth Organization, and Scouts, building on the same concept, use peer counseling to influence young people to assume responsible actions and healthy life-styles. The community health nurse participates in and supports existing programs in addition to counseling and referring young people needing help.

Stress control programs for children and adolescents do not exist in any great numbers, yet they are needed. Many of the health problems discussed in this chapter relate to the emotional health of young people. Reckless driving, suicide, homicide, unwanted pregnancy, smoking, alcoholism, drug misuse, obesity, anorexia nervosa, and bulemia, as well as other problems — all signal the presence of some kind of stress and coping skills inadequate to handle it. Crisis intervention programs and services that treat a problem

395

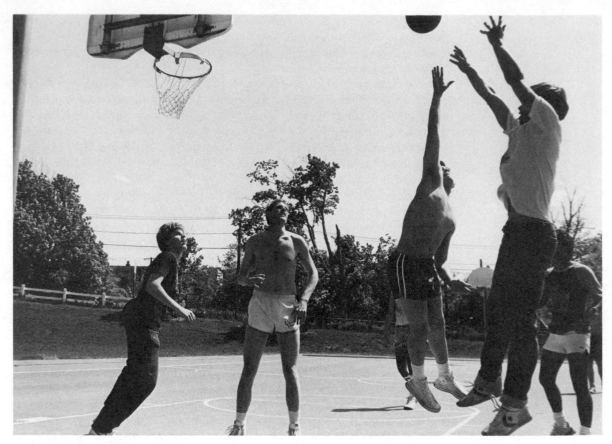

Figure 14-5
Vigorous exercise that promotes fitness and self-discipline is an important contributor to young people's health. Team sports further enhance the development of social skills and healthy relationships.

after it occurs are helpful and can prevent problems from developing further. More needed, however, for this population group are programs that build coping skills early, including self-help and mutual support activities. Programs offered in a group context, such as those mentioned earlier — 4-H, Scouts, various character-building clubs, and organizations like Outward Bound — have proven most effective. For the nurse, recognition of young people at risk, counseling, and early referral to sources of help can prevent problems from arising. Reduction of stresses in the family and community environments can further enhance this group's health.

Community Health Nursing Interventions for Children's Health

The previous description of programs addressing children's health problems also points out areas of deficiency in services. Community health nurses face the challenge of continually assessing each population group's current health problems as well as determining available and needed services. Some gaps can be filled by nursing interventions. Others must be referred to various members of the community health team with whom the nurse may sometimes collaboratively develop services.

Community health nursing interventions with preschool and school-age populations are those outlined in the basic conceptual model discussed in Chapter 3: education, engineering, and enforcement. We have seen examples of each mentioned in the previous discussion. For instance, the nurse uses educational interventions when teaching proper nutrition, family planning, physical and psychological effects of drug abuse, safety precautions, or weight control. Each of these involves providing information and encouraging client groups to act on that information in a responsible manner that is health enhancing. Engineering interventions, those strategies in which the nurse uses a greater degree of persuasion or positive manipulation, are evident in conducting voluntary immunization programs, encouraging use of contraceptives, counseling for stress reduction, identifying and treating STD sexual contacts, or encouraging use of safety devices, for example, stairway guards. The nurse uses enforcement interventions, those activities employing some form of coercion, when requiring immunizations, which are mandated by law, or when reporting illegal drug use, child abuse, or environmental health standards violations, such as rat infestation of a home.

School Health

In community health practice, nursing service to a school-age population requires a special mind-set. Nurses must shift from a focus entirely on individual schoolchildren or small groups of children to one that includes aggregates. In order to show how this shift can be made, let us consider what your role as school nurse would involve.

Imagine that you, a community health nurse, recently became school nurse for Keeler Elementary School. You have been working with families and groups in the community for several years, but you have not done school nursing before. Since it is summer and school has not yet started, you take time to get acquainted with the school and the nurse's role.

Mrs. Murray, the principal, is happy to talk with you. She comments that she expects the nurse to keep the children as healthy as possible and be the major consultant on health matters in the school. Because she is very busy with administrative concerns, she prefers that you carve out your own role, although she wants to be kept informed of your plans. She describes the school to you. Built 40 years ago, Keeler has 353 students in grades kindergarten through sixth. With 14 teachers, its pupil-teacher ratio is 25:1. The teachers give some health instruction to their classes. Mr. Jones, a fourth-grade teacher, was a medical corpsman in the army and handles first-aid problems for the school when the nurse is not there. Two PTA mother-volunteers keep the student health records in order. You can ask for more help if you need it. Mrs. Murray gives you material to read that describes school health services generally.

NURSING SERVICES

You learn that school health services incorporate three functions: health services, health education, and improvement of the school environment (Schaller, 1981). Health services include programs such as vision and hearing screening, psychological testing, health examinations, emergency care, and referrals. There are special correction and training services for speech, hearing, or mental health problems. Student and family counseling are important components; there is a program of communicable disease control. School health services also include health appraisal and services for school personnel.

The health education function of school health services involves planned and incidental teaching of health concepts; classes in health science and healthful living; and use of educational media, library resources, and community facilities. These activities aim to integrate health information with students' daily living experiences, to build positive attitudes toward health, and to establish sound health practices.

The third function of school health services is the promotion of healthful school living. Emphasis on a healthful physical environment includes proper selection, design, organization, operation, and maintenance of the physical plant. Consideration should be shown for areas such as adaptability to student needs; safety; visual, thermal, and acoustic factors; aesthetic values; sanitation; and safety of the school bus system. Healthful school living also emphasizes planning a daily schedule that monitors healthful classroom experiences, extra class activities, school lunches, emotional climate, program of discipline, and teaching methods. It also seeks to promote the physical, mental, and emotional health of school personnel.

HEALTH TEAM

You are impressed with all that can be done in school health and explore the subject further through reading and interviewing school personnel. It quickly becomes apparent that school health, like all health programs in the community, requires a team effort. Although the school nurse plays a central role, she collaborates with many other individuals. The school principal influences all phases of the school health program. Mrs. Murray, for example, can promote good school health through actively supporting all the school's health services, setting policies, and tapping community resources. She can reinforce positive efforts, ranging from health teaching to good housekeeping by the custodian, within the school. Because of the principal's influential position, it is absolutely essential that the nurse maintain a positive working relationship with her.

Teachers, whether they are involved in regular instruction, physical education, or special education classes, play a major role in school health. Because they spend so much time with students, their observations, health teaching, and personal health habits have a profound effect on student health and the quality of school health services. Nurse and teachers must collaborate constantly.

Other health team members, such as health educators, health coordinators, psychologists, audiologists, counselors, dentists, dental hygienists, social workers, or health aides, may be present depending on the size and financial resources of the school. All team members, including students, parents, and the custodian, have a specialized role complementary to that of the school nurse. Consultation and referral between team members are crucial to implementing the school health program (Fig. 14-6).

The school physician may work full-time, part-time, or be available on a consultation basis. This role focuses largely on advising and consulting in policy and medical-legal matters. The physician often serves as liaison with the community and other health agencies and consults with those who plan and develop school health programs. The physician may also become involved in some student health appraisal and health problem intervention (Schaller, 1981). A good working relationship between the school nurse and school physician is important. The nurse's role, while complementary to and unique from the physician's, nonetheless may need clarifying and interpreting to maximize the effectiveness of their collaboration.

You want to learn more about the school nurse's role. You consult with

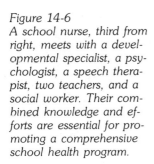

Figure 14-6
A school nurse, third from right, meets with a developmental specialist, a psychologist, a speech therapist, two teachers, and a social worker. Their combined knowledge and efforts are essential for promoting a comprehensive school health program.

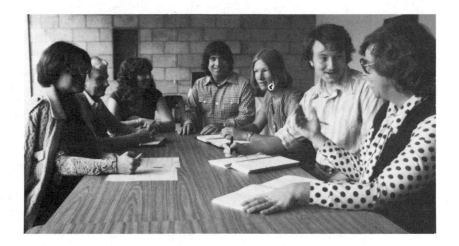

your nursing supervisor who explains the difference between specialized school nursing and the generalized school nursing that you will be expected to practice.

Specialized and Generalized Nursing Roles

School nurses operate from one of two administrative bases. In many localities, school nurses are hired through the public school system and maintain a specialized, school-based service. There is growing conviction that such nurses should work under the jurisdiction of the board of health rather than the board of education. With professional instead of educational supervision, better utilization of the nurse and greater quality of health care service would be ensured (Humes, 1975). An advantage of the specialized school nurse role is that the nurse can concentrate all her time and effort on the school health program and thus develop specialized skills in school health assessment and intervention. A disadvantage is that school nurses' practice is often limited to the school setting. A specialized role may prevent the school nurse from assessing preschoolers, providing health service to families of school-children, or making broader community assessments and contacts.

School nurse practitioners, nurses with advanced preparation and experience in child care and school health, assume an even more specialized and expanded role — that of identifying and managing many of the health problems of schoolchildren. They have made a significant contribution to the provision of primary health care to schoolchildren. They have an important but different function from that of school nurses who are community health nurses.

Generalized school nurses work within the framework of generalized community health nursing, serving private and sometimes public schools as part of their caseloads. The advantage of a generalized school nurse role is the broader community base from which the nurse can operate. This base allows contact with preschoolers and families, strengthened knowledge of the community and its resources, and integration of in-school and out-of-school care (Freeman & Heinrich, 1981). Humes (1975, p. 396) also argues, ''A public health nurse working in the schools tends to have more of a working knowledge of the general health needs of the community. With this kind of background information she is better able to view student health problems in a community context.'' A disadvantage of the generalized role, however, is that the nurse often has less time to meet school health needs.

Whether specialized or generalized, the primary functions of the school nurse are to prevent illness and to promote and maintain the health of the school community. A philosophy of school nursing, adopted in Minnesota, is suggested by your supervisor as a basis for your school nursing practice (Minnesota Nurses Association, 1974, p. 3):

All children and their families have a right to education which guides them toward self-awareness and self-realization in meeting the needs of complex living. The focus of public health school nursing is the self-motivation of individuals and families to seek and maintain optimum health. The partnership of public health school nursing and education is essential for increasing high level wellness of students, their families, school personnel, and the community.

The community health nurse not only serves individuals, families, and groups within the context of school health, but also the school as an organization and its membership (students and staff) as population groups.

School has started, and the three days a week you spend at Keeler never seem to be enough time to finish all there is to do. You have already looked through student records to determine children with health problems and followed up on your findings. You sent five children home with notes recommending dental work; sent little Norma, a new kindergartner, to the audiologist after testing her hearing; and referred Jimmy Hansen for psychological testing. You found out that Tommy Sandberg had a convulsive disorder but did not take his medication regularly. You visited his family, explained the need for consistent treatment and medical supervision, had him start on a regular treatment program, and gave him his medication during school hours. Many individual children in your school show signs of improved health as a result of your efforts. Several families of children in the school are now part of your regular caseload. The group you started with sixth graders on how to become good baby-sitters is going well. Yet there are so many children you have not assessed. Moreover, what about the teachers' needs? You know that you are not really providing service to the whole school community. You realize that you must shift your focus.

Nursing Goals

Previously your primary goal as a school nurse had been to assess and promote the health of the preschool and school-age child. Changing your focus means you now adopt a broader set of goals for school nursing that involve the school organization and population levels. You want to include the individual, family, and group levels. Basing your goals on those outlined by the Minnesota Nurses Association (1974), you aim to do the following:

1. Assess the health and developmental status of the preschool and school-age child
2. Promote and maintain optimal health of students, families, and school personnel
3. Implement an appropriate plan for the education and care of each exceptional and each handicapped child

At these levels, you concentrate on selected individuals, selected families, or special groups needing nursing or other professional intervention. Many of these clients will be referred to other community resources for assistance. You plan to get to know personally each member of the school family and staff, including the secretary and the custodian, in order to cultivate their good will, sharpen their observation skills regarding the students, and assess their own health needs. A faculty or staff member who is not well physically or emotionally may significantly influence the health of the school community.

ORGANIZATIONAL LEVEL

At the organizational level, you aim to fulfill the following responsibilities (Minnesota Nurses Association, 1974):

1. Establish and revise school and district health policies, administration, and philosophy pertaining to school health services.
2. Develop and maintain a system of emergency care.
3. Provide for school safety and a healthful school environment.
4. Facilitate comprehensive community health care planning and resources development to include the health needs of the preschool and school-age populations and their families.

This level requires more attention than you have given to it in the past. True, you have worked out a system with Mr. Jones to handle basic first aid for injuries and have updated physician orders to cover emergencies. Now you make certain everyone understands what to do and where to go in the event of an emergency such as a tornado. Some school safety issues have been addressed, but now you need to examine the overall safety of the building and check with administration about safety of the school buses. You look into the effectiveness of fire drills and alternate routes for emptying the building. You oversee the handling of dangerous materials in the science laboratories.

The school environment needs more careful assessment. You start checking the nutritional value of the school lunches and the ventilation of classrooms. You begin to analyze seating arrangements in each classroom while observing students and consult with teachers about your observations. The dingy halls of the old building soon take on a new cheerful appearance through the work of your volunteer paint crew from the PTA.

As an organization, Keeler Elementary School is functioning fairly well, you decide. The pupil-teacher ratio is slightly high by some standards, but a class of 25 students is generally considered a manageable load. To provide students with more individual attention, you suggest adding more teacher aides. Faculty on the whole get along well with with each other and with Mrs. Murray. There is open communication and positive feedback. Working conditions are pleasant, and faculty requests are answered in a reasonable amount of time. There is also adequate space, equipment, personnel assistance, and support for your school health program.

To influence school health policy and resource planning, you volunteer to serve on a district committee that meets once a month. Meeting other professionals concerned about school health broadens your understanding of school and community needs and also gives you ideas on intervention strategies and how to tap community resources.

POPULATION GROUP LEVEL

At the population group level, you aim to achieve the following goals (Minnesota Nurses Association, 1974):

1. Assess the collective needs of preschool and school-age children and school personnel.
2. Identify existing and potential health problems in the school population (and in the larger community affecting it), determine those at greatest risk, develop a plan, and intervene to minimize or prevent problems.
3. Promote and maintain optimal health of the student body and the school personnel population.
4. Prevent and control communicable disease in the student population (in order to protect the well-being of students and the community).
5. Evaluate and upgrade the contribution of the school nurse role toward promoting the health of the school community.

During a conference with your community health nursing supervisor, you review the new goals and make plans for conducting a broader assessment of the school population's health. Journal articles and discussion with other school nurses give you additional ideas. For example, one school nurse, instead of performing a routine physical examination on every child, developed a systematic method of classroom assessment. She evaluated an entire class of 25 to 30 children at one time through regular observation of their behavior and developmental status and through close consultation wtih teachers that alerted them about special student behaviors to observe (Withrow, 1979). You decide to try this method in combination with further data gathering on selected children through screening, interviews, and family visits. The yearly vision and hearing screening, which you are required to give students, offers another opportunity to observe them closely for signs of child abuse, malnutrition, or other physical or emotional problems that might be prevalent among this population group.

You assess preschool-age children who will be starting kindergarten next year by holding a Saturday afternoon preschool fair. Invitations are sent out to all the families in the community with four-year-old children. PTA volunteers help you organize games and refreshments and conduct school tours. Registered nurse volunteers from the community assist you in cursory physical exams that include vision and hearing screening. You notify parents immediately if children need follow-up care.

While conducting this preschool assessment, you keep in mind that you want a profile of this population of four-year-olds, not just each individual child's health picture. You look for recurring problems that are common to the group, such as skin rashes, orthopedic defects, headaches, eating or respiratory difficulties, and signs of communicable diseases. Such population screening has sometimes uncovered widespread community health problems. For instance, recognition of common symptoms among Love Canal residents in New York led to a discovery that the river was contaminated with poisonous industrial wastes. In 1980, a community in Memphis, Tennessee, whose incidence of miscarriages, cancer, and infant deaths had markedly increased, discovered that nearby chemicals buried many years previously were the cause. Identifying common problems among the preschool or school-age populations enables you to take corrective action on a broader scale and thus to help many children at once as well as to take preventive action.

You begin to collect data on the needs of the school personnel population by observing and talking informally with faculty and staff. You discover that some of the teachers seem on the verge of burning out. They do not enjoy their teaching, feel tired most of the time, take piles of work home with them every night, do not sleep well, and often feel irritable toward the children. With school administration's approval, you plan a workshop to prevent teacher burnout. Expert consultants help the teachers learn to recognize symptoms and how to avoid burnout. During the workshop the teachers develop specific plans to help them cope with their present situations and design strategies for alleviating future stress.

The three sets of goals for school nursing have helped you refocus your thinking and expand your service to include not only individual, family, and group levels of nursing intervention but school organization and school population group levels as well.

Summary

Children are an important population group. Community health nurses need to understand children's health problems and how they can be addressed.

Mortality rates for children have decreased dramatically since the early 1900s. Causes of death have also changed. Infectious diseases used to be the leading threat to the lives of children; now accidents are the leading cause of death for children over one year of age. Morbidity rates among children, in contrast to their mortality rates, remain high. Children are still vulnerable to many illnesses, injuries, and emotional problems.

404

Infant life and health is most threatened by low birth weight and congenital anomalies. Infant deaths are most often caused by respiratory distress, sudden infant death syndrome, and premature delivery. For preschoolers, the major threat to life and health is accidents (falls, drownings, burns, and poisonings). Other health concerns include acute illnesses, particularly respiratory illness, and nutritional, dental, and emotional needs. Motor vehicle accidents are the leading cause of death for school-age children. Further health problems for this group include respiratory illnesses, injuries, infectious diseases, digestive conditions, emotional and behavioral problems, handicaps, and nutritional problems. Mortality rates for adolescents are twice as high as those for younger children. Violent deaths and injuries are the leading threats to life and health in this population group. Accidents (motor vehicle and other), homicides, and suicides are the three major causes of death. Other health problems include alcohol and drug abuse, unwanted pregnancies, STDs, and poor nutrition.

Health services for children span three categories: preventive, health protecting, and health promoting. The community health nurse plays a vital role in each. Preventive services include prenatal care, immunization programs, parental support services, family planning programs, services for those with STDs, and alcohol and drug abuse prevention programs. Health protection services include accidents and injury control, programs to reduce environmental hazards, control of infectious diseases, services to protect children from child abuse, and fluoridation of community water supplies to protect children's dental health. Health promotion services include programs in early childhood development; nutrition and weight control; exercise and physical fitness; smoking, alcohol, and drug abuse education; and stress control.

Community health nurses use three basic interventions while serving children's health needs. With educational interventions, such as nutrition teaching, nurses provide information and encourage clients to act responsibly on behalf of their own health. With engineering interventions, such as encouraging use of contraceptives, nurses employ persuasive tactics to move clients toward more positive health behaviors. With enforcement interventions, such as reporting and intervening in child abuse, nurses practice some form of coercion to protect children from threats to their health.

Nursing of the school age population involves providing health services and health education and ensuring a healthful school environment. School nurses may be generalized or specialized but overall they seek to improve the health of school children as an aggregate.

Study Questions

1. What is the major cause of death among school-age children? What community-wide interventions could be initiated to prevent these deaths?

Select one intervention and describe how you and a group of community health professionals might develop this preventive measure.

2. Describe one health promotion program you, as a community health nurse, could initiate and carry out to improve the health of children in a day care center.

3. How can environmental health protection programs affect the future health of infants? Why is control of environmental hazards important for any age child? List three things a nurse can do to protect children against environmental hazards.

4. A 14-year-old girl from a middle-class family and a 14-year-old girl from a poor family both come to the family planning clinic where you work. The girls have similar symptoms that possibly indicate gonorrhea. Would your assessment and interventions be the same or different with each girl? What are your values and attitudes toward people with diseases that are sexually transmitted? Does social class, race, age, or sex make any difference in how you feel about them? What is one action the community health nurse can take to prevent such diseases in this population group?

References

Alcohol, Drug Abuse, and Mental Health Administration. (1980). *The alcohol, drug abuse, and mental health national data book* (DHEW Publication). Rockville, MD: U.S. Government Printing Office.

Avery, J. (1980). The safety of children in cars. *Practitioner, 224,* 816–821.

Bell, M., Ternberg, J., & Bower, R. (1980). Low velocity vehicular injuries in children — Runover accidents. *Pediatrics, 66,* 628–631.

Child homicide — United States. (1982). *Morbidity and Mortality Weekly Report, 31,* 292–294.

Children's Bureau. U.S. Department of Health, Education and Welfare. (1963). The abused child — Principles and suggested language for legislation on reporting of the abused child. Washington, D.C.: U.S. Government Printing Office.

Children's Defense Fund. (1979). *America's children and their families: Basic facts.* Washington, D.C.: Author.

Comstock, G. (1981). Influence of mass media on child health and behavior. *Health Education Quarterly, 8,* 32.

Freeman, R., & Heinrich, J. (1981). *Community health nursing practice* (2nd ed.). Philadelphia: W. B. Saunders.

Hanlon, J., & Pickett, G. (1984). *Public health: Administration and practice* (8th ed.). St. Louis: Times Mirror/Mosby.

Humes, C. W., Jr. (1975). Who should administer school nursing services? *American Journal of Public Health, 65,* 394.

Jonides, L. (1982). Childhood obesity: A treatment approach for private practice. *Pediatric Nursing, 8,* 320–322.

Kleinman, J. (1981, November). Trends and variations in birth weight. Paper presented at the annual meeting of the American Public Health Association, Los Angeles.

Langford, R. (1981). Teenagers and obesity. *American Journal of Nursing, 81,* 556–559.

Maltreatment of children: Recommendations of Committee on the Infant and Preschool Child of the American Academy of Pediatrics. (1966). *Pediatrics, 37,* 377.

Merritt, T., Laurence, R., & Naeye, R. (1980). The infants of adolescent mothers. *Pediatric Annals, 9*(3), 32.

Minnesota Nurses Association, Special Committee, School Nurse Branch. (1974). *Goals of school nursing: An interpretive tool.* St. Paul, MN: Minnesota Nurses Association.

National Center for Health Statistics. (1983, December). Health — United States 1983 (HHS Publication No. PHS 84-1232). Washington, DC: U.S. Government Printing Office.

Newacheck, P., Budetti, P., & McManus, P. (1984). Trends in childhood disability. *American Journal of Public Health, 74,* 232–236.

Pilliteri, A. (1981). *Child health nursing: Care of the growing family* (2nd ed.). Boston: Little, Brown.

President's Commission for a National Agenda for the Eighties. (1981). Helping families — to help themselves. *International Journal of Family Therapy, 3,*(3), 208–233.

Public Health Service. (1979). *Healthy people: The surgeon general's report on health promotion and disease prevention* (DHEW Publication No. 79-55071). Washington, D.C.: U.S. Government Printing Office.

Schaller, W. (1981). *The school health program* (5th ed.). Philadelphia: Saunders College.

Tyrell, S. (1981). Accidents will happen. *Health and Social Science Journal, 9,* 263–265.

Withrow, C. (1979). The school nurse takes a look at her charges. *Nursing '79, 1,* 48–51.

Selected Readings

American Public Health Associations. (1980). Health of school-age children (Resolution No. 7905). *American Journal of Public Health, 70,* 304–305.

Avery, J. (1980). The safety of children in cars. *Practitioner, 224,* 816–821.

Blum, R. (Ed.). (1982). *The clinical practice of adolescent medicine.* New York: Academic Press.

Budetti, P., Butler, J., & McManus, P. (1982). Federal health program reforms: Implications for child health care. *Milbank Memorial Fund Quarterly, 60*(1), 155.

Children's Defense Fund. (1979). *America's children and their families: Basic facts.* Washington, D.C.: Author.

Committee on School Health. (1981). School health: A guide for health professionals. Evanston, IL: American Academy of Pediatrics.

Comstock, G. (1981). Influence of mass media on child health and behavior. *Health Education Quarterly, 8*(1), 32.

Cushner, I. (1981). Maternal behavior and perinatal risks: Alcohol, smoking, and drugs. *Annual Review of Public Health, 2,* 201.

Daniel, W. (1977). *Adolescents in health and disease.* St. Louis: C. V. Mosby.

Daniel, W. (1981). Overview of adolescent health problems. *Southern Medical Journal, 74,* 569.

Doyle, K., & Cassell, C. (1981). Teenage sexuality: The early adolescent years. *Obstetrics and Gynecology Annual, 10,* 423.

Freeman, R., & Heinrich, J. (1981). *Community health nursing practice* (2nd ed.). Philadelphia: W. B. Saunders.

Green, L., & Iverson, D. (1982). School hearlth education. *Annual Review of Public Health, 3,* 321.

Hanlon, J., & Pickett, G. (1984). *Public health: Administration and practice* (8th ed.). St. Louis: Times Mirror/Mosby.

Holt, S., & Robinson, T. (1979). The school nurse's family assessment tool. *American Journal of Nursing, 79,* 950.

Jonides, L. (1982). Childhood obesity: A treatment approach for private practice. *Pediatric Nursing, 8,* 320–322.

Langford, R. (1981). Teenagers and obesity. *American Journal of Nursing, 81,* 556–559.

Long, G., Whitman, C., Johansson, M., Williams, C., & Tuthill, R. (1975). Evaluation of a school health program directed to children with history of high absence — A focus for nursing intervention. *American Journal of Public Health, 65,* 388–393.

McAlister, A. (1981). Social and environmental influences on health behavior. *Health Education Quarterly, 8*(1), 25.

Merritt, T., Laurence, R., & Naeye, R. (1980). The infants of adolescent mothers. *Pediatric Annals, 9*(3), 32.

Newacheck, P., Budetti, P., & McManus, P. (1984). Trends in childhood disability. *American Journal of Public Health, 74,* 232–236.

O'Brien, M., Manley, M., & Heagarty, M. (1975). Expanding the public health nurse's role in child care. *Nursing Outlook 23,* 369–373.

Pipes, P. (1981). Nutrition in infancy and childhood (2nd ed.). St. Louis: C. V. Mosby.

Porter, P. (1981). Realistic outcomes of school health service programs. *Health Education Quarterly, 8*(1), 81.

President's Commission for a National Agenda for the Eighties. (1981). Helping families — to help themselves. *International Journal of Family Therapy, 3*(3), 208–233.

Public Health Service. (1979). *Healthy people: The surgeon general's report on health promotion and disease prevention* (DHEW Publication No. 79-55071). Washington, D.C.: U.S. Government Printing Office.

Schaller, W. (1981). *The school health program* (5th ed.). Philadelphia: Saunders College.

Schlechter, F. (1981). An experiment in group adolescent weight loss guidance. *Journal of School Health, 51*(2), 123–124.

408

School-age day care: Developing a responsive curriculum. (1980, January). *Child Care Information Exchange*, pp. 17–20.

Silver, G. (1981). Redefining school health services: Comprehensive child health care as the framework. *Journal of School Health, 51*(3), 157–162.

Tyrell, S. (1981). Accidents will happen. *Health and Social Science Journal, 9*, 263–265.

Withrow, C. (1979). The school nurse takes a look at her charges. *Nursing '79, 1*, 48–51.

Wold, S. (1980). *School nursing: A framework for practice.* St. Louis: C. V. Mosby.

Zabin, L., & Clark, S. (1981). Why they delay: A study of teenage family planning clinic patients. *Family Planning Perspective, 13*(5), 205.

15

The Nature of Families

Imagine that you are employed as a community health nurse by an agency in Los Angeles. In a single day you might visit five families, each with different health problems. A young single mother seeks help in caring for her sick infant. Another family has an elderly parent recently discharged from the hospital after a stroke. The third family, Vietnamese refugees, needs instruction on the purchase and preparation of food. In the other two visits, you will check the progress of a serious burn on the arm of a ten-year-old, develop a contract for weight control with his mother, and assist a recently retired couple in adjusting to their new stage of life.

As you set out for a day of work, what kinds of things will you need to know? You will have to deal with specific health problems such as strokes, burns, and retirement. You need to know your goals — the promotion of health and self-care. You will have to rely on your knowledge of cultural differences when working with the Vietnamese family and perhaps other clients. You will need to know how to use certain tools such as problem solving and contracting. You will need to understand communication and know how to develop a helping relationship.

But do you need to know something about the nature of families? What should be known about the five families you will visit, apart from their individual members and problems? Do families, as basic units of a community, have characteristics that affect community health nursing service? The answer is an unqualified yes. As a community health nurse, your effectiveness depends on knowing how to work with families as a unit.

Characteristics of Families

Let us begin with three observations. First, all families are unique. The five families you will visit have their own distinct problems and strengths. None will be exactly like any other family. As you approach the door of a large house or ring the doorbell of an apartment, you cannot assume that you know what the family inside will be like. Consequently, you will have to gather information about each particular family in order to achieve your nursing objectives.

Second, every family is like every other family. The five families you visit do have certain features that they share with all families. These universal characteristics provide an important key to understanding each family's uniqueness. Five of the most important family universals for community nursing are listed below:

1. Every family is a small social system.
2. Every family has its own cultural values and rules.
3. Every family has structure.
4. Every family has certain basic functions.
5. Every family moves through stages in its life cycle.

No matter how many families you might visit in the course of a year, each one will have these universal features. It will be important to know how the social system, cultural values, structure, function, and stage of development affect health care provision. These five universals of family life provide the framework of this chapter.

Third, some families are more alike than others. Between the extremes of complete uniqueness and universal features, certain similarities among some families permit a classification of subtypes. For example, although all families have structure, the five you visit may consist of four types — two nuclear families (husband, wife, children), one nuclear dyad (husband and wife), one multigenerational family, and one single-parent family. Knowing the range of variation within the family universals will help prepare you for the families you encounter. As we consider the universals of family life, we will also discuss those subtypes that characterize our own society; if we took a worldwide perspective, subtypes in family life would greatly proliferate, although the universals would still exist.

Families as Social Systems

All of us fall into the trap of viewing families merely as a collection of individuals. Caused partly by our cultural value of strong individualism, this error also occurs because we encounter families through the individual members. When a community health nurse sits in a living room talking with a young mother about her new infant, it is difficult to realize that all the other family members are present by way of their influence. We can see this by examining the nature of families as social systems.

Interdependence among Members

First, all the members of a family, because they are units within a system, are interdependent. One member's actions affect the other members. For example, the community health nurse cannot expect a father's change in life-style to reduce his risk of coronary heart disease not to affect the rest of the family. If he cuts back on working overtime, the family's income will be reduced. If he begins to eat different foods, food preparation and eating patterns in the family will be altered. A new exercise program may upset other family routines. Furthermore, as this one member adjusts to the demands of a change in life-style, his ability to carry out his usual roles as husband and father may be affected.

This interdependence involves a set of internal relationships that influences the effectiveness of family functioning. There is a complex network of communication patterns among family members. It is possible to diagram the network as a family map of all the dyads, triads, and combinations of interactions that occur within families (Satir, 1972). The way parents relate to each other, for instance, influences the quality of their parenting. When the lines between them are strong and nurturant, they have more to offer their children. Marital, parent-child, and sibling relationships all significantly influence family functioning (Fig. 15-1). They determine how well the family as a system handles conflict, provides a support system for its members, copes with crises, solves daily problems, and capitalizes on its own resources.

Family Boundaries

Second, families, as systems, set and maintain boundaries. Family closeness, which results from shared experiences and expectations, links family members together in a bond that excludes the rest of the world. Witness an example of family unity as the Pedrocelli extended family gathers for a Sunday afternoon backyard picnic. Witness, too, the distinctiveness of this family from all the others in the neighborhood. Because of the things they have in common, the Pedrocellis set and maintain boundaries that unite them and also differentiate them from others.

Families, however, are not closed systems. Their boundaries are semipermeable, providing protection and preservation of family unity and autonomy while also allowing selective linkages with external associations. The Pedrocellis, like any family, need and have reciprocal relationships with other social systems, such as schools and work. In some instances, the outside contact

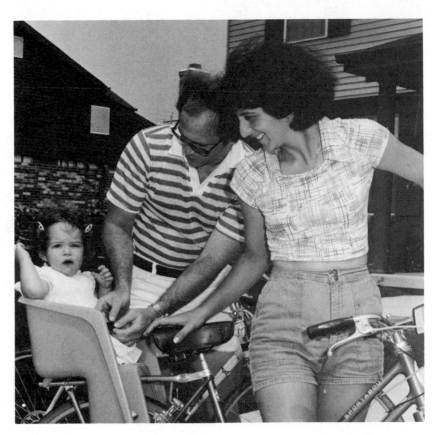

Figure 15-1
*Enjoying activities together
contributes to family unity
and strengthens positive
relationships.*

is minimal and not reciprocal. Troubled families, for example, may have limited ability to reach for and utilize the resources around them; they certainly have little, if anything, to give to others in return. Their external relationships depend primarily upon the community extending itself to them. Other families, to varying degrees, establish contact with the community. They develop patterns of giving and receiving that provide them with resources in times of need. Because families are not closed systems, they also contribute to community enrichment.

Adaptive Behavior

Third, families are equilibrium-seeking and adaptive systems. In accordance with their very nature, families never stay the same. They shift and change in response to internal and external forces. Internally, the family composition changes as new members are added. Roles and relationships change as members advance in age and experience, and normative expectations change

413

as members resolve their tensions and differing points of view. Externally, families are bombarded by influences from sources such as school, work, peers, neighbors, church, and government; consequently, they are forced to accommodate to new demands. Adapting to these influences may require a family to change its behavior, goals, and even its values. Like any system, the family needs a state of quasi equilibrium in order to function. Thus, with each new set of pressures, the family shifts and accommodates as a means of regaining balance and a normal life-style. There are times when a family's capacity for equilibrium seeking and adaptation is taxed beyond its limits. At this point the system may be in danger of disintegrating; that is, family members will leave because of unresolved conflict. It is then that families may need some form of intervention, such as extended family mediation or external professional help, to provide a supplemental resource for restoring family equilibrium.

Goal-directed Behavior

Finally, families as social systems are goal directed. Families exist for a purpose — to establish and maintain an environment that promotes the development of their members. In order to accomplish this goal, a family must perform basic functions such as providing love, security, identity, a sense of belonging, preparation for adult roles in society, and maintenance of order and control. In addition to these functions, each family member engages in tasks to maintain the family as a viable unit. We shall examine these functions and tasks in more detail shortly.

Family Culture

Shared Values and Their Effect on Behavior

Because every family has its own set of values and rules for operation, we can speak of family culture. Although families share many broad cultural values, they also develop unique variants. Some values will be explicitly stated: "Family matters must always stay within the family." Such values may give rise to specific operating rules: "Don't tell any of your friends how much money Daddy earns."

However, like all cultural values, many will remain at a tacit level, outside the conscious awareness of family members. These values become powerful determinants of what the family believes, feels, thinks, and does. A family that values free expression for every member engages comfortably in loud, noisy debates, while another family that values quietness, order, and control will not tolerate its members raising their voices. One family uses birth control based on beliefs about human life and parental responsibility; another family chooses not to use birth control because it holds a different set of values.

414

How a family views education, health care, life-style, child rearing, sex roles, or any of the myriad other issues requiring choices depends upon the cultural values of that family.

Family values include those beliefs transmitted by previous generations, religious influences, immediate social pressures, and the larger society. The combination of all these influences may lead a family to decide, perhaps unconsciously, that it is important to compete and succeed. Conversely, it may feel it is important to "hang loose" and never worry about tomorrow. Values become an integral part of a family's life and are very difficult to change.

Prescribed Roles

Roles, the assigned or assumed parts that members play during day-to-day family living, are bestowed and defined by the family. That is, the family determines who will play which roles and generally what each role will comprise. For instance, in one family the father role assigned to the male adult may be defined as an authoritative one that includes establishing rules, judging behavior, and administering punishment for violation of rules. In another family, the father role may be defined primarily as loving benefactor. If there is an absence of an immediate male parent, a grandfather, uncle, friend, or mother may take over the father role. Families distribute among the roles all the responsibilities and tasks necessary to conduct family living (Fig. 15-2). The responsibilities of breadwinner and homemaker, for example, with their accompanying tasks, may belong to husband and wife, respectively, or may be shared if both husband and wife work.

Family members often play several roles at the same time (Satir, 1972). A woman, for instance, may play the role of wife to her husband, daughter to her mother living in the same home, and mother to each of her children. Even her mother role may involve wearing several different hats because it varies slightly with each child. A single-parent family often combines the roles of father and mother in one person but may distribute responsibilities and tasks more widely. A grandmother or children may thus relieve the demands placed on the single parent. Among families, there is great variation in expectations for each role and the degree of flexibility in role prescriptions. Consequently, a family may place great demands on some members, although at the same time, members may interpret their roles differently. Confusion and conflict can develop unless roles are clarified.

Power System

Power, the possession of control, authority, or influence over others, assumes different patterns in each family. In some families, power is concentrated primarily in one member, while in others it is distributed on a more egalitarian

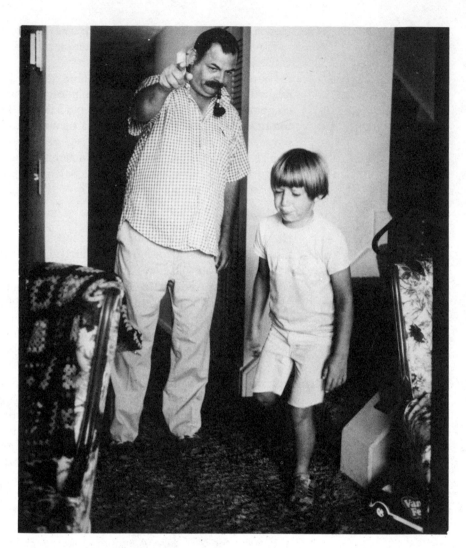

Figure 15-2
The role of disciplinarian is often difficult, but it is necessary to guide a child's socialization.

basis. The traditional patriarchal family, in which the father holds absolute authority over the other members, is rare in American society. However, the pattern of husband as head of the household and dominant member of the family is still frequently seen. Whether male or female, the dominant partner holds the majority of the decision-making power, particularly over the more important family affairs, such as employment, financial matters, and sexual activity. Other areas of decision making, including choices about vacations, housing, leisure activities, household purchases, and child rearing may be shared or delegated. However, with changing societal influences,

416

the present trend among American families is toward egalitarian power distribution. Many families now practice joint decision making and equal participation by all members.

Roles often influence power distribution within the family. Along with the responsibilities attached to a role, a family may assign decision-making authority. The mother role frequently includes decision-making power regarding household management. A responsibility related to a son's role, such as lawn mowing, may empower him to decide when and how often he does the job.

Family power structure is also influenced by the amount of personal power residing in each member (Robischon & Smith, 1977). A mother or eldest son, for example, may exercise considerable influence over the family by virtue of personality and position rather than delegated authority. Even the child who throws temper tantrums may wield considerable power in a family.

We have viewed families as social systems. We have examined the cultural dimensions of families. We know that a family is tied biologically through kinship and probably socially through choice. We know that it exists for a purpose. How, then, does one define family? Duvall's definition nicely summarizes these aspects of the family: "The family is a unity of interacting persons related by ties of marriage, birth, or adoption, whose central purpose is to create and maintain a common culture which promotes the physical, mental, emotional, and social development of each of its members" (Duvall, 1972, p. 5).

Family Structures

For many people, the term *family* evokes a picture of a husband, wife, and children living under one roof with the male as breadwinner and the female as homemaker.

This nuclear family is often seen as the norm for everyone. Variations from this pattern have generally been treated as deviant and abnormal, even in recent studies of the family (Olsen, McCubbin, & Associates, 1983). The traditional nuclear family has been sacrosanct because it is such a fundamental part of our cultural heritage, an ideal reinforced by religion, education, and other influential social institutions. Recent changes in the nuclear family have led some to predict the demise of the family itself, yet reality insists that the nuclear model is not the only valid family form. The pressures of social conditions such as emerging new life-styles, increasing significance of work for women, and changing sexual roles have effected changes in the American family. We now see a growing number of households of cohabiting adults, single parents, and single persons. Although the classic family form continues to, and most likely always will, exist, there are now many variations of the nuclear model as well as emerging new patterns of family structure. Each requires recognition and acceptance by the professionals who wish to help actualize family health potential.

Families come in many shapes and sizes. We can place these varying family structures into two general categories, traditional and nontraditional.

Traditional Families

Traditional family forms are the forms most familiar to us. There is generally no question that these are families; society sanctions their legitimacy. The most obvious are husband, wife, and children living together (nuclear family), or husband and wife living together alone, either childless or with children launched (nuclear dyad). Community health nurses also work with many families that have one parent as a result of divorce, separation, or death. The nurse may visit an elderly man living alone in a high-rise apartment (single-adult family) or a home where a grandmother and a divorced older granddaughter with her baby are living with the daughter's nuclear family (multigenerational family). Sometimes, particularly among ethnic groups, we find a group of relatives that consists of several nuclear families who live close to each other and share goods and services. Perhaps they own and run a family business together, sharing income and expenses, eat many meals together, and all have some responsibility for raising the children (kin network). Table 15-1 lists traditional family structures.

Career patterns, particularly for women, further characterize traditional family structures. Scanzoni (1983, p. 85) distinguishes between three types of nuclear families in which women and men are either "workers," "achievers," or "partners." In the first type, husband and wife are both earners; each holds a full- or part-time job. The second type describes couples in which both partners have careers and are usually employed full-time. Equal partners, the third type, refers to a shared, interdependent relationship in which "all work and domestic arrangements are open to negotiation and continual renegotiation." Nuclear dyads may be any of these three types. Some single-parent families include a working adult; others may have a single parent, such as a woman deserted by her husband and without any employable skills, who has no career. These variant structures remind us that even traditional families can assume many forms.

Nontraditional Families

Nontraditional family structures include all the newly emerging family forms; some of these forms are accepted by society and others are strongly questioned on the basis of illegitimate union. Table 15-1 lists some of the prominent nontraditional structures. One of the more well known nontraditional family forms is composed of several unrelated, monogamous (married or committed

418

Table 15-1
Traditional and Nontraditional American Family Structures

Structure	Participants	Living Arrangements
Traditional		
Nuclear family	Husband Wife Children	Common household
Nuclear dyad	Husband Wife	Common household
Single-parent family	One adult (separated, divorced, widowed) Children	Common household
Single adult	One adult	Living alone
Multigenerational family	Any combination of the first four traditional family structures	Common household
Kin network	Two or more reciprocal households (related by birth or marriage)	Close geographic proximity
Nontraditional		
Commune family	Two or more monogamous couples Shared children	Common household
Group marriage commune family	Several adults "married" to each other Shared children	Common household
Group network	Reciprocal nuclear households or single members	Close geographic proximity
Unmarried single-parent family	One parent (never married) Children	Common household
Unmarried couple	Two adults (heterosexual, same sex, homosexual)	Common household
Unmarried couple and child family	Two adults (as above) Children	Common household

Source: Adapted from M. B. Sussman (1971).

to one person) couples living together and collectively rearing their children (commune family). A variation of the commune family is the common household in which several adults are all "married" to each other; they share everything, including sex and child rearing (group marriage). Occasionally a group of nuclear families, not related by birth or marriage but bound by a common set of values such as a religious system, live close to each other and share goods, services, and child-rearing responsibilities (group network). Some commune and group network families select one of their members, usually a male, to be their leader, or head.

Some nontraditional families clearly form outside marriage. One example, seen more and more in community health, is the single, unmarried parent (most often a young, unwed mother) and child (Fig. 15-3). Many adult couples form a family alliance outside marriage or through a private ceremony not legally recognized as marriage (unmarried couple). They may range from young adults living together to an elderly couple sharing their lives outside of marrige to avoid tax penalties. Such cohabiting couples may be heterosexual, homosexual, or the same sex without a sexual relationship. In some instances, these couples have their own biologic or adopted children (unmarried couple and child family).

Nontraditional families make up an increasing proportion of the American population. For instance, in 1960, legally married couples made up 75 percent of American households. That figure had declined to 65 percent by 1975, and by 1990, based on current trends, analysts project that figure to drop to 55 percent (Masnick & Bane, 1980, p. 49). Less than 20 percent of American families now have the traditional model of a working father, a full-time homemaker mother, and one or more children (*A Growing Crisis*, 1983). The number of couples who share a household without marrying more than doubled between 1970 and 1979 (Cherlin, 1981, p. 12). Approximately 24 percent of all families in the United States have a woman as head of the household (children present but no male adult), and that figure is projected to increase to 29 percent by 1990. The number of households headed by men (children present but no female adult) is increasing and from 11 percent in 1975 is projected to reach 16 percent by 1990 (Masnick

Figure 15-3
The single, unmarried parent with a child is a family form seen frequently by community health nurses. Each type of family structure has its own unique set of resources and needs.

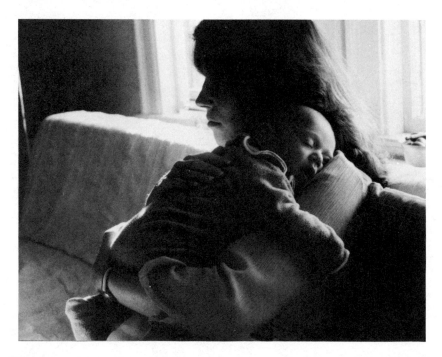

& Bane, 1980, p. 49). Divorce is also changing family frameworks: "Two out of every five marriages end in divorce (higher for teenage marriages) and approximately 50 percent of all children can expect to live in one-parent homes at some time during their childhood" (Pearce & McAdoo, 1981).

Varying family structures raise three important issues to consider. First, community health nurses can no longer hold to the myth that idealizes the traditional nuclear family (Cogswell, 1975). Societal changes force them (and all who work with families) to accept many variations in family forms as valid and functional. Unless community nurses adopt this posture and avoid judging by standards appropriate to the idealized nuclear family, they are in danger of creating even more problems for the families they attempt to serve. To hold to an ideal that parents must meet all their children's needs, for example, can lead to a conclusion that parenting is defective when children have personality deficits. This expectation may be unrealistic and unattainable for dual-career and, perhaps even more so, for single-parent families, who require supplemental resources to meet children's needs.

Second, the structure of an individual's family may change several times over a lifetime. A girl may be born into a kin network, shift to a nuclear family when her parents move and become part of a single-parent family when her parents are divorced. As she matures, she may choose to become a single adult living alone, later to become a part of a cohabiting couple, and still later to marry and form a nuclear family. For the individual, each variant family form involves changes in roles, interaction patterns, socialization processes, and linkages with external resources (President's Commission, 1981).

Finally, each type of family structure creates different issues and problems that, in turn, influence a family's ability to perform its basic functions. (Scanzoni, 1983, p. 187). Each particular structure determines the kind of support needed from nursing or other human service systems (Sussman & Cogswell, 1972). A single adult living alone, for instance, may lack companionship or a sense of being needed by other family members. A kin network family provides broad, extended family support and security but may have problems in power distribution and decision making. An unmarried couple raising a child may be parenting well but not receiving needed external support from the community in the form of recognition, approval, or assistance. Variations in structure, then, create differing family strengths and needs, an important consideration for community nurses.

Family Functions

Families in every culture throughout history have engaged in the same basic functions. From one society to the next the manner in which these tasks were performed varied. Nonetheless, families reproduced children, physically maintained their members, and provided social placement, socialization, emotional support, and social control (Goode, 1977). Some societies have experimented with separation of these functions, allocating activities such as child care, socialization, or social control to a larger group. The Israeli kibbutz and Chinese commune are examples. Yet, for most peoples, the individual family unit (in its variant forms) persists, accompanied by most of the same basic functions. In American society, certain social institutions perform some aspects of traditional family functions. Schools, for example, help socialize children; professionals supervise health care; and churches influence values. Thus we see some modifications in patterns of functioning. Six functions are typical of American families today. Families provide (1) affection, (2) security, (3) identity, (4) affiliation, (5) socialization, and (6) controls (Duvall, 1977; Sussman, 1971; Zelditch, 1964).

Affection

The family functions to give members affection and emotional support (Fig. 15-4). Love brings couples together initially in our society and later produces children. In some cultures affection comes after marriage. Continued affection creates an atmosphere of nurturance and care for all family members that is necessary for health, development, and survival (Aldous, 1978). It is common knowledge that infants cannot survive without love. Indeed, human beings of any age require love as sustenance for growth and find it primarily in the family. Families, unlike many other social groups, are bound by affectional ties whose strength determines family happiness and closeness. Consider how the sharing of gifts on a holiday or the loving concern of a family for a sick member draws the family together. Positive sexual identity and sexual fulfillment are also influenced by a loving atmosphere. Early students of the family emphasized sexual access and procreation as basic family functions (Zelditch, 1964). Now we recognize that families exist not only to regulate the sex drive and perpetuate the species but also to sustain life and foster human potential through a strong, affectional climate.

Security

Families meet their members' physical needs by providing food, shelter, clothing, health care, and other necessities; in so doing, they create a secure environment. Members need to know that these basics will be available and that the family is committed to providing them.

The stability of the family unit also gives members a sense of security. The family offers a safe retreat from the competition of the outside world, especially when members are accepted for themselves. They can learn, make mistakes, and grow in a secure environment. Where else does the toddler, after repeated falls, receive the encouragement to keep trying to walk; or

422

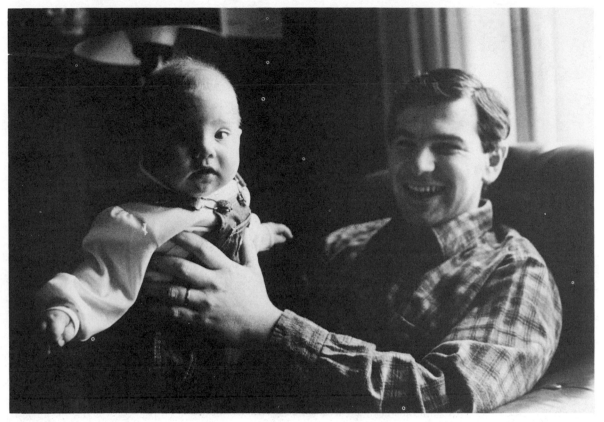

Figure 15-4
An important family function is to demonstrate affection in order to promote members' growth. A child, recognizing his father's love, responds with confidence.

the child, teased by a bully, regain his courage; or a parent, feeling burned out on a job, find comfort and renewal? The dependability of the family unit promotes confidence and self-assurance among its members, contributing to their mental and emotional health and equipping them with the skills necessary to cope with the outside world.

Identity

The family functions to give members a sense of social and personal identity. From infancy on, the individual gains a sense of identity and worth from the family. Like a mirror, the family reflects back to its members a picture of who they are and how valuable they are to others. Positive reflections provide the individual with a sense of satisfaction and worth, such as that experienced by a girl when her family applauds her efforts in a swimming meet. Need fulfillment in the home determines satisfaction in the outside world; it particularly affects other interpersonal relationships and career choices.

423

Roles learned within the family also give members a sense of identity. A boy growing up and learning his family's expectations for the male role soon develops a sense of the kind of person he must strive to be; often, he is expected to be strong, competitive, successful, and unemotional.

Families influence their members' social placement. That is, as a result of genetics, social class, race, economic position, and many other factors, families determine where their members will be placed in the social order. Social placement is a way of telling members who they are. For example, the members of a wealthy, influential family will be expected to follow in that family's tradition of attending Ivy League schools, mixing in upper-class social circles, and selecting high-status careers. A poor family, with its contrasting value system and social heritage, may influence its members to receive very little formal education and move into a trade at an early age. In fact, families influence their members' physical characteristics, intellectual abilities, educational experiences, social positions, economic levels, and religious and political affiliations. All these factors help to shape member identity.

Affiliation

The family functions to give members a sense of belonging throughout life. Because families provide associational bonds and group membership, they help satisfy their members' needs for belonging. We all know that we are integral, that we belong, to our families. However, the quality of a family's communication influences its closeness. If communication patterns are effective, then affiliation ties are strong and belonging needs are met. One family handles conflict over financial expenditures, for instance, by discussing differences and making compromises. A second family never resolves its financial conflicts. Instead, one member makes a selfish purchase and another member retaliates with an equally expensive personal expenditure. The healthier interactional pattern of the first family contributes to its strong sense of affiliation.

The family, unlike other social institutions, involves permanent relationships. Long after friends from school, the old neighborhood, work, or church have come and gone, we still have the family. The family provides its members with affiliation and fellowship that are unbroken by distance or time. Even when scattered across the country, family members will gather to support each other and to share in a holiday, wedding, graduation, or funeral. After separation, there is no need to reestablish ties; it is taken for granted that we belong and that we can take up where we left off. It is to the family we turn in times of happiness or need. We know we can freely share our distress and joy, call at any time, and borrow a shoulder to cry on or money to get us out of a financial bind. The durability of this affiliation remains a resource for life.

Socialization

The family functions to socialize the young. Families transmit their culture, that is, their values, attitudes, goals, and behavior patterns, to their members. Members, socialized into a way of life that reflects and preserves that cultural heritage, pass that heritage on, in turn, to the next generation (Fig. 15-5). From infancy on, we learn to control our bowels, eat with utensils, dress ourselves, manage our emotions, and behave according to sociocultural prescriptions for our age and sex. Through this process, we learn our roles in the family. Our life-styles, the foods we prefer, our relationships with other people, our ideas about child rearing, and our attitudes about religion, abortion, equal rights, or euthanasia are all strongly influenced by our families. Although experiences outside of the family also have a strong influence on roles, they are filtered through the perceptions we acquired during early socialization.

Figure 15-5
This little boy learns early that sports are an important part of the male role.

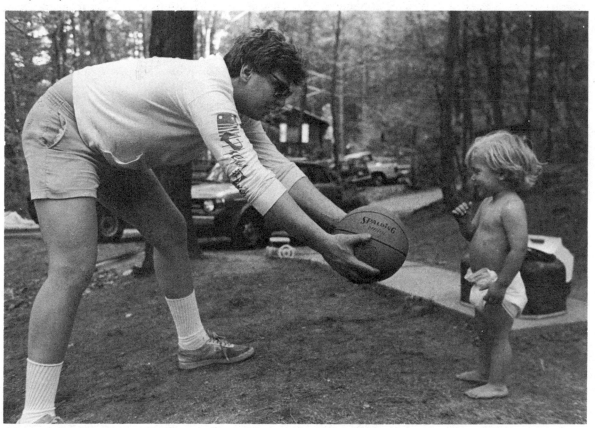

The socialization process also influences the degree of independence experienced by growing children. Some families release their maturing members by degrees, preparing them early for adult roles. Other families promote dependent roles and find release painful and difficult.

Controls

The family functions to maintain social control. Families maintain order through establishment of social controls both within the family and between family members and outsiders. Members' conduct is controlled by the family's definition of acceptable and nonacceptable behaviors. From minor points such as elbows off the table to larger issues, such as standards of home cleanliness, appropriate dress, children's proper address of adults, or a teen-ager's curfew, the family imposes limits. Then it maintains those limits by a system of rewards for conformity and punishment for violation. Children growing up in a family quickly learn what is "right" and what is "wrong" by family standards. Gradually family control shifts to self-control as members learn to discipline their own lives; later on, they will adopt or modify many of the same standards to use with their own children.

Division of labor is another aspect of the family's control function. Families allocate various roles, responsibilities, and tasks to their members in order to assure provision of income, household management, child care, and other essentials (Fig. 15-6).

Families also regulate the way internal and external resources are used.

Figure 15-6
Family members all have assigned responsibilities. Older children often help with the care and training of their younger siblings. Here a young girl reads a bedtime story to her little sister.

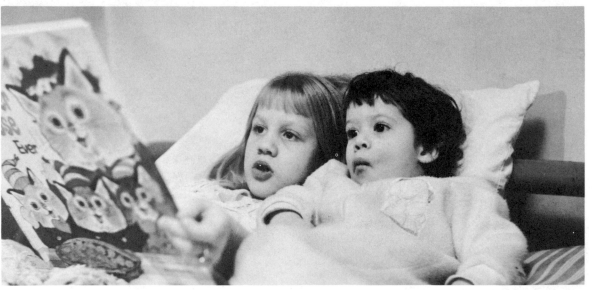

Table 15-2
Family Functions and Tasks

Family Functions	Associated Developmental Tasks
Affection	Establishment of climate of affection Promotion of sexuality and sexual fulfillment Addition of new members
Security	Maintenance of physical requirements Acceptance of individual members
Identity	Maintenance of motivation Self-image and role development Social placement
Affiliation	Development of communication patterns Establishment of durable bonds
Socialization	Internalization of culture (values and behavior) Guidance for internal and external relationships Release of members
Controls	Maintenance of social control Division of labor Allocation and utilization of resources

The family identifies internal resources, such as member abilities, financial income, or material assets, and decides how they will be utilized. For instance, a man with artistic skills may be the member to landscape the yard, and a woman with mechanical aptitude the member to repair appliances. This same family may choose to drive an old car in order to spend a fair portion of its income on entertainment like eating in restaurants or going to movies. Families also determine the external resources used by their members. Some families take advantage of the many religious, health, and social services available to them in the community. They seek regular medical care, encourage their children to participate in scouting programs, become involved in church activities, or join a bowling league. Other families, not recognizing or valuing external resources, limit their members' use of them.

Each of the six functions just described is an ongoing family responsibility, essential for the maintenance and promotion of family health (Duvall, 1977). Incorporated into these functions are specific tasks that a family must do to promote its growth and development. These activities are a family's developmental tasks, summarized in Table 15-2.

Family Life Cycle

Our examination of their nature has shown that families are social systems with cultural values, structures, and functions. Another way to understand families is to view them developmentally.

Families, while maintaining themselves as entities, change continuously. These changes occur in a sequential pattern known as the family life cycle, sometimes called the "family career" (Aldous, 1978). Families inevitably grow and develop as individuals mature and adapt to the demands of successive life changes. A family at its inception has a different composition, set of roles, and network of interpersonal relationships than at later points in time.

Consider the following example. The Jordans, a young married couple, concentrated on learning their respective roles of husband and wife and building a mutually satisfying marriage relationship. With the birth of their first child, Scott, the family composition and relationships changed, and role transitions occurred. The Jordans were not only husband and wife but father, mother, and son; the family had added three new roles. Within the next four years, two daughters, Lisa and Tammy, were born. The introduction of each new member not only increased family size but significantly reorganized family living. As a result, Duvall (1977, p. 32) points out, "no two children are born into exactly the same family." One by one the children entered school; Mrs. Jordan went to work for a florist; and soon Scott was leaving for college. The Jordans, like every family, were moving through the family life cycle and, in so doing, were experiencing developmental change.

Developmental Stages

Family development through the life cycle occurs in a predictable pattern of recognizable stages. Gross examination of family development shows two broad stages: *expansion* of the family as new members are added and roles and relationships are increased and *contraction* of the family as members leave to start lives of their own. Within this framework of the expanding-contracting family are more specific stages that mark changing patterns in family growth and development. Duvall (1977) outlines eight stages in the family life cycle, which begins when a couple marries and first forms their own family, continues through the years of having, rearing, and launching children, to the empty nest, retirement, and finally death of both spouses. Figure 15-7 depicts these stages.

In this model the age of the oldest child serves as a criterion for demarcation between stages. A family enters the preschool stage, for instance, when the oldest child is 2½ years of age and moves into the school stage when the oldest child is 6 years of age, even though the family may have other younger children. The size of each wedge in the circle reflects that stage's relative length. As a result of societal changes, particularly increased life span and changing roles and career patterns for women, families are having fewer children, the child-rearing period is shorter and the median length of marriage has increased to 43.6 years (Aldous, 1978). As a result, couples are spending

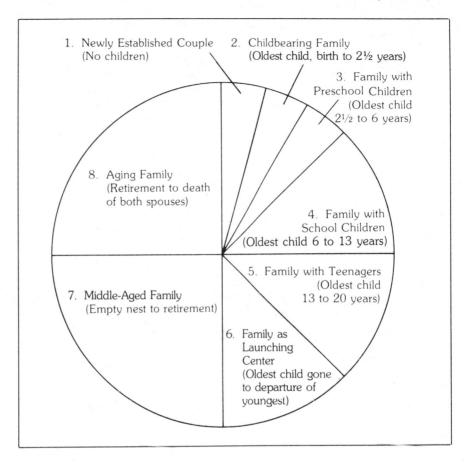

Figure 15-7
Eight stages of the nuclear family life cycle.

a longer portion of their lives together alone, thus expanding stages, 1, 7, and 8.

To progress through the stages of the life cycle, a family must carry out its basic functions and the developmental tasks associated with those functions (see Table 15-2). Unlike individual developmental tasks, which are specific to each age level, family developmental tasks are ongoing throughout the life cycle. All families, for instance, must provide for the physical needs of their members at every stage. The manner and degree to which each function is carried out will vary, however, depending on how well members are meeting their individual developmental tasks and on the demands of each particular stage. Physical maintenance, for example, will be affected by parents' ability to accept responsibility and seek out the necessary resources to provide food, clothing, and shelter for their children. At early stages, children will usually be dependent on their parents for meeting these needs; at the school, teenage, and launching stages, however, children may increasingly contribute to home management and family income. The responsibility for these tasks shifts from parents to other family members as well.

Some functions require greater emphasis at certain stages. Socialization, for example, consumes much of a family's time during the early years of member development. These same functions and their associated developmental tasks can be further broken down into actions specific to certain stages. A family, for example, while carrying out its function of maintaining controls, sets clearly defined limits for children at the preschool stage. "Do not cross the street," "You may have dessert only after you finish your vegetables"; Bedtime is at 8:00 P.M. During the school stage, control activities may center around allocating responsibilities and division of labor within the family: "Feed the dog"; "Clean your room"; "Take out the trash." When a family reaches the teenage stage, its control function increasingly focuses on the relationships between family members and outsiders. It may regulate some activities through means such as setting a "home by midnight" limit. In other areas, such as moral conduct, controls may use family values and thus be more subtle. A family at this stage must recognize the need for young people to assume increasing responsibility for their own behavior as well as realize its own diminishing control over members. Duvall (1977) describes these activities as "stage-critical" family developmental tasks (see Table 15-3).

Nonnuclear Families

Up to this point, our discussion of the family life cycle has focused on the nuclear family. Since we encounter many nuclear families in community health, the family life cycle provides a useful means for analyzing their growth and development. However, other family structures, such as single adults living alone, single-parent families, or couples who never have children, follow different life cycle patterns. They do not fit the framework just presented and require different criteria for analysis. Researchers in family theory have yet to describe nonnuclear family stages in any systematic fashion. Stein (1981) suggests the notion of a "life-spiral" rather than a life cycle pattern to more realistically describe the fluctuations of contemporary nontraditional families. Aldous (1978) has suggested, as one example, the following stages for families of divorced women who do not remarry.

Stage 1 Establishment of the single parent family
Stage 2 Women institute or reinstitute their work-life career
Stage 3 Women with adolescents
Stage 4 Women with young adults
Stage 5 Women in the middle years
Stage 6 The retirement of women from work-life career or parental responsibilities

430

Table 15-3
Selected Stage-Critical Family Developmental Tasks

Stage of Family Life Cycle	Family Position	Stage-Critical Family Developmental Tasks
Married couple	Wife Husband	Establishing a mutually satisfying marriage Adjusting to pregnancy and the promise of parenthood Fitting into the kin network
Childbearing	Wife-mother Husband-father Infant daughter, or son, or both	Having and adjusting to infants, and encouraging their development Establishing a satisfying home for both parents and infant(s)
Preschool-age	Wife-mother Husband-father Daughter-sister Son-brother	Adapting to the critical needs and interests of preschool children in stimulating, growth-promoting ways Coping with energy depletion and lack of privacy as parents
School-age	Wife-mother Husband-father Daughter-sister Son-brother	Fitting into the community of school-age families in constructive ways Encouraging children's educational achievement
Teenage	Wife-mother Husband-father Daughter-sister Son-brother	Balancing freedom with responsibility as teenagers mature and emancipate themselves Establishing outside interests and careers as growing parents
Launching center	Wife-mother-grandmother Husband-father-grandfather Daughter-sister-aunt Son-brother-uncle	Releasing young adults into work, military service, college, marriage, etc., with appropriate rituals and assistance Maintaining a supportive home base
Middle-aged parents	Wife-mother-grandmother Husband-father-grandfather	Rebuilding the marriage relationship Maintaining kin ties with older and younger generations
Aging family members	Widow or widower Wife-mother-grandmother Husband-father-grandfather	Coping with bereavement and living alone Closing the family home or adapting it to aging Adjusting to retirement

Source: Adapted from Duval (1977).

Carter and McGoldrick (1980) suggest phases for divorce and remarriage and propose that each phase is accompanied by emotional transitions and certain developmental concerns. Tables 15-4 and 15-5 show these phases.

Summary

Community health nurses' effectiveness in working with families depends on their understanding of the nature of families.

Every family is unique; its needs and strengths are different from every other family. At the same time, each family is alike because all share certain

Table 15-4
Life Cycle Phases in Divorce

Phase	Emotional Transitions	Developmental Issues
Divorce		
1. Decision to divorce	Accepting of inability to resolve marital tensions	Acceptance of one's own part in the failure of the marriage
2. Planning breakup of the system	Supporting viable arrangements for all parts of the system	a. Working cooperatively on problems of custody, visitation, finances b. Dealing with extended family about the divorce
3. Separation	a. Willingness to continue cooperative coparental relationship b. Work on resolution of attachment to spouse	a. Mourning loss of intact family b. Restructuring marital and parent-child relationships; adaptation to living apart c. Realignment of relationships with extended family; staying connected with spouse's extended family
4. Divorce	More work on emotional divorce: Overcoming hurt, anger, guilt	a. Mourning loss of intact family: giving up fantasies of reunion b. Retrieval of hopes, dreams, expectations from the marriage c. Staying connected with extended families
Post-Divorce Family		
1. Single-parent family	Willingness to maintain parental contact with ex-spouse and support contact of children with ex-spouse and his or her family	a. Making flexible visitation arrangements with ex-spouse and his or her family b. Rebuilding own social network
2. Single-parent (Noncustodial)	Willingness to maintain parental contact with ex-spouse and support custodial parent's relationship with children	a. Finding ways to continue effective parenting relationships with children

Source: Carter & McGoldrick (1980).

universal characteristics. Five of these universals have particular significance for community health nursing.

First, every family is a small social system. All the members within a family are interdependent; what one does affects the others and, ultimately, influences total family health. Families, as social systems, set and maintain boundaries that unite them and preserve their autonomy while also differentiating them from others. Because these boundaries are semipermeable, families can link with external resources. Families are equilibrium-seeking and adaptive systems that strive to adjust to internal and external life changes. Also, like other systems, families are goal directed. They exist for the purpose of promoting their members' development.

Second, every family has its own culture, its own set of values and rules for operation. Family values influence member beliefs and behaviors. These same values prescribe the types of roles that each member assumes. A family's culture also determines its power distribution and decision-making patterns.

Table 15-5
Life Cycle Phases in Remarriage

Steps	Emotional Transitions	Developmental Issues
1. Entering new relationship	Recovery from loss of first marriage (adequate "emotional divorce")	Recommitment to marriage and to forming a family with readiness to deal with the complexity and ambiguity
2. Conceptualizing and planning new marriage and family	Accepting one's own fears and those of new spouse and children about remarriage and forming a stepfamily Accepting need for time and patience for adjustment to complexity and ambiguity of a. Multiple new roles b. Boundaries: space, time, membership, and authority. c. Affective Issues: guilt, loyalty conflicts, desire for mutuality, unresolvable past hurts	a. Work on openness in the new relationships to avoid pseudomutuality. b. Plan for maintenance of cooperative coparental relationships with ex-spouses c. Plan to help children deal with fears, loyalty conflicts, and membership in two systems. d. Realignment of relationships with extended family to include new spouse and children. e. Plan maintenance of connections for children with extended family of ex-spouse(s).
3. Remarriage and reconstitution of family	Final resolution of attachment to previous spouse and ideal of "intact" family; Acceptance of a different model of family with permeable boundaries	a. Restructuring family boundaries to allow for inclusion of new spouse-stepparent. b. Realignment of relationships throughout subsystems to permit interweaving of several systems. c. Making room for relationships of all children with biological (noncustodial) parents, grandparents, and other extended family. d. Sharing memories and histories to enhance stepfamily integration.

Source: Carter & McGoldrick (1980).

Third, every family has structure that can be categorized as either traditional or nontraditional. The most common traditional family structure is the nuclear family, consisting of husband, wife, and children living together. Other traditional structures include husband and wife living together alone, single-parent families, single-adult families, multigenerational families, and kin networks. Nontraditional family structures incorporate many newly emerging family forms, some recognized as legitimate by society and others not easily accepted. These variations include commune families, group marriages, group networks, an unmarried single-parent family, and an unmarried couple living together alone or with children.

Variant family structures remind us that the nuclear family is no longer the only viable family form, that people experience many family structures during their lifetimes, and that a family's ability to perform its basic functions is influenced by its structure.

Fourth, every family has certain basic functions. A family gives its members affection and emotional support. It promotes security through provision of an accepting, stable environment in which physical needs are maintained. A family gives members a sense of social and personal identity as well as influences their placement in the social order. It provides members with affiliation, a sense of belonging. It socializes its members by teaching basic values and attitudes that determine their behavior. Finally, the family maintains order through establishment of social controls.

Fifth, every family moves through stages in its life cycle. Families develop in two broad stages: a period of expansion when they add new members and roles and a period of contraction when members leave. More specific developmental stages within this expanding-contracting framework can also be identified. For the nuclear family we see eight stages ranging from the newly established couple through childbearing, child rearing, and child launching to middle and old age.

While advancing through each developmental stage in the life cycle, a family must continue to perform all of its basic functions. It must also accomplish certain tasks specific to each stage. Life cycle stages and developmental tasks will vary for families with differing structures.

Study Questions

1. Select a family (other than your own) that you know well and analyze it, answering the following questions:
   a. If the major breadwinner in this family became permanently disabled and unable to work, how would the family most likely respond — immediately and in the long run?
   b. What are some of this family's rules for operating and the values underlying those rules?
   c. Structurally, what kind of family is it?
   d. What are the strongest and weakest functions performed by this family and why do you think so?
   e. In what developmental stage is this family and how does that affect its functioning?
2. Describe the major differences that you see between a nuclear family and a single-parent family. How do these differences affect the families' roles and functions?
3. Discuss the pros and cons of a married couple both working at full-time careers. Should they have children? In what ways could a community health nurse assist this couple? Whose values should be considered in making decisions about their family life?

References

A growing crisis: Disadvantaged women and their children. (1983). Washington, D.C.: U.S. Commission on Civil Rights.

Aldous, J. (1978). *Family careers: Developmental change in families.* New York: Wiley.

Carter, E. A., & McGoldrick, M. (Eds.) (1980). *The family life cycle.* New York: Gardner Press.

Cherlin, A. J. (1981). *Marriage, divorce, remarriage.* Cambridge, MA: Harvard University Press.

Cogswell, B. (1975). Variant family forms and life styles: Rejection of the traditional nuclear family. *Family Coordinator, 24,* 391.

Duvall, E. M. (1977). *Marriage and family development* (5th ed.). Philadelphia: Lippincott.

Goode, W. J. (1977). The family as a social institution. In W. J. Goode (Ed.), *Principles of sociology.* New York: McGraw-Hill.

Hymovich, D., & Barnard, M. (Eds.). (1973). *Family health care.* New York: McGraw-Hill.

Masnick, G. & Bane, M. J. (1980). *The nation's families: 1960–1990.* Boston: Auburn.

Olson, D., McCubbin, H. I., & Associates. (1983). *Families: What makes them work.* Beverly Hills, CA: Sage.

Pearce, D. M., & McAdoo, H. (1981). *Report of the National Advisory Commission on Economic Opportunity.* Washington, D.C.: U.S. Government Printing Office.

President's Commission for a National Agenda for the Eighties. (1981). Helping families — To help themselves. *International Journal of Family Therapy, 3,* 208–233.

Robischon, P., & Smith, J. A. (1977). Family assessment. In A. Reinhardt & M. Quinn (Eds.), *Current practice in family-centered community nursing.* St. Louis: C. V. Mosby.

Satir, V. (1972). *Peoplemaking.* Palo Alto, CA: Science and Behavior Books.

Scanzoni, J. (1983). *Shaping tomorrow's family: Theory and policy for the 21st century.* Beverly Hills, CA: Sage.

Stein, P. J. (Ed.). (1981). *Single life: Unmarried adults in social context.* New York: St. Martin's.

Sussman, M. B. (1971). Family systems in the 1970s: Analysis, policies, and programs. *Annals of the American Academy, 396,* 216–235.

Sussman, M. B., & Cogswell, B. (1972). The meaning of variant and experimental marriage styles and family forms. In M. B. Sussman (Ed.), *Non-traditional family forms in the 1970's.* Minneapolis, MN: National Council on Family Relations.

Zelditch, M. (1964). Family, marriage, and kinship. In R. E. Faris (Ed.), *Handbook of modern sociology.* Chicago: Rand McNally.

Selected Readings

Aldous, J. (1978). *Family careers: Developmental change in families.* New York: Wiley.

Bould, S. (1977). Female-headed families: Personal fate control and the provider role. *Journal of Marriage and Family, 39,* 339–348.

Cherlin, A. J. (1981). *Marriage, divorce, remarriage*. Cambridge, MA: Harvard University Press.

Cogswell, B. (1975). Variant family forms and life styles: Rejection of the traditional nuclear family. *Family Coordinator, 24,* 391.

Cogswell, B., & Sussman, M. (1972). Changing family and marriage forms: Complications for human service systems. In M. Sussman (Ed.), *Nontraditional family forms in the 1970's*. Minneapolis, MN: National Council on Family Relations.

Crawford, C. O. (Ed.). (1971). *Health and the family: A medical-sociological analysis*. New York: Macmillan.

Duvall, E. M. (1977). *Marriage and family development* (5th ed.). Philadelphia: Lippincott.

Getty, C., & Humphreys, S. (1981). *Understanding the family: Stress and change in American family life*. New York: Appleton-Century-Crofts.

Glasser, P. H., & Glasser, L. N. (1970). *Families in crisis*. New York: Harper & Row.

Glick, P. C. (1975, February). A demographer looks at American families. *Journal of Marriage and Family, 37,* 15–26.

Goode, W. J. (1971, November). World revolution and family patterns. *Journal of Marriage and Family, 33,* 624–635.

Goode, W. J. (1977). The family as a social institution. In W. J. Goode (Ed.), *Principles of Sociology*. New York: McGraw-Hill.

Haley, J. (Ed.). (1971). *Changing families*. New York: Grune & Stratton.

Hill, R. B. (1971). *The strengths of black families*. New York: Emerson Hall.

Hogan, P. (1975). Creativity in the family. In *Series on creative psychology, No. 2* (pp. 1–32). Ardsley, NY: Geigy Pharmaceuticals.

Howard, J. (1978). *Families*. New York: Simon & Schuster.

Hymovich, D., & Barnard, M. (Eds.). (1973). *Family health care*. New York: McGraw-Hill.

Kanter, R. M. (1972). Getting it all together: Some group issues in communes. *American Journal of Orthopsychiatry, 42*(4), 72.

Knafl, K. A., & Grace, H. K. (1978). *Families across the life cycle*. Boston: Little, Brown.

Marciano, T. D. (1975). Variant family forms in a world perspective. *Family Coordinator, 24,* 407.

Martin, E. P., & Martin, J. M. (1978). *The black extended family*. Chicago: University of Chicago Press.

Masnick, G., & Bane, M. J. (1980). *The nation's families: 1960–1990*. Boston: Auburn.

McCubbin, H. I. (1979). Integrating coping behavior in family stress theory. *Journal of Marriage and Family, 41,* 237–244.

Mendes, H. A. (1979). Single-parent families: A typology of lifestyles. *Social Work, 24,* 193.

Miller, J. R., & Janosik, E. H. (1980). *Family-focused care.* New York: McGraw-Hill.

Minuchin, S. (1974). *Families and family therapy.* Cambridge, MA: Harvard University Press.

Olson, D., McCubbin, H. I., and Associates. (1983). *Families: What makes them work.* Beverly Hills, CA: Sage.

Otto, H. A. (1973). A framework for assessing family strengths. In A. Reinhardt & M. Quinn (Eds.), *Family-centered community nursing.* St. Louis: C. V. Mosby.

Pratt, L. (1976). *Family structure and effective health behavior: The energized family.* Boston: Houghton Mifflin.

President's Commission for a National Agenda for the Eighties. (1981). Helping families — to help themselves. *International Journal of Family Therapy, 3,* 208–233.

Rapoport, R., & Rapoport, R. N. (1975). Men, women, and equity. *Family Coordinator, 24,* 421.

Robischon, P., & Smith, J. A. (1977). Family assessment. In A. Reinhardt & M. Quinn (Eds.), *Current practice in family-centered community nursing.* St. Louis: C. V. Mosby.

Rossi, A. S. (1968). Transition to parenthood. *Journal of Marriage and Family, 30,* 26.

Safilios-Rothschild, C. (1976). Dual linkages between the occupational and family systems: A macrosociological analysis. *Signs, 1,* 51.

Satir, V. (1967). *Conjoint family therapy.* Palo Alto, CA: Science and Behavior Books.

Satir, V. (1972). *Peoplemaking.* Palo Alto, CA: Science and Behavior Books.

Scanzoni, J. (1983). *Shaping tomorrow's family: Theory and policy for the 21st century.* Beverly Hills, CA: Sage.

Schulman, G. (1981). Divorce, single parenthood, and stepfamilies: Structural implications of these transitions. *International Journal of Family Therapy, 3,* 87–112.

Skolnick, A., & Skolnick, J. (1974). *Intimacy, family, and society.* Boston: Little, Brown.

Skolnick, A., & Skolnick, J. (1977). *Family in transition: Rethinking marriage, sexuality, child rearing, and family organization* (2nd ed.). Boston: Little, Brown.

Stein, P. J. (Ed.). (1981). *Single life: Unmarried adults in social context.* New York: St. Martin's.

Sussman, M. B. (Ed.) (1972). *Non-traditional family forms in the 1970's.* Minneapolis, MN: National Council on Family Relations.

Sussman, M. B. (Ed.). (1974). *Sourcebook on marriage and the family* (4th ed.). Boston: Houghton Mifflin.

Sussman, M. B., & Cogswell, B. (1972). The meaning of variant and experimental marriage styles and family forms. In M. B. Sussman (Ed.), *Non-traditional family forms in the 1970's*. Minneapolis, MN: National Council on Family Relations.

Van Dusen, R. A., & Sheldon, E. B. (1976). The changing status of American women: A life cycle perspective. *American Psychology, 31,* 106–116.

Zelditch, M. (1964). Family, marriage, and kinship. In R. E. Faris (Ed.), *Handbook of modern sociology*. Chicago: Rand McNally.

16

Family Health: Assessment and Practice

Community health nursing has a long history of concern for family health. During the nineteenth century, public health nurses became aware through home visits of the significant influence that the family had on individual health. For example, many of the sick poor failed to recover because they lacked resources and support from their families. These nurses began to view client care from the more holistic perspective of family care. Nursing educators, as early as 1919, were introducing concepts of family care into curricula (Ford, 1973). By 1932, the National Organization of Public Health Nursing strongly declared that *family* health was the cardinal concern of all public health nursing practice.

Although nursing continues to emphasize the family as the unit of service, a gap exists between theory and practice (Freeman & Heinrich, 1981). The problem derives in part from a health care system that fosters an individualistic orientation, often to the exclusion of the family. We have a proliferation of programs geared to individuals in specific age groups or with specific health problems. Many third-party payers and reimbursement policies impose limits on the kinds of services funded, most of which are for individuals. Even public health agencies tend to organize their services around individuals. Often in response to governmental requirements, they may keep statistical records on specific disease or service categories, thus reflecting an individual rather than a family orientation. Although nurses may subscribe to the value of a family and community orientation, their experience with acute care based on the medical model often leads them to practice individualistic nursing in community health.

Importance of Family Health

The Family as an Entity for Service

Despite these obstacles, family nursing persists. Three major reasons underlie its continuing importance for community health. First, the family as a unit is a target for service. Much research has demonstrated that families behave as units and need to be viewed in totality for therapy to be effective (Satir, 1967). The family does not simply provide the context for understanding and giving care to individuals. As we saw in chapter 15, it is a separate entity with definite structure, functions, and needs. The total family can be viewed as the client. In every society throughout history, the family is the most basic unit; so too in community health (Pratt, 1976). It is the family more than any other societal institution, that nurtures and shapes a society's members. Since community health practice serves population groups, we now focus on this basic societal unit, one in a series of increasingly larger communities.

Effect of Family Health on Individual Health

Second, family health and individual health strongly influence each other. The health of each member affects the other members and contributes to the total family's level of health. Following her husband's stroke, for example, a woman may successfully cope with the resulting physical and emotional demands of his care but have inadequate reserves to meet effectively the needs of her children. The level at which a family functions — how well it is able to solve problems and help its members reach their potential — significantly affects the individual's level of health. A healthy family will foster individual growth and resistance to ill health and sustain its members during times of crisis. On the other hand, a family with limited capacity for problem solving and self-management is often unable to promote the potential of its members or assist them in times of need. Consider a family with an abused child. That family's level of functioning is generally very low, and the physical, emotional, and social health of each member suffers as a result.

Family health standards influence members' health practices. For instance, many individuals, even as adults, adhere to family patterns of eating, exercise, and communication. Family values influence decisions about health services such as whether or not a child receives immunizations or the mother uses birth control. Family decisions determine the kind of health care a member receives. For example, will sick members only receive care at home or will the family seek professional help? If professional advice is received, to what

440

degree will the family carry it out? It is clear that individuals influence family health and that the family can either obstruct or facilitate individual health. The family, then, becomes an important focus for community health nursing assessment and intervention.

Effect of Family Health on Community Health

Third, family health affects community health. Rarely do families live in isolation from one another. Even in the most uncommunicative of neighborhoods, one family's noisy children, another family's trash-littered yard, and another's barking dog all have an impact on the surrounding families. The level at which each family functions determines whether or not it can promote a healthier community and support other families and groups rather than merely remain a liability.

Healthy families influence community health positively. Some families, for example, have temporarily housed Southeast Asian or Cuban refugees and assisted them in finding employment. Others have formed community groups to encourage neighborhood safety and beautification. Many families are regularly involved in church, scouting programs, parent-teacher-student associations, or other civic activities that promote the common good.

Conversely, families with a low level of health have a negative influence on community health. Because they lack the resources to manage their own affairs, they frequently create problems and even health hazards for others. Garbage left to accumulate in a backyard, for example, attracts rats; abandoned appliances may become death traps for playing children. Regardless of socio-economic level, a poorly functioning family becomes a drain on community resources and a threat to community health. Consider the large proportion of tax dollars and private funds that go into remedial programs for children with learning and behavior difficulties caused by problems at home, for adults with mental health problems, for the chemically dependent, and for victims of family violence — groups signficantly influenced by unhealthy families. Since family health affects the health of other families, groups, and communities, nurses who help families develop and maintain positive health patterns and practices are also promoting community health.

Characteristics of Healthy Families

You ring the doorbell and wait. Soon someone opens the door and ushers you into the living room. You explain, in response to their quizzical expressions, that you are here to help this family sustain or raise its level of health. Of course you do not say it quite that way. Perhaps you say, "I understand you have a new baby. I'm the community nurse, and I would like to assist you in any way that I can." Or you may say, "I have come to see how you are getting along since your surgery." However, your job extends far beyond simply teaching infant care or postsurgical rehabilitation. This is a family, an interdependent group of people who function as a unit. That individual, the precipitating cause of the referral, is only one part of the total group upon whom you should focus. How can you sustain or raise this family's level of health? How do you determine that level?

From our discussion in chapter 15, we learned that families, to be healthy, must accomplish certain basic functions that they must adapt to their unique structure, environment, and needs. To develop a clearer frame of reference for understanding family health, let us consider two families in particular.

The Murphys live in a modest two-story house that is clean, comfortable, and homey. There are seven of them — Jack, Bev, and their five children. Jack, now 43 years of age, has worked with the local Ford agency since high school, starting out as a mechanic and moving up to his present position of shop foreman. Bev, 41 years old, stayed home to care for the children until all were in school and then took a job as checker at a nearby supermarket. Because Bev had new responsibilities, Jack and the children took over many of the housekeeping tasks. As the Murphy children grew up, each assumed additional chores around the house as well as found jobs in the community. Two children now have paper routes, one baby-sits, one does yard work, and the oldest boy bags groceries at the market where his mother works. Each family member feels encouraged toward independence; at the same time, each member also feels supported and loved.

As a family, the Murphys do many things together. When the children were younger, they had "family night" every Friday; they played games, ate homemade goodies, and went on outings together. Church activities, baseball, and PTA functions now involve the family as a unit. Trips to the grandparents' farm in the neighboring state are delightful ways to spend the holidays or part of a summer vacation. Harmony does not always prevail with the Murphys, however. There are many disagreements over family rules, financial decisions, and other areas of family life. However, since they are accustomed to talking things over, they resolve these conflicts without difficulty. Jack and Bev together usually make the major family decisions, such as buying a car or deciding where to go on vacation. Frequently they involve the children in making decisions and encourage them to think for themselves. Around the dinner table, the Murphys often discuss current events, report on their activities, or debate various issues.

On the whole, they have had very few illnesses. There were some childhood diseases, a scattering of colds and flu, and a few broken bones over the years. Until Bev's cholecystectomy three years ago, none of them had undergone surgery. The family belongs to a prepaid health care plan through Jack's job and therefore is able to visit a clinic for regular checkups, immunizations, and early treatment of problems without feeling undue financial stress from health care costs. At home the Murphys eat well, and most of them are involved in some kind of exercise; even Bev, who has to watch her weight, swims regularly at the YWCA with a group of her friends from church.

The Stone family lives in the same town as the Murphys. Their sprawling rambler house in the suburbs is the center of much activity. John, 44 years old, is a professor at the community college located four blocks away. Because his office is so close, John often eats lunch, studies, and holds some of his classes in his home. Students also drop by frequently. Shirley, 45 years of age, became a social worker three years ago after going back to school. She has a heavy caseload and takes her clients' problems so much to heart that many of her evenings are spent on the phone or making extra visits. The Stones have two daughters and one son. Their 19-year-old daughter attends the community college and continues to live at home. Now the proud owner of his own car, the 17-year-old son, a junior in high school, has turned the family driveway into an auto repair shop where he and his friends spend hours tinkering with their cars. The youngest girl, a 14-year-old cheerleader in her junior high school, has a frenetic social life. The family's pets, two German shepherds and three cats, run loose and create confusion.

John has always believed that the father is the head of the house and that his responsibility is to make the rules. He expects Shirley to enforce them. Shirley, however, is disorganized and unable to discipline herself or the children; thus, assigned tasks are not done, rules are not observed, meals are almost never eaten together, and the house is never clean. John retreats to his study while Shirley spends longer hours on the job and the children go their separate ways, unconcerned about helping at home. Communication among them is infrequent. In earlier years John and Shirley were close even though Shirley always had difficulty managing the home. Since she returned to school and then to work, Shirley has been unable to keep up with the dual demands of career and homemaking. The family still expects her to do all the shopping, cooking, cleaning, and laundry. John is supportive of her professional efforts as long as they do not require him to make any adjustments in his routine and life-style. Shirley has a cleaning woman come once a week, but the house quickly resumes its perpetual disarray.

The Stones spend very little time together as a family, and consequently know almost nothing about each other's activities, interests, or needs. John, frustrated at not getting a promotion this year, has become more reclusive and has begun to drink heavily. Feeling inadequate about her inability to manage her life, Shirley has stepped up her work activities, drinks coffee excessively, and takes two or three Valium each day. Their son, kicked off the football squad for violating training rules, uses his car as an outlet for aggression and to attract attention. Unbeknownst to her parents, the younger daughter has been smoking marijuana for the past six months.

Some families, like the Murphys, are healthy. Others, like the Stones, are not. Still others are somewhere in between. In fact, family health, like individual health, ranges along a continuum from wellness to illness. A family may be at one point on that continuum now and at a much different point six months from now. Family health refers to the health status of a given family at a given point in time. What is it that tells us the Murphys are a healthy family and the Stones are not?

A cursory view shows that the Murphys are accomplishing their basic functions. We see indications of a loving, nurturing climate (affection). The family provides consistently for its members' physical and emotional needs (security). Each member appears to be growing in independence and successfully adding new roles (identity). The family is close and utilizes effective communication patterns (affiliation). Members' behavior appears consistent with family values (socialization), and division of tasks and use of resources are flexible and adapted to changing family needs (controls).

The Stones, on the other hand, are not accomplishing these functions. At an earlier stage, they were a close, loving family, but now the members have drifted apart. There is little evidence of an affectional climate. Physical and emotional needs are met only minimally, if at all, which contributes to lack of security and inadequate identity development. Communication patterns are poor; there is little sense of affiliation. Because guidance of values and behavior is almost nonexistent now, the family has little influence on members' socialization or social control. At this point in time, we see a poorly functioning family, an unhealthy family.

Analysis of a family in terms of how it meets these basic functions, however, does not give us a satisfactory picture of its health status. More definitive criteria are needed. Over the years, research on families, and particularly on family health behavior, gives us a growing body of data with which to assess family health.

One means of viewing family health is by examining family strengths. Olson & Associates (1983, p. 93) identify seven major family strengths important for family functioning and coping with crises: family pride, family support, cohesion, adaptability, communciation, religious orientation, and social support. This list builds on work done by earlier family researchers who saw family strengths as important and untapped resources. Otto (1963) emphasized the following family abilities:

To provide a sense of family unity, loyalty, and interfamily cooperation
To provide support and security
To perform roles flexibly
To maintain constructive relationships with the community

Other researchers have identified various characteristics, such as good communication patterns, spending time together, having a strong religious orientation, dealing with crises positively, a sense of unity and commitment to

444

one another, and respect and appreciation for one another (Beam, 1979; Stinnett, 1981; Stinnett & Saur, 1977). Results from the White House Conference on Families survey defined "strong" families as (1) families that highly value their relationships and (2) families whose members support each other through good and bad times (Tanner-Nelson and Banonis, 1981). The literature on families describes healthy families as having six important characteristics (Olson, McCubbin, & Associates, 1983; Otto, 1973; Pratt, 1976; Robischon & Smith, 1977):

1. There is a facilitative process of interaction among family members.
2. They enhance individual member development.
3. Their role relationships are structured effectively.
4. They actively attempt to cope with problems.
5. They have a healthy home environment and life-style.
6. They establish regular links with the broader community.

Let us examine these characteristics more closely.

Facilitative Interaction among Members

Healthy families communicate. Their patterns of interaction are regular, varied, and supportive. Adults communicate with adults, children with children, and adults with children. These interactions are frequent and assume many forms. Healthy families use frequent verbal communication. Like the Murphys, they discuss problems, confront each other when angry, share ideas and concerns, and write or call each other when separated. They also communicate frequently through nonverbal means, particularly those families from cultural or subcultural groups that are less verbal. There are innumerable ways — smiling encouragingly, embracing warmly, frowning disapprovingly, being available, withdrawing for privacy, doing an unsolicited favor, serving tea, giving a gift — to convey feelings and thoughts without words. The family that has learned to communicate effectively has members who are sensitive to each other. They watch for cues and verify messages in order to assure understanding. This kind of family recognizes and deals with conflicts as they arise. Its members have learned to share and to work collaboratively with each other (Figure 16–1).

Effective communication is necessary for a family to carry out its basic functions. To demonstrate affection and acceptance, to promote identity and affiliation, and to guide behavior through socialization and social controls, family members must communicate. Like the correlation between a high degree of communication and a high degree of effectiveness in organizational functioning, families' facilitative communication patterns promote the health and development of their members (Pratt, 1976).

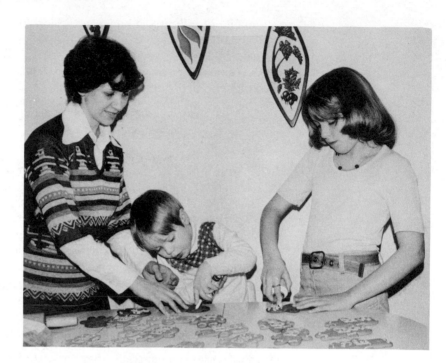

Figure 16-1
Healthy families have fun together and engage in activities that promote their members' growth.

Enhancement of Individual Development

Healthy families are responsive to their individual members' needs and provide the freedom and support necessary to promote each member's growth: "The level of health will be greater in families which support their members' personal needs and interests, assist the members' efforts to cope and function, and tolerate and encourage members' moves toward self-actualization" (Pratt, 1976, p. 125). If a father in a healthy family loses his job, his family will work to support his ego and help him use his energy constructively to adjust and find new work. The healthy family recognizes the growing child's need for independence, which it fosters through increasing opportunities for the child to try new things alone. This kind of family can tolerate differences of opinion or life-style. It is able to accept each member unconditionally and respect each one's right to be his or her own self. Within an appropriate framework of stability and structure, the healthy family encourages freedom and autonomy for its members. Patterns for promoting individual member development will vary from one family to another, depending on its cultural orientation. The way autonomy is expressed in an Italian-American family will differ from its expression in a Chippewa Indian family, yet each family can promote freedom and autonomy. The result of

446

promoting individuality is an increase in competence, self-reliance, social skills, intellectual growth, and overall capacity for self-management among family members (Pratt, 1976).

Effective Structuring of Relationships

Healthy families structure their role relationships to meet changing family needs over time (Holman, 1983, p. 29). In a stable social context, some families may establish member roles and tasks, such as breadwinner, primary decision maker, and homemaker, which are maintained as workable patterns throughout the life of the family. Families in rural areas, isolated communities, or religious and subcultural groups are more likely than others to retain role consistency because they face few, if any, external pressures or needs to change. The Amish communities in the midwest have maintained marked differentiation in family roles for more than 100 years.

However, in a technologically advanced industrial society such as ours, most families must adapt their roles to be consistent with changing family needs created by external forces. As women choose to or must enter the work force, for instance, family roles, relationships, and tasks need to change to meet the demands of the new situation (Safilios-Rothschild, 1976). Many husbands assume more homemaking responsibilities; fathers engage in child rearing; children, along with the adults in their families, assume shared decision making and a more equal distribution of power. The latter may be essential for the survival of a single-parent family in which the children must assume adult responsibilities while the parent is working to support the family (Mendes, 1979).

Changing life cycle stages require alterations in the structuring of relationships. (Olson, McCubbin, & Associates, 1983). The healthy family recognizes its members' changing developmental needs and adapts parenting roles, family tasks, and controls to fit each stage. Jobs around the house increase in complexity and responsibility as children are capable of handling them. Rules of conduct relax as members learn to govern their own behavior.

Active Coping Effort

Healthy families actively attempt to overcome life's problems and issues. When faced with change, they assume repsonsibility for coping and seek energetically and creatively to meet the demands of the situation. (Olson, McCubbin, & Associates, 1983). One family dealt with the increased cost of food, for example, by raising all their own vegetables, doing home canning and freezing, cutting down on meat, substituting other protein foods, and eating at restaurants less. The result was a 25 percent decrease in their overall food expenses. Healthy families are open to innovation. Their coping ability is enhanced by receptivity to new ideas and means for solving problems (Fig. 16-2). The family that responds to gas shortages and increased gas prices by deciding to cut down on daily travel may only be adding to their difficulties. On the other hand, a family facing the same problem may solve it by exploring new ways to reach destinations. These might include increased use of public transportation and car pools; walking, bicycling, or skiing to school or work; rearranged schedules to avoid frequency of trips to regular destinations; and shopping ahead to avoid last minute trips to stores. In contrast to those who passively and fatalistically limit themselves to working with only the most obvious aids, healthy families actively seek and use a variety of resources to solve problems. They may discover these resources within the family or they may find them externally; they engage in self-care. For example, a professional couple who were faced with the expense of daytime baby-sitting arranged their schedules so that they could take turns staying home with the baby. Later, they joined a cooperative preschool that allowed their child to attend daily but required parental participation only one day a week. After having additional children, the parents, more financially able, hired live-in help. They were able to help themselves as well as accept outside help.

Healthy Environment and Life-style

Another sign of a healthy family is a healthy home environment and life-style. Healthy families create safe and hygienic living conditions for their members. For instance, the healthy young family removes the potential hazards of exposed electric outlets and cleaning solvents from the reach of crawling infants. Older families recognize a greater potential for falls, resulting from poor eyesight and coordination; they install good lighting and sturdy railings. These same families are concerned about cleanliness as a means of reducing infections and the spread of disease-causing organisms. Healthy families promote a healthy family life-style by encouraging an appropriate balance of activity and rest; they foster a nutritionally sound diet and promote regular exercise. The emotional climate of a healthy family is positive and supportive of member growth (Fig. 16-3). Contributing to this healthy emotional climate is a strong sense of shared values, often combined with a strong religious orientation (Olson, McCubbin, & Associates, 1983, p. 93). Such a family, like the Murphys, demonstrates caring, encourages and accepts expression of feelings, and respects divergent ideas. Members can express their individuality in the way they dress or decorate their rooms. The home environment makes family members feel welcome and accepted. As a result of all these emphases, individual members in a healthy family engage in positive personal health practices that range from regular toothbrushing all the way to coping effectively with a death in the family.

448

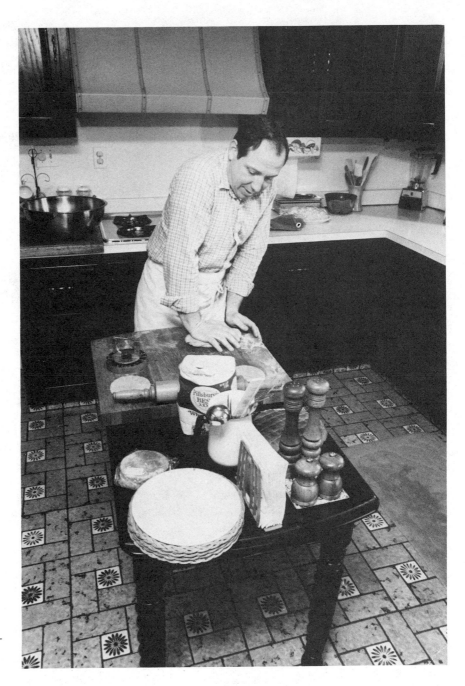

Figure 16-2
Many men today assume responsibility for home maintenance tasks, particularly in dual-career or single-parent families.

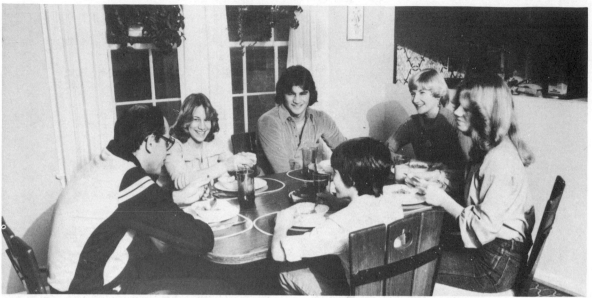

*Figure 16-3
A positive, supportive
emotional climate is a sign
of a healthy family.*

Regular Links with the Broader Community

Healthy families maintain dynamic ties with the broader community. They participate regularly in external groups and activities, often in a leadership capacity. We may see them join in local politics, participate in a church bazaar, or promote the school's paper drive to raise money for science equipment. They use external resources suited to their family's needs (Fig. 16-4). For example, a farm family with teenagers, recognizing the importance of peer group influence on adolescents, became very active in the 4-H club. Another family, in which the father was out of work, joined a job transition support group. The Murphys chose a health care plan that met their family's health care needs. Healthy families also know what is going on in the world around them. They show an interest in current events and attempt to understand significant social, economic, and political issues. This ever-broadening outreach give families knowledge of external forces that might influence their lives. It exposes them to a wider range of alternatives and a variety of contacts, which increases their options for finding resources and strengthens their coping skills.

Family Health Assessment

A family's level of health may be elusive unless the nurse has some means for assessment. As with the Stones and the Murphys, the community health nurse may have a general idea or intuitive sense about whether or not a

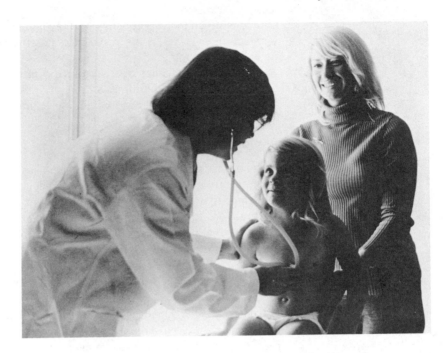

Figure 16-4
Healthy families seek out
and use external resources
such as regular health care.

family is healthy. More difficult is knowing *how* healthy. What is that family's level of health? Assessing family health in a systematic fashion requires two tools: (1) a conceptual framework upon which to base the assessment and (2) a method for measuring a family's level of functioning within that framework.

Conceptual Frameworks

Several conceptual frameworks have been used historically to study families. Three, in particular, continue to be used today: interactional, structural-functional, and developmental. (Broderick, 1976; Christensen, 1964; Hill and Hansen, 1960). The interactional framework describes the family as a unity of interacting personalities. It emphasizes communication, roles, conflict, coping patterns, and decision-making processes — all internal relationships — but neglects the family's interaction with the external environment.

The structural-functional framework describes the family as a social system relating to other social systems in the external environment, such as church, school, work, and health care system. This framework examines the interacting functions of society and the family on each other as well as their structures and how the structure affects their functioning.

The developmental framework studies families from a life-cycle perspective by examining members' changing roles and tasks in each progressive life cycle stage. This framework incorporates elements from the interactional and

451

structural-functional approaches so that family structure, function, and interaction are viewed in the context of the environment through each stage of family development.

The six characteristics discussed in the previous section provide us with a description of healthy families that serve as one framework for assessing family health using interactional and structural-functional concepts.

Assessment Tools

Many different tools are used to assess families. These tools serve to generate information about selected aspects of family structure and function; thus the tool must match the purpose for assessment.

Three well-known tools are the ecomap, the genogram, and the family sculpture (Holman, 1983). The ecomap is a diagram of the connections between a family and the other systems in its ecological environment. It could be useful, for instance, to examine the various factors present (and possibly contributing to) a child abuse situation. Developed by Dr. Ann Hartman in 1975 to help child welfare workers study family needs, the tool visually depicts the dynamic family-environment interactions. The nurse involves family members in the map's development. They draw a center circle representing the family and then smaller circles on the periphery to represent people and systems, such as school or work, whose relationships with the family are significant. The map is used to discuss and analyze these relationships (Hartman, 1978; Holman, 1983, p. 62). Figure 16-5 displays an ecomap.

The genogram provides information about a family's history over a period of time, usually three or more generations. It diagrams family relationships by listing the family genealogy accompanied by significant life events (birth, death, marriage, divorce, illness), identifying characteristics (race, religion, social class), occupations, and places of family residence (Holman, 1983, p. 68). Again, this tool is used jointly with the family. It encourages family expression and sheds light on family behavior and problems. Figure 16-6 shows a sample genogram.

Family sculpture is a dynamic process that engages the family in creating a live family portrait (Holman, 1983, p. 75). Family members assume postures and spatial relationships that represent their behaviors and feelings toward one another and their environment. Various members serve as sculptor, "molding" the family into the picture that they perceive as reality. The nurse uses this tool to help the family understand its relationships and to form a basis for nursing care planning and intervention.

Community health nurses also use a variety of family assessment guides that may be used to gather data on family structure, functions, development, or combinations of all three (Kandzari, Howard, & Rock, 1981). Public health nursing agencies generally develop their own instruments often in the

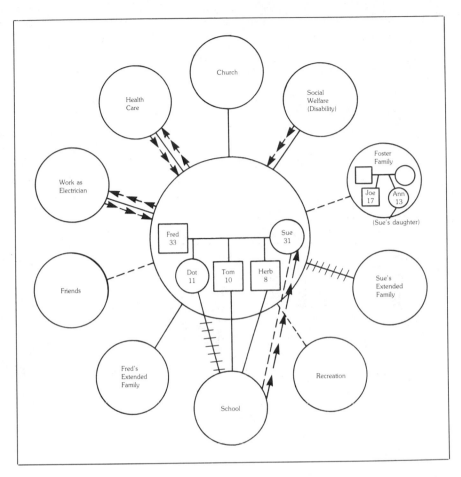

Figure 16-5
Ecomap of a family's relationship to its environment. Lines indicate types of connections: solid lines, strong; dotted lines, tenuous; lines with cross bars, stressful. Arrows signify energy or resource flow, and absence of lines indicates no connection.

form of a questionnaire, checklist, or interview guide. The format varies to fit organizational needs. For example, many agencies are changing to computerized information management systems and are adjusting data collection to be technologically compatible. Two sample assessment guides (Figs. 16-7, 16-8) are presented in this chapter.

Other tools, such as videotaping family interaction, structured observation, or analysis of life-changing events using the Holmes-Rahe scale (Holmes and Rahe, 1967) are all useful adjuncts. Tools are often used in combination to enhance breadth of data collection and understanding of the family. Any assessment tool should be applied in the context of the five guidelines for assessing family health discussed below.

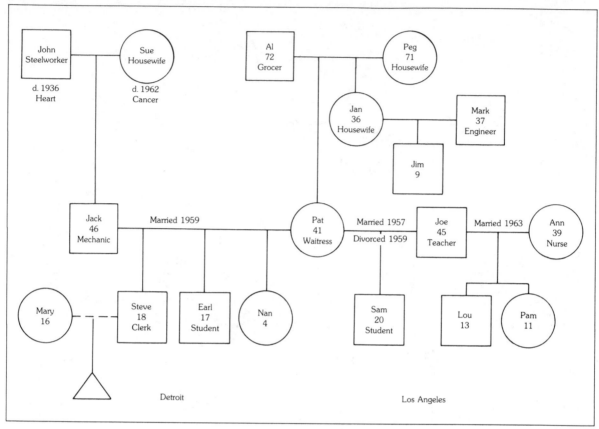

Figure 16-6
A genogram depicting three generations of family history.

Guidelines for Family Health Assessment

FOCUS ON THE FAMILY, NOT THE MEMBER

Family health is more than the sum of its individual members' health. If we were to rate the health of each person in a family and then combine those scores, we would still not know how healthy that family was. To assess a family's health, we must consider that family as a single entity and appraise its aggregate behavior. As we consider each criterion in the assessment process, we ask, "Is this typical of the family as a whole?" Assume that you are assessing the communication patterns of a family. You notice that there is supportive interaction between two members in the family. What about the others? Further observation shows good communication among all but one member. You may decide that, in spite of that one person, the family as a whole has good communication. When individual member behavior

454

deviates from the aggregate picture, you will want to note these differences. They can influence total family functioning and will need to be considered in nursing care planning.

UTILIZE ASSESSMENT QUESTIONS

The activities of any investigator, if fruitful, are guided by goal-directed questions. When solving a crime, a detective has many specific questions in mind. So, too, does the physician attempting a diagnosis, the teacher trying to discern a student's knowledge level, or the mechanic repairing a car. Similarly, the nurse determining a family's level of health has specific questions in mind. It is not enough to make family visits and merely ask members how they are. If relevant data are to be gathered, relevant questions must be asked. Figure 16-7 provides a set of questions that community health nurses may use to assess a family's health. Built upon the framework of the characteristics of a healthy family, these questions guide thinking and observations. They direct attention to specific aspects of family behavior in order that the goal of discovering a family's level of health can be achieved. Consider the characteristic "Active Coping Effort." When visiting a family as the community health nurse, you watch for signs of their response to change and their problem-solving ability. You ask yourself, "Does this family recognize when it needs to make a change?" or "How does it respond when a change is imposed?" Perhaps a health problem has arisen: for instance, the baby has diarrhea. Does the family assume repsonsibility for dealing with the probelm? Do family members consider a variety of ways to solve it? How do they respond to your suggestions? Do they seek out resources on their own, such as reading about causes of infant diarrhea or consulting with you, their doctor, or a clinic? How well do they use resources, once identified? Do they take a problem, try creative methods for solving it, and see it through to resolution? As you focus on these behaviors, you are asking yourself goal-directed questions aimed at finding out the family's coping skills. This investigation will be one part of your assessment of the family's total health picture.

The set of questions presented in Figure 16-7 is one useful way to appraise family health. Another, more open-ended format is used by some community health nursing agencies. This approach, displayed in Figure 16-8, proposes assessment categories as a stimulus for nursing questions. When exploring family support systems, for example, you will ask, "What internal resources or strengths does this family have?" "Who, outside of the family, can they and do they turn to for help?" "What agencies, such as churches, clubs, or community services, do they use?" The open-ended style of this assessment tool allows you to raise a variety of questions aimed at determining family health.

Family Assessment

Family Name _____

Family Constellation

Member	Birth Date	Sex	Marital Status	Education	Occupation	Community Involvement

Financial Status _____

Using the following scale, score the family based on your professional observations and judgment:

0 = Never   3 = Frequently
1 = Seldom   4 = Most of the time
2 = Occasionally   N = Not observed

	score	date	score	date	score	date	score	date

Facilitative Interaction among Members
- a. Is there frequent communication among all members?
- b. Do conflicts get resolved?
- c. Are relationships supportive?
- d. Are love and caring shown among members?
- e. Do members work collaboratively?

Comments _____

_____

Totals

Enhancement of Individual Development
- a. Does family respond appropriately to members' developmental needs?
- b. Does it tolerate disagreement?
- c. Does it accept members as they are?
- d. Does it promote member autonomy?

Comments _____

_____

Totals

	score	date	score	date	score	date	score	date

Effective Structuring of Relationships
   a. Is decision making allocated to appropriate members?
   b. Do member roles meet family needs?
   c. Is there flexible distribution of tasks?
   d. Are controls appropriate for family stage of development?

Comments _____

_____ Totals

Active Coping Effort
   a. Is family aware when there is a need for change?
   b. Is it receptive to new ideas?
   c. Does it actively seek resources?
   d. Does it make good use of resources?
   e. Does it creatively solve problems?

Comments _____

_____ Totals

Healthy Environment and Life-style
   a. Is family life-style health promoting?
   b. Are living conditions safe and hygienic?
   c. Is emotional climate conducive to good health?
   d. Do members practice good health measures?

Comments _____

_____ Totals

Regular Links with Broader Community
   a. Is family involved regularly in the community?
   b. Does it select and use external resources?
   c. Is it aware of external affairs?
   d. Does it attempt to understand external issues?

Comments _____

_____ Totals

Figure 16-7
Family assessment using questions.

457

```
┌──────────────────────────────────────────────────────────────────────────┐
│                          FAMILY ASSESSMENT                                 │
│                                                                            │
│  Family Name                                                               │
│                                                                            │
│  Family Constellation                                                      │
│                                                                            │
│  Member names              Occupation              Educational background  │
│                                                                            │
│                                                                            │
│                                                                            │
│                                                                            │
│  Significant change in family life                                         │
│                                                                            │
│  Coping ability of family                                                  │
│                                                                            │
│  Energy level                                                              │
│                                                                            │
│  Decision-making process within the family                                 │
│                                                                            │
│  Parenting skills                                                          │
│                                                                            │
│  Support systems of the family                                             │
│                                                                            │
│  Use of health care (include plans for emergencies)                        │
│                                                                            │
│  Financial status                                                          │
│                                                                            │
│  Other impressions                                                         │
│                                                                            │
│  Signature of Nurse _____ Date _____      │
└──────────────────────────────────────────────────────────────────────────┘
```

Figure 16-8
*Open-ended family
assessment.*

ALLOW ADEQUATE TIME FOR DATA COLLECTION

Accurate family assessment takes time. An appraisal done on the first or second visit will most likely give only a partial picture of how that family is functioning. You need time to accumulate observations, make notes, and see all the family members interacting together in order to make a thorough assessment. To appraise family communication patterns, for instance, you will want to observe the family as a group, perhaps at mealtime or during some family activity. They will need to feel comfortable in your presence in order to respond freely; it takes time and patience for such an ambience to develop.

Consider one nurse's experience. Joe Burns had talked with the Olson family twice, first in the clinic and then at home. Since Mr. Olson had not

458

been present either time, Joe asked to see the family together and arranged an evening visit. The Olsons were receiving nursing service for health promotion. They were particularly interested in discussing discipline of their young children and contracted with Joe for six weekly visits to be held in the late afternoon when Mr. Olson was home from work. Joe's assessment began on his first contact with the Olsons. He made notes on their chart and, guided by questions similar to those in Figure 16-7, he kept a brief log. After the fourth visit, he filled in an assessment form to keep as a part of the family record. It was not until then that Joe felt he had enough data collected to make valid judgments about this family's level of health.

ASSESSMENT CAN BE QUANTITATIVE AS WELL AS QUALITATIVE

Any appraisal of family health must be qualitative. That is, you must determine the presence or absence of essential characteristics in order to have a data base for planning nursing action. To guide planning more specifically, you can also determine degrees of the presence or absence of these signs of health. This is a quantitative measure. You are not just asking whether a family does or does not engage in some behaviors, you are asking how often. Is this behavior fairly typical of the family, or does it occur infrequently? Figure 16-7 demonstrates one way to measure quantitatively. If you were to use this tool to assess the Murphy family's ability to enhance individuality, for example, you could score their behavior on a scale from zero to four, zero meaning never and four meaning most of the time. After several observations, you would probably conclude that they responded appropriately to the members' developmental needs (a. under "Enhancement of Individual Development") most of the time. Opposite a. on the assessment form, you would place the numeral 4 and the date of assessment.

The value of developing a quantitative measure is to have some basis for comparison. You can assess a family's progress or regression by comparing its present score with its previous scores. Had you conducted a family health assessment six months ago on the Stones, for instance, and compared it with their present level of health, you would probably have discovered a drop in their scores in several areas. Many of their communication patterns, role relationships, and coping skills, in particular, would show signs of deterioration. A scored assessment gives you a vivid picture of exactly which areas need intervention. For this reason, it is useful to conduct periodic assessments. Some have suggested that assessments be conducted every three months (Hott, 1977). In this manner, you can monitor the progress of high-risk families through the early introduction of particular preventive measures, should you see a trend or regressive behavior in some area. Periodic quantitative assessments also provide a means of evaluating the effectiveness of nursing action. You can point to documented signs of growth.

Quantitative data serve another useful purpose. You can compare one

459

family's health status with that of another family in your caseload as a basis for priority setting and nursing care planning. The difference in the levels of health between the Stones and the Murphys tells you that the Stones need considerably more attention right now.

USE FAMILY ASSESSMENT TOOLS WITH CAUTION

Although nurses seek to validate data, their assessment of families is still based primarily on their own professional judgment. Assessment tools can guide observations and even quantify those judgments, but ultimately any assessment is subjective. Even though you observe that the Murphys make good use of their prepaid health plan, your decision that the use of this external resource is contributing to their health is still a subjective one. This decision is not bad. Indeed, effective health care practice depends on sound professional judgment. However, nurses must, at the same time, be cautious about overemphasizing the value of an assessment tool. It is not infallible. It is only a tool and should be used as a guide for planning, not as an absolute and irrevocable statement about a family's health status. This caution is particularly important when dealing with quantitative scores, which may seem to be objective.

Ordinarily, it is best to conduct assessment of a family unobtrusively. The tool is not a questionnaire to be filled out in the family's presence; its purpose is to guide observations and judgments. Before going into a family's home, the community health nurse may wish to review the questions while sitting in the car. The nurse may find it helpful to keep the assessment tool in a briefcase for easy reference during the visit. Depending upon the nurse's relationship with a family, notes may be made during or immediately after the encounter. Like Joe, the nurse may choose to keep a short log — an accumulation of notes — until enough data has been collected to complete the assessment form.

Occasionally, a family with high self-care capability may be involved in the assessment. The nurse will want to introduce the idea carefully and use professional judgment to determine when the family is ready to engage in this kind of self-examination.

Family Health Practice Principles

Family nursing is a kind of nursing practice in which the family is the unit of service. It is "not merely a family-oriented approach in which family concerns that affect the health of the individual are taken into account" (Robischon & Smith, 1977). But how does one provide health care to a collection of people? Although there are some who claim such service cannot be done (Kinlein, 1978), we have increasing scientific evidence that supports

460

its feasibility and, in fact, its necessity. It does not mean that nursing must relinquish its service to individuals. On the contrary, one of the distinctive contributions of nursing as a profession is its holistic approach to individual needs. Community health nurses rise to the challenge of adding a unique kind of service, one that has been neglected for too long — service to population groups that include families.

Several principles can clarify our understanding of family nursing and guide practice with families.

Work with the Family Collectively

To practice family nursing, nurses must adopt a different mind-set. For the moment, they need to set aside the usual focus on individuals and remind themselves that several people together have a collective personality, collective interests, and a collective set of needs. Viewing a group of people as one unit becomes less difficult when we examine the way we often think. We often speak, for instance, of an organization as conservative or liberal. We say that a group has taken a stand on abortion or that a business needs to become better organized. In each case, we view the group collectively, as a single entity with attributes and activities in common. So it is with families. A family has its own personality, interests, and needs.

Working with several people at the same time is not as difficult as it may initially seem. We have all experienced being part of a group that was treated as a single unit. A coach admonishes his team, "Let's practice the pivot turn one more time." A teacher says to a group of 12-year-olds, "Now, class, I'd like you to divide into groups of four each and prepare a three-page paper on how we can enjoy winter. This will be due in one week." A mother addresses her family, "This house has got to be cleaned before Grandma gets here." The church school teacher, during final Christmas play rehearsal, begs the cast members to review their lines. In each instance, the group as a whole is addressed. Group action is expected. Evaluation of the outcomes will be based on what the group does collectively.

With families, the approach is very similar. As much as possible, community health nurses want to involve all the members during nurse-client interaction. This approach reinforces the importance of each individual member's contribution to total family functioning. Nurses want to encourage everyone's participation in the work that the nurse and the family jointly agree to do. Like the coach, the nurse wants to help them work together as a team for their collective benefit.

Consider how you might work with the Stone family collectively. An initial contact by phone call or home visit could be used to determine whether the Stones were interested in family nursing. If not, individual members might want service, and a family focus could be introduced later. If the Stones did want family care, you would ask to meet with the entire family to discuss what the service had to offer and what they would hope to gain from it. You would explain that each person must be involved and committed to the agreed-upon goals; that, like a team of oarsmen, the family would have to pull together to accomplish the purpose of the visits. To help the Stone family improve its health status, you might jointly decide to work first on family communication patterns. A session of brainstorming could uncover many causes of poor communication. More brainstorming might suggest solutions and plans for action. On each visit you would view the Stones as a group. You would expect group responses and actions. Evaluation of outcomes would be based on what the family did collectively.

Start Where the Family Is

When working with families, community health nurses begin at their present, not their ideal, level of functioning (Kinlein, 1978). Although you may recognize that the Stones need to develop more facilitative interaction, the family may not wish to, or be ready for, work on its communication patterns. To discover where a family is, community health nurses act in two ways. First, they conduct a family assessment to ascertain the members' needs and level of health. Concurrently, they determine their collective interests, concerns, and priorities.

The Kegler family illustrates this principle. Marcia Kegler brought her baby to the well-child clinic once but failed to keep further appointments. Concerned that the family might be having other difficulties, the community health nurse made a home visit. The mobile home was cluttered and dirty; the baby was crying in his playpen. Marcia seemed uninterested in the nurse's visit. She listened politely but had little to say, only repeating that everything was OK and that the baby was doing fine. He was just fussy now because he was teething, she explained. As they talked, Marcia's husband Bob, a delivery van driver, stopped by to pick up a sports magazine to read on his lunch hour. The three of them discussed the problems of inflation and how expensive it was to raise a child. The nurse reminded them that the clinic was free, and that they could at least get good health care without extra cost. They agreed without enthusiasm. After Bob left, the nurse spent the remainder of the visit discussing infant care with Marcia, particularly emphasizing regular checkups and immunizations.

The next visit also focused on the baby, but the nurse had an uncomfortable feeling that this family was not really interested in her help. After consulting her supervisor, the nurse did what she wished she had done in the first place. She asked to talk with Marcia and Bob together and explained frankly why she had first come to their home and what she could offer in the way of counseling, teaching, support, and referral to other community resources. She then asked them what, if anything, would they like. What were their concerns? The Keglers were more than responsive. There followed a listing of financial difficulties so long that sometimes they had felt like giving up. Yet the Keglers believed they would eventually overcome their problems if they just had "someone to lean on," as they put it. Their greatest concern at this point in time was for friends. They were new in the city, and both their families lived some distance away on farms. The neighbors were friendly but not close enough to confide in.

Now the nurse could start where this family was. In addition to providing needed support herself by focusing on the parents instead of the baby, the nurse also introduced them to a young couples' group which met at the community center. She had learned that, although their baby's health should be a concern, the Keglers' present social needs were greater and required her attention first.

Fit Nursing Intervention to the Family's Stage of Development

Although every family engages in the same basic functions, the tasks to accomplish these functions vary with each stage of the family's development. A young family, for instance, will appropriately meet its members' affiliation needs by establishing mutually satisfying relationships and meaningful communication patterns. As the family enters later stages, these bonds change with the release of some members into new families and the loss of others through death. Awareness of the family's developmental stage enables the nurse to assess the appropriateness of the family's level of functioning and to tailor intervention accordingly.

A nurse's work with the Roberts family exemplifies this principle. The Roberts, a couple in their midsixties, had recently moved to a retirement complex. They had received nursing visits following Mrs. Roberts' stroke three years previously but requested service now because Mr. Roberts was feeling "poorly" all the time. He thought that perhaps his diet and lack of activity might be the causes and hoped the nurse would have some helpful suggestions. The couple had eagerly awaited Mr. Roberts' retirement from teaching, planning to be lazy, travel, visit all their children, and do all those things they never had time to do when they were young. Now neither of them seemed to have any energy or capacity to enjoy their new life. The move from their home of 28 years had been difficult; they were still trying to find space in the tiny apartment for their cherished books and mementos, many of which had had to be given away.

The nurse recognized that Mr. and Mrs. Roberts were experiencing a situational crisis (leaving their home of 28 years) and a developmental crisis (entering retirement and the aging stage). Many of the Roberts' expectations for this new life stage were unrealistic; they had not adequately prepared themselves for the adjustments that the loss of their home and retirement would demand. Through discussion, the nurse was able to help the Roberts understand their situation and feelings. They decided on a series of nursing visits focused on adapting to retirement and aging as well as agreed that the Roberts needed a support group of other persons who were experiencing some of the same difficulties. Such a group was currently meeting in the retirement center; they joined it. Because this nurse was able to help the Roberts through the crisis in a supportive and nonjudgmental manner, she found them receptive later to discussing preparation for the inevitable loss and bereavement that would occur when one of them died. She was suiting her nursing intervention to this family's stage of development.

Recognize the Validity of Family Structural Variations

Many families seen by community health nurses are nontraditional in structure, particularly single-parent families and unmarried couples. Other families are organized around nontraditional patterns; for example, both parents may have careers or a husband may care for children at home while his wife financially supports the family. There are reasons for these variant structures and organizational patterns. They result from social change — change in employment practices, welfare programs, economic conditions, sex roles, status of women and minorities, birth control, divorce, war, and many other influences. Such variations in family structure and organization lead to revised patterns of family functioning. Member roles and tasks often differ dramatically from our expectations, as in a family with a single parent who works full-time while raising children or a dual-career marriage in which both partners have undifferentiated roles. Community health nurses, many of whom are accustomed to traditional family patterns, may find such variations difficult to understand or accept unless they recognize their validity.

There are two important aspects to consider in this principle. First, what is normal for one family is not necessarily normal for another. Each family is unique in its combination of structure, composition, roles, and behaviors. As long as a family carries out its functions effectively and demonstrates the characteristics of a healthy family, we must agree that its form, no matter how variant, is valid.

Second, families are constantly changing. Marriage transforms two people into a married couple without children. Adding children changes this family's structure. Divorce again alters structure and roles. Remarriage with the addition of children from another family changes the family again. Children grow up and leave the home while the parents, together or singly, are left to adjust to yet another family structure. And so it goes. Throughout the life cycle, a family seldom stays the same for very long. Each of these changes forces a family to adapt to its circumstances. Consider the young woman with a baby whose husband deserts her. She has no choice but to assume a single-parent role. Each change also creates varying degrees of stress and demands considerable adaptation energy on the family's part. Many family changes are predictable; they are part of normal life cycle growth. Some are not.

The nurse's responsibility is to help families cope with the changes while remaining nonjudgmental and acceptant of the variant forms encountered.

Homosexual unions are difficult for some nurses to deal with. Because homosexual families are not always recognized as a valid family form for religious or other resons, the nurse may feel uncomfortable relating to them. Yet the nurse's responsibility remains the same. Like any family, homosexual couples need to carry out basic functions and develop characteristics that promote their collective health. The nurse can view these, and all families, as unique groups, each with its own set of needs, whose interests can best be served through unbiased care.

Emphasize Family Strengths

Too often, without meaning to derogate, community health nurses focus their attention on family weaknesses, referring to them as needs or problems. It seems to suit their role as helper to look for things that need help. This negative emphasis can be devastating to a family and demolish any hopes of a truly therapeutic relationship. No one likes to be criticized, people with a lowered self-image (composing a large share of the community health nurse's caseload) least of all. Instead, families need their strengths reinforced.

Emphasizing a family's strengths makes that group of people feel better about themselves. It fosters a positive self-image and promotes self-confidence. It energizes the family to cope more effectively with life. This is not to say that nurses should ignore problems. On the contrary, their assessment should explore all aspects of family functioning to determine both strengths and weaknesses. The nurse needs a total picture to achieve adequate perspective in nursing care planning, and begin work on problems when the family is ready and chooses to. Yet, even as the nurse becomes aware of a family's various behaviors, the emphasis should stay on the positive ones. Emphasizing strengths says, in effect, "Proof that you are important to me is that I see many good things about you."

Family strengths, according to Hill (1971), are "those traits which facilitate the ability of the family to meet the needs of its members and the demands made upon it by systems outside the family unit." Not all traits that appear positive are necessarily strengths, however. Before the nurse selects a trait to emphasize, it is important first to examine it closely and ask whether or not that behavior is actually facilitating family functioning. A strong work orientation may be a strength when balanced with play and relaxation, but a family obsessed by work is experiencing this trait as a weakness. Hott (1977) suggests that the differentiating factor between whether a trait is a strength or a weakness is the amount of free choice, as opposed to compulsive drive, exercised.

Some traits a nurse may consider possible strengths to emphasize are basic family functions, family developmental tasks, and characteristics of family health. For instance, a nurse might wish to commend a family that meets its members' physical, emotional, and spiritual needs; shows respect for various members' points of view; or fosters self-discipline in its children (Otto, 1973).

We see a vivid illustration of this principle in the family nursing care of the Stevensons. The community health nurse made an initial home visit after referral by an outpatient physician who was concerned about possible child abuse. Alice Stevenson had brought her baby to the emergency room for treatment of a head laceration. He had fallen off the table while she was changing him, she claimed. Bruises on his arms made the physician suspicious, but Alice explained those as caused by his older brother's rough play. The nurse opened the visit by stating she was simply following up on the emergency room treatment and wanted to see how they were progressing. She made no mention of child abuse. She observed the mother and children closely, looking for small things to compliment Alice on while learning all she could about the family background. Because the nurse appeared approving rather than suspicious or judgmental, Alice agreed to further visits.

During a later session Alice admitted to the nurse that she had dropped the baby on purpose. She could not get him to stop crying, no matter what she did; she just could not endure it any longer. There had been other times when she had physically abused him, too. She had not wanted this baby at all; her husband had gotten her pregnant and then left her shortly before the baby was born. Like many abusive parents, Alice had unrealistic expectations for her children's behavior as well as very inadequate self-esteem (Kempe & Helfer, 1972). Realizing that Alice would be particularly vulnerable to any criticism, the nurse concentrated on her strengths. She complimented her on how well she managed her home and dressed the children, on maintaining her job, and on reading stories to the three-year-old boy. It took many visits before Alice trusted the nurse, but in time they were able to discuss her feelings frankly and work toward improving this family's health. Emphasizing strengths had provided a bridge for the Stevensons into a helping relationship.

Summary

The family as the unit of service has received increasing emphasis in nursing over the years. Today family nursing has an important place in nursing practice, particularly in community health nursing. Its significance results from recognition that the family itself must be a target of service, that family health and individual health strongly influence each other, and that family health affects community health.

Healthy families demonstrate six important characteristics:

1. There is a facilitative process of interaction among family members.
2. They enhance individual member development.
3. Their role relationships are structured effectively.
4. They actively attempt to cope with problems.
5. They have a healthy home environment and life-style.
6. They establish regular links with the broader community.

To assess a family's health systematically, the nurse needs a conceptual framework upon which to base the assessment and an instrument for measuring the family's level of functioning within that framework. The six characteristics of a healthy family provide a framework that community health nurses can use. This chapter discusses two instruments, an assessment tool using questions and an open-ended assessment form, which can facilitate specific assessment of family health.

During assessment, the nurse focuses on the family rather than the individual member, utilizes relevant assessment questions, allows adequate time for data collection, considers collection of quantitative as well as qualitative data, and uses the assessment instruments with caution.

Community health nurses enhance their practice with families by observing five principles:

1. Work with the family collectively.
2. Start where the family is.
3. Fit nursing intervention to the family's stage of development.
4. Recognize the validity of family structural variations.
5. Emphasize family strengths.

Study Questions

1. Construct an ecomap of a family that you know well. Ask a colleague to help you with this task. Make it a simulated interview and alternate role playing the part of the nurse and the client family. Afterward, assess the balance between the family and the resouces in its environment.
2. Draw a genogram of your family and ask a colleague to role-play the part of the community health nurse while you play the client. Make your drawing of the genogram as complete as possible. Then analyze your thoughts and feelings (Holman, 1983, p. 74):
   How did you feel while tracing your family history?
   Did you learn anything new about your family?
   Did any family trends or traits appear?
   Did any uncomfortable or suppressed information come to the surface?
   Do you have any new insights about your family?

3. Assess a family (other than your own) that you know well by completing a family assessment guide. You may use one of the forms in this chapter or a form available to you from some other source. Based on your assessment, determine one nursing intervention that could be used to promote this family's health.

References

Beam, W. W. (1979). College students' perception of family strengths. In N. Stinnett, B. Chesser, & J. De Frain (Eds.), *Building family strengths: Blueprints for action.* Lincoln, NE: University of Nebraska Press.

Broderick, C. B. (1967). In D. H. Olson (Ed.), *Treating relationships.* Lake Mills, IA: Graphic.

Christensen, H. T. (Ed.). (1964). *Handbook of marriage and the family.* Chicago: Rand McNally.

Ford, L. C. (1973). *The development of family nursing.* In D. Hymovich & M. Barnard (Eds.), *Family health care.* New York: McGraw-Hill.

Freeman, R. B., & Heinrich, J. (1981). *Community health nursing practice.* Philadelphia: W. B. Saunders.

Hartman, A. (1978). Diagrammatic assessment of family relationships. *Social Casework 59*(10), 59–64.

Hill, R. B. (1971). *The strengths of black families.* New York: Emerson Hall.

Hill, R., & Hansen, D. (1960). The identification of conceptual frameworks utilized in family study. *Marriage and Family Living, 22,* 299–311.

Holman, A. M. (1983). *Family assessment: Tools for understanding and intervention.* Beverly Hills, CA: Sage.

Holmes, T., & Rahe, R. (1967). The social readjustment rating scale. *Journal of Psychosomatic Research, 11,* 213–217.

Hott, J. R. (1977). Mobilizing family strengths in health maintenance and coping with illness. In A. Reinhardt & M. Quinn, *Current practice in family-centered community nursing.* St. Louis: C. V. Mosby.

Kandzari, J. H., Howard, J. R., & Rock, M. (1981). *The well family: A developmental approach to assessment.* Boston: Little, Brown.

Kempe, C. H., & Helfer, R. E. (Eds.). (1972). *Helping the battered child and his family.* Philadelphia: Lippincott.

Kinlein, M. L. (1978). Point of view on the front: Nursing and family and community health. *Family and Community Health, 1*(1), 57.

Mendes, H. A. (1979). Single-parent families: A typology of life-styles. *Social Work, 24,* 193.

Olson, D., McCubbin, H. I., & Associates. (1983). *Families: What makes them work.* Beverly Hills, CA: Sage.

Otto, H. A. (1963). Criteria for assessing family stength. *Family Process, 2*(2), 329–337.

Otto, H. A. (1973). A framework for assessing family strengths. In A. Reinhardt & M. Quinn (Eds.), *Family-centered community nursing: A socio-cultural framework.* St. Louis: C. V. Mosby.

Pratt, L. (1976). *Family structure and effective health behavior: The energized family.* Boston: Houghton Mifflin.

Robischon, P., & Smith, J. A. (1977). Family assessment. In A. Reinhardt & M. Quinn (Eds.), *Current practice in family-centered community nursing.* St. Louis: C. V. Mosby.

Safilios-Rothschild, C. (1976). Dual linkages between the occupational and family systems: A macrosociological analysis. *Signs, 1,* 51.

Satir. V. (1967). *Conjoint family therapy.* Palo Alto, CA: Science and Behavior Books.

Stinnett, N. (1981). In search of strong families. In N. Stinnett, B. Chesser, & J. De Frain (Eds.), *Building family strengths: Blueprints for action.* Lincoln, NE: University of Nebraska Press.

Stinnett, N., & Saur, K. H. (1977). Relationship characteristics of strong families. *Family Perspective, 11*(4), 3–11.

Tanner-Nelson, P. & Banonis, B. (1981). Family consensus and stress identified in Delaware's White House Conference on the family. In N. Stinnett, J. DeFrain, K. King, P. Knaub, and G. Rowe (Eds.). *Family strengths* III: Roots of well being (pp. 43–60). Lincoln, NE: University of Nebraska Press.

Selected Readings

Archer, S. E. (1975). Family: A model of an open system. In S. E. Archer & R. Fleshman (Eds.), *Community health nursing: Patterns and practice* (pp. 30–37). North Scituate, MA: Duxbury Press.

Bould, S. (1977). Female-headed families: Personal fate control and the provider role. *Journal of Marriage and the Family, 39,* 339–348.

Choi, T., Josten, L., & Christiansen, M. L. (1983). Health-specific family coping index for noninstitutional care. *American Journal of Public Health, 73,* 1275–1277.

Crawford, C. O. (Ed.). (1971). *Health and the family: A medical-sociological analysis.* New York: Macmillan.

Darrill, J., & Hyde, J. (1975). Working with high-risk families: Family advocacy and the parent education program. *Children Today, 4,* 23.

Ford, L. C. (1973). The development of family nursing. In D. Hymovich & M. Barnard (Eds.), *Family health care.* New York: McGraw-Hill.

Gelles, R. J. (1976). Demythologizing child abuse. *Family Coordinator, 25,* 135.

Glasser, P. H., & Glasser, L. N. (1970). *Families in crisis.* New York: Harper & Row.

Hill, R. B. (1971). *The strengths of black families.* New York: Emerson Hall.

Hogan, P. (1975). Creativity in the family. In *Series on creative psychology, No. 2* (pp. 1–32). Ardsley, NY: Geigy Pharmaceuticals.

Holman, A. M. (1983). *Family assessment: Tools for understanding and intervention.* Beverly Hills, CA: Sage.

Hott, J. R. (1977). Mobilizing family strengths in health maintenance and coping with illness. In A. Reinhardt & M. Quinn (Eds.), *Current practice in family-centered community nursing.* St. Louis: C. V. Mosby.

Hymovich, D., & Barnard, M. (Eds.) (1973). *Family health care.* New York: McGraw-Hill.

Kandzari, J. H., Howard, J. R., & Rock, M. (1981). *The well family: A developmental approach to assessment.* Boston: Little, Brown.

Kempe, C. H., & Helfer, R. E. (Eds.). (1972). *Helping the battered child and his family.* Philadelphia: Lippincott.

Knafl, K. A., & Grace, H. K. (1978). *Families across the life cycle.* Boston: Little, Brown.

Lockhart, C. A. (1975). Family assessment of coping ability. In S. E. Archer & R. Fleshman (Eds.), *Community health nursing: Patterns and practice* (pp. 333–336). North Scituate, MA: Duxbury Press.

Martin, E. P., & Martin, J. M. (1978). *The black extended family.* Chicago: University of Chicago Press.

McCubbin, H. I. (1979). Integrating coping behavior in family stress theory. *Journal of Marriage and the Family, 41,* 237–244.

Mendes, H. A. (1979). Single-parent families: A typology of life-styles. *Social Work, 24,* 193–199.

Miller, J. R., & Janosik, E. H. (1980). *Family-focused care.* New York: McGraw-Hill.

Minuchin, S. (1974). *Families and family therapy.* Cambridge, MA: Harvard University Press.

Murphy, N. (1978). Training professionals to support and increase the competence of young parents. *Journal of Nursing Education, 17*(7), 41–49.

Murray, R., & Zentner, J. (1975). *Nursing assessment and health promotion through the life span.* Englewood Cliffs, NJ: Prentice-Hall.

Olson, D., McCubbin, H. I., & Associates. (1981). *Families: What makes them work.* Beverly Hills, CA: Sage.

Otto, H. A. (1973). A framework for assessing family strengths. In A. Reinhardt & M. Quinn (Eds.), *Family-centered community nursing.* St. Louis: C. V. Mosby.

Pratt, L. (1976). *Family structure and effective health behavior: The energized family.* Boston: Houghton Mifflin.

President's Commission for a National Agenda for the Eighties. (1981). Helping families — to help themselves. *International Journal of Family Therapy, 3,* 208–233.

Robischon, P., & Smith, J. A. (1977). Family assessment. In A. Reinhardt & M. Quinn (Eds.), *Current practice in family-centered community nursing.* St. Louis: C. V. Mosby.

Rossi, A. S. (1968). Transition to parenthood. *Journal of Marriage and Family, 30*(2), 26–39.

Satir, V. (1967). *Conjoint family therapy*. Palo Alto, CA: Science and Behavior Books.

Satir, V. (1972). *Peoplemaking*. Palo Alto, CA: Science and Behavior Books.

Skolnick, A., & Skolnick, J. (1977). *Family in transition: Rethinking marriage, sexuality, child rearing, and family organization* (2nd ed.). Boston: Little, Brown.

Smiley, O. R. (1973). The family-centered approach — A challenge to public health nurses. *International Nurses Review, 20*(2), 49–50.

Sobol, E. G., & Robischon, P. (1975). *Family nursing: A study guide* (2nd ed.). St. Louis: C. V. Mosby.

Steward, R. F. (1973). The family that fails to thrive. In D. Hymovich & M. Barnard (Eds.), *Family health care*. New York: McGraw-Hill.

Sweeney, B. (1970). Family-centered care in public health nursing. *Nursing Forum, 9,* 169–176.

Tapia, J. A. (1972). The nursing process in family health. *Nursing Outlook, 20,* 267–270.

Watts, R. J. (1979). Dimensions of sexual health. *American Journal of Nursing, 79,* 1568–1572.

17

Health of the Working Population

Elaine Richard
Barbara W. Spradley

One of the largest population groups of concern to community health is the working population. In the United States it is made up of 113 million people, 40 percent of whom are women. This aggregate is composed of generally well adults whose health and safety at work, until a few decades ago, were viewed as their own responsibility. In recent years we have come to recognize that safety and health in the workplace have a major influence on the public's health and that employers and others must share in the responsibility for workers' safety and health on the job. Potential or actual injuries and illnesses associated with the workplace are the focus of the field known as occupational health.

This chapter examines selected aspects of occupational health. First it defines who the working population is and the impact of the work environment on this group's health. Then it reviews and summarizes historical perspectives and legislation affecting the health of the working population. Finally, it describes the health needs of workers, ways to meet those needs, and the community health nurse's contribution to the health of the working population.

Defining the Working Population

What is the working population? When we think of workers we generally think of people who are gainfully employed, and we visualize the most obvious types: an executive in a three-piece suit carrying a briefcase, a

472

professional person in uniform, a jeans-clad worker with a lunch pail. In actuality there is an almost infinite variety of types of workers and jobs encompassing nearly every conceivable activity. Most are paid monetarily for what they do. Others, such as housewives and volunteers, also work but are not identified in the labor (worker) statistics. Yet all these workers have health needs that should be addressed by community health practitioners.

The working population shares in common that it is made up of people who work, and it includes most of the country's well adults. At the federal level it is appropriate to consider the total working population as a single group whose need for safe and healthful working conditions can be enhanced through public education and enabling legislation. We shall discuss these efforts in a later section. For assessment of needs and health services provision, however, the community health nurse must view this aggregate in terms of smaller groups or subpopulations. That is, the nurse must assess the health and safety needs of a specific group of workers and the hazards associated with their work environments, whether assembly line workers in a plant, bank tellers, farmers, or operators of video display terminals, and then design health interventions and mechanisms for service provision appropriate to that working group. Let us look more closely at the work environment and factors in it that affect worker health.

The Work Environment

The healthy adult working population, although scattered throughout the nation in a myriad of urban and rural settings, still shares characteristics of its work environment in common. We shall examine five environmental factors common to every work setting and discuss their potential impact on the health of workers. The five factors are (1) physical, (2) chemical, (3) biologic, (4) ergonomic, and (5) psychosocial.

Physical factors are structural elements of the workplace that influence worker health and productivity. Various features on the job form an assemblage of parts that defines the physical work environment. These include such factors as work space, temperature, lighting, noise, vibration, color, radiation, pressure, and soundness of building and equipment construction. The quality of such elements can make an impact on worker health. Excessive noise, for example, may disrupt concentration; interfere with on-the-job communication, job performance, and safety; and, over a period of time, cause hearing loss (Olishifski, 1979, p. 9). Extremes of temperature are another example. Field laborers, road construction crews, or persons working around furnaces may experience heat extremes that, if compounded by excessive physical exertion, can cause heatstroke. Excessive levels of electromagnetic and ionizing radiation found in certain manufacturing operations or hospitals may also create serious deleterious effects. Pressure extremes, experienced by deep-sea divers or by persons working at high altitudes or in tunneling operations, may cause improper gas exchange and tissue damage affecting ears, sinuses, and teeth (Olishifski, 1979, p. 16). Many physical factors can threaten safety, such as lack of protection from acetylene torch sparks, sharp or falling objects, or weak scaffolding.

Chemical factors are the chemical agents present in the work environment that may threaten worker health and safety. Numerous chemicals are found in the raw materials and production processes of manufacturing and in the day-to-day operations of industries and businesses, such as dry cleaning, painting, food companies, photography, automobile manufacturing, plastics, farming, pharmaceuticals, and hospitals. In recent years, chemical agents have become an increasing menace to the health of the working population (Public Health Service, 1979, p. 102). The giant petroleum industry followed by the modern chemical industry have introduced new chemicals at the alarming number of 1,000 new compounds a year, subjecting workers to unknown hazards. Chemicals are present in many forms. Frequently chemicals are associated with gases; however, they are also present in the form of solvents, mists, vapors, dusts, and solids. Depending on their form and structure, chemicals enter the human body through the lungs, gastrointestinal tract, and the skin. Therefore, an understanding of the toxicology of chemicals is essential for identifying (1) the amount of chemical exposure that produces toxicity, (2) the routes through which chemicals enter the body, and (3) the appropriate personal protection for workers. For example, lead enters the body through the gastrointestinal tract and the lungs. Workers exposed to toxic levels must maintain good hand-washing practices, avoid eating on the job to prevent the ingestion of this chemical, and at the same time employ appropriate respiratory protection to prevent inhaling this agent.

Many toxic chemicals such as insecticides are taken for granted in daily use, and their toxicity frequently ignored. Careless handling and needless exposure can lead to serious burns, poisoning, asphyxia, tissue damage, or even cancer. Some inert, nontoxic industrial materials, such as resins and polymers, may decompose and form toxic byproducts when heated. Workers need to be warned and protected from all potential hazards associated with the materials they must use on the job. With proper handling and protection, many toxic conditions can be prevented. Ideally, all toxic substances would be eliminated through substitution of nontoxic agents, when such chemicals exist.

Biologic factors are the biologic organisms and potential contaminants found in the work environment. These include bacteria, viruses, rickettsias, molds, fungi, parasites of various types, insects, animals, and even toxic plants that may be present. Potential biologic hazards, such as infectious or parasitic diseases, may derive from exposure to contaminated water or to insects. Other vehicles include improper waste or sewage disposal, unsanitary work environments, improper food handling, and unsanitary personal practices.

474

Workers in every setting have their own unique set of potential biologic hazards. Agricultural workers, for instance, are subject to a condition called "farmer's lung" that comes from inhaling fungi-contaminated grain dust. Staphylococcal and other infectious agents threaten hospital workers. Brucellosis (undulant fever) and Q fever from infected cattle are a threat to slaughterhouse workers. Outdoor workers, such as builders, forest rangers, or environmental specialists, face the hazards of insect and animal attack as well as contact with toxic plants, such as poison oak and ivy.

Ergonomic factors also affect workers' well-being. The term *ergonomics* means "the customs, habits, and laws of work " (Olishifski, 1979, p. 17). Ergonomics has become a field of study in occupational health and is described by the International Labor Office as "the application of human biological science in conjunction with the engineering sciences to achieve the optimum mutual adjustment of man and his work, the benefits being measured in terms of human efficiency and well-being" (cited in Olishifski, 1979, p. 17). In short, it deals with people interacting with their work environments.

For our purposes in describing the elements of the work environment, ergonomic factors are the customs, laws, design, and expectations of the work itself. They include all the physiological and psychological demands (and potential stressors) that the job makes on the worker. The design of necessary tools, work space, physical positions workers must assume and motions they must make to do the job, standards and habits associated with carrying out the work — all these have an impact on the worker's health. (Figure 17-1). Health problems can arise from improper lifting habits, inadequate or unsafe tools, or unrealistic job demands; from a work design that promotes interruptions, provides inadequate space, and offers only poor ventilation; or from any other stress-producing working conditions. For example, Mexican field laborers in some southwestern states as recently as 1984 were required to use short-handled hoes to speed production and maximize crop yield. Hours of stooping over plants in this doubled-up position, however, caused serious skeletal and internal injuries, some of which were permanent.

Psychosocial factors are all the responses and behaviors that workers exhibit on the job based on the attitudes and values learned from their cultural backgrounds and life experiences. They are the workers' response to the work. Some people may appear (and feel) fatigued, tense, bored, angry, depressed, or agitated. Others may be enthusiastic and energized. Similar work conditions can evoke different responses from people. Repetitive work for some may be boring, but for others it offers an opportunity for reflection. Certain types of work can be challenging for some, not challenging enough for others.

The nature of the work itself evokes worker responses as much as the work conditions do. Work that is time pressured or that conflicts with personal values may create tremendous stress for employees. Ethical dilemmas, such as promoting a product whose sales will benefit the company (and preserve

475

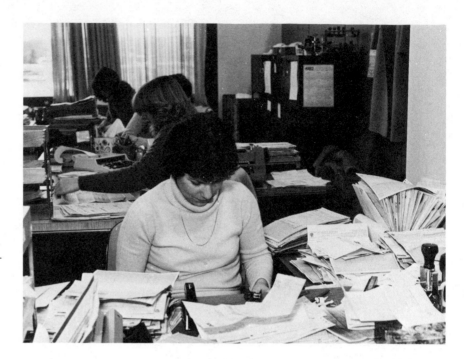

Figure 17-1
Ergonomic factors can cre-
ate stressful working condi-
tions that affect employee
health. Several studies
have demonstrated that
secretaries are among the
most highly stressed
workers.

the employee's job) but whose use may be injurious to the public, can tear people up emotionally. Peer pressure can create another set of stressors as is evident in the personal conflict experienced by many workers during a strike. Yet another psychosocial factor that can make the work situation hazardous to employee health involves unrealistic personal expectations on the part of workers for what they can and hope to accomplish on the job. Unattainable aspirations can lead to chronic stress and fatigue and eventual burnout (Veninga & Spradley, 1981).

Depending on the work setting, the presence of these five factors will vary in intensity and potential for threat to worker health. They present a core of critical data for occupational health assessment and planning. Table 17-1 summarizes these five environmental factors.

Health and the Workplace: Historical Perspectives

The work setting clearly presents many hazards to worker health; nonetheless, conditions in the work setting have improved considerably from previous years. Modern occupational health is an outgrowth of the nineteenth-century Industrial Revolution in England. Deplorable work conditions and exploitation of workers created a growing public concern and spawned the development

476

Table 17-1
Factors Influencing Health and Productivity in the Work Environment

Variable	Physical	Chemical	Biologic	Ergonomic	Psychosocial
Definition	Structural elements of workplace	Chemical agents present in work environment	Biologic organisms and potential contaminants in work environment	Customs, rules, design, and expectations of the work itself	Workers' values, attitudes, and responses
Selected Types	Radiation Noise Vibration Light Temperature Space Color Pressure Construction	Mists Vapors Gases Solids Liquids Dusts Solvents	Viruses Insects Molds Fungi Bacteria Animals Plants Parasites Rickettsias	Design of work space Design of job Work habits Required motions Design of tools Work standards Work flow	Emotional Boredom Anger Depression Behavioral Fatigue Tension Cultural Values Norms
Illustrative Potential Hazards	Excessive noise Electromagnetic radiation Excessive ionizing radiation Temperature extremes Excessive vibration Pressure extremes Unsafe objects or structures	Excessive airborne concentrations Topical irritants Toxic absorption through skin Toxic ingestion	Contaminated water or food Improper waste or/sewage disposal Unsanitary work environment Improper food handling Insect or animal attack Unsanitary personal practices	Improper lifting Poor motions or positions Improper tools Inadequate space to do work Interruptions Unrealistic work expectations Repetitive motion	Boring work Unchallenging work Time pressure Conflicts with worker values Group dissatisfaction Unrealistic personal expectations Peer pressure

of many protective laws. This influence was felt in the United States whose early agricultural character in the 1800s was rapidly being replaced by industrialization. By 1900 the United States supplied more than one-third of the world's annual demand for iron and steel (Lee, 1978, p. 65). As industrial growth escalated, immigrants poured into the United States, forming a large portion of the labor force. Workers, adults and children, commonly worked 12- to 14-hour shifts, seven days a week, under unspeakable conditions of grime, dust, physical hazards, smoke, and noxious fumes. People accepted work-related illnesses and injuries as necessary risks and expected to live shorter lives, into the forties and fifties, death being common in the thirties for workers in some trades (Lee, 1978).

The connection between work conditions and health was ignored. Employers attributed employees' poor health and early deaths to the workers' own personal habits on the job or their home living conditions. Physicians, uneducated in the relationship between work and health, blamed industrial-related diseases, like silicosis, lead poisoning, and tuberculosis, on other causes. But the evidence was there. In the early 1900s the Public Health Service conducted one of the first scientific studies in occupational hazards by investigating dust conditions in mining, cement manufacturing, and stone cutting. Other studies followed. Lead poisoning was as high as 22 percent among a group of pottery workers studied. A 1914 study of garment workers showed a high incidence of tuberculosis related to poor ventilation, overcrowding, and unsanitary work conditions. Other investigations revealed phosphorous poisoning among workers in the match industry (1912), radium poisoning in the watch industry (1920s), and mercury poisoning in the felt hat industry (1930s) (Lee, 1978). The public was awakening to the effect of work conditions on people's health.

With development of the labor movement came the demand for healthful and safe working conditions. Workers' compensation laws provided for occupational injury and disease coverage, and other efforts were made to protect workers against the health hazards of the workplace. The health of American workers is better today than it has ever been, but health hazards still exist and new ones continue to develop as technology and environmental influences change. Occupational health faces the challenge of continued protection and promotion of worker health and improvement of the work environment.

Significant Legislation Affecting the Health and Safety of Workers

The preceding historical summary clearly emphasizes the need for public awareness and understanding before changes could occur to improve the health of the working population. Such understanding has resulted from knowledge based on experience and research.

The earliest systematic study of occupational disease was recorded in 1700 by Bernardino Ramazzini, now known as the "father of occupational medicine" (Lee, 1978, p. 77). This Italian physician had the foresight, when attempting a diagnosis, to ask what occupation the patient was engaged in. Despite his influence, interest in and information concerning worker health evolved slowly. A few classic studies, some of which are mentioned in the previous section, influenced the gradual development of protective legislation. Futher influence came from disastrous events in the workplace. One notable event was the Triangle Waist factory fire in New York City in 1911 in which 154 workers, mostly young women, died. Fire escapes ended in midair and the factory doors were locked. This tragic event resulted in the first serious safety laws to protect working people (Morris, 1976). Today a growing body of legislation exists to protect the health and safety of workers. Current laws that employers must implement include the following.

The Workmen's Compensation Act of 1911 was enacted in several states

478

initially and finally in all states by 1948. This law requires employers to carry employee insurance that provides compensation for wages lost and costs of medical and rehabilitative care associated with work-related diseases and injuries. Application of the law varies from state to state. A trend across all states, however, is to emphasize early intervention and rehabilitation.

Second Injury Funds, established under most state workers' compensation laws, encourage employers to hire the handicapped. Employees who acquire a "second injury" (for example, loss of a limb or an eye, or a worsened chronic condition) from their work are covered. When the second injury results in permanent, total disability, the employer is then liable only for the amount of disability directly attributable to the worker's employment while the funds cover the difference to which the employee is entitled. Again, coverage varies with each state. The Department of Labor enforces the provision of these funds.

The Federal Coal Mine Health and Safety Act of 1967 is a unique law in that it is the only federal program that deals with a specific occupational disease. The act originally provided for the establishment of health standards in coal mines and medical examinations for actively employed underground coal miners. Through the Social Security Administration, it also provided black lung benefits. Specifically, it required all exposed workers to have radiographic examinations and provided federal funds to compensate mine victims and survivors of deceased miners. The subsequent Federal Mine Safety and Health Ammendments Act of 1977 retains most of the original provisions.

The Occupational Safety and Health Act of 1970 has had tremendous significance for the working population. Generally it seeks to provide workers with protection against personal injury and illness resulting from hazardous working conditions. More specifically, its purpose and functions are "to assure safe and healthful working conditions for working men and women; by authorizing enforcement of the standards developed under the Act; by assisting and encouraging the States in their efforts to assure safe and healthful working conditions; by providing for research, information, education, and training in the field of occupational safety and health; and for other purposes" (Lee, 1978, p. 80).

The act created two federal agencies. The Occupational Safety and Health Administration (OSHA), housed in the Department of Labor, became its regulatory branch. Its research branch became the responsibility of the National Institute for Occupational Safety and Health (NIOSH), based in the Public Health Service (under the Department of Health and Human Services). Specifically, OSHA responsibilities include the following (Lee, 1978, p. 81):

Development and updating of mandatory occupational safety and health standards.
Enforcement of regulations and standards

Requirement of employers to keep accurate records on work-related injuries, illnesses, and hazardous exposures

Maintenance of an occupational safety and health statistics collection and analysis system (collaborating with NIOSH)

Supervision of worker education and training to identify and prevent unsafe or unhealthy working conditions (collaborating with NIOSH)

Provision of grants to states to assist in compliance with the Act

NIOSH responsibilities include the following (Hanlon & Pickett, 1984, p. 357):

Research on occupational safety and health problems

Hazard evaluation

Toxicity determinations

Work force development and training

Industry-wide studies of chronic or low-level exposures to hazardous substances

Research on psychologic, motivational, and behavioral factors as they relate to occupational safety and health

Training of occupational safety and health professionals

The Privacy Act of 1974 ensures that only necessary information be collected on individuals by federal agencies. Futhermore, this information, such as medical history, education, or financial and employment history, must be maintained so that the individual's privacy is protected (Lee, 1978, p. 83).

The Toxic Substances Control Act of 1976 serves to ensure that chemical substances do not present an "unreasonable risk of injury to health or the environment" (Lee, 1978, p. 83). The act requires that certain chemical substances and mixtures be tested and their use restricted. It is also concerned with the manufacture, processing, commercial distribution, and disposal of such substances. The Environmental Protection Agency enforces the Act.

Worker Right-to-Know Legislation, enacted in at least one-third of the states, ensures that workers are adequately informed regarding hazards in their places of work. A growing sentiment in the nation says that workers should know what risks they face on the job.

Health Needs of the Adult Population

The working population, as mentioned previously, is made up of adults whose health determines the productivity and well-being of our communities and our nation. For all American adults, aged 25 to 64, the major causes of death are heart disease. cancer, accidents, stroke, and cirrhosis of the liver. Table 17-2 shows the ten leading causes of death for this population group.

Chronic diseases pose the most significant threat to the health of American adults (Public Health Service, 1979, p. 53). More than one-third of all deaths

480

Table 17-2
Ten Leading Causes of Death for American Adults Aged 25–64 Years per 100,000 Population

Cause of Death	Total	Male	Female
Heart disease	729.1	539.9	189.2
Cancer	669.7	373.8	295.9
Accidents	169.4	130.5	38.9
Cerebrovascular diseases	100.0	55.1	44.9
Chronic liver disease and cirrhosis	89.0	60.8	28.2
Chronic obstructive pulmonary diseases	73.0	36.0	37.0
Suicide	64.3	47.7	16.6
Homicide	54.6	44.8	9.8
Diabetes mellitus	40.6	20.9	19.7
Pneumonia and influenza	31.2	20.7	10.5

Source: U.S. Bureau of the Census (1984). Statistical Abstract of the United States 1984, 104th ed. Washington, DC: U.S. Government Printing Office.

among adults aged 25 to 64 are due to cardiovascular diseases, primarily coronary artery (heart) disease and stroke. Heart disease has been the leading cause of death for men above age 40. Women, on the other hand, prior to menopause have only one-third the heart disease rate of men. After that the incidence in women increases. By age 70 it is nearly the same, and by age 85 the rates are equal.

In addition to its impact on mortality rates, heart disease has a tremendous impact on worker health. It is the "greatest cause of permanent disability claims among workers under 65. . . . [it is] responsible for more days of hospitalization than any other single disorder. And it is the principal cause of limited activity for some 2.5 million Americans under age 65" (Public Health Service, 1979, p. 56).

Strokes, too, in addition to being a significant cause of death (almost 10 percent of the total mortality rate), leave many American adults disabled with paralysis, speech problems, and memory loss. Furthermore, "nearly 10 percent of nursing home admissions in people under 65 are because of strokes" (Public Health Service, 1979, p. 56). Blacks between the ages of 25 and 64 are more than twice (2.5 times) as susceptible to strokes as whites, largely because of the high prevalence and incidence of hypertension among black Americans.

The most important preventable risk factors affecting heart disease are smoking, hypertension, cholesterol, and diabetes (Public Health Service, 1979, p. 57). Others include overweight, physical inactivity, personality factors affecting stress perception, genetic influence, and use of oral contraceptives. The likelihood of heart disease or stroke occurring multiplies with the increasing number of risk factors present.

The second most common cause of death among adults is cancer, a disease that strikes one out of every four Americans (Public Health Service, 1979, p. 60). Lung, large intestine, and breast cancers cause the most fatalities among this age group. An increasing number of these are occupational and smoking-related malignancies whose direct etiology often remains unclear since there may have been repeated and prolonged exposure to several carcinogenic agents over many years.

Major preventable risk factors contributing to cancer are smoking, alcohol, diet, radiation, sunlight, occupational exposure, water and air pollution, and heredity (Public Health Service, 1979, p. 62). For the working population, occupational exposure presents an increasing set of health hazards as new chemicals and other potential cancer-causing materials are produced and used every year. In addition, known carcinogenic agents, such as asbestos and vinyl chloride continue to threaten the health of workers who, without adequate protection, develop malignancies not commonly found in the general population. Mesothelioma, a lung cancer related to asbestos exposure, has even been documented among people whose only known exposure was to the contaminants carried home on the shoes and clothes of the worker (Lee, 1978, p. 74). It has been estimated that up to 20 percent of total cancer deaths may be due to occupational hazards (Public Health Service, 1979, p. 8) (Figure 17-2).

Three other problems posing major threats to the health of American adults, and thus to the working population, are accidents, alcohol abuse, and mental illness. Each has taken a tremendous toll in lives lost and health and productivity diminished. The surgeon general's report on health promotion and disease prevention states a compelling case for the preventability of these problems (Public Health Service, 1979).

Work-Related Health Problems

What are the health problems of the working population specifically? American workers are exposed to numerous safety and health hazards in the work environment, which we examined earlier in this chapter. Their impact on worker health has led to identification, by NIOSH (1983), of the ten leading work-related health problems:

1. Occupational lung disease
2. Musculoskeletal injuries
3. Occupational cancer
4. Fractures, amputations, eye losses, and traumatic deaths
5. Cardiovascular diseases

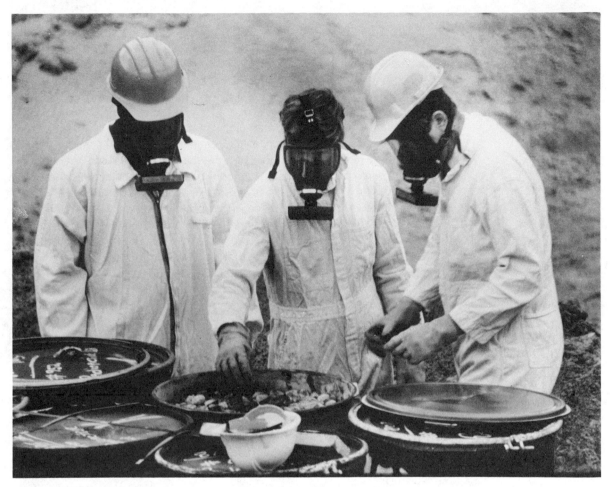

Figure 17-2
Some workers must deal with known carcinogenic agents on the job. Adequate protection is essential for their health and safety.

6. Reproductive problems
7. Neurotoxic illness
8. Noise-induced hearing loss
9. Dermatologic problems
10. Psychological disorders

Each year 13,000 adults lose their lives to work-related injuries, and approximately 100,000 die from work-related illnesses (Public Health Service, 1979, p. 107). We are seeing a gradual decline in occupational injury rates, a decline attributable, largely, to better protective and preventive action. However, reported occupational illnesses may increase. While the incidence of some of these diseases will diminish through preventive efforts, epidemiologic research will continue to shed new light on the nature, causes, and linkages of occupational diseases contributing to a likely increase in their reporting (Hanlon & Pickett, 1984, p. 351).

Collection of occupational disease data has been difficult since the lag time is so great between exposure and onset of the disease and actual clinical evidence. Silicosis, for example, takes 15 years to develop. Some cases of mesothelioma have not become evident until 25 years after the worker was last exposed to asbestos (Hanlon & Pickett, 1984, p. 352). Many workers who have moved on to other jobs or retired are only now discovering disease that may be connected to previous employment. Documenting this connection poses problems. Nonetheless, more sophisticated epidemiologic methods and an improved data base are enabling public health and industrial researchers to demonstrate linkages and make more accurate predictions. They estimate, for instance, that of the 6,000 current and previous uranium miners, approximately 600 to 1,100 will die of lung cancer in about 20 years because of radiation exposure (Key, Henschel, Butler, Ligo, & Tabershaw (Eds.), 1977). More than 12 percent of active coal miners have radiographic evidence of pneumoconiosis (APHA, 1975), and workers exposed to heavy metals, such as lead, mercury, and arsenic, will likely develop related diseases. Researchers have also demonstrated the relationship between cotton mill dust and byssinosis, a lung disease formerly thought not to exist in the United States. Epidemiologists are studying the connections between skin diseases and materials used on the job, a problem of considerable magnitude since dermatologic problems are among the most common of occupational diseases. It is estimated that seven million industrial workers have exposure to noise levels that cause impaired hearing (Hanlon & Pickett, 1984, p. 352). As the knowledge base regarding occupational illnesses increases, nurses will be better equipped to design more effective protective and preventive measures.

A final set of health problems affecting workers encompasses all the psychological stresses that workers experience on the job or bring to the job from their personal lives. There is some evidence that up to 30 percent of absenteeism is due to emotional disturbances (Hanlon & Pickett, 1984, p. 354). Pressures at work to be more productive or a physically stressful work environment, for example, excessive noise, heat, or vibration, can send a worker home to take out his or her frustrations through such outlets as domestic or alcohol abuse. Problems at home, like financial or interpersonal difficulties, can, on the other hand, affect the worker's performance on the job. Either source of stress creates a vicious cycle perpetuating and escalating the problems in both settings with the potential for unsafe practice at work and harm to self or family at home. Clearly workers' mental health influences their safety, their productivity, and their level of health.

Occupational Safety and Health Programs

What efforts are being made to address the above problems and to promote the health of the working population? Of primary concern to occupational health and safety professionals are the factors in the work environment that have an impact on workers' health and safety. Clearly the business of occupational health is the prevention of work-related hazards, the protection of workers from known health risks, and the promotion of fitness and productivity among workers.

Occupational health programs, generally speaking, have grown tremendously since World War II. Many manufacturing plants, service organizations such as the Kansas Farm Bureau, and commercial establishments, including department stores, have instituted some kind of health program for employees. Many programs still concentrate on providing emergency care, but others are beginning to recognize the importance of prevention and health promotion. For example, Sperry Univac of St. Paul, Minnesota, has held an Employee Health Promotion Day, and Ball Electronics keeps employees fit with exercise breaks. The Resource Trust Company of Minneapolis, Minnesota, pays the initial fee and half the weekly dues of any employee who attends Weight Watchers. As an added incentive, the firm reimburses the other half of the costs to employees when they meet their weight objectives (*Wellness Gazette*, 1980).

Because the nature of work differs from one business to another. as well as the number and type of workers employed, the potential hazards and the need and type of on-site health programs varies. For example, construction and mine workers are a high-risk group for certain types of injuries and illnesses. These workers require an aggressive surveillance program that focuses on prevention and personal protection. On the other hand, professionals, such as lawyers and accountants, who in general do not encounter physical safety and health hazards on the job but may experience psychological stresses, would benefit more from a health promotion program that includes emphasis on stress management and physical fitness.

In order to determine the priorities for intervention and the appropriate health goals and objectives for an aggregate of workers, it is essential that an environmental and workers' assessment be conducted. Knowledge of workers' job classifications, materials handling, and exposures will provide clues to potential hazardous substances and working conditions. This information, together with data on the characteristics of the aggregate in terms of age, sex, race, and existing health conditions, should be compiled. In addition, one should examine workers' compensation claims and occupational safety and health reports to identify subpopulations at risk for occupational illness and injury.

The two professionals who generally provide the on-site services are the occupational health nurse (OHN) and the safety specialist. Other members of the interdisciplinary team may include an industrial hygienist, ergonomist, toxicologist, and occupational health physician. However, these specialists are generally employed by large corporations or they provide only selected part-time services on a contractual basis. Therefore, the occupational health nurse position in a company setting is the cornerstone to occupational health.

Because the working population is primarily composed of healthy adults, the goal of occupational health is to provide a healthy and safe work environment and to promote personal health behaviors of workers in an attempt to maintain a healthy, productive work force. Thus, occupational health programs encompass the entire spectrum of the health continuum involving the practice components of disease prevention, health protection, and health promotion (White, 1982). Table 17-3 describes these practice priorities.

The practice priority of prevention holds primary importance in occupational health because work-related injuries and illnesses are frequently not reversible. Limb loss or mesothelioma from asbestos exposure are conditions for which there are no cures. Interventions, therefore, are aimed at eliminating the hazards by such methods as redesigning the equipment to provide safety guards and to substitute materials that are effective but less toxic. The surgeon general's report points out, "Once these occupational hazards are defined,

Table 17-3
Practice Priorities in Occupational Health

Goal and Function	Prevention	Protection	Promotion
Goal	Elimination of hazardous substance or condition	Avoidance of injury or illness of high-risk workers	Attainment of an optimal level of personal health
Function	Job analysis Preplacement exams Hazard communication Materials handling and training Industrial hygiene sampling Health surveillance Safety measures on equipment Safety work procedures Walk-through evaluations	Personal safety measures Hard hats Ear muffs or plugs Safety glasses Respirators Foot protection Skin barrier creams Legislation and regulation OSHA standards Employees right-to-know laws	Wellness Physical fitness Smoking cessation Nutritional awareness Stress management Screening Health risk appraisal Cancer detection Diabetes and hypertension screening Health policy formulation Smoking Alcohol Healthful foods in cafeteria

486

they can be controlled. Safer materials may be substituted; manufacturing processes may be changed to prevent release of offending agents; hazardous material can be isolated in enclosures; exhaust methods and other engineering techniques may be used to control the source; special clothing and other protective devices may be used (Figure 17-3); and efforts can be made to educate and motivate workers and managers to comply with safety procedures" (Public Health Service, 1979, p. 8).

The practice priority of protection becomes essential when hazardous

Figure 17-3
A welder wears protection against ultraviolet light.

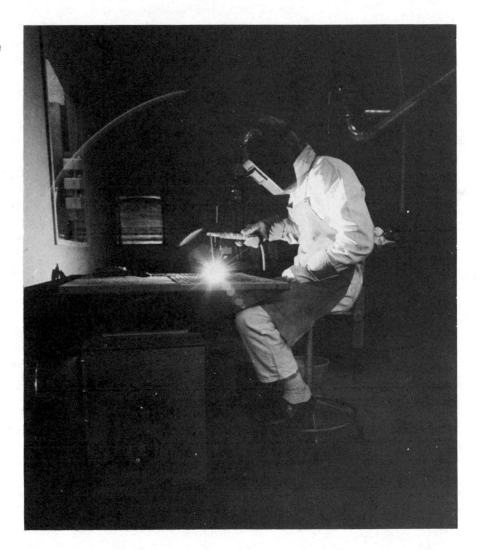

exposures cannot be eliminated. Construction workers, for example, wear hard hats and steel-toed safety shoes to protect themselves from falling objects. Protection of workers is frequently achieved through legislation and regulation. The Occupational Safety and Health Act of 1970, discussed previously, provided the impetus for worker protection. More recently, employee right-to-know legislation has passed in several states, focusing on training of employees who are working with potentially hazardous agents. The enforcement of such regulations will continue to be the key intervention for ensuring that workers are adequately protected on their jobs.

Occupational safety programs available in many industries include plant surveillance, safety violation reporting, and worker safety education. Genetic screening, present in a few settings, identifies workers with sensitivity to specific hazards; however, it is a controversial program. criticized by labor and civil rights groups as an invasion of privacy. It may be more appropriate to protect all workers from those hazards (Hanlon & Pickett, 1984, p. 355).

The practice priority of health promotion has appropriately received much attention and activity in the workplace over the past decade. The workplace is an ideal setting to conduct health promotion efforts for two important reasons: (1) the vast majority of the healthy population may be reached at the worksite, and (2) employers have viewed wellness programs as legitimate, worthwhile employee benefits to promote and support.

Of significance for community health is the fact that health promotion activities in the workplace can involve long-term interventions that will allow for a variety of educational and motivational strategies to be employed as well as a systematic plan for on-going monitoring and evaluation of programs. The work environment itself can serve as a model healthy community. The adoption of positive health policies on such issues as smoking, cafeteria meal planning, alcohol, and seat belt use will establish health norms for company personnel. Many of these positive health behaviors could also have an impact on the employees' home and family.

Typical health promotion programs include exercise, weight loss, smoking cessation, and nutrition education. There is growing evidence that wellness efforts are effective. Some research indicates that, as a result of wellness promotion, employees have shown increased self-esteem, improved job performance and job satisfaction, decreased absenteeism, and less use of company health services (Azarow & Cardy, 1981; Jaffe, 1977; McGill, 1979). Health promotion programs in the workplace have the potential for providing a significant contribution to adult health as well as to research and development in this new arena of wellness. Cost and production incentives increasingly cause greater receptivity among employers to methods that enhance employee wellness. More research is needed to demonstrate the correlation between healthy employees and increased productivity on the job. Health promotion will continue to be a vital area of emphasis for the working community.

Nonoccupational Health Programs

Although employers are not required to provide treatment of nonoccupational (not incurred as a result of being on the job) injuries and illnesses, many companies do provide such services. One reason is that the location in which some health problems, such as muscle strain, influenza, and minor rashes, are acquired cannot easily be determined, thus making it simpler to provide service regardless of source. The on-site treatment of minor acute injury and illness as well as employee counseling is dependent on the philosophy of the company, the employment of an OHN, and the company's prior experience with offering these services as an employee benefit.

From the nurse's perspective, the advantages of offering nonoccupational health services are the following:

1. The OHN develops rapport with employees and can detect health problems early.
2. Loss of employee productive time is minimized when treatment is given on-site.
3. The OHN, through triage, can decide which cases require medical attention and which can be managed by the nurse (Figure 17-4).
4. The OHN can provide needed on-going personal health education and counseling in the context of a more holistic view of the worker.
5. On-site chronic disease management, such as hypertension monitoring,

Figure 17-4
Early detection of warning signs that might lead to coronary artery disease or other illness is an important part of the occupational health nurse's preventive program.

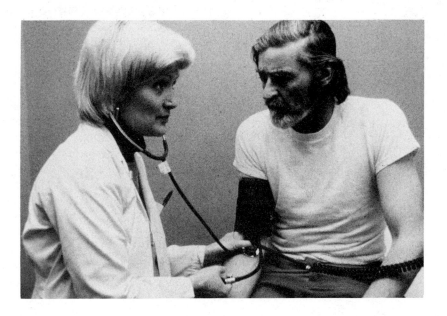

increases compliance thereby saving costs of physician visits and complications associated with noncompliance with treatment.

6. The OHN provides employees with personal contact — a valued commodity in our high-technology work environments.

A concern expressed by a number of OHNs is that too much time can be spent in nonoccupational illness management to the neglect of a more aggressive occupational health surveillance program. As OHNs learn more concerning the environmental factors that threaten the health of this population group, they will likely spend less time with illness management and move more aggressively into primary prevention, protection, and health promotion efforts.

Occupational Health: Nursing's Contribution and Challenge

Community health nurses have a long history of involvement in occupational health. In 1895, the Vermont Marble Company hired the first industrial nurse in the United States to care for its employees and their families. It was an unusual demonstration of interest in employee welfare at that time. The nursing service, consisting almost entirely of home visiting and care of the sick, was free to employees and their families. Gradually this nursing role changed. By World War II there was a striking increase in employment of industrial public health nurses who practiced illness prevention and health education among employees at work. In addition to emergency care and nursing of ill employees, the activities of many industrial nurses involved safety education, hygiene, nutrition, and improvement of working conditions. Yet a significantly high number of industrial injuries and sick employees kept many nurses too busy to do anything but illness care. They might see as many as 75 or more patients a day in the plant dispensary, where they provided first aid and medications (Kalisch & Kalisch, 1978). More recently, as we have seen, employee health programs have improved as socioeconomic and political pressures have created improved safety and health standards for the work environment. These changes have caused the role of the nurse to expand and change also.

As we examine occupational health and the role of the occupational health nurse, we must remind ourselves that traditional nursing practice with individuals and groups of employees is very different from aggregate nursing. We must again broaden our perspective to include the health needs of working population groups.

In 1979, Arthur D. Little, Inc. conducted a study of occupational health nursing. The findings revealed that occupational health nursing services contributed positively to employee health and morale. The study also concluded that on-site services were cost-effective by reducing (1) lost work time, (2) insurance premiums, and (3) medical costs (Little, 1980).

The nurse's role in occupational health, as previously mentioned, has traditionally focused on illness and injury care. This has been the direct result of the knowledge and skills obtained in basic nursing education. During the last decade, a number of nursing education programs (primarily on the graduate level) have developed a specialty focus in occupational health. In addition, many continuing education programs provide OHNs with updated information and skill training for identifying and assistance in managing the physical, chemical, biologic, ergonomic, and psychosocial factors in the work environment that contribute to the health and safety of workers. As a result, the OHN's role is not universal; it is dependent on the type and philosophy of the company, type and number of workers, the health professionals involved, exposures and potential hazards in the work environment, and the knowledge and skills of the nurse.

Nurses who select the field of occupational health and safety will encounter significant differences from employment in the acute care setting. In order to make the adjustment, the nurse should be aware of the factors that make practice in occupational health unique.

The *setting*, unlike hospitals or ambulatory care centers, is in a nonhealth care institution where production or service (not health care) is the goal of the organization. The OHN participates in the organization's goals through activities that will contribute to a productive work force.

The *position* of the OHN in the organization is as staff (versus being a line employee). Although the nurse is generally responsible for the management of the occupational health unit, the OHN serves in the capacity of health consultant to line management personnel. Therefore, the power to effect change is not in any position of authority but in the OHN's expertise.

The *location* of the OHN contributes to isolationism. It is estimated that more than 65 percent of OHNs are the only health professionals in the industrial setting (Jacobson & Richard, 1982). This lack of on-site supervision and direction requires OHNs to be comfortable, competent, and independent decision makers. Because of their isolation, OHNs need to network with other nurses and professional organizations in the community for peer support and setting of appropriate occupational health standards (Jacobson & Richard, 1982, p. 116).

The *client* served in occupational health is a well population with whom long-term contact is possible. For this reason, OHNs know their clients well and have opportunities to work with them through various stages of personal as well as health service-related incidents. Exposure to this continuum of health care challenges OHNs to utilize all the community health nursing model interventions — education, engineering, and enforcement — described in chapter 3.

491

Finally, the *practice focus* is aggregate oriented; the nurse serves a worker population group. Environmental factors significantly influence the health and safety of workers. Therefore, OHNs need to constantly monitor the work environment and assess the health needs of the entire worker population in order to identify populations at risk and develop prevention, promotion, and protection programs. Nurses with community health experience, an aggregate focus, and strong managerial skills are in the best position to meet the needs of this population.

Community-based Occupational Health

Agencies external to business and industry also provide occupational health nursing services. Historically, public health nurses of visiting nurse associations made home visits to sick employees and their families. In subsequent years, public health agencies provided part-time nursing services to small companies. These services included supervising the work environment, conducting health examinations, keeping records, teaching health, health counseling, providing first aid, giving immunizations, and referring workers to community resources. More recently, community health nursing services have offered health screening and health promotion programs. Furthermore, OHN consultants based in state departments of health provide consultation and continuing education programs to nurses employed in occupational health settings.

Hospital-based occupational health programs, large medical-industrial health clinics, and insurance companies also provide occupational health nursing services. These services may be in the form of direct care (rehabilitation of an injured worker) or indirect care (consultation on implementing regulations regarding record keeping or compiling health data statistics).

A continuing unmet public health need is the health of workers in smaller companies (approximately 100 or fewer employees). These companies have more hazards because equipment and controls are often inadequate. They seldom, if ever, have a health professional on site, nor has the community provided health services that would meet their needs. Attempts have been made by some communities, but no sustained efforts exist. Community health nurses are in a position to accept this challenge and develop a system that will ensure ongoing service to this high-risk population.

Community health nurses continue to have a significant role in occupational health — directly and indirectly. Let us consider how you as an OHN might practice nursing with the working community.

Employee Health Case Study

You have just been hired, let us imagine, as a full-time OHN for Allied Electronics, a firm that manufactures and sells electronic components and equipment. Allied's 450 employees are scattered through its sprawling five-acre plant located on the edge of the city. At present, Allied's health program consists of several components. The health service, run by the nurse, provides emergency care for employees who are injured or become ill on the job. An on-call physician has left standing orders for the nurse to use in emergencies and sick care. Regular checking for real or potential hazards in the work environment is done through the safety division by the plant safety engineer. Allied pays for a large percentage of employee health care through its health benefits program; this is precisely why Allied has hired you. Health insurance premiums per employee have skyrocketed, and managers are looking for alternative solutions to lower health provision costs. They would like you to develop a new approach to employee health.

Nursing Goals

A broad goal for occupational health is "the promotion and maintenance of the highest degree of physical, social, and emotional well-being of workers in all occupations" (Tinkham, 1977, p. 7). In actual practice, this goal is only beginning to be realized in selected instances. Nevertheless, it is a worthy and, more important, an essential objective in the realization of an energized and productive working community.

We can address this goal more specifically through the following four working goals that guide occupational health nursing practice. These goals summarize a comprehensive listing of occupational health nursing competencies developed by M. J. Keller. For a complete presentation of the competencies with suggested nursing actions, see Keller in association with W. T. May (1971).

1. Assess the health needs of employees and intervene to promote and maintain their highest possible level of wellness.
2. Study factors in the work environment that are a real or potential hazard to employee health, and take action to minimize their impact or prevent their occurrence.
3. Provide early diagnosis and prompt treatment for injury or illness on the job.
4. Provide programs for employees with disease or disability aimed at restoring and maintaining their maximum level of functioning.

Health Team

Even as you consider these goals, you realize that you will not be pursuing them alone. Like most community health efforts, your work will require collaboration with others. Company management and administrative personnel will be important partners with you in this venture. As Keller (1979, p. 414) points out, "The philosophy and vision of these administrative persons can make or break the contribution of the nurse and the development of her full potential." Collaboration may take time but will be worth the investment. Your goal is to gain the respect and trust of management and establish open communication lines in order that you may influence company policies regarding the nature and scope of its health program.

The company physician is another important health team member with whom the nurse collaborates. Whether working as a full-time, part-time, or on-call staff member, the physician has a strong influence on the company's health policies and programs. Development of a positive ongoing working relationship with the physician gives the nurse a powerful supporter of proposals and program efforts.

Based in health service, usually a part of personnel services, the nurse works closely with other professional, technical, and clerical personnel, particularly those from the safety, engineering, and industrial hygiene departments. Any comprehensive assessment of employee health and safety problems, as well as any health promotion program, would require cooperation and assistance from many individuals of various departments within the organization.

Finally, the occupational health team is not complete without the workers themselves. You will want to encourage employees to identify problems and needs. They can also contribute to decision making regarding health programs. Their cooperation in implementing and evaluating programs is essential for an effective health protection and promotion effort.

As the only nurse at Allied, you will particularly need skills in effective communication, leadership, change management, and assertiveness. These tools will be crucial to effectively interpreting your role and promoting your ideas. Your goal is to establish positive working relationships with the other team members, on whom your success depends.

Nursing Services

Nurses involved in occupational health have a unique opportunity to help shape the health profile of the working population. The degree of that influence depends on how the nurse defines her role. Also, the nurse must be able to overcome the many obstacles incurred in the occupational setting, including restrictive company policy, misunderstanding of the nurse's role, and lack of time for innovative program development. The nurse's role in occupational health, therefore, still varies considerably. It ranges from only providing emergency care for injuries or illness on the job to establishing comprehensive policy and programs covering health promotion, accident and disease prevention, and innovative care for disease and disability.

MEETING EMPLOYEE NEEDS

Occupational health nursing applies the philosophy and skills of nursing and community health to protecting and promoting the health of people in the

494

context of their employment (Brown, 1981; Jacobson & Richard, 1982; Keller, 1979). In other words, the OHN relies on in-depth nursing preparation as well as a strong community health background to provide the tools and perspectives necessary for meeting the challenges of occupational health. Many nurses in occupational health acquire additional physical assessment and management skills as well.

Specifically, some of your typical nursing activities in the new job will include history taking, partial physical examinations, ordering of tests, and emergency care. You will refer many employees for further treatment and follow-up care. Keeping health records will be an expected part of your job, but it can be largely delegated to clerical help. You will participate in conducting health education and health counseling sessions for groups as well as for individual employees. Health assessment, screening, and monitoring are also important aspects of your role.

In order to keep a proper perspective on your goals and also to begin developing a more innovative approach to meeting the employees' health needs (the reason you were hired), you do some strategic planning. You review your four main goals, develop specific objectives for each one, and schedule times when the activities to meet those objectives will be done.

Meeting most of the individual and group needs of employees can be accomplished by scheduling health service hours, classes, and counseling sessions. You plan time to visit departments, observe, and interview selected personnel as part of your health assessment process.

You know there is a relationship between the health of the employees (a population group) and the health of Allied Electronics (an organization). Consequently, you keep a running log of observations on how the company functions and what its effects are on the employees. For example, you notice that some departments seem to place greater stress on their workers than other departments. Among these workers there is a higher incidence of hypertension, headaches, gastrointestinal disturbances, and other somatic complaints. You collect data on the working conditions in those departments. Is there high production pressure? Are there any opportunities to relieve stress on the job? Do workers receive any positive feedback about their work? Could the symptoms be caused or aggravated by some environmental factor such as chemical gases, or noise? (See Figure 17-5.)

ASSESSMENT STRATEGIES

To assess the health needs of the total employee population and selected smaller population groups within the company, you use several approaches. You first enlist the assistance of the company computer services, compile the results of individual health histories and physical examinations, and analyze the findings. A picture emerges of dominant health problems among the employees and of the workers at greatest risk for other problems.

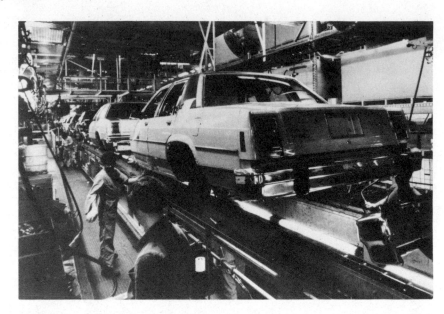

Figure 17-5
The work environment can contribute to or detract from employees' health. Effects of hazards, noise, and toxic chemicals are examples of the nurse's concerns for the workers in this auto assembly plant.

It appears that hypertension, overweight, excessive smoking, and inadequate exercise are the major problems common to Allied's employee population. You can attack these problems on several fronts. You start a regular program of blood pressure monitoring. The employee health education program can be upgraded with new videotapes and literature to make workers more health conscious and show them how to improve their health. Specifically, they learn how to lose weight, manage stress, stop smoking, and maintain an exercise program. More important than information, however, is motivation. You convince management that company inducements, such as Resource Trust Company's payment for Weight Watchers' costs, are important in stimulating employee participation. You tell them about the Speedcall Corporation of Hayward, California, which pays its workers a seven-dollar weekly bonus if they do not smoke on the job. After two years on this program, 20 of 24 smokers had quit smoking on the job (*Minnesota Council on Health Newsletter,* 1979, Jan.). Ball Electronics gives workers time for exercise breaks (*Wellness Gazette,* Jan., 1980). A number of Milwaukee, Wisconsin, companies, some of them splitting the cost between employer and employee, have enrolled employees in the Milwaukee YMCA fitness programs. Allied's management agrees to give time for exercise breaks, a weekly bonus to employees who stop smoking on the job, and a quarterly bonus to those whose blood pressure readings are within normal limits.

Another approach that you use to assess the health needs of the employee population is to conduct an environmental survey of health hazards. Using data from the safety division's regular spot checking, you collaborate with the division on systematic observations of working conditions and interviews of workers. In addition, you post suggestion boxes and gain management's approval to give any employee half a day off with pay for suggesting a safety or health improvement that is implemented into the health program. You gain further ideas from other companies' measures. For example, Scherer Brothers Lumber Company in Minneapolis has removed cigarette machines and stocked other vending machines with nutritionally beneficial foods, such as granola bars, yogurt, and fruit drinks. The company provides fresh fruit instead of sweet rolls to its employees without charge. It has reduced its noise levels, provided a health maintenance organization medical insurance option to encourage illness prevention, and initiated a committee of employees to plan wellness activities (*Minnesota Council on Health Newsletter,* 1979, October).

To assess employee population health further, you participate in a committee composed of the company physician and other personnel to analyze accidents, injuries, and illnesses. The findings reveal a high percentage of injuries and absenteeism. One possible solution is to offer incentive pay similar to the programs instituted by other companies. Parsons Pine Products, Inc., an Ashland, Oregon, manufacturing plant, had a high rate of accidents and absenteeism. Management offered incentive pay to encourage employee wellness. For each month that workers were not absent or late they received eight hours of extra pay. In addition, if they had no injury accidents during the quarter, they received two more hours of pay per month. As a result, absenteeism was reduced by 30 percent, accident rates dropped from 86 percent above average to almost zero, and the company's medical insurance costs dropped (*Minnesota Council on Health Newsletter,* 1978, September). Scherer Brothers also uses "wellness pay." For each month that employees are not absent from work because of illness, they receive two hours of extra pay (*Minnesota Council on Health Newsletter,* 1979, October).

Another problem uncovered in your analysis is a rising incidence of back injuries among Allied's production workers. You learn that Ball Electronics has a similar problem, and you consider its approach. Ball has instituted a voluntary exercise program. Once or twice a day, assembly line workers engage in five-minute limbering and strengthening exercises near their work stations. They are also invited to use the company exercise room, attend optional exercise classes offered at break times (lasting five extra minutes for employees on company time) and after work, and join the company running club. The program has already resulted in improved productive efficiency and job satisfaction but has not been in effect long enough to measure direct impact on back injuries (*Minnesota Council on Health Newsletter,* 1979, October). In the meantime you offer literature on backache prevention and present two classes, one at noon and the other at the beginning of the afternoon shift, on ways to strengthen back muscles and prevent injuries.

Each set of data gathered through the various assessment approaches gives you material to guide your planning and development of health programs. An important dimension in this process is accurate record keeping. Exact figures on incidence and prevalence of health problems in the company give you ammunition to justify your programs and data with which to compare the result when you evaluate program outcomes.

Occupational health nursing demands a great deal from the nurse. Individual needs in the workplace will always compete for the nurse's time and attention with aggregate needs, often to the detriment of the latter. To maintain a proper focus on aggregate needs requires discipline and commitment, commitment based on a different mind-set and the realization that health and productivity of workers is interrelated with the health of the community. The factors that contribute to the health of workers, namely the workplace and the community-at-large, are a responsibility of all who serve as community health nurses.

Summary

The working population, composed of well adults, makes up the majority of the American people. The profile of this aggregate is changing from an industrialized labor force to a greater proportion of white-collar workers and professionals.

Five types of environmental factors, common to all work settings, can influence worker health or safety. Physical, or structural, elements include such things as temperature and noise extremes. Chemical factors are the potentially hazardous chemical agents present. Biologic organisms, such as viruses, bacteria, and fungi, may contaminate the work environment and cause disease. Ergonomic factors include the customs, design, and expectations of the job that influence the way people interact with their work environment. Psychosocial factors are the workers' feelings and behaviors in response to the job. Assessment of all these is critical in determining appropriate occupational health interventions.

Worker health has only recently become a target for health intervention. Historically, workers have suffered unhealthy, dangerous working conditions and contracted debilitating, often fatal, diseases and injuries directly attributable to their employment. The labor movement and workmen's compensation laws turned the tide in favor of workers' rights in the early 1900s. Several important laws affecting worker health and safety have been passed since 1911. Two of the more significant of these are the Occupational Safety and Health Act of 1970 and the more recent worker-right-to-know legislation taking hold in an increasing number of states.

Chronic diseases are the prime threat to the health of the adult working population. Heart disease ranks highest in mortality rates, cancer second, and stroke third. Leading work-related health problems include occupational lung disease, injuries, and occupational cancers.

Programs designed to serve the health needs of the working population vary with occupational site and assessment of needs unique to that setting. Occupational health services encompass the three public health practice priorities — prevention, protection, and health promotion. Preventive programs seek to eliminate potential hazards to worker health and safety. Protective services shield workers from remaining hazards. Health promotion, or wellness, programs seek to maintain and improve the personal health of workers. Health services for workers may also cover nonoccupational illness.

OHNs practice in settings where the production of goods and services is the goal of the organization. The OHN's role requires management skills and expertise in environmental and adult health. OHNs generally work independently and serve population groups on a long-term basis. Community health nurses based in other agencies may also serve occupational health clients, often on a contractual basis with the company.

Occupational health nursing applies the philosophy and skills of nursing and community health to protecting and promoting the health of people in the context of their employment. The nurse must view the client population as a whole, work with other company professionals to assess worker health needs and the needs associated with the work environment, and then design, implement, and evaluate the services.

Study Questions

1. The hospital work environment poses many potential threats to its employees' health. Select a unit in the hospital with which you are familiar, and identify one health hazard for each of the five factors described in this chapter.
2. What is one method of control (protection or prevention) that you would suggest for each of the five factors identified above?
3. If you were asked to offer a weight control program for a local industry of 100 employees, what steps would you consider taking to develop such a program?

References

American Public Health Association (1975). *Chart book: Health and work in America.* Washington, DC: U.S. Government Printing Office.
Azarow, J., & Cardy, W. (1981, November). Health on the job: Change the worker

or change the workplace. Paper presented at the Annual Meeting of the American Public Health Association, Los Angeles.

Brown, M. L. (1981). *Occupational health nursing: Principles and practice*. New York: Springer.

Hanlon, J., & Pickett, G. (1984). *Public health: Administration and practice* (8th ed.). St. Louis: Times Mirror/Mosby.

Jacobson, R., & Richard, E. (1982). Occupational health nursing: A public health perspective. In B. Spradley (Ed.), *Readings in community health nursing* (2nd ed.). Boston: Little, Brown.

Jaffe, R. (1977, November). Science and wellness: The new medicine. Paper presented at the 105th Annual Meeting of the American Public Health Association, Washington, DC.

Kalisch, P., & Kalisch, B. (1978). *The advance of American nursing*. Boston: Little, Brown.

Keller, M. (1979). Health needs and nursing care of the labor force. In M. J. Fromer (Ed.), *Community health care and the nursing process*. St. Louis: C. V. Mosby.

Keller, M. J., in association with May, W. T. (1971). *Occupational health content in baccalaureate nursing education*. Cincinnati, OH: National Institute of Occupational Safety and Health.

Key, M., Henschel, A., Butler, J., Ligo, R., & Tabershaw, I. (Eds.) (1977). *Occupational diseases: A guide to their recognition* (rev. ed.) (DHEW [NIOSH] Pub. No. 77-181). Washington, DC: U.S. Government Printing Office.

Lee, J. (1978). *The new nurse in industry: A guide for the newly employed occupational health nurse* (DHEW [NIOSH] Pub. No. 78-143). Cincinnati, OH: U.S. Government Printing Office.

Little, A. D. (1980). *Costs and benefits of occupational health nursing*. (DHEW [NIOSH] Pub. No. 80-140). Cincinnati, OH: U.S. Government Printing Office.

McGill, A. M. (Ed.). (1979). *Proceedings of the National Conference on Health Promotion Programs in Occupations Settings*. DHHS, Office of the Assistant Secretary for Health. Washington, DC: U.S. Government Printing Office.

Minnesota Council on Health Newsletter. (1978, September). Minneapolis, MN: Minnesota Council on Health.

Minnesota Council on Health Newsletter. (1979, January). Minneapolis, MN: Minnesota Council on Health.

Minnesota Council on Health Newsletter. (1979, October). Minneapolis, MN: Minnesota Council on Health.

Morris, R. B. (Ed.). (1976). *The United States Department of Labor bicentennial history of the American worker*. Washington, DC: U.S. Government Printing Office.

National Institute for Occupational Safety and Health. (1983). *Program plan by program areas for FY 1983* (DHHS Pub. No. 83-102). Washington, DC: U.S. Government Printing Office.

Olishifski, J. B. (Ed.). (1979). *Fundamentals of industrial hygiene* (2nd ed.). Chicago: National Safety Council.

Public Health Service. (1979). *Healthy people: The surgeon general's report on health promotion and disease prevention* (DHEW Publication No. 79-55071). Washington, DC: U.S. Government Printing Office.

Tinkham, C. W. (1977). The Catherine R. Dempsey memorial lecture: Occupational health nursing in the 1980s. *Occupational Health Nursing, 25,* 7–13.

Veninga, R., & Spradley, J. (1981). *The work stress connection*. Boston: Little, Brown.

Wellness Gazette. (1980, January). Minneapolis, MN: Minnesota Council on Health.

White, M. S. (1982). Construct for public health nursing. *Nursing Outlook, 30,* 527–530.

Selected Readings

American Public Health Association (1975). *Chart book: Health and work in America.* Washington, DC: U.S. Government Printing Office.

Brennan, A. J. (1982). Health promotion in business: Caveats for success, *Journal of Occupational Medicine.*

Brown, M. L. (1981). *Occupational Health Nursing: Principles and Practice.* New York: Springer.

Ciliska, D. K. (1982). Lifestyle education and modification in the occupational health setting. *Occupational Health Nursing.*

Clement, J., & Gibbs, D. (1983). Employer consideration of health promotion programs: Financial variable, *Journal of Public Health Policy.*

Dean, D. H. (1981). Bringing health promotion to the worksite: Issues, opportunities and a developing model, *Health Education Quarterly.*

Fielding, J., & Breslow, L. (1983). Health promotion programs sponsored by California employers. *American Journal of Public Health* 73(5): 538–542.

Hanlon, J., & Pickett, G. (1984). *Public health: Administration and practice* (8th ed.). St. Louis: Mosby.

Jacobson, R., & Richard, E. (1982). Occupational health nursing: A public health perspective. In B. Spradley (Ed.), *Readings in Community Health Nursing* (2nd ed.). Boston: Little, Brown.

Keller, M. (1983). Health needs and nursing care of the labor force. In M. J. Fromer, *Community health care and the nursing process* (2nd ed.). St. Louis: C. V. Mosby.

Key, M., Henschel, A., Butler, J., Ligo, R., & Tabershaw, I. (Eds.). (1977). *Occupational Diseases: A Guide to their Recognition* (rev. ed.). Washington, DC: U.S. Government Printing Office, DHEW (NIOSH) Publication No. 77-181.

Laughlin, J. A. (1982). Wellness at work: A seven-step 'dollars and sense' approach, *Occupational Health Nursing.*

Lee, J. (1978). The new nurse in industry: A guide for the newly employed occupational health nurse. Cincinnati, OH: U.S. Government Printing Office, DHEW (NIOSH) Publication No. 78-143.

Little, A. D. (1980). Costs and benefits of occupational health nursing. Cincinnati, OH: U.S. Government Printing Office, DHEW (NIOSH) Publication No. 80-140.

McGill, A. M. (Ed.). *Proceedings of the National Conference on Health Promotion Programs in Occupations Settings.* DHHS, Office of the

Assistant Secretary for Health. Washington, DC: U.S. Government Printing Office.

Morris, R. B. (Ed.). (1976). The United States Department of Labor bicentennial history of the American worker. Washington, DC: U.S. Government Printing Office.

National Institute for Occupational Safety and Health (1983). Program Plan by Program Areas for FY 1983. Washington, DC: DHHS Publication No. 83-102.

Olishifski, J. B. (Ed.) (1979). Fundamentals of industrial hygiene (2nd ed.). Chicago: National Safety Council.

Public Health Service. (1979). *Healthy people: The surgeon general's report on health promotion and disease prevention* (DHEW Publication No. 79-55071). Washington, DC: U.S. Government Printing Office.

Richter, E., & Kretzmer, D. (1980). Prevention through pre-review in occupational health and safety. *American Journal of Public Health, 70*(2), 157–159.

Rutstein, D., et al. (1983). Sentinel health events (occupational): A basis for physician recognition and public health surveillance. *American Journal of Public Health 73*(9), 1054–1062.

Salmon, J. (1983). Injuries grow as USA exercises, USA TODAY.

Serafini, P. (1976). Nursing assessment in industry. *American Journal of Public Health 66,* 755.

Veninga, K. A. (1983). How to establish a nutrition education program. *Occupational Health Nursing,* 34–38.

Veninga, R., & Spradley, J. P. (1981). The work stress connection. Boston: Little, Brown.

Webb, S. R. Jr. (1975). Objective criteria for evaluating occupational health programs. *American Journal of Public Health 65,* 31.

18

Health of the Elderly

The elderly constitute a large and growing population group in our country. They make up a group whose health needs we do not fully understand, and we have yet to offer the full complement of services they require and deserve.

For community health nursing, this population group poses a special challenge. The increasing number of elderly people in the community multiplies the need for health-promoting and preventive services to maximize their ability to remain independent and contributing citizens. This group's greater longevity add another dimension of concern replete with all the problems brought on by diminishing functional capacity and increasing chronic disease and disability. Significant economic, environmental, and social changes create a demand for greater protective and preventive services for older adults in addition to requiring adjustments in health care provision patterns. The challenge is clear. Nursing must study the needs of this group and respond with appropriate, effective interventions.

Our focus in this chapter is on population-based nursing for the elderly. There are four fundamental requirements for effective nursing of any population:

1. Know the characteristics of the population.
2. Set aside stereotypes based on misconceptions of the population.
3. Know the health needs of the population as a basis for nursing intervention.

503

4. View the population from an aggregate, public health perspective that emphasizes health protection and promotion and disease prevention.

In this chapter we first examine the characteristics of the aging population and then some misconceptions about the elderly. Next we explore the health needs of older adults. Finally, we discuss population-based health services and nursing interventions applied to the health of the aging population.

Characteristics of the Elderly Population

Never before in the history of our society has the population of elderly people been so large. Moreover, it is increasing in size. Nearly 27 million people in the United States, 11.6 percent of the country's population, are over 65 years of age, and by 2040 that number is expected to double to more than 55 million (Spiegel, 1983). Women outnumber men in the older population because they live an average of 8 years longer. In fact, "women outlive men every place in the world where women no longer perform backbreaking physical labor and where adequate sanitation and a reduced maternal mortality are present" (Butler & Lewis, 1977, p. 5). In the United States, there are 6.5 million more women than men, a proportion of approximately 106 women for every 100 men.

People are living longer. In 1900 the average life expectancy in the United States was 47 years, and only 4 percent of the population was over 65 years of age. Now, as a result of improved health care, a reduction in infant mortality, and new medical discoveries, the average life expectancy has increased to 74 years (71 for men, 78 for women). For those who reach age 65, the life expectancy becomes even higher by an average of 15 or more additional years; men can expect to live an average of 13 additional years, and women an average of 17 additional years. The average life expectancies (as of 1977) for blacks (63.8 years), Hispanics (mid-50s), and American Indians (47 years), however, are considerably lower.

Within the elderly population, the number of people living into "older" old age has increased. Almost half of the elderly are over 75 years of age, more than 1 million are 85 or more years of age, and more than 110,000 claim to be over 100 years of age. The 75-years-and-over age group is the most rapidly growing segment of the entire U.S. population. As the number of "older" elderly increases, so too does the size of the group needing assistance with activities of daily living. Dressing, eating, toileting, and bathing become more and more difficult for the over-85 group whose dependency and activity limitations predictably grow with age. Public health observers predict that "with more and more people living through their seventh and eighth decades of life, the size of the potentially dependent population may increase even more dramatically" (Hanlon & Pickett, 1984, p. 434). In the past, women in this age group have been more dependent than men. By the time they reach 85 and over, these women are also likely to outnumber older men two to one, adding to the potential care needs of this population group.

Other facts about the elderly are also useful for community health nurses to know. Most elderly men are married and thus have some companionship. Two-thirds of elderly women are widows. Most senior citizens live in the central part of the cities (about 60 percent), and the remainder in rural areas (5 percent on farms, 35 percent in small towns). Some speculate that in 15 or 20 years this demographic picture will change, and more elderly will be living in the suburbs. Nearly 25 percent of older Americans are poor, many of them living in profound poverty, unable to afford clothing, recreation, transportation, or other assets that younger people consider necessary for mental health, social status, avoidance of isolation, and personal growth.

Misconceptions About the Elderly

All of us have had personal experiences with the elderly. We have watched an older person cross the street; we have observed elderly relatives and neighbors; we have seen older people shopping in the supermarket. During professional training, nurses encounter many sick elderly people. These past experiences with individuals often become the data upon which we base our assumptions about this population. When we generalize our knowledge about a few older persons to the entire aging population, we are stereotyping. Many people, including health professionals, have misconceptions about the elderly. These misconceptions often arise from negative personal experiences. Practitioner bias can interfere with effective practice and prevent the kind of service aging persons need or deserve. Below are some of the more common misconceptions (Butler & Lewis, 1977).

It is not true that most old people are dependent. On the contrary, 95 percent of the elderly live in the community, outside formal institutions. Approximately 70 percent live in families, and 25 percent live alone or with nonrelatives. Of those living alone or with nonrelatives, some live in boarding homes or personal care homes where assistance is provided in the activities of daily living. The majority of the elderly are vigorous and functioning independently. Of the total elderly population, 45 percent (49.1 percent for males, 43.9 percent for females) has some limitations in activity, usually caused by physical handicaps such as arthritis, heart conditions, or vision or hearing loss. Only 5 percent live in formal institutions such as nursing homes, long-term care facilities, supervised living facilities, and mental institutions. And not all of these are permanent residents. Many are recovering from illnesses and will go back to the community.

It is not true that chronological age determine "oldness." One 75-year-old woman is actively involved in community organizations, drives her own car, and plays golf. She still has some dark hair and has few wrinkles. Another 75-year-old woman is stooped, wrinkled, slow, and confined to her room. Most old people are quite distinct from one another, and they age at widely disparate rates (Public Health Service, 1979, p. 71). Physical, social, and mental health parameters, life experiences, as well as genetic traits all combine to make aging an individualized process.

It is not true that most old people are senile. Senility, while not an actual medical term, is widely cited by health professionals and laymen alike to denote deteriorating mental faculties associated with old age. Such stereotypical labeling often provides an easy escape for practitioners impatient with an older person's complaints. It interferes with proper diagnosis and treatment. Senility, or dementia, may in actuality have its etiology from some other source (Public Health Service, 1979, p. 75):

> Among the many causes of apparent senility which can be treated to reverse the condition are drug interactions, depression, metabolic disorders (thyroid, kidney, liver, and pituitary malfunction, as well as hypercalcemia and Cushing's Syndrome), chronic subdural hematoma, certain tumors, alcohol toxicities, chemical intoxications (arsenic and mercury), nutritional deficiencies, sensory deprivation due to social isolation or failing sight or hearing, chronic infections, hypoxia or hypercapnia associated with chronic lung disease, and anemia.

Certainly arteriosclerosis and senile brain disease may cause mental disorders among the elderly. But many so-called senile cases, compounded by anxiety, loss, grief, or psychosomatic problems, are treatable and sometimes preventable.

It is not true that all old people are content and serene. The tranquil picture of Grandma sitting in her rocker with her hands folded in her lap is misleading. It is true that many older people have learned to accept rather than fight the hardships and vicissitudes of life. Yet, for most people, old age brings increasing problems — physical, emotional, social, and financial — to harass and worry them. Depression, sometimes confused with dementia because the symptoms of disorientation, failing memory, and eccentric behavior are similar, is a frequent problem among the elderly.

It is not true that old people cannot be productive or active. More than 3 million Americans over 65 years of age work full- or part-time, and many others, not counted in labor statistics, work but do not report their earnings because of Social Security restrictions. Healthy old people do not disengage; rather, they are active and involved (Figure 18-1). Butler and Lewis (1977) emphasize that activity instead of disengagement produces the best psychological climate for the elderly.

It is not true that most older people have diminished intellectual capacity. Studies show that intelligence, learning ability, and other intellectual skills do not decline with age (Butler & Lewis, 1977). Intelligence is more directly affected by health; poor health and near death cause a drop in intellectual

506

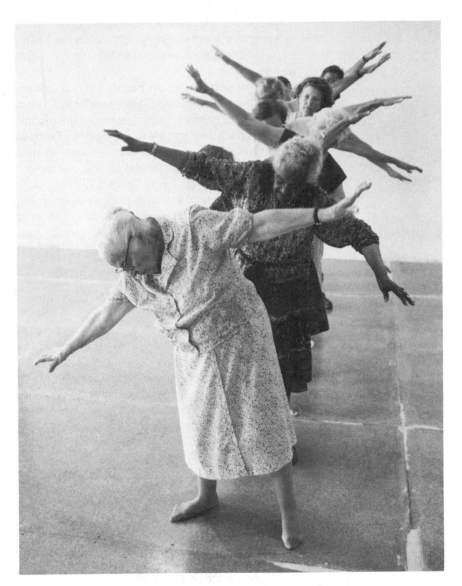

Figure 18-1
These senior citizens in Washington, DC have turned to modern dance as a form of creative expression. Their active involvement in a meaningful activity signals healthy aging.

functioning (Jarvik, Eisdorfer, & Blum, 1975). Speed of reaction tends to decrease with age, but basic intelligence does not. In fact, some abilities, such as judgment, accuracy, and general knowledge, may increase with age. Most older people are largely capable of making their own decisions; they want and need the freedom to make choices and to be as independent as their limitations will allow.

Misconceptions about their intelligence often lead to the treatment of older

507

people as children. Practitioners who infantilize their approaches to and programs for the elderly may create self-fulfilling prophecies: old age may indeed resemble a second childhood if the elderly are stripped of their rights and dignity.

It is not true that all old people are resistant to change. In a study of nursing home residents, Carp (1966) concluded that rigidity is not intrinsic to aging but rather tends to result from difficult social or physical situations. When these pressures are lifted, the rigidity disappears. The elderly have spent a lifetime adapting to change, with varying measures of success. The ability to change does not depend on age but rather on personality traits acquired throughout life (Butler & Lewis, 1977). An older person's apparent resistance to change may be a factor of her established personality. Then again, her conservatism may be caused by socioeconomic pressures. Financial concern, for example, may cause an older property owner to vote against a school levy that would increase her taxes.

Characteristics of the Healthy Elderly

To counter these misconceptions, we need to ask instead, "What does it mean to age successfully?" What is healthy old age? This has been a topic of growing interest among gerontologists. The Andrus Gerontology Center at the University of Southern California and others have been conducting research in this area for many years. We don't know conclusively all the variables that influence healthy old age, but we do know that a lifetime of healthy habits and circumstances, a strong social support system, and a positive emotional outlook all have a major influence on the resources people bring to their later years. Most of us recognize a healthy older person when we meet one. Let us meet such a person.

CASE EXAMPLE

Minerva Blackstone, affectionately called Minnie by her friends, is a lively 87-year-old woman who enjoys life. Every day, except in bad weather, she walks the half mile to the house of her granddaughter, Karen, for a visit. There she works on the quilt, stretched on a frame, that she is making for Karen. Twice a week Minnie takes the city bus to the senior citizens' center to join her friends in an exercise class. Although her eyesight has failed somewhat, Minnie enjoys reading in the evening and crocheting while she watches TV. Mysteries and comedies are her favorite kinds of stories. She is not content, however, unless she has kept up on the latest political developments. She always has opinions on current events and expresses them with vigorous shakes of her curly white hair at her monthly group meeting on women and politics. She has a good appetite and generally sleeps well. Minor arthritis does not hamper her activities, nor does the hypertension that she controls by taking her medication with conscientious regularity. Minnie is enjoying healthy, successful old age.

What is healthy old age? As we said earlier, the vast majority (95 percent) of the elderly, like Minnie Blackstone, are living outside institutions and maintaining relative independence, even those with chronic diseases and other disabilities. They are able to function. The ability to function is a key indicator of health and wellness and is an important factor in understanding healthy aging. Good health in the elderly means maintaining the maximum degree of physical, mental, and social vigor of which one is capable. It means being able to adapt, to continue to handle stress, and to be active and involved. In short, healthy aging means being able to function with, and despite, disabilities, with no more than ordinary help from others (Public Health Service, 1979).

Wellness among the elderly population varies considerably. It is influenced by many factors such as personality traits, life experiences, current physical health, and current societal supports. Some elderly people, like Minnie Blackstone, demonstrate maximum adaptability, resourcefulness, optimism, and activity. Others, often those from whom we tend to draw our stereotypes, have disengaged and present a picture of dependence and resignation. Most of the elderly population is somewhere in between these two extremes. Although the level of wellness varies among the elderly, that level can be raised. The challenge in community health nursing is to maximize the wellness potential of the elderly. Nurses must analyze and capitalize on the elderly's strengths, not focus only on their problems. As Butler and Lewis (1977) so poignantly describe it, the goal is to enable older people to thrive, not merely survive.

Health Needs of the Elderly

The third requirement for working with any population is to know that group's health problems and needs. Aging in and of itself is not a health problem. Rather, aging is a normal, irreversible physiological process. Its pace, however, can sometimes be delayed, researchers are discovering (Rosenfeld, 1976), and many of the problems associated with aging can be prevented (Hanlon & Pickett, 1984, p. 442). The aging process is subtle, gradual, and lifelong. One can see remarkable differences between individual's rates of aging; even in a single individual, various systems of the body age at different rates. Thus, chronological age cannot serve as an indicator of health needs; "nevertheless, the proportion of people with health problems increases with age and, as a group, the elderly are more likely than younger persons to suffer from multiple, chronic, and often disabling conditions" (Public Health Service, 1979, p. 71).

The leading causes of death among the age 65 and over population are heart disease, cancer, and stroke followed by influenza and pneumonia, arteriosclerosis, and diabetes mellitus (National Center for Health Statistics,

1981). Deaths in the group aged 65 to 74 years have declined, but the sharpest rise occurs for those over age 85. While most of the elderly population is healthy, 80 percent have at least one chronic condition causing nearly half of the elderly population to experience some kind of activity limitations (Mundinger, 1983, p. 171). A small proportion are dependent and disabled, requiring more extensive care.

The most frequent health problems experienced by older people in the community are arthritis, reduced vision, hearing losses, heart conditions, and hypertension. Acute illness, such as influenza and pneumonia, or injuries, such as burns and those from falls, occur less frequently and can often be prevented.

A significant health problem for the elderly arises from adverse drug effects. Older people's bodies handle drugs differently than those of younger people on whom most clinical trials take place. Thus, overprescription of medications or complicated drug regimens for many older persons lead to unexpected and dangerous drug interactions. The elderly need education about the drugs they take and their possible effects. They also need proper supervision of their overall medication intake.

Depression, too, is a difficult problem for older adults. Loss of a spouse, loss of friends, economic problems, physical disease and disability, loneliness, or drug side effects can make elderly people feel that life holds no meaning. Social and emotional withdrawal often occurs as does suicide.

In addition to these problems, elderly people have specific health needs. At all stages of life, people have the same basic needs. We know that the elderly, like any age group, have physiological, safety, love and belonging, esteem, and self-actualization needs. Their physical, emotional, and social needs are complex and interrelated. As community health nurses assess the health of the elderly population, however, some needs in particular demand extra attention.

Among these is the need for *good nutrition*. People who have maintained sound dietary habits throughout life need change little in old age. Many have not established such habits but may wish to. One study of an elderly population group revealed their desire for help with weight control, cooking, and shopping for good nutrition (Archer, Kelly, & Bisch, 1984, p. 166). Older people need to maintain their optimal weight by eating a generally low-fat, moderate-carbohydrate, and high-protein diet. They should avoid habitual use of laxatives, adding instead more fiber and bulk to their diet. Loss of teeth will cause some to need foods that are easier to chew. Eating should be a pleasurable experience, preferably taking place in the company of other people.

Older people continue to need *exercise* (Fig. 18-2). Aging does not and should not involve passivity; instead, physical activity and movement contribute to quality of intellectual and physical performance in old age. Exercise, such as a daily walk, can keep muscles in good tone, enhance circulation, and

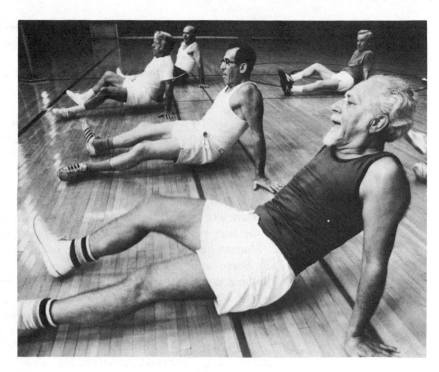

Figure 18-2
Community health nurses must learn the needs of each population group, such as elderly persons' need for physical fitness. Here a group of senior citizens exercise in their community center gymnasium.

promote mental health. Exercise may occur in connection with such activities as homemaking chores, gardening, hobbies, or recreation and sports. Often such physical outlets are done in the company of other people (Fig. 18-2), meeting social and emotional needs as well.

Economic security is another major need for older adults. Worry over finances is often one of the most debilitating factors in old age. Fearing the potential costs of major illness and not wanting to be a burden on family or friends, many older people will conserve their limited financial resources by eating cheaply, using health resources sparingly, and spending little on themselves: "Too often, the fear — let alone the reality — of financial straits prevents elderly people from leading the full and active lives of which they are capable" (Public Health Service, 1979, p. 77). Putting older people in touch with appropriate community resources can do much to relieve this source of stress.

Older people need *independence*. As much as possible, the elderly need to make their own decisions and manage their own lives. Even those with activity limitations because of disability can still exercise decision-making options about many, if not most, aspects of their daily living. The need for autonomy — to be able to assert ourselves as separate individuals — is great for all of us. With life's restrictions ever increasing for the elderly person, this need is all the greater. Independence helps to meet another need, that

511

of self-respect and dignity. The elderly need to have their ideas and suggestions heard and acted upon and to be addressed by their preferred names in a respectful tone of voice. Respect for the old is not a strong value in our culture, but one that needs to be cultivated. Older people represent a rich resource of wisdom, experience, and patience that we are generally wasting in our country.

Older people need *companionship and social interaction,* particularly when they live alone. The company of other people as well as the companionship of a household pet offers an avenue for expression and response and adds meaning to life. Many studies of mortality patterns demonstrate that older adults living together have a greater survival rate and retain their independence longer than those who live alone (Hanlon & Pickett, 1984, p. 436). The problem is of greatest significance for women who outnumber men considerably in the later years and who live alone more frequently (Figure 18-3).

Meaningful activity is another need of the elderly. It too adds purpose to life. Some kind of active role in community life is essential for mental health, satisfaction, and self-esteem. It can range from involvement in hobbies, such as gardening or crafts, to volunteer work or even full-time employment. One current example is the federally supported Foster Grandparents and Senior Companions program that engages the help of more than 18,000 seniors. These older adults work 20 hours a week offering companionship and guidance to 63,500 handicapped children across the country. Another program, the Foundation for Grandparenting in New York, plans to use grandparent volunteers to work with schoolchildren on a long-term relationship basis ("America's forgotten resource: Grandparents," 1984, p. 77).

A final need of the elderly, and one that is receiving increasing attention, is that of a *dignified death.* Quality of life has become an important issue, and as Kübler-Ross (1975) describes it, death is the final stage of growth, deserving that same measure of quality. A dignified death — as free as possible from pain, humiliation, discomfort, or financial concerns — can be the end product of a quality aging process. For most elderly persons this means having a choice, whenever possible, about where and under what circumstances death will occur. Freedom from financial worries, knowledge that their affairs and family members are taken care of, opportunity for spiritual counseling, and peaceful surroundings, preferably at home with the support of loved ones, are all important quality considerations.

Community Health Perspective

Another requirement for nursing of the elderly as a population group is to view them from a broad, community health perspective. In general, we can divide nursing service to the elderly into two approaches. One approach emphasizes the science of geriatrics; the other, the science of gerontology.

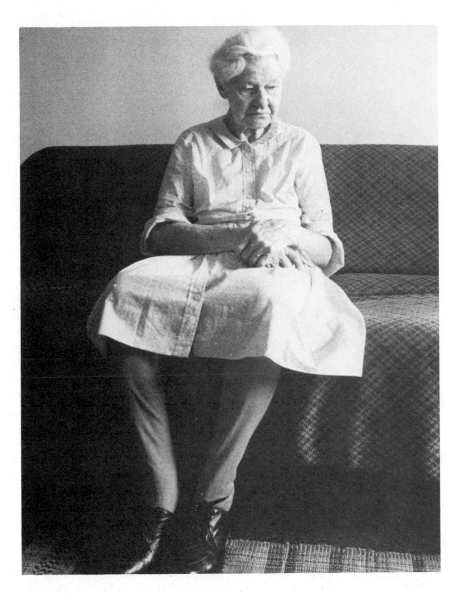

Figure 18-3
Many elderly people, particularly women, live alone. Without the company and stimulation of other people their days can be long, lonely, and empty of meaning.

Although these fields overlap, they tend to differ in at least one significant way. Geriatrics is the study of diseases of old age, while gerontology studies the broader phenomena of aging itself (Burnside, 1976). Geriatric nursing in the past has been oriented primarily toward care of the sick aged. Gerontological nursing, a broader practice, concentrates on preventing illness and promoting the health and maximum functioning of older adults (Davis, 1975). While both are important dimensions of nursing practice, a community health perspective emphasizes the gerontological approach.

513

Community health nurses work with many elderly people. In one instance, the nurse may promote and maintain the health of a vigorous 80-year-old man who lives alone in his home. As another example, the nurse may give postsurgical care at home to a 69-year-old woman, teach her husband how to care for her, and help them contact needed community resources for shopping, meals, housekeeping, and transportation services. Perhaps the focus is on teaching nutrition and a healthful life-style to a family, including the 73-year-old grandmother who lives with them. Yet again, the nurse may lead a support group for senior citizens who have recently lost their spouses through death.

A large portion of the community health nurse's work with the elderly is at the individual, family, and group levels. However, a community health perspective also leads to concern for and work with large aggregates of the elderly. There are many population groups composed of elderly persons. All the seniors attending an adult day-care center, belonging to a retirement community, living in a nursing home, or using Meals on Wheels are some examples. Others include residents of a senior citizens' high-rise apartment building, retired business and professional women, elderly residents in a community at risk for glaucoma, the elderly poor, and skid row alcoholics.

Having a community perspective means that the nurse sees the "forest," not just the "trees." Problems in individual segments of a population group can negatively effect the rest of the group. Witness the spread of influenza when people are unprotected. Conversely, health-promoting and disease-preventing measures aimed at an entire population group enhance the health of the individuals involved. For example, a positive life-style emphasis in a retirement community or a comprehensive nutrition and meal-planning program in a senior day care center can have far-reaching health benefits for the older adults who make up each of those populations. A community health "forest thinker" keeps the big picture in mind and designs interventions for the public good.

Health Services for the Elderly Population

How well are we meeting the needs of our older adults? To answer this question, we must first raise other questions. Do health programs for the elderly encompass the full range of needed services? Are they close enough that they can be reached easily when needed? Do they encourage elderly clients to function independently? Do they treat senior citizens with respect and preserve their dignity? Do they recognize older adults' need for companionship, economic security, and social status? When appropriate, do they promote meaningful activities instead of overworked games like bingo and shuffleboard? Games can be useful diversions but must be balanced with opportunities for creative outlets, continued learning, and community service.

Several criteria emerge from this list of questions that describe an effective community health service delivery system for the elderly. Four, in particular, deserve our attention.

CRITERIA FOR EFFECTIVE SERVICE

Comprehensive

An effective community health service delivery system for the elderly should be comprehensive. Many communities provide some programs, such as limited health screening or selected activities, but do not offer a full range of services that would more adequately meet the needs of their senior citizens. Gaps and duplication in programs most often result from poor or nonexistent community-wide planning. Furthermore, such planning should be based on thorough assessment of elderly people's needs in that community. A comprehensive set of services should provide the following:

Health care services (prevention, early diagnosis and treatment, rehabilitation)
Health education (including preparation for retirement)
Recreation and activity programs
Adult day care programs
Specialized transportation services
In-home services
Adequate financial support

Coordinated

A second criterion for a community service delivery system for the elderly is coordination. Often older persons go from one agency to the next. After visiting one place for food stamps, they may go to another for answers to Medicaid questions, another for congregate dining, and still another for health screening. Such a potpourri of services reflects a system organized for the convenience of providers rather than consumers. It encourages nonuse or misuse. Instead, there should be coordinated, community-wide assessment and planning. Communities must consider alternatives such as multiservice agencies that can meet many needs in one location. As a surgeon general's report indicates, "Many elderly people . . . need a range of services — dietary guidance, eye care, foot care, dental care, and social assistance, as well as routine medical care. And these are best provided at one center" (Public Health Service, 1979, p. 76).

A coordinated information and referral system provides another needed link. Most communities need a better information network. A directory of all resources and services for the elderly with the name and telephone number of a contact person for each listing is available in some communities and should be developed in those without one. A simplified information

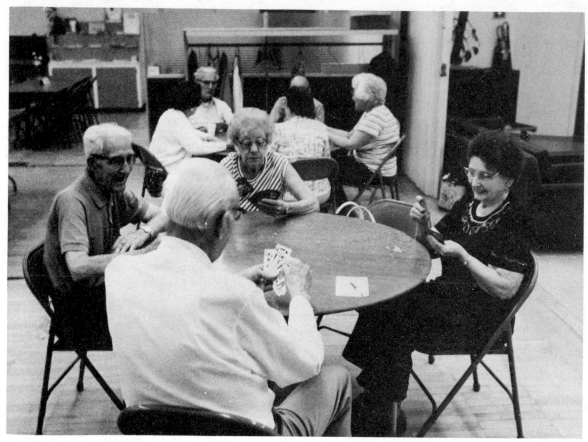

Figure 18-4
Senior citizens are a group whose needs must also be viewed from an aggregate perspective if community health services are to be effective. Recreational activities are one of many programs included in a comprehensive system serving the elderly population.

and referral system — a system that includes one number to call to find out what resources and services are available and how to get them — is particularly helpful to older people.

Accessible

A third criterion is accessibility. Too often, services for the elderly are not conveniently located or are prohibitive in cost. Some communities are considering multiservice community centers that would bring programs and services for the elderly closer to home. More convenient and perhaps specialized transportation services and more in-home services, such as Meals on Wheels, may further solve accessibility problems for many older adults. Federal, state, and private funding sources can be tapped to ease the burden on the already economically pressured elderly population.

516

Quality

Finally, an effective community service system for older people promotes quality programs. By that is meant services that truly address the needs and concerns of a community's senior citizens. Evaluation of the quality of a community's services for the elderly is closely tied to their assessed needs. What are this specific population group's needs in terms of nutrition, exercise, economic security, independence, social interaction, meaningful activities, and preparation for death? Planning for quality community services depends on having adequate, accurate, and current data. Periodic needs assessment is a necessity to ensure updated information and to promote quality services. Unfortunately, in most communities this is not done with any regularity or thoroughness, if at all. Many agencies in a given community are involved in delivering services for the elderly. Collaboration and surveys of seniors, perhaps spearheaded by community health nurses as was done in northern California (Archer, Kelly, & Bisch, 1984), can provide that information so vital for planning the needed quality programs.

INSTITUTIONAL CARE

While only 5 percent of the elderly population live in formal institutions, such organizations remain the most visible type of health service for older adults. Of these, nursing homes make up the largest portion. More than 1.5 million elderly persons live in nursing homes, and despite government attempts to protect these individuals and contain costs through admission and care standards, costs have increased along with questions about quality of care.

There is widespread fear and despair associated with nursing homes. Too many older people and their families have been exploited by an industry that frequently puts profit ahead of meeting this group's needs. The book *Tender Loving Greed* (Mendelson, 1974) graphically describes the problem. Even in institutions where the quality of care is acceptable, costs are so high that family resources are soon depleted. Although Medicaid and Medicare pay for most (close to 60 percent) of nursing home costs, life savings that older parents had hoped to leave for their children may be quickly consumed, forcing them into indigence and dependence on public funds. Dread of nursing homes arises, too, from dehumanizing institutional regulations, such as segregation of sexes, strict social policies, and overuse of tranquilizers and demeaning or even abusive conditions that promote institutional control rather than the clients' well-being.

Institutions housing the dependent elderly involve several levels of nursing care. Those involving the highest level are called skilled nursing facilities. Less costly are intermediate care facilities that still provide health care but decrease the amount and type of care given. Medicare generally only pays for skilled nursing facilities services. Medicaid pays for care in skilled as well as intermediate care facilities. Personal care homes, a third level, offer basic social supports, such as bathing and grooming, without medical services. Payment may come from private funds, Title XX (Social Security Act) funds, old age assistance, or aid to the disabled. Boarding homes, a fourth level, house elderly persons needing meal service and light housekeeping but who can manage their own personal care. Government funds are not available to support these institutions. Congregate care and group homes are an alternative for specific elderly populations, such as alcoholics or developmentally disabled, and are often subsidized by concerned community organizations.

DEINSTITUTIONALIZATION

"Deinstitutionalizing" people, or promoting their living outside institutions, has received considerable emphasis recently. The trend started several decades ago when it became evident that tuberculosis patients improved more readily and cost of care was less if they were treated on an outpatient basis. Care of the mentally ill began to be deinstitutionalized in the 1950s for the same reasons, and treatment of the developmentally disabled followed suit. For the elderly population we now see an increasing emphasis on avoidance of needless institutionalization and maintenance of functional independence.

The trend toward deinstitutionalized care for the elderly stems from several incentives. The potential for cost saving appears to be much greater if dependent older people can be discharged from institutions and maintained at home. We know that many nursing home residents are there needlessly (Hanlon & Pickett, 1984, p. 440) and could manage outside the institution given adequate assistance. Deinstitutionalization encourages functional independence as well as emotional well-being.

On the other hand, deinstitutionalization is not the panacea that many believe it to be. Although some studies have demonstrated cost savings, others have shown that community-based systems are more expensive (Toff, 1981). We do not have complete data yet for comparisons. Research has not yet fully assessed the costs to the community for health and social services incurred in maintaining deinstitutionalized dependent people. Nor have most studies been able to determine the change in functional level of people being deinstitutionalized (Hanlon & Pickett, 1984, p. 440). Furthermore, services for the dependent elderly in the community are often fragmented, inadequate, and inaccessible with little or no maintenance of standards or quality control. Institutions, despite their problems, are at least regulated and must be accountable for their clients' safety and care.

There is a solution. The dependent elderly need someone in the community to assess their particular needs, assemble and coordinate the appropriate resources and services, and serve as their advocate. It is a role most appropriately filled by the community health nurse. This case management approach tailors services to fit the needs of clients and enables them to function longer outside of institutions (Hanlon & Pickett, 1984, p. 440).

Various techniques are available to assess the needs of older adults. A comprehensive one, the Older Americans Resources and Services Information System (OARS), developed by Duke University, established baseline data on clients' well-being, available economic and social resources, physical and mental health status, and clients' capacity for self-care (Pfeiffer, 1978; Fillenbaum & Smyer, 1981). The clients' capacity for self-care is assessed by means of the Capacity for Self-care Index, which ascertains clients' ability to go outdoors, climb stairs, move about their homes, bathe, dress, and cut toenails (Shanas, 1980). Other techniques, like the Activities of Daily Living (ADL) survey (Katz, et al., 1970), determine an elderly person's physical, psychological, and social needs. A frequently overlooked area for assessment is elderly clients' spiritual needs. Religious dedication and spiritual concern often increase in later years. Limited ability or lack of transportation may prevent older people from attending religious services or engaging in spiritually enhancing activities. Self-health ratings, including clients' reporting on their spiritual needs, is another useful assessment technique.

The case management concept has been practiced by community health nurses for many years with their own clients with a primary focus on health needs. Social workers use case management to address their clients' problems with their assessment focusing on social needs, including financial problems. Some health maintenance organizations provide a coordinated system of services for their enrolled clients. Unfortunately, many elderly people in the community have no such advocate; a more comprehensive, community-wide system is needed in many localities to serve the total elderly population. Such a system could be based on establishment of an agency specifically designed to serve as case manager, or "agent," to assess client needs and assemble existing agencies and services to meet those needs (Kodner & Feldman, 1981).

Other alternatives to institutionalization include home services and partial day care services. Home care provides services, such as skilled nursing care, physical or speech therapy, homemaker services, and dietetic counseling. Day care can offer shelter, social activities, nutrition, nursing care, and physical and speech therapy. Both alternatives are useful for families unable to care for an elderly member during work or school hours.

SERVICES FOR THE WELL ELDERLY

Services for the other 95 percent of the elderly population should have as their primary goals the avoidance of needless institutionalization and the maintenance of functional independence. Needs assessment, using techniques such as OARS or the ADL survey mentioned in the previous section, forms

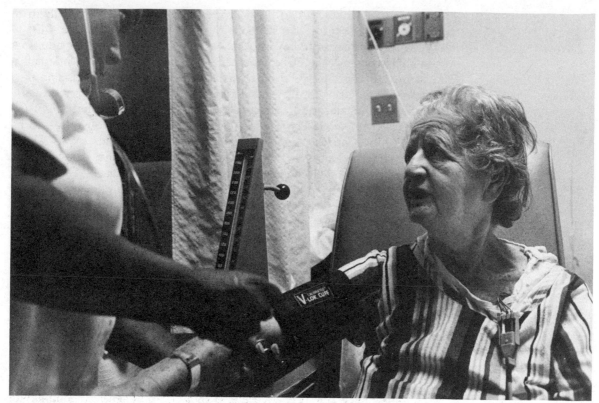

Figure 18-5
Having her blood pressure taken, part of geriatric screening, can lead to early detection of health problems and be reassuring to this elderly woman.

the basis for determining appropriate services. Although most of the well elderly can assess their own health status, many are reluctant to seek needed help. Thus, *outreach programs* serve an important function in many communities. They locate elderly persons in need of health or social assistance and refer them to appropriate resources.

Geriatric screening is another important program for early detection and treatment of health problems among older adults. Conditions in particular to watch for include hypertension, glaucoma, hearing disorders, cancers, diabetes, anemias, depression, and nutritional deficiencies. At the same time, assessment of elderly clients' socialization, housing, and economic needs with proper referrals can prevent further problems from developing that would influence their health status.

Health maintenance programs may be offered through a single agency, such as a health maintenance organization, or coordinated by a case management agency with referrals to other providers. These programs should cover a wide range of health services needed by the elderly, such as those given below (Public Health Service, 1979, pp. 76–78):

Dietary guidance and food services like Meals on Wheels or group meal
    services
Dental care
Podiatry
Vision testing and eyeglasses
Hearing screening and hearing aid assistance
Exercise and fitness programs
Speech or physical therapy
Home health services, including skilled nursing and home health aide services
Routine medical care
Medical supplies or equipment
Health education
Medication supervision

Social assistance services may well be offered in conjunction with health
maintenance programs since the two are so interrelated. The elderly have
many needs in this area. They include the following:

Financial aid and counseling
Safe and affordable housing
Transportation services
Home maintenance assistance (housekeeping, chores, repairs)
Recreation and educational programs
Religious ministries
Community centers for social opportunities
Communication services (phones, access to health professionals)
Legal aid and counseling
Volunteer and employment opportunities
Library services, including talking books and large-print publications
Escort and protective services
Friendly visiting and companions
Senior citizen discounts (food, drugs, transportation, recreation)

Respite care is a service receiving increasing attention and is aimed primarily
at care giver needs. Many elderly persons at home are cared for by a
spouse or other family member. The demands of such care can be exhausting
unless the care giver can get some relief, or respite — thus the name of
this service. Respite care may be available through an agency that provides
volunteers to relieve care givers, giving them time away on a regular basis
or permitting a periodic vacation. Some hospitals and nursing homes provide
extra rooms to give temporary institutional housing for the elderly while care
givers take a break. Elderly clients may also need a change from the constant
interaction with their care givers.

Hospice care may be offered through an institution such as a hospital, or it may be a program providing services that enables dying persons to stay at home. Its purpose is to make the dying process as dignified, free from discomfort, and emotionally, spiritually, and socially supportive as possible. Some community health nursing agencies offer hospice programs staffed by their nurses. For the elderly, it is a service that has been well received, meets important needs, and is growing in use.

Implications for Community Health Nursing

Community health nurses can make a significant contribution to the health of the elderly population. Because these nurses are in the community and already have contact with many older adults, they are in a prime position to begin needs assessment and planning for the health of this group. Though many of the services named above are not within the scope of nursing's practice, the case management role can and often should be a critical aspect of the nurse's contribution to this population.

The health care scene in terms of services available for the elderly is changing dramatically. The numbers and types of home care services, for example, are mushrooming. Many entrepreneurs, recognizing the potential of this growing market, are offering goods and services targeted for older adults. Nursing must keep abreast of these changes — aware of new developments, new programs, new regulations, new social and economic forces (like prospective payment) and their potential impact on the provision of health services. Even more important, community health nurses will need to be proactive, designing interventions that maximize nursing's resources and provide the greatest benefit to elderly clients. For example, community health nurses could develop a case management program for older adults as a community-wide assessment, information, and referral service. Such a program might contract with existing agencies to serve as a clearinghouse for the elderly and channel clients to appropriate services. Financing of such a program might be based on tax dollars (if a public agency), grants, or some innovative fee-for-service reimbursement system.

Many of the elderly population's health problems can be prevented and their health promoted. Change to a healthier life-style is one of the most important preventive measures the nurse can emphasize. Examples include stopping smoking, eating regular and well-balanced meals, exercising regularly, keeping weight within 15 pounds of normal for body build, consuming no or only moderate amounts of alcohol, getting proper rest, and maintaining a healthy emotional outlook. Educating the elderly about their health conditions and use of their medications is another important focus that can prevent problems. Influenza and pneumonia can be prevented through regular health maintenance and immunizations. Other problems associated with environmental conditions and the aging process, such as arthritis, diabetes, and some cancers, can be diagnosed early, treated, and their influence diminished in terms of their effect on functional independence.

With an elderly population that is increasing in size and age, community health nurses face a serious challenge in addressing its needs. At the same time nursing can be on the forefront of developing innovative health services for this group, rising to meet the opportunity and the challenge.

Summary

The elderly population is increasing in size and age. Accompanying these changes are this group's escalating health needs with concomitant requirements for new and improved services. Community health nursing has an opportunity to accept the challenge, study the needs of older adults, and develop effective, population-based nursing interventions. Population-based nursing requires four emphases: (1) know the characteristics of the population, (2) avoid misconceptions about them, (3) know the group's health needs, and (4) maintain an aggregate perspective.

The number of adults 65 and over is growing. Their percentage of the total popualtion is increasing. Women still live longer than men, and more women are alone in their later years. Given these facts, the potential for a growing number of dependent elderly is great.

Misconceptions or practitioner bias about older adults can interfere with effective community health nursing practice. Contrary to some beliefs, most (95 percent) of the elderly live outside institutions and are relatively independent. Chronological age does not determine "oldness." Senility is not a problem for most older people, but depression and worry often are. Many elderly people are active in the community, most maintain their intellectual ability, and many adapt well to change.

Healthy aging involves the ability to function as independently as possible. It means maintaining the maximum degree of physical, mental, and social vigor of which one is capable. It includes the ability to adapt, to handle stress and change, to be meaningfully active and involved.

The health needs of the elderly center around chronic, often progressive, and disabling conditions. Leading causes of death are heart disease, cancer, and stroke. The most frequent health problems are arthritis, vision and hearing losses, heart conditions, and hypertension. Acute illnesses common to the elderly, primarily influenza and pneumonia, are preventable. Other health problems of older adults include drug reactions and depression.

To promote and maintain health and prevent illness, elderly people need good nutrition, exercise, economic security, independence, companionship and social interaction, and meaningful activity. They also deserve, when possible, a dignified and peaceful death.

An aggregate, community health perspective means that the nurse sees and seeks to serve the entire population of older adults, not just individuals. This is enhanced by examining what services are available and needed, and analyzing their effectiveness when used. Effective community health services for the elderly should be comprehensive, coordinated, accessible, and of high quality, targeted to the specific needs of the older population.

Institutions house 5 percent of the elderly. Most of these are nursing homes where elderly residents require skilled nursing care. Intermediate care facilities, personal care homes, and boarding homes offer decreasing amounts and levels of care.

A trend toward deinstitutionalization is creating many more alternatives for older adults to maintain functional independence at home. It has the potential for being more cost-effective but poses new problems with evaluating quality and coordinating services. A solution can be application of the case management concept, which offers a centralized system for assessing the elderly population's needs and matching those needs with appropriate services.

Services needed by the well elderly include outreach programs, geriatric screening, health maintenance programs that cover a wide range of health services, social assistance services, respite care, and hospice care.

Community health nurses can promote and preserve the health of the elderly by practicing from a perspective of population-based nursing, by developing more effective services such as comprehensive case management, and by promoting healthy life-styles and activities among older adults.

Study Questions

1. Picture in your mind an elderly person whom you know well or know a great deal about. Make a list of characteristics that describe that person. How many of these characteristics fit your picture of most senior citizens? What are your biases about the elderly?

2. If you were Minnie Blackstone's community health nurse, what interventions would you consider using to maintain and promote her health? Why?

3. As part of your regular community health nursing work load, you visit a senior day care center one afternoon a week. You take the blood pressures of several people who are on hypertensive medications and do some nutritional counseling. The center accommodates 60 senior clients, and you would like to serve the health needs of the entire aggregate. What are some potential health needs of this group? What actions might you consider taking that would be at an aggregate level?

4. Assume you have been asked by your local health department to determine the needs of the elderly population in your community. How would you begin conducting such a needs assessment? What data might you want

to collect? How would you find out what services are already being offered and whether or not they are adequate?

References

America's forgotten resource: Grandparents (1984, April 30). *U.S. News & World Report*, pp. 76–77.

Archer, S. E., Kelly, C. D., & Bisch, S. A. (1984). Senior life-style survey. In S. E. Archer, C. D. Kelly, & S. A. Bisch (Eds.), *Implementing change in communities: A collaborative process*. St. Louis: C. V. Mosby.

Burnside, I. M. (Ed.). (1976). *Nursing and the aged*. New York: McGraw-Hill.

Butler, R. N., & Lewis, M. I. (1977). *Aging and mental health: Positive psychosocial approaches* (2nd ed.). St. Louis: C. V. Mosby.

Carp, R. M. (1966). *A future for the aged: Victoria Plaza and its residents*. Austin: University of Texas Press.

Davis, B. A. (1975). Gerontological nursing comes of age. *Journal of Gerontological Nursing, 1,* 6.

Fillenbaum, G. G., & Smyer, M. A. (1981). The development, validity, and reliability of the OARS multidimensional functional assessment questionnaire, *Journal of Gerontology, 36*(4), 428.

Hanlon, J. J., & Pickett, G. E. (1984). *Public health: Administration and practice* (8th ed.) St. Louis: Times Mirror/Mosby.

Jarvik, L. F., Eisdorfer, C., & Blum, J. E. (Eds.). (1975). *Intellectual functioning in adults*. New York: Springer Verlag.

Katz, S., et al. (1970). Progress in the development of the index of ADL. *The Gerontologist, 10,* 20–27.

Kodner, D. L., & Feldman, E. S. (1981). The service coordination/delivery dichotomy: A critical issue to address in reforming the long-term care system. Paper presented at annual meeting of the American Public Health Association, Los Angeles.

Kübler-Ross, E. (1975). *Death: The final stage of growth*. Englewood Cliffs, N. J.: Prentice-Hall.

Mendelson, M. A. (1974). *Tender loving greed*. New York: Knopf.

Mundinger, M. *Home care controversy: Too little, too late, too costly*. Rockville, MD: Aspen.

National Center for Health Statistics, Statistical Abstracts Division of Vital Statistics. (1981). Hyattsville, MD, U.S. Department of Health and Human Services.

Pfeiffer, E. (Ed.). (1978). *Multidimensional functional assessment: The OARS methodology* (2nd ed.). Durham, NC: Duke University Center for Study of Aging and Human Development.

Public Health Service. (1979). *Healthy people: The surgeon general's report on health promotion and disease prevention* (DHEW Publication No. 79-55071). Washington, DC: U.S. Government Printing Office.

Rosenfeld, A. (1976). *Prolongevity*. New York: Avon Books.

Shanas, E. (1980). Self-assessment of physical function: White and black elderly in the United States. In S. Haynes & M. Feinleib (Eds.), *Epidemiology of aging* (NIH Pub. No. 80-969). Washington, DC: U.S. Department of Health and Human Services.

Spiegel, A. D. (1983). *Home healthcare: Home birthing to hospice care.* Owings Mills, MD: National Health Publishing.

Toff, G. E. (1981). *Alternatives to institutional care for the elderly: An analysis of state initiatives.* Washington, DC: Intergovernmental Health Policy Project.

Selected Readings

Archer, S. E., Kelly, C. D., & Bisch, S. A. (1984). Senior-life style survey. In S. E. Archer, C. D. Kelly, & S. A. Bisch (Eds.), *Implementing change in communities: A collaborative process.* St. Louis: C. V. Mosby.

Archer, S. E., Kelly, C. D., & Bisch, S. A. (1984). Senior resources survey. In S. E. Archer, C. D. Kelly, & S. A. Bisch. *Implementing change in communities: A collaborative process.* St. Louis: C. V. Mosby.

Birenbaum, A., Aronson, M., & Seiffer, S. (1979). Training medical students to appreciate the special problems of the elderly. *The Gerontologist, 19,* 575–579.

Branch, L., Katz, S., Kneipmann, K., & Papsidero, J. (1984). A prospective study of functional status among community elders. *American Journal of Public Health, 74,* 266–268.

Burnside, I. M. (Ed.). (1976) *Nursing and the aged.* New York: McGraw-Hill.

Butler, R. N., & Lewis, M. I. (1977). *Aging and mental health: Positive psychosocial approaches* (2nd ed.). St. Louis: C. V. Mosby.

Clemons, B. (1982). Teaching longevity. *Friendly Exchange, 3*(1), 21.

Cohen, C., & Sokolvsky, J. (1980). Social engagement versus isolation: The case of the aged in SRO hotels. *The Gerontologist, 20,* 36–43.

Collins, R. (1982). Toward a theory of gerontological nursing. *Nursing and Health Care, 3,* 550–556.

de Tornyay, R. (1980). Public health nursing: The nurse's role in community-based practice. *Annual Review of Public Health, 1,* 83.

Eisdorfer, E., & Wilke, F. (1976). Research in aging. In A. Hoffman (Ed.), *Daily needs and interests of older people.* Springfield, IL: Charles C Thomas.

Ekerdt, D., Baden, L., Bossé, R., & Dibbs, E. The effect of retirement on physical health. *American Journal of Public Health, 73,* 779–783.

Fahey, C. (1981). Some political, economic, and social considerations. In R. Morris (Ed.), *Allocating health resources for the aged and disabled.* Lexington, MA: D. C. Heath.

Fowles, D. (1978). *Some prospects for the future elderly population: Statistical reports on older Americans.* Washington, DC: U.S. Department of Health, Education and Welfare, Office of Human Development, National Clearinghouse on Aging.

Fries, J., & Crapo, L. (1981). *Vitality and aging: Implications of the rectangular curve.* San Francisco: W. H. Freeman.

Hanlon, J. J. & Pickett, G. E. (1984). Public health: Administration and Practice (8th ed.). St. Louis: Times Mirror/Mosby.

Hayter, J. (1983). Modifying the environment to help older persons. *Nursing and Health Care, 4,* 265–269.

Hickey, R., & Douglass, R. (1981). Mistreatment of the elderly in the domestic setting: An exploratory study. *American Journal of Public Health, 71,* 500.

Kane, R. A., & Kane, R. L. (1981). *Assessing the elderly.* Lexington, MA: Lexington Books.

Kane, R. L., & Kane, R. A. (1980). Long-term care: Can our society meet the needs of its elderly? *Annual Review of Public Health, 1* 227.

Managan, D., Wood, J., Heinichen, C., Hoffman, M., Hess, G., & Gillings, D. (1974). Older adults: A community survey of health needs. *Nursing Research, 23,* 426.

Muller, C. Health status and survival needs of the elderly. *American Journal of Public Health, 72,* 789–790.

Olson, I. (1982). Attitudes of nursing students toward aging and the aged. *Gerontology and Geriatrics Education, 2,* 233–236.

Pfeiffer, E. (Ed.) (1978). *Multidimensional functional assessment: The OARS Methodology* (2nd ed.). Durham, NC: Duke University Center for Study of Aging and Human Development.

Schrock, N. (1980). *Holistic assessment of the healthy aged.* New York: Wiley.

Shanas, E. (1980). Self-assessment of physical function: White and black elderly in the United States. In S. Haynes & M. Feinleib (Eds.), *Epidemiology of aging* (NIH Pub. No. 80-969). Washington, DC: U.S. Department of Health and Human Services.

Seigel, J. (1980). Recent and prospective demographic trends of the elderly population and some implications for health care. In S. Haynes and M. Feinlein (Eds.), *Epidemiology of aging* (NIH Pub. No. 80-969). Washington, DC: U.S. Department of Health and Human Services.

Stefl, B. (1976). Prevention measures and safety factors for the aged. In I. M. Burnside (Ed.), *Nursing and the aged.* New York: McGraw-Hill.

Stone, V. (1977). Nursing of older people. In E. Busse & E. Pfeiffer (Eds.), *Behavior and adaptation in late life* (2nd ed.). Boston: Little, Brown.

Training materials guide: Community care for the aging. (1981). Washington, DC: The Washington School of Psychiatry, Special Projects Division.

U.S. Department of Health , Education and Welfare, Public Health Service. (1969). *Working with older people: A guide to practice* (Vol. 1). Arlington, VA: Author, Division of Health Care Services.

19

Home Health Care

Barbara W. Spradley
Beverly Dorsey

There are people of all ages who need health services at home. Handicapped children, postsurgical patients, diabetics, quadriplegics, cancer patients, disabled elderly — all are part of a population group needing home health care. Often this group is referred to as the homebound population. It is true that many people are, in fact, confined to their homes. Others, who can leave with assistance, also need home services, although they are not technically homebound. An additional group of well people have also traditionally utilized home health services. Among them are new mothers and babies receiving infant care and postpartum follow-up, families receiving mental health counseling or parental guidance, and elderly people receiving assistance with medication supervision or nutritional counseling. Both homebound and well clients represent long-standing targets for community health nursing service in the home.

The picture in home health care is changing, however. New home care provision structures are emerging along with dramatic shifts in financing and provider roles. These changes are having a profound and continuing impact on community health nursing practice. In addition, the population needing home services is growing dramatically for several reasons. The number of dependent elderly is increasing with a corresponding rise in the incidence of chronic illnesses. Earlier hospital discharges, driven by cost-containment pressures, are creating an escalating number of people of all ages needing care in the community. Public awareness and demand for home services as an alternative to institutional care, broader third-party payment coverage for home care, along with greater physician acceptance of this phenomenon further enlarges the size of the group utilizing home health care. Finally, more acutely ill clients of all ages, who previously would have remained hospitalized or institutionalized, can be maintained outside the hospital or other institution because of sophisticated technological advances that allow such complex procedures as intravenous chemotherapy to be provided routinely at home.

This chapter examines the nature of home health services — how they have evolved and what they are today. It explores the needs of the population utilizing home health care, the services available to meet those needs, and community health nursing's role in home health care.

What Is Home Health Care?

Home health care, broadly defined, refers to all the services and products that maintain, restore, or promote physical, mental, and emotional health that are provided to clients in their homes. Its purpose is to maximize clients' level of independence and minimize the effects of existing disabilities through noninstitutional, supportive services (Lundberg, 1984; Stewart, 1979). In other words, a primary aim of care in the home is to prevent institutionalization (Mundinger, 1983).

The generally accepted definition of home health care has been stated by Warhola (1980):

> Home health care is that component of a continuum of comprehensive care whereby health, social and support services are provided to individuals and families in their places of residence and in the community for the purpose of promoting, maintaining or restoring health, or of maximizing the level of independence, while minimizing the effects of disability and illness, including terminal illness. Services appropriate to the needs of the individual and family are planned, coordinated, and made available by providers organized for the delivery of home care through the use of employed staff, contractual arrangements, or a combination of the two patterns.

Because the population utilizing home health care is so varied in age and needs, home health care covers a broad range of services. They include nursing; medical and dental care; pharmaceutical services; social services counseling; physical therapy; speech therapy; occupational therapy; laboratory testing; nutrition advice; homemaker or home health aide services; medical equipment and supplies provision; chore services; and transportation (Warhola, 1980). These services consist of two basic types: professional and support.

Home health care aims to accomplish the following (Home Care Guidelines, 1981):

1. Support families and individuals to avoid premature or inappropriate admission to an institutional care setting
2. Provide respite for families and responsible caretakers from continuous care and supervision of elderly and physically impaired persons and to assist caretakers in providing appropriate services
3. Maintain or restore elderly and physically impaired persons to optimal functional potential and to retard physical and emotional deterioration
4. Provide for support and follow-up services to persons residing in their own or a family member's home
5. Facilitate appropriate release of elderly and physically impaired persons from acute and long-term care facilities to family care or to other community-based programs
6. Provide home-based services to the terminally ill and their families in cooperation with other community-based health and social services.

These goals are not easily accomplished without an effective, coordinated home care system. Recent changes are forcing community health nurses and other providers to reexamine how this can be done. Home health care today has changed dramatically from its beginnings. Let us examine those changes and the forces shaping home health practice today.

Historical View of Home Health Services

Early home health services in the United States were organized and administered by laypersons in the late 1800s. They provided nursing care and taught cleanliness and home care techniques to the ill and their families. In 1877, the Women's Branch of the New York City Mission was the first group to employ a graduate nurse to deliver home care (Spiegel, 1983). Since that time nurses have played a primary role in home care.

The Visiting Nurse Service of New York City, established in 1893 by Lillian Wald, was the first U.S.-organized home nursing service. Through Lillian Wald's influence, the Metropolitan Life Insurance Company began a home nursing service for its New York City policyholders in 1909 that later became a model for other insurance companies in the 1920s. This included full coverage for home services (Mundinger, 1983, p. 37). The first government health department offering visiting nurse care was the Los Angeles Health Department established in 1898 (Spiegel, 1983).

Home care continued to be a part of nursing practice as the nursing profession developed. Twenty visiting nurse agencies serving the urban poor were operating by 1900, and in 1912 the Red Cross initiated a visiting nurse service for rural communities. Service was provided to the sick, well babies, and to schoolchildren. County health departments, too, were soon providing home nursing care in rural areas, enhanced by the development of automobiles.

Physicians were actively involved in home care before World War II. The war, however, created a physician shortage, and for the sake of efficiency, patients came to physicians. The cost-effectiveness of this pattern prompted its continuance, leaving a gap in home care that was filled by a growing number of visiting nurse associations.

The first hospital-based home care program was founded in 1947 by Dr. E. M. Bluestone at Montefiore Hospital in New York City. This program was prompted by the fact that many people with chronic illnesses were hospitalized for excessive periods of time. A team approach was utilized for posthospital acute care and was the beginning of the concept of convalescent care in the home. The program was also unique in that services were not limited to the poor or the elderly. The first paraprofessional home services — homemakers — were instituted then also. By 1958, this program had added therapy, nutrition, and X-ray and laboratory services to the initial team of physicians, nurses, and social workers. Housekeeping and chore services were provided indirectly through community resources (MacNamara, 1982).

The passage of the Medicare and Medicaid legislation in 1965 drastically changed the home care delivery system. Before Medicare was created, most home care was provided by voluntary visiting nurse associations (VNAs). The majority of home care clients were elderly persons, suffering from various chronic conditions, whose greatest need was for nursing care complemented by some health aide and homemaker services. According to Mundinger (1983, p. 39), "A typical visit included bathing the patient, reviewing self-care (nutrition, elimination), and attending to such tasks as vitamin or insulin injections or dressings for chronic ulcers." Payment came either from welfare or from personal payment based on a sliding fee scale subsidized by charity.

With the advent of Medicare, not only did the payment source change but client eligibility, the provision of home care and the purpose of that care changed as well. For more than 70 years before Medicare, ever since Lillian Wald's establishment of the first visiting nurse service, nurses had successfully provided home care on their own to the sick, the disabled, and children. Prior to federal payment, "it was not seen as necessary or even appropriate for physicians to direct home care" (Mundinger, 1983, p. 40). The need for some kind of gatekeeper to ensure provision of services to those who truly needed them as well as political pressures from medical groups concerned about Medicare's impact on medical practice led the federal government to appoint physicians to direct the traditionally nonmedical home services. Home care became more narrowly defined as a substitute for costly, extended hospitalization, and it changed to a medical-based model of practice (Mundinger,

531

1983, p. 39). Eligibility for Medicare payment of home care was based on patients' acute care conditions; they must be homebound, in need of skilled care (medically directed service given by a nurse or other professional), and under the treatment of a physician. Furthermore, the referring physician must plan, review, and certify as necessary the care to be given.

The medical model radically changed what had been historically the mission of home health care. Previously home services sought to provide nursing care, assistance, and support. Community health problems, after Medicare's advent, were viewed as medical problems whose solution was disease eradication. Home care became medical care. This view overlooked the need for preventive and health-promoting services and discounted the clear need of homebound clients for support services. Physicians and policymakers did not seem to be truly aware of the range of health needs clients had in the home. Somehow there was an assumption that if people could go home from the hospital they could manage meals, laundry, shopping, cleaning, and psychosocial support without supplemental assistance. Home services during these years still included health promotion, health teaching, and holistic family care. Medicare and Medicaid, however, did not cover these services; instead, public health agencies through their nurses provided the services without charge.

The passage of Medicare also influenced the structure of home care services. For the first time, home care agencies, in order to be certified for Medicare reimbursement, were required to provide one other service in addition to nursing. This service could be physical therapy, occupational therapy, speech therapy, social services, or home health aide services. About 250 of the existing 1,163 agencies qualified for Medicare participation in 1966. The total number of home care agencies declined after the implementation of Medicare, many smaller voluntary organizations going out of business because they could not develop the service scope and complexity required. This led to the growth of public home health agencies, proprietary agencies, and hospital-based agencies. During the first decade after passage of Medicare, those that met the standards increased by 71 percent to about 430. The most growth was in hospital-based agencies.

From a historical perspective, the escalation in home health care would seem to suggest that we are back where we started. New Mexico Democratic Senator Jeff Bingaman commented in testimony at budget committee hearings in 1984: "Health care in America has come full circle. Health care originated in the home and moved to the hospital with the advent of technology and improved diagnostic and treatment methodologies. Now a new emphasis is being placed on the home to control costs," ("Legislative Round Up," 1984, p. 5). Although home care is back in the spotlight, its mission, services, financing, and providers have all changed. Let us examine some of those changes.

Home Health Services

Who Uses Home Health Services?

What groups utilize home health services and how can we be certain that programs address their needs? The first part of the question is more readily answered than the second.

The largest subpopulation in the United States using home care is the elderly. According to *Research News* (1984, p. 12), in 1983, the National

Figure 19-1
The care and support of family members play a critical role in enabling the homebound population to avoid institutionalization.

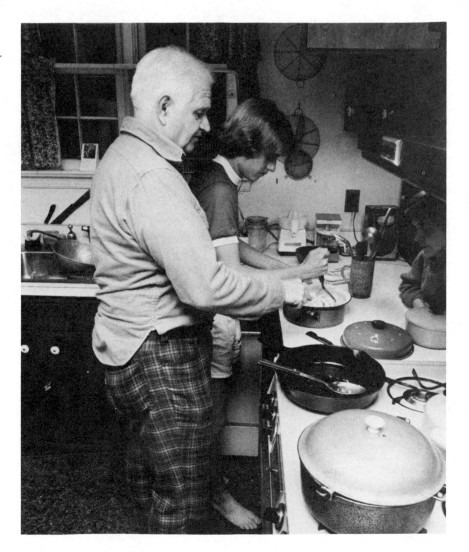

Center for Health Statistics reported that, in 1979, "4.9 million adults living in communities needed the help of another person in carrying out everyday activities." The report went on to say that "4.1 million adults needed or received the help of another person for shopping, household chores, preparing meals, or handling money." Of the total number reported, 2.9 million were 65 years or over, and the need for assistance rose sharply with age. In the 65 to 74 age group, less than one in ten needed help, but of those 85 years and over, four in ten needed help. Bakken (1983) adds that these elderly could avoid institutionalization if they received support for their personal care.

According to another national study, an estimated 5.8 million persons make up the noninstitutionalized long-term care population. This figure includes persons of all ages and diagnoses who "due to a long-lasting condition, require or receive human help in personal care, mobility, household activities or home delivered health care services" ("Research News," 1984, p. 13). This study, too, showed that dependency increases with age, dramatically so after age 75. Among older adults, the most likely to be dependent were nonwhite females. White males were slightly more dependent than white females under age 75, but after 75, white males were the least likely to be dependent for personal care ("Research News," 1984, p. 13). Two other studies, describing Medicare patients receiving home health care, showed that of all home care patients, two-thirds are women and that approximately one-third of all home care patients live alone (*Home Health*, 1979). We can conclude from the above reports that approximately 4.9 million adults and 1.1 million children need some type of home health services.

Besides the elderly and long-term care populations, another group needing home care is made up of discharged acute care patients. Although exact figures on the size of this group are not available, we know that it is increasing rapidly. Rising hospital costs and prospective payment incentives, in conjunction with dramatic technological advances that make it possible for complicated procedures to be administered in the home, contribute to an enlarging population receiving home care. Many of these are elderly persons who have been hospitalized with an episode of acute illness or disability and need convalescent home care. Others include babies and children with disabilities or individuals sent home with monitors, medications, IVs, and various therapies (See Figure 19-2).

Another subpopulation receiving home services is what one health planner calls the "wellness home care market" (Louden, 1983, p. 109). These people do not need medical care but have concerns about their health and well-being and are receptive to health promotion and illness prevention strategies. They use services such as diagnostic testing and screening (for example, blood pressure monitoring); educational counseling (for example, nutrition information); support for daily living, including home maintenance and

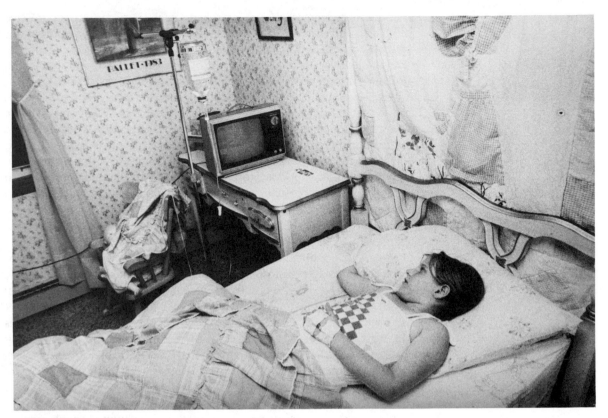

Figure 19-2
Intravenous therapy and other treatments now can be routinely administered in the home serving the needs of a home care population that spans all ages.

housekeeping; and illness prevention (for example, information about exercise and stress management). People of all ages make up this group, and it includes a good portion of the elderly population, many of whom are well elderly persons whose functional dependency has increased to the point of needing support for activities of daily living.

The distinctions between these four groups are blurred, and their members overlap, particularly in the case of the elderly. Combined, however, they form a large population that utilizes home care and is rapidly expanding.

Needs of Home Health Recipients

The majority of home health service recipients are elderly. Their home health needs fall into six categories described by Mundinger (1983, pp. 171–175):

1. *Chronic illness and disability care.* The most common diagnoses of elderly home care clients are cancer, diabetes, and cardiovascular disease. Each

is chronic, degenerative, and disabling. Each can lead to progressive pathology and deterioration with increased possibility of complications and growing dependency care needs. The large majority (80 percent) of older adults over 65 live with at least one chronic illness, and many with a mixture of several acute and chronic illnesses and disabilities (Fedder, Abrams, & Lamy, 1984, p. 28). Many clients, for example, have arthritis and hypertension in addition to cancer or diabetes. The complexity of their conditions leads to a greater variety of home care service needs.

2. *Social networks.* Meaningful contact with other people is a basic human need, and the elderly homebound, many of whom live alone, especially need this. Social supports are a vital component of home care. When social supports are present, research demonstrates, clients live longer and are happier (Weissert, 1980) — a reflection on the quality of life for home care clients that should consume more of home care providers' attention.

3. *Sheltered or congregate housing.* As more families are scattered geographically and unable to care for their elderly members and as more older persons live longer, group living for the mostly independent elderly fills an important need. Minor supervision or assistance with activities of daily living are available in sheltered or congregate housing. Residents can assist one another with tasks, meals may be taken in the company of other people, if desired, and a nurse is often available or on call. This family-type housing enables older people to maintain their independence for a longer period of time.

4. *Personal services.* We have already seen that a large number of elderly persons need assistance with personal care. This includes preparing meals, doing laundry, shopping, bathing, housecleaning, and being transported to community care centers, such as the physician's office, dentist's office, or hair dresser's salon. Many elderly people in institutions would be living at home if their personal care needs could be met there (Gary, 1979; Kane & Kane, 1978). Sometimes these needs are met voluntarily by family members, a spouse, or friends. Without these resources, elderly people are forced to use up their own funds before becoming eligible for public monies, but by then they may have lost the home in which to live independently: "Requiring the independent and economically stable elderly to become dependent if they are to receive assistance is a financially foolish and socially questionable policy" (Mundinger, 1983, p. 173).

5. *Payment for drugs, eyeglasses, preventive podiatry, and dentistry.* All of these represent ongoing needs of elderly persons whose limited resources frequently prevent them from being met. Mundinger (1983) points out that the increasing number of accidents among the elderly (causing a greater number of referrals for home care than illness in her study population) may well be due to lack of proper glasses, medications, or other necessary care. Poor vision, inadequate medication for hypertension or

536

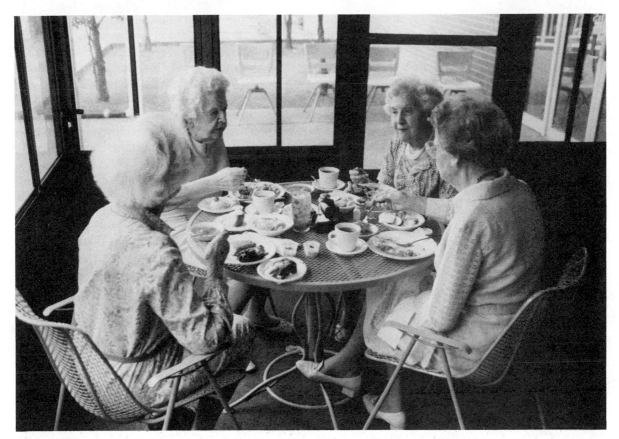

Figure 19-3
Congregate dining in a home-like atmosphere enables these elderly friends to enjoy a meal together and strengthen their social networks.

arthritis, improper foot care, or dental disease can cause accidents or illness leading to institutionalization.

6. *Day care.* Many elderly persons living at home are cared for by family members whose schedules require them to be away during the day. Day care for the elderly frees family members for work or recreation and gives elderly persons a social outlet as well. It may be the deciding factor in living at home versus institutionalization.

All home health service recipients, including the elderly, have needs, varying with their ages and the demands of their health conditions. Both long-term and acute care conditions require assistance that can be divided into two categories: one is services and the other is supplies and equipment (Louden, 1983). The professional services of nurses, physicians, aides, and physical, respiratory, speech, and occupational therapists, meeting the homebound's first category of needs, are a major component of home health care. An interdisciplinary team is necessary to meet the many and complex

537

needs of this population whose major needs, more than medically related care, are in areas of health teaching, psychological and social support, and prevention or reduction of disability (Mundinger, 1983). Social support personnel (such as social workers, ministers, family members) and nutritional services (such as Meals on Wheels and congregate dining) fill other vital areas of need. Important additional services may include data and claims processing, equipment service, and home telemetry.

The second category of need is for supplies and equipment. An increasing number of new products are availavble to maintain ill or disabled people at home. They include oxygen and respiratory devices; durable medical equipment, such as wheelchairs, lifts, and walkers; rehabilitation equipment, such as an exercise "horse" or hand grips; nursing care supplies, such as dressings, decubiti cushions, or catheters; drug therapy supplies, such as disposable syringes and intravenous therapy supplies, oxygen concentrator, or needleless insulin injector; nutritional supplies (including oral and total parenteral nutrition); and home kidney dialysis equipment and supplies.

"Wellness" home services recipients have a different set of needs. Their concerns focus on health-promoting and illness-preventing activities. Services used by this group have already been discussed. They include diagnostic screening, educational counseling and information, daily living support services, and illness prevention services (like exercise guidance and weight and stress control). This group uses certain supplies and equipment such as products for self-diagnostics and screening and for self-treatment, vitamin and nutritional supplements, exercise equipment, products that assist in the activities of daily living, and communications and security devices (Louden, 1983).

Designing Relevant Home Health Services

Assessment of home health clients' needs is essential for appropriate program development. A growing body of research data is shedding light on this area, and nurses should review this information. Further research and community needs assessment should be conducted to make home care services appropriately focused. Mundinger (1983), for example, has demonstrated that home health care, when efficiently organized with good backup services, is a highly cost-effective way of caring for the elderly. She also demonstrated that many critically needed services, such as home safety assessment, extensive family medications review, care adapted to the home setting, coordination of care with medical and other community resources, were nonreimbursable (Mundinger, 1983). This is one of many studies pointing out deficiencies in the reimbursement system for home health services.

The U.S. Department of Health and Human Services has published a quantitative formula for analyzing community need for home care services that is helpful in program development (Warhola, 1980). It enables the home service planner to estimate the number of potential home care users in a given service area by examining the elderly population, the acute care discharged patients, and those inappropriately placed in skilled or intermediate care nursing facilities.

Planning for effective home health services must take into account that the majority of clients have chronic conditions compounded by periodic acute episodes. A diversified service system is necessary to meet this range of needs. Figure 19-4 lists the four major components necessary to provide a full range of home care services. The VNA of Dallas has developed a system of services that provides a useful alternative model (Holt, 1984). It includes three service divisions — home health care, hospice, and long-term care. Each division offers a variety of specialty services. For example, home health care includes nursing services, extended (24-hour) services, patient education, medical social services, homemaker and home health aides, nutritional consultation, durable medical equipment, and rehabilitative services such as physical therapy. Hospice services include care, support, and mobilization of resources for clients in the final stage of life and their families. Hospice benefits cover such things as continuous care, respite care, and bereavement counseling. Long-term care includes meals delivered to the home, family care, and primary home care (personal care, housekeeping, meal preparation, and other home chores). A major contributing factor in the success of this VNA is its community-based planning and partnership with community care contract providers and appropriate state agencies and legislators. All were "committed to finding alternatives to institutionalization" (Holt, 1984, p. 53). This home service agency packaged a diversified set

Figure 19-4
Components of a local home health care system.

Day Care
Home Health Care

nursing	social work
medical	nutrition
homemaker/home health aide	pharmaceutical services
homemaker services	other services:
attendant services	inhalation therapy
physical therapy	renal therapy
occupational therapy	mental health
speech pathology	lab & diagnostic
	supplies/equipment

Hospice
Respite
Other Service Components

call-in assurance	home delivered meals
chore services	housekeeping services
congregate meals	night care
family subsidies	sheltered housing
financial & legal counseling/services	special transportation/escort services
friendly visitor	

Source: *Minnesota Community Health Services Home Care Guidelines*, Office of Community Development, Minnesota Department of Health, February, 1981.

of services that met a much broader range of home care clients' needs than "the traditional medically-oriented, single purpose skilled services offered by home care agencies under Medicare" (Holt, 1984, p. 53).

Ideally, home health services are centrally coordinated by health professionals and operated by means of a case management system based on assessed clients' needs (Warhola, 1980). A case manager may or may not provide direct care and serves as "broker" to see that clients receive needed home care and supportive services (National Association for Home Care, 1984, p. 32). Providing continuity of care between institutions, such as the hospital, nursing home, or long-term care facility, and the home is one emphasis of this case management approach along with assignment of appropriate services and resources.

Current Status of Home Health Services

Home health services are on the cutting edge of change in health care provision. Spurred on by multiple forces (Louden, 1983; Moxley, 1984; Mundinger, 1983; Spiegel, 1983), home care is growing rapidly. One major force is cost-containment pressures by government and third-party payers and employers who appreciate home care's lower costs. Another is the expanding aging population that has increasing dependency needs. In addition, hospitals and nursing homes will eventually be unable to handle the load created by the rise in the number of elderly people needing medical attention. Fewer family care givers are available since more women work outside the home. Consumers have increased health awareness and concern. Patients are demanding greater satisfaction and quality of life to which care in the home contributes. A final force of growing significance in home health care is the impact of medical and computer technology. Advanced equipment design, electronics, and communication systems have the potential for enabling the ill and disabled to live near-normal lives outside institutions with home services as the sustaining intermediary.

As the demand for home health care increases, so too do the number and variety of agencies providing services. No longer is home care the sole province of public health nursing agencies and VNAs. Palley & Oktay (1983) state that by 1981, according to a Health Care Financing Administration report, there were 3,136 home health agencies certified by Medicare in the United States. Of these, 1,231 were governmental, 544 were private and nonprofit, 436 were hospital-based nonprofit programs, 515 were run by VNA's, and 297 were proprietary agencies. By 1984 there were approximately 5,000 home health agencies, 4,000 of which were certified by Medicare. In addition, there were 5,000 homemaker–home health aide agencies and 1,200 hospices. Nearly half of the hospices were based in home health agencies (Brown, 1984).

540

Today one of the fastest growing types of home health care agencies is the hospital-based agency. The number of not-for-profit hospitals offering home care services increased by 67 percent between 1976 and 1982 (Louden, 1983, p. 110). Escalating costs and a declining census are forcing many hospitals to explore alternative revenue sources; expansion into home care is viewed as a logical extension of hospital services (Lundberg, 1984). One argument is that continuity of care can be maintained for patients. Another is that hospital staff are better trained to handle the demands of highly technological and skilled care now required in many home care situations. We will see many more hospitals developing home care programs in the near future.

Proprietary, for-profit agencies form the other fastest growing group moving into home care. The number of privately owned home health agencies grew from 3,100 to 3,700 between 1980 and 1983 and the proprietary companies have managed to create a business where they now supply the majority of home care personnel throughout the nation (Spiegel, 1983). Pharmaceutical companies, insurance companies, temporary staffing agencies, nursing homes, and many others have entered the competitive and mushrooming field of home care. Even some durable medical equipment and supply companies have expanded into providing skilled nursing and other comprehensive services in the home. Companies such as Abbott Laboratories of Chicago, American Hospital Supply Corporation of Evanston, Illinois, Baxter Travenol Laboratories, Inc., of Deerfield, Illinois, and Johnson & Johnson of New Brunswick, New Jersey, are offering home care services along with their home care product businesses (Louden, 1983).

Home care services in the past were generally provided by not-for-profit agencies while the for-profit sector sold home care equipment and supplies. These patterns are changing. The traditional equipment and supply companies see an opportunity for financial profit in offering services and the not-for-profit providers find the supply and device market, which offers even higher profit margins, financially attractive (Louden, 1983). Hospitals are important customers of supply companies. Consequently, to avoid competing with them, many supply companies are attempting various joint ventures with hospitals.

Products and services that are frequently used in the home care market include incontinence products, self-diagnostic or treatment products, and supplies or services for home parenteral nutrition, intravenous therapy, chemotherapy, kidney dialysis, and respiratory therapy.

Total parenteral nutrition (TPN) is one of the fastest growing high-tech procedures being performed in the home. Home TPN was introduced about ten years ago as a technique to facilitate hospital discharge of those patients whose primary reason for hospitalization was parenteral nutrition support. Nearly 3,000 patients in the United States have been involved in such home care programs since their introduction (Ament, 1983). TPN is a method of intravenous feeding used to sustain people who have intestinal obstructions, malabsorption syndromes or other digestive disorders, or anorexia nervosa and occasionally for those who during the postoperative period following gastrointestinal surgery need feeding. At first patients needed to be connected to intravenous equipment for 24 hours a day, but technological advances in the early 1970s permitted more rapid infusion of the nutritional solutions so that clients can now be free from tubes and solution bags for more than 16 hours a day. Between 0.3 percent and 5.5 percent of all patients hospitalized in the United States are now receiving TPN. In 1982, 2,200 clients received TPN intravenous feedings in their homes, compared with 1,200 in 1980. By 1985 this number was expected to increase to 4,100 (News Briefs, 1982).

Home administration of many complex high technology procedures is proving to be cost-effective. One study showed a reduction in costs for TPN from $200 per day to $65 per day (Ament, 1983). Others demonstrated significant reductions in the cost of home intravenous antibiotic administration (News Briefs, 1982; *Hospital Peer Review*, 1983). A home intravenous cancer chemotherapy program in Houston estimated a cost savings of more than half a million dollars in one year *Hospital Peer Review*, 1983).

Numerous problems have yet to be resolved in providing home care services. While cost savings have been clearly demonstrated in studies of home care, studies have not addressed all the questions that need answering. For example, care of a severely disabled person in the home may appear less costly than in a nursing home, but what is it costing the family or the community? It may be prohibitive in terms of the drain on physical and emotional as well as financial resources (Figure 19-5). In some instances nursing home care may be less costly than maintaining people at home. Utilization of home care benefits under Medicare and Medicaid is increasingly subject to fraud and abuse (Mundinger, 1983). Costs to the federal government of subsidizing home health care are increasing at a shocking rate (31 percent annually for Medicare from 1972 to 1982 and 23 percent annually for Medicaid from 1977 to 1982) (*Home Health Journal*, 1983). Some studies show that home health services are simply add-ons. There is little evidence that these services have contributed to decreased hospital stays or have substituted for extended institutionalization (Hammond, 1979). Health and Human Services Secretary Margaret Heckler commented in 1983: "The issue is not whether the per-visit cost of home care is lower than the per-diem cost of inpatient care, but the degree to which home care substitutes for more expensive institution care. Overall costs may well increase unless expanded home care is targeted to individuals who would otherwise require institutional care" (*Home Health Journal*, 1983).

A further problem in home care is the quality issue. With so many proprietary agencies entering the field, many uncertified by Medicare and not subject to any standards of care, the potential for reduced quality of services is

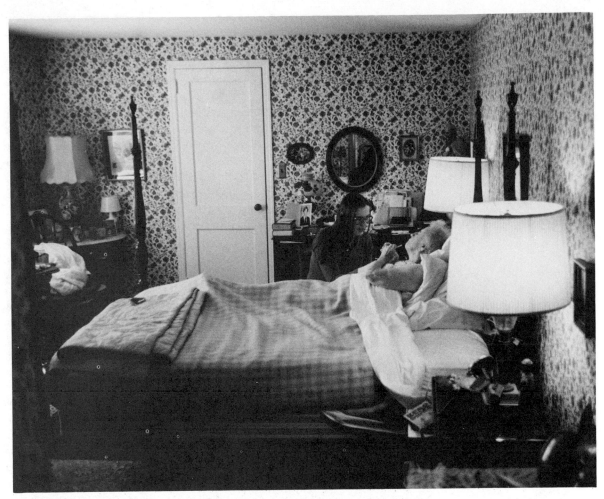

Figure 19-5
Although care at home has many benefits for home-bound clients, the demands on family care givers' physical, emotional, and financial resources can be heavy.

great. Closely tied to quality is the problem of fragmented and overlapping services, emphasizing the need for coordination and case management.

Community Health Nursing and Home Care

The changing picture in home health services has significantly affected community health nursing. Formerly the sole providers of home health care, community health nursing agencies now find hospitals, once their primary referral sources, serving those clients themselves. Medicare and other reimbursements for home care used to generate a sizable portion of community health nursing agencies' budgets. With decreased referrals those revenues are diminishing. Furthermore, home care providers, whether operating for profit or not will often refer clients to public agencies when Medicare benefits or third-party coverage has run out, requiring taxes or charity to subsidize the care.

The changing financial structure of home health services poses a dilemma for community health nursing agencies faced with a conflict in values between the competition model and basic public health values (described in chapter 2). Although hospitals and other technologically skilled home care providers can offer important and necessary services to clients at home, their personnel are not usually oriented to giving holistic, family-focused, preventive, and health-promoting care so essential for the health of this client population, nor do most home care providers wish to offer this broader range of services because of their added expense.

The solution appears to lie in new forms of public-private partnerships. Some innovative programs are already proving successful, such as the VNA of Dallas (Holt, 1984) cited earlier in this chapter. This agency's partnership with public agencies and diversified services offered along a continuum of care place it in a better position for government reimbursement. Some agencies are forming coalitions to work collaboratively for referrals and case management. Minnesota has a preadmission screening program that assesses persons before they enter nursing homes to determine their ability to remain in the community. This comprehensive screening, done in part by community health nurses, provides revenue for the agency and is a potential source of new referrals for home care.

Community health nurses face new challenges and new roles in home care. The home care client population still has the same basic needs, but the changing health care delivery structure requires that nurses develop creative new ways of meeting them. One role that community health nurses are particularly suited for is case management. Coordination of needed services and resources with provision of continuity of care are critical elements of an effective home health program.

Community health nurses are demonstrating the value of assessment of client health status using functional level as a predictor of need rather than gauging need by diagnostic category. Both the VNS of Omaha, Nebraska, and the Ramsey County Nursing Service of St. Paul, Minnesota, have been using a function code system for determining client health status and ability to manage the activities of daily living. It underscores a problem that providers and legislators have been debating for some time and that is the inappropriateness of applying a classification system like Medicare's diagnosis-related group categories to community health clients. Research in home care client assessment is an area for greater community health nursing involvement.

Summary

A large group of people of all ages make up the population receiving home health services. Home health care, broadly defined, refers to all the services provided to clients at home that maintain, restore, or promote their health. Historically these services have been provided primarily by public health nurses who combined illness care in the home with comprehensive family care and health promotion. The passage of Medicare and Medicaid legislation drastically changed the home care system in terms of payment source, client eligibility, provision of home care, and the purpose of the care. Physicians were appointed gatekeepers of the system, and home care became medical care. Traditional preventive and health-promoting services continued as separate programs delivered by community health nurses.

The major target population for home health services are the elderly, the disabled (those needing noninstitutionalized long-term care), discharged acute care patients, and those interested in wellness and self-care. Needs of the elderly home care population include chronic illness or disability care, social networks, sheltered or congregate housing, personal services, payment for drugs, glasses, preventive podiatry and dentistry, and day care. All home care recipients need a variety of services from a multidisciplinary group of professionals and support personnel. They also use a large variety of equipment and supplies.

A relevant system for home health services requires a proper needs assessment, and providers should plan diversified services to accommodate the complex and wide-ranging needs of this population. A full range of services includes day, home health, hospice, and respite care. Case management is a critical factor for coordinating continuity of care.

Many forces are influencing the current and future status of home health services. Among them are cost-containment pressures, an increasing elderly population, demands for consumer satisfaction, and advanced technology. In addition to the traditional VNAs and public health nursing agencies, a variety of other agencies offers home health services. The fastest growing of these are the hospital-based and the proprietary for-profit home care programs. As the home care market expands, so does the competition for providing services and products.

Many problems exist in the home care field, including misuse of home care funding, not enough research to demonstrate its cost-effectiveness, and the difficulty of providing quality service to those who need it most.

Community health nursing faces a critical time of challenge and opportunity. Competing home health agencies are greatly influencing the number and type of clients that community health nurses normally serve. Changing financial structures and costs require that community health nursing develop new partnerships and innovative service delivery patterns. A critical service they can provide is using case management in addition to developing more effective ways to measure home care client needs and health status.

Study Questions

1. Assume you have been assigned to provide home care to a 75-year-old woman with arthritis, hypertension, and chronic leukemia who lives alone. What are some general areas of information you will need to gather before beginning to plan her care? Contrast what her care will involve now with what it might have been forty years ago.
2. As part of your community health nursing agency planning team, you are concerned about developing a comprehensive home health services system. What elements should you consider including in it? How would you determine the exact programs to include?
3. From the home care client population's point of view, quality of care is probably the most important criterion for home health services today. What are the needs of the elderly homebound and what actions might you take to ensure that these needs are met? Design a hypothetical home care program for an agency's elderly population.

References

Ament, M. (1983). The economic growth of the total parenteral nutrition. *Nutrition and the M.D., 9*(6), 11.

Bakken, K. L. (1983). Integrated health care: The whole person in community. *Nursing Economics, 1*(2), 178–180.

Brown, K. (1984, January-February). Speakers stress home health agency diversification. *Home Care/Rehabilitation Product News,* p. 10.

Fedder, D., Abrams, M. K., & Lamy, P. (1984). The pharmacist in home health care: Part I — Drugs and the elderly. *Caring, 3*(5), 28–31.

Gary, L. R. (1979). Home health care regulation: Issues and opportunities. New York: Hunter College.

Hammond, J. (1979). Home health care cost effectiveness: An overview of the literature. *Public Health Reports, 94*(4), 305–311.

Holt, S. W. (1984). Continuity of care in the home: Building a diversified service system that works. *Caring, 3*(5), 49–56.

Home care guidelines. (1981). Minnesota Community Health Services, Office of Community Development, Minneapolis, MN: Minnesota Department of Health.

Home health and other in-home services. (1979). Department of Health, Education and Welfare. Report to Congress. Washington, DC: U.S. Government Printing Office.

Home Health Journal. (1983, Nov.), *4*(11), 9–11. Jacksonville, FL: Home Care Management Consulting, Inc.

Hospital Peer Review. (1983, April, June; 1984, January), *8*(4), *8*(6), *9*(1). Atlanta: American Health Consultants, Inc.

Kane, R., & Kane, R. (1978). Care of the aged — An old problem in search of new solutions. *Science, 200,* 913–918.

Legislative round up: Durenberger sees home care prospective payment near. (1984). *Caring, 3*(5), 5–6.

Louden, T. L. (1983). Opportunities — and competition — in home healthcare are on the rise. *Modern Healthcare. 13*(12), 109–112.

Lundberg, C. J. (1984). Home health care: A logical extension of hospital services. *Topics in Health Care Financing, 10*(3), 22–32.

MacNamara, E. (1982). Home care: Hospitals rediscover comprehensive home care. *Hospitals, 16*(21), 60–66.

Moxley, J. H., III. (1984). New opportunities for out-of-hospital health services. *New England Journal of Medicine, 310*(3), 193–197.

Mundinger, M. (1983). *Home care controversy: Too little, too late, too costly.* Rockville, MD: Aspen Systems.

National Association for Home Care. (1984). *Position paper on legislative and regulatory issues: A blueprint for action.* Washington, DC: Author.

News Briefs. (1982). Home health care may help hospitals live with 7.9% caps. *Modern Health Care, 12*(12), 9.

Palley, H. A., & Oktay, J. S. (1983). In-home and other supportive community-based services for the chronically limited elderly: Problems, prospects, and proposals. *Home Health Care Services Quarterly, 4*(2), 3–9.

Research news: Studies on elderly show need for home care. (1984). *Caring, 3*(5), 11–13.

Speigel, A. D. (1983). *Home health care: Home birthing to hospice care.* Owings Mills, MD: National Health Publishing.

Stewart, I. E. (1979). *Home health care.* St. Louis: C. V. Mosby.

Warhola, C. (1980). *Planning for home health services — A resource handbook* (DHHS Pub. No. [HRA] 80-14017). Washington, DC: U.S. Government Printing Office.

Weissert, N. (1980). Effects and costs of day care and homemaker services for the chronically ill elderly. Bethesda, MD: National Center for Health Services Research.

Selected Readings

Bakken, K. L. (1983). Integrated health care: The whole person in community. *Nursing Economics, 1*(2), 178–180.

Ballard, S. & McNamara, R. (1983). Quantifying nursing needs in home health care, *Nursing Research, 32,* 236–241.

Berkman, L., & Syme, S. (1979). Social networks, host resistance, and mortality. *American Journal of Epidemiology, 110*(5), 583–589.

Brook, R., & Lohr, K. (1981). Quality of care assessment: Its role in the 80s. *American Journal of Public Health, 81,* 681–682.

Brown, K. (1984, January-February). Speakers stress home health agency diversification. *Home Care/Rehabilitation Product News,* p. 10.

Callahan, J. (1980). Responsibilities of families for their severely disabled elders. *Health Care Financing Review, 4,* 29–48.

DeCrosta, T. (1984). Home health care: It's red hot and right now. *Nursing Life, 2,* 54–60.

Donlan, T. G. (1983, March 21). No place like home. *Barron's,* pp. 6, 7, 32.

Gary, L. R. (1979). *Home health care regulation: Issues and opportunities.* New York: Hunter College.

Hammond, J. (1979). Home health care cost effectiveness: An overview of the literature. *Public Health Reports, 94*(4), 305–311.

Holt, S. W. (1984). Continuity of care in the home: Building a diversified service system that works. *Caring, 3*(5): 49–56.

Home health and other in-home services. (1979). Department of Health, Education and Welfare. Report to Congress. Washington, DC: U.S. Government Printing Office.

Home health care: Its utilization, costs and reimbursement. (1977). New York: Health Services Agency of New York City.

Home health: the need for a national policy to better provide for the elderly. (1977). Department of Health, Education and Welfare. Report to Congress. Washington, DC: U.S. Government Printing Office.

Inui, T., Stevenson, K., Plorde, D., & Murphy, I. (1980). Needs assessment for hospital-based home care services. *Research in Nursing and Health, 3*(3), 101–106.

Kane, R., & Kane, R. (1978). Care of the aged — An old problem in search of new solutions. *Science, 200,* 913–918,

Kuntz, E. F. (1983). Hospitals move into home care by striking partnership deals. *Modern Healthcare, 13*(12), 116–118.

Louden, T. L. (1983). Opportunities — and competition — in home healthcare are on the rise. *Modern Healthcare, 13*(12), 109–112.

Lundberg, C. J. (1984). Home health care: A logical extension of hospital services. *Topics in Health Care Financing, 10*(3), 22–32.

MacNamara, E. (1982). Home care: Hospitals rediscover comprehensive home care. *Hospitals, 16*(21), 60–66.

Moxley, J. H., III. (1984). New opportunities for out-of-hospital health services. *New England Journal of Medicine, 310*(3), 193–197.

Mundinger, M. (1983). *Home care controversy: Too little, too late, too costly.* Rockville, MD: Aspen Systems.

National Association for Home Care. (1984). *Position paper on legislative and regulatory issues: A blueprint for action.* Washington, DC: Author.

Pegels, C. (1980). *Health care and the elderly.* Rockville, MD: Aspen Systems.

Powell, D. J. (1984). Nurses — "High touch" entrepreneurs. *Nursing Economics, 2*(1), 33–36.

Public Health Nursing Section. (1982). *Assessment of health risks in the home environment: A manual designed to assist public health nurses perform an environmental assessment.* Minneapolis, Minnesota Department of Health.

Somers, A. (1978). The high cost of health care for the elderly: Diagnosis, prognosis, and some questions for therapy. *Journal of Health Policy, Politics & Law, 4*(2), 163–180.

Somers, A., & Bryant, N. (1975). Home care: Much needed, much neglected, *Annals of Internal Medicine, 82,* 111–112.

Spiegel, A. D. (1983). *Home healthcare: Home birthing to hospice care.* Owings Mills, MD: National Health Publishing.

Trager, B. (1980). *Home health care and national policy.* New York: Hawthorne Press.

U.S. General Accounting Office. (1982). The elderly should benefit from expanded home health care but increasing these services will not insure cost reductions (Pub. No. GAO/IPE-83-1). Gaithersburg, MD: Author.

Vladek, B. (1980). *Unloving care.* New York: Basic Books.

Warhola, C. (1980). *Planning for home health services — A resource handbook* (DHHS Pub. No. [HRA] 80-14017). Washington, DC: U.S. Government Printing Office.

Widmer, G., Brill, R., & Schlosser, A. (1978). Home health care services and cost. *Nursing Outlook, 26,* 488–493.

four

Expanding the Nurse's Influence

20

Leadership and Managing Change

Leading people to change their beliefs and practices about health lies at the heart of all community health nursing. This aim characterizes work at every level, from individual clients to large organizations and communities. At all levels, to influence change requires knowledge and skill in two closely related areas: leadership and management of change.

How do nurses carry out their roles as both leader and change agent at the community level? With such rapidly expanding opportunities, it is possible to give several examples. One community health nurse becomes a member of the Governor's Commission on the Handicapped. In addition to understanding the entire state as a community and the handicapped as a special population, she urges the commission to formulate new plans for meeting the needs of the handicapped. Another nurse, as a member of a metropolitan health planning board, works to improve health care for a group of Hmong immigrants from Southeast Asia. In a rural community of farms and small towns, another nurse organizes a grass-roots committee concerned about a nearby nuclear generating plant. The committee works to develop an emergency evacuation plan in case of radiation leaks from the plant. All three of these nurses are involved in leadership and change at the community level. They are working to change people's beliefs regarding health and health activities and to involve them in creating organized responses to community problems.

Community health nurses also lead people to change at the organizational level. Let us say that you are a staff nurse in a public health nursing agency. Like the other staff members, you feel overburdened by paperwork. You may feel burned out and lack clear goals for your daily tasks. Setting priorities is difficult. Rather than blaming yourself, you recognize that other staff feel the same way; it is an organizational problem. During a staff meeting, you bring up the problem of job stress and suggest that everyone read an article on the subject to discuss at the next staff meeting. The first discussion is so successful that others follow. At your prompting, a regular staff development meeting evolves with rotating leadership. As the months pass, a new sense of direction emerges among the staff. People feel more competent to cope with job stress, and morale improves. Although you worked informally, you acted as a leader to bring about organizational change. The result not only left individuals feeling better able to cope with their jobs, but also improved the health of the organization.

Community health nurses also seek to influence families to achieve new levels of health. One nurse assists a family in improving its communication; another leads a family through the stress caused by incest and helps its members to change and move to a new level of health. You can act in a leadership capacity with groups, perhaps negotiating a contract with a group to quit smoking or to develop a school program on battered children. The list goes on and on, but in every case the pattern of assuming leadership in order to promote change in health practices is the same. Even with individuals you will seek to influence change. You may teach a young mother to care for her handicapped child. You may negotiate a contract regarding regular exercise with a man recovering from a heart attack. Hardly a day goes by for most community health nurses without deep involvement in leadership and change activities at every level of practice.

The roles of leader and change agent both require specialized knowledge and skills to be effective. This chapter examines leadership and the management of change. We will see how they are inextricably linked and how community health nurses incorporate them into practice.

Leadership

Many nurses do not see themselves as leaders nor do they wish to become leaders. All too often, leadership for these nurses has come to mean they must assume a formal position of being in charge. As leaders, they would have to tell other people what to do. Some nurses feel it means being alone at the top of a group or organization, taking all the risks and being held accountable for the outcomes. Many of these conceptions of leadership, however, are based on false premises.

Leadership is *an interpersonal process in which one person influences the activities of another person or group of persons toward accomplishment of a goal in a specific situation* (Hersey & Blanchard, 1977, and Moloney, 1979). In its simplest terms, leadership involves setting the pace, going first, and guiding and directing the way people think and act. It is accomplishing goals with and through people (Hersey & Blanchard, 1977). To lead requires interacting with other people to influence them to achieve the goal. Let us look at three major characteristics of leadership implied in this definition.

Leadership Characteristics

First, leadership is purposeful: it always has a goal. No act of leadership exists without a reason. A mayor wants low-cost housing for the poor; a community nurse wants to see a family change its nutritional habits; a minister wants transportation that is accessible to all the physically handicapped. In each instance, the leader has a purpose and hopes that others will come to share that purpose. A leader will work to achieve goals by making them clear, attainable, specific, and agreeable to the follower constituency.

Second, leadership is interpersonal. It is a social exchange, a transaction between the two parties of leader and follower (Merton, 1969). These parties share information in a variety of patterns. An authoritarian army general gives direct orders to his military personnel; the president of a garden club makes informal suggestions to club members. In both cases, however, the leader and followers must maintain a relationship that fosters ongoing communication and facilitates the goal-seeking process.

Third, leadership means influencing. In one small community that existed in a larger city, a nurse received reports of several children who had been bitten by rats. A casual survey revealed alleys with piles of garbage and trash that attracted rats. The nurse, as a leader, wanted to influence members of this community to eliminate a public health problem. She could not clean up all the refuse herself, nor would city maintenance crews undertake the responsibility. In order to mobilize the local citizens to achieve this goal, she needed to influence them. She began with the parents of children bitten by rats, influencing them to call their neighbors together. At that meeting, she spoke about the potential health hazard with a resulting need for eliminating the garbage and trash from alleys. She quietly listened to the discussion and offered suggestions when the group decided to form a committee and hold a clean-up day. As a leader, she offered guidance and direction, thus influencing the ideas and activities of this group of followers.

Leadership, then, in community health means to influence people toward development of an optimally healthy life-style and environment. Any purposeful effort to influence behavior is an example of leadership; thus, every community health nurse can act as a leader (Hersey & Blanchard, 1977). Moreover, according to Moloney (1979), all nurses should exercise leadership. She bases her rationale on the fact that nurses must accept responsibility for revitalizing and upgrading professional nursing practice and for improving health services. She declares: "Accountability for professional practice implies that nurses are functioning as leaders in health care. If nurses are to become accountable for practice, they must broaden their view of what responsible leadership entails" (Moloney, 1979, p. 3). Nurses have many opportunities to exercise leadership. In community health, they may lead citizens; in practice, they may lead clients toward optimal health; as nurse managers, they may lead colleagues to improved practice; and as nurse faculty, they may lead students toward future leadership (Moloney, 1979).

Leadership Functions

Leadership functions occur at many levels, each with its own set of activities and sphere of influence. A captain's leadership functions will differ from a corporal's, a governor's from a school board member's, and a corporation president's from an assembly line inspector's. Within community health nursing, the functions of leadership also vary depending upon the nurse's position and work situation. Take, for example, a large community health nursing agency. Listed below are some areas of influence associated with various positions:

Director	Influences organizational policy and decision making
Associate director	Influences management of specific aspects of the organization
Supervisor	Influences structure and process of providing care
Team leader	Influences day-to-day quality of nursing practice
Staff nurse	Influences client health, behavior, and environment

In other settings for community health nursing practice, such as rural or occupational environments, there may be only one nurse present to provide leadership that encompasses many, if not all, of these activities. Beyond the agency itself, the leadership role of each nurse extends to influencing those community attitudes, programs, and environmental factors that affect community health. Each nurse must assess the situation and determine the kind and extent of leadership needed.

What are the functions of leadership in community health nursing? Argyris (1976, p. ix) summarizes several functions: "Leaders . . . know how to discover the difficult questions, how to create viable problem-solving networks to invent solutions to these questions, and how to generate and channel human energy and commitment to produce the solutions." More specifically, five essential functions are required for effective leadership at any level: (1) the creative function, (2) the initiating function, (3) the risk-taking function, (4) the integrative function, and (5) the instrumental function. These functions do not occur in any particular order; rather, they operate simultaneously throughout the leadership process.

CREATIVE FUNCTION

Nurse leaders must be able to envision new and better ways to solve problems. This first step in creativity is then followed by developing methods and activities for carrying out the solutions. This function requires ingenuity, innovation, vision, and a future orientation. For instance, a nurse in a rural agency recognized that the home health aides or homemakers could potentially meet more client needs, find their jobs more fulfilling, and better serve the agency through an expanded role. She revised their job descriptions and instituted an expanded role-training program (Hennes, 1979). The creative leadership function is one that includes generating ideas and developing designs for action.

INITIATING FUNCTION

As a leader, the nurse introduces change and sets its process in motion. This function includes convincing clients or followers of the need for change, starting the problem-solving process, and launching the activities needed to carry out the plan. Like all the other leadership functions, it requires decision-making skills. For example, after seeing an increased number of pregnancies, a nurse who works in a high school convinces the girls to start a prenatal counseling group and originates a series of sex education seminars. The initiating function begins the process toward goal accomplishment. It is the stimulus or "push" that starts clients or followers on their course of action.

RISK-TAKING FUNCTION

Every leader is faced with uncertainty, and to proceed under uncertain conditions is to take risks. What nurse, working with a family or group in the community, has not encountered a number of unpredictable variables during the process of planning with clients for health goals? Will this diet control the disease? Will client self-disclosure in this group therapy lead to group acceptance and understanding or to open ridicule and a deteriorated self-image? Will the new drug counseling clinic significantly reduce the problem, or will county funds have been spent needlessly, thus jeopardizing future funding requests? Leaders cannot guarantee outcomes. The leadership process requires careful planning based on all available data and the creation of scenarios in order to predict all possible obstacles and outcomes. It even requires preparation of alternative courses of action, should earlier plans fail. Nevertheless, some variables cannot be predicted beyond a certain point, and leaders must be willing to take chances. They have to be willing to go out on a limb, to expose themselves to possible failure and embarrassment. Taking chances also means they will expose clients or followers to potential negative outcomes. No leader throughout history has operated without taking risks. Effective leaders, however, take calculated risks; they weigh the pros and cons and potential consequences of each action before proceeding. Their concern is to minimize harmful exposure to followers.

INTEGRATIVE FUNCTION

This aspect of the leadership role focuses on strengthening collective ties and uniting clients or followers through a strong sense of purpose. The leader reminds the followers of their goals, encourages pride in their group identity, stablizes intragroup relations, and mediates interpersonal conflict. Community health nurses working with families and groups frequently find members at odds or cross-purposes with one another. Individuals in any group setting tend to have their own hidden agendas and separate needs. One of the nurse leader's jobs is to keep the client group on target by clarifying and reinforcing the goals they have mutually identified. The integrative function requires good interpersonal skills for establishing positive relationships with, as well as between, followers. This function supports the aim of promoting member commitment and cooperation.

INSTRUMENTAL FUNCTION

Leaders must also keep followers moving in the right direction, the purpose of the instrumental or facilitative function. As Schaefer (1975, p. 16) puts it, a leader is "capable of moving others in the direction the leader is moving." For nurse leaders, this function involves good communication. They must keep in constant touch with clients or followers, make certain that goals and activities are understood and agreed upon, and encourage both negative and positive feedback. Leaders further stimulate followers to progress toward achievement of goals by reinforcing desired behaviors and by setting the pace themselves. The latter is particularly important for gaining followers' respect and sustained commitment. To set the pace means nurse leaders must demonstrate competence, practice what they preach, and show followers that they believe in them and in what they are asking followers to accomplish.

Areas of Influence

Community health nurses exercise the functions of leadership in ever-widening spheres of influence, as is shown in Figure 20-1. The central aim of this leadership role is to influence community health. The first area of focus is to improve the immediate environment, which includes physical, psychological,

558

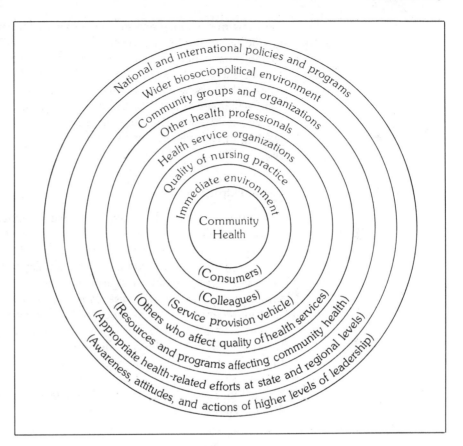

Community
Health

(Consumers)

(Colleagues)

(Service provision vehicle)

(Others who affect quality of health services)

(Resources and programs affecting community health)

(Appropriate health-related efforts at state and regional levels)

(Awareness, attitudes, and actions of higher levels of leadership)

National and international policies and programs

Wider biosociopolitical environment

Community groups and organizations

Other health professionals

Health service organizations

Quality of nursing practice

Immediate environment

Figure 20-1
Areas of potential leader-
ship influence within com-
munity health nursing
practice.

social, and spiritual factors, by influencing consumer health-related behavior. Community health nurses exercise leadership when they influence the quality of nursing practice of their co-workers through, for instance, peer consultation and review. They may also influence the service provision vehicle, the agency or organization through which care is offered, by accepting a high-level position or by serving on committees and taking an active part in quality control. Other professionals involved in the health provision system are an additional target of community health nurses' leadership influence. Ongoing communication with colleagues from other disciplines may serve to stimulate these professionals' awareness of health needs and facilitate development of appropriate services. Community health nurses may influence groups and organizations that affect community health, such as clubs, churches, or the legislature, by keeping them informed about health problems and suggesting ways they can improve community health levels. Extending their leadership influence even wider, community health nurses may focus on the wider biosociopolitical environment of the city, county, state, or region. For example, the nurse may support anti-smoking programs or campaign for proper disposal of nuclear waste. Finally, community health nursing leadership may extend to influencing national and international policies and programs that affect health, such as those of the World Health Organization. Participating in citizens' lobbies, serving on national committees, or contacting senators and representatives of the U.S. Congress are some of the many possible actions nurses could take. The number of spheres in which the nurse exercises a leadership role varies, depending on health needs, the work situation, the nurse's abilities, and time.

Leadership Styles

Some nurses effectively influence people's behavior. Others do not. What causes the difference? What accounts for effective leadership? Some researchers, assuming that certain individuals acquire or are born with leadership qualities, have sought to identify the personality traits of leaders. These efforts have been unsuccessful in establishing any one group of traits that would predict leadership effectiveness (Moloney, 1979).

More recent research has focused on the behavior of leaders during interaction with followers. This approach views leader behavior, rather than leader personality, as the chief determinant of leadership effectiveness. From this research, several taxonomies of leadership styles have evolved. We will first consider one that identifies three styles: (1) autocratic leadership, (2) participative leadership, and (3) laissez-faire leadership (Hersey & Blanchard, 1977, Moloney, 1979, & Uris, 1964).

LEADER BEHAVIOR

Autocratic Style

The autocratic style is authoritarian. Leaders who adopt this style use their power (usually the power of their position) to influence their followers. The autocratic leader gives orders and expects others to obey without question. Suggestions from followers are not, as a rule, invited or accepted. The leader is dominant; the followers have little power or freedom of choice. In times of extreme crisis, an autocratic style may enhance survival. Sometimes a nurse finds that members of a group will expect to be led in an autocratic style. They may see the nurse as the qualified expert among them.

Participative Style

The participative style, a supportive approach, is sometimes called the democratic style. This form of leadership has become increasingly popular in recent years as leaders have sought to involve followers in the decision-making process. This style tends to promote followers' self-esteem and to increase motivation and productivity (Fig. 20-2). Leaders utilizing this style

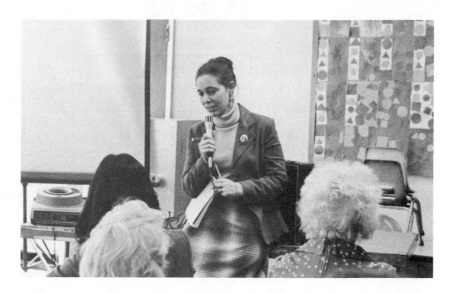

Figure 20-2
As a leader, the nurse seeks to influence clients toward a healthier state. Here the nurse involves a class of senior citizens in a discussion about their health. She uses a partici-pative leadership style.

sometimes find it difficult to maintain control and prevent followers from taking charge while remaining democratic. Some participative leaders permit their followers more freedom and power than others. Generally, however, this leadership style allows followers considerable freedom to make choices.

Laissez-faire Style
The laissez-faire style means giving the followers free rein to do whatever they wish. The leader maintains a hands-off policy that gives complete freedom of choice to the group members, who set their own goals, carry out their own activities, and are essentially independent of the leader. This style may be effective in a group whose members have both the motivation and competence to achieve the goals. Although someone is formally the leader, this style uses little or no direct influence, and some people would argue against its classification as a style of leadership.

TASK- AND RELATIONSHIP-ORIENTED LEADERSHIP

We discussed earlier that leadership is accomplishing goals with and through people. Consequently, leaders must be concerned with tasks (in order to achieve goals) and with relationships (to show concern for people) (Hersey & Blanchard, 1977). These two dimensions, tasks and relationships, become opposite points of emphasis on a continuum of leader behavior, as is illustrated in Figure 20-3. Research has shown that autocratic leaders tend to be concerned about goals and are task oriented, whereas participative leaders are concerned about people and emphasize relationships. These two emphases

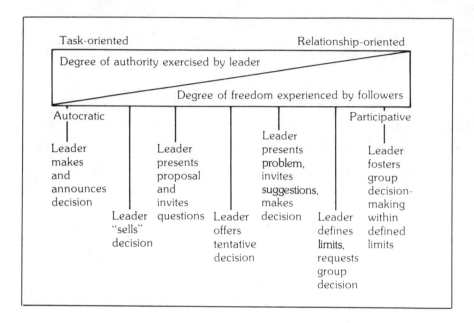

Figure 20-3
Leadership behavior
continuum.

have led to a new taxonomy of leadership styles as either task oriented or relationship oriented (Hersey & Blanchard, 1977).

Leader behavior research has demonstrated that leadership style has a significant influence on leadership effectiveness. However, since many variables, such as leader personality, follower needs and resources, and the situation, influence effectiveness, no one style can be advocated as best.

SITUATIONAL-ORIENTED LEADERSHIP

The situational approach to study of leadership behavior has yielded the most promising results. Based on a recognition that leadership is a relationship between leader, followers, and the situation, it is unrealistic to assume a single, ideal type of leader behavior. A participative style of leadership used in one organization is not always successful in another, similar organization. An integrated style that shows high concern for both tasks and relationships might be appropriate in one setting but not in another. Researchers pursuing the situational approach have concluded that the situation dictates the style of leadership one should use. Because every situation is unique, leadership becomes a dynamic process of adapting one's style to the demands of the situation. Hersey and Blanchard (1977, p. 101) refer to this process as "adaptive leader behavior." Its implications for community health nursing can be stated thus: the more nurses adapt their style of leader behavior to meet the particular situation and the needs of clients or followers, the more effective they will be in reaching health-related goals.

562

The most effective leadership style, then, is an adaptive one. Nurses will need to determine the most appropriate style by assessing the unique qualities of each situation, followers' needs and degree of independence, and their own personalities and abilities.

Conditions for Effective Leadership

The ultimate test of nurse leadership is in the outcomes. Are goals met? What did the leader accomplish? To reach a successful outcome involves certain factors. Adherence to these factors will contribute to positive results, but violation of one or more of them will create negative results. They form the conditions necessary for leadership to be effective.

1. Followers must understand the suggestion, advice, or directive in order to make compliance possible.
2. Followers must be able to carry out the suggestion. They must have or be supplied with the needed resources or abilities.
3. The required action must be consistent with the followers' personal values and interests.
4. The required action must be consistent with the followers' collective purposes, values, and norms; that is, followers must be in tune with group or organizational goals.

Central and most important to effective leadership is a relationship of trust, respect, and mutual exchange between leader and followers. It is through this transactional relationship that community health nurses can satisfy the conditions for effective leadership and accomplish positive outcomes.

Nature of Change

"To lead means to effect change" (Moloney, 1979, p. 87). When nurses suggest that postcoronary clients adopt a new, healthier pattern of living, they are asking them to change. Teaching diabetic children how to give themselves insulin is introducing a change. Revising home health aide/home-makers' responsibilities, again, requires that those individuals change. Since community health nursing's responsibility is to accomplish health goals and thus promote change, nurses cannot lead without introducing change. Therefore, it becomes imperative for community health nurses to understand the nature of change, how people respond to it, and how to manage it.

What is change? For some analysts, change means that things are out of balance; they refer to it as an upset in a system's equilibrium (Bennis, Benne, Chin, & Corey, 1976). For instance, when the mother of a family becomes ill, that family's normal functioning is thrown off balance. Adjustments are required; new patterns of behavior become necessary. Others view change as the process of adopting an innovation (Spradley & McCurdy, 1980). Something different, such as a new diet, is introduced; change occurs when the innovation is accepted, tried, and integrated into daily living. Lippitt (1973, p. 37) defines change as "any planned or unplanned alteration of the status quo in an organism, situation, or process," thus reminding us that change may occur either by design or by default. Still others view change in terms of its effect on behavior. They say change is both the altering of a situation and, depending upon how people define the new situation, the way behavior is altered to fit it (Zaltman & Duncan, 1977). We can see that change requires adjustment in thinking and behavior and that people's responses to change vary according to their perceptions of it. Change threatens the security that people feel when following established and familiar patterns. It generally requires the adoption of new roles. Change is disruptive.

Kinds of Change

The way people respond to change depends, in part, on the kind of change it is. We can describe the change process as occurring along a continuum between two opposites, evolutionary change and revolutionary change (Gerlach & Hine, 1973).

EVOLUTIONARY CHANGE

Evolutionary change tends to be gradual and requires adjustment on an incremental basis. It modifies rather than replaces a current way of operating. Becoming parents, stopping smoking by gradually cutting back on the number of cigarettes smoked each day, and losing weight by eliminating desserts and sweets are examples of evolutionary change. Since it is gradual, this kind of change does not require radical shifts in goals or values; in fact, it may enhance current goals or values. Less threatening and more readily adopted than revolutionary change, evolutionary change is sometimes considered reform. It resembles variations on a musical theme.

REVOLUTIONARY CHANGE

Revolutionary change, in contrast, is more rapid, drastic, and threatening. It may completely upset the balance of the system. It involves different goals and perhaps radically new patterns of behavior. This kind of change resembles a whole new musical theme. Sudden unemployment, stopping smoking overnight, losing the town's football team in a plane accident, or suddenly removing a child from abusive parents are examples of revolutionary change. In each instance, the people affected have little or no advance warning and time to prepare. High levels of psychic energy and rapid behavior change

564

are required in adapting to revolutionary change; as a result, incapacitation, resistance, or denial of the new situation frequently occurs.

The impact of a proposed change on a system will clearly depend on the degree of its evolutionary or revolutionary qualities, a factor to be considered in planning for change. Some situations lend themselves better to one kind of change than the other. A community in need of improved facilities for the handicapped, such as ramps and wider doors, can introduce this change on an evolutionary, incremental basis; whereas a community involved in an unsafe, intolerable, or life-threatening situation, such as a serious epidemic, may require revolutionary change.

Stages of Change

The process of change occurs in three stages described by Lewin (cited in Lippitt, Watson, & Westley, 1958) as unfreezing, moving, and refreezing.

UNFREEZING

Unfreezing, the first stage, occurs when a need for change develops. People are motivated to change either intrinsically or by some external force. During this stage the need for change creates disequilibrium in the system. A system in disequilibrium is more vulnerable to change. People have a sense of dissatisfaction; they feel a void that they would like to fill. Like an amputee eager to use a prosthesis or a community concerned about safe intersections, they are ready for change. Thus, the unfreezing stage involves initiating the change.

Unfreezing may occur spontaneously. A family requests help in solving a problem with alcoholism; a group seeks help in adjusting to retirement. However, the nurse–change agent may need to initiate the unfreezing stage by attempting to motivate clients to see the need for change.

MOVING

Moving, the second stage of the change process, occurs when people examine, accept, and actually try out the innovation. For instance, this is the period when participants in a prenatal class are learning exercises or when the elderly in a senior citizens center are discussing and trying out ways to make their apartments safe from falls. During the moving stage, people experience a series of attitude transformations ranging from early questioning of the innovation's worth to full acceptance and commitment to accomplishing the change. The change agent's role during this stage is to help clients see the value of the change, encourage them to try it out, and assist in adopting it for use.

REFREEZING

Refreezing, the third and final stage in the change process, occurs when the change is established as an accepted and permanent part of the system. The rest of the system has adapted to it. Since it is no longer viewed as disruptive, threatening, or even new, people no longer feel resistant to it. As the change is integrated, the system becomes refrozen and stabilized. We know that refreezing has occurred when weight loss clients, for instance, are regularly following their diets and losing weight, or when the senior citizens have installed grab bars in their bathrooms and removed the scatter rugs, or when the community has erected stop signs and established crosswalks at dangerous intersections.

Refreezing involves integrating or internalizing the change into the system and then maintaining it. Simply because a change has been accepted and tried does not guarantee that it will last. Often there is a tendency for old patterns and habits to return; consequently, the change agent must take special measures to assure maintenance of the new behavior. We will discuss ways to stabilize a change in the next section.

Planned Change

Planned change can be defined as a purposeful, designed effort to effect improvement in a system with the assistance of a change agent. Several characteristics in this definition distinguish planned change from unplanned change. First, the change is purposeful and intentional; there are specific reasons or goals prompting the change. These goals give the change effort a unifying focus and a specific target. Unplanned change occurs haphazardly, and its outcomes are unpredictable. Second, the change is by design, not by default. Thorough, systematic planning provides structure for the change process, a map to follow toward a planned destination. Third, planned change in community health aims at improvement. That is, it seeks to better the present situation, to promote a higher level of efficiency, satisfaction, or productivity. Just as not all movement is forward, not all change is positive or growth producing. Planned change, however, aims to facilitate growth. Finally, the change is accomplished by means of an influencing agent. The change agent serves as a catalyst in developing and carrying out the design; the change agent's role is a leadership role.

Planned Change Process

Before initiating planned change, community health nurses need to consider the dynamics of change in the context of system functioning. Any system seeks to achieve and maintain a relative state of equilibrium. It is in the

566

nature of a system to seek this stability in order to maximize its ability to function. Yet the internal and external forces acting upon every system create new needs that, in turn, demand change in order to restore the system to a new level of functioning and equilibrium. For example, toxic fumes emanating from a derailed freight train forced community residents in a southern town to flee. The introduction of this external force upset the community's equilibrium and ability to function. Every effort was made to remove the source of danger and restore the community to normal functioning. The creation of a new need (to eliminate the toxic fumes) led to a change effort (the cleanup process) in order to restore system balance (normal community living). Community health nurses, as change agents, are responsible for seeing that the needs of clients are met through some kind of change and that a new equilibrium is achieved as soon as possible. They can meet those needs, effect change successfully, and restore clients to a stable state by conducting planned change.

Planned change involves a systematic sequence of activities that utlilizes the nursing process. We shall consider eight basic steps to follow in the successful management of change (Spradley, 1980). They are (1) recognize the symptoms, (2) diagnose the need, (3) analyze alternative solutions, (4) select a change, (5) plan the change, (6) implement the change, (7) evaluate the change, and (8) stabilize the change. Figure 20-4 shows how forces acting on a system create a need for change. When we recognize that need, we have begun the change process. This model also illustrates what happens when the nurse fails to respond to the need for change. The need remains and, in fact, may increase. The client system (those involved and affected by the change) and the change agent must work together throughout the entire planned change process. Their respective roles will vary depending upon the situation, but no planned change will be truly effective without recognition and utilization of this helping relationship. The model depicts the client system as variable and vacillating (wavy arrow) because the client system is generally composed of a number of people. It may be an entire community. Thus it will experience many fluctuations in its involvement with the change process. The change agent (straight arrow), as a good leader and manager, analyzes the situation thoroughly, plans carefully, and sets a steady course for effecting the change.

STEP 1. RECOGNIZE THE SYMPTOMS

The first step in managing change is to realize that there is a need for change by listing all the need's indicators. In this step, one should gather and examine the presenting evidence, not diagnose or jump ahead to treatment. For instance, let us say that several clients request help with parenting. Before we can diagnose or plan, we must determine all the indicators of a need. We cannot assume that these clients feel inadequate in the parent role, nor

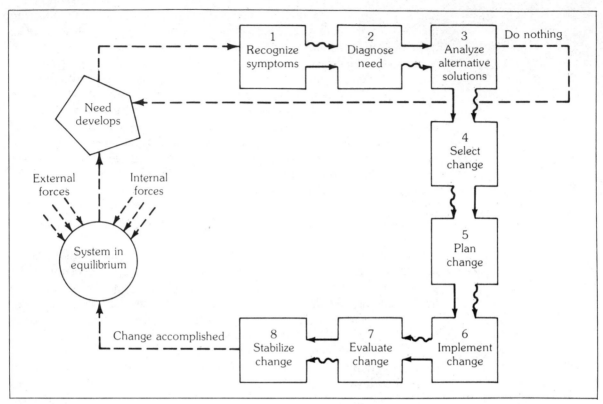

Figure 20-4
Planned change model.
The change agent (solid line) and the client system (wavy line) must work together to effect change.

can we assume that they lack information about parenting or are having difficulty with their children. One, all, or perhaps none of these assumptions may be true. Therefore, we first look for symptoms and discover that some of the parents have trouble talking to their teenagers, others wonder if their children's behavior is normal, a few question how strictly they should set limits, and still others are not certain about how to handle punishment. These symptoms are pieces of evidence that we will diagnose in the next step. It is an assessment phase. Before moving on, however, we need to ask ourselves as change agents what our motives are for pursuing this change. Inappropriate motives, such as wanting to be needed, can cloud judgment and interfere with effective management of change.

STEP 2. DIAGNOSE THE NEED

Diagnosis means to analyze the symptoms and reach a conclusion about what, if anything, needs changing. First, describe the situation as it is now (the real) and compare it to the way it should be (the ideal). For example,

568

you may notice a great deal of loud arguing and conflict among members of a client family. Although your ideal may be quiet harmony, noisy conflict may be normal, functional behavior for this family. In that case, there is no discrepancy between the real and the ideal and therefore no need for change. If, however, there is a discrepancy between the real and the ideal, then a need exists and a change effort is justified (Hersey & Blanchard, 1977). From speaking with the parents, we recognize that their behavior and concerns indicate a possible lack of information about and confidence in the parenting role. A gap clearly exists between their present and ideal situations; therefore, there is a need.

Next, determine the exact nature and cause of the need. Gathering data by means such as questioning clients, checking the literature, or seeking consultation is important for making a more accurate diagnosis. We question the parents in more detail about the difficulties they are having with their children. How do they feel about being parents? What are the most difficult aspects of parenting for them? Have they read any books or used any other resources to help them in their parenting activities? Who do they talk to, if anyone, about parenting problems? When they have a problem handling the raising of their children, how do they usually solve it? We also seek secondary data by checking the literature ourselves to determine the most effective approaches to solving parenting problems. We consult an expert on family life to get ideas about what this group of parents might need, given the symptoms we have seen. We need to come to a conclusion about what specific changes are needed for these parents. Unless the diagnosis is made accurately, the entire change effort may be addressing its attention to the wrong problem. Also, when possible, the client system should help diagnose. We ask the parents to help us determine what, exactly, it is that they need.

Finally, we must narrow the findings down to a single diagnostic statement that also includes the cause. The parents, we discover after data collection, are insecure in their parenting roles. They believe the insecurity is caused partially by lack of knowledge about how to carry out parental responsibilities. Primarily, however, they are convinced that the cause is lack of a supportive reference group. Most of them live some distance from relatives or no longer maintain close ties with relatives. Our diagnosis for these parents is insecurity in the parenting role. We define the cause to be lack of support as well as some lack of knowledge.

STEP 3. ANALYZE ALTERNATIVE SOLUTIONS

Once we know the diagnosis and its cause, we are ready to identify solutions or various alternative directions to follow. Like the physician who has studied the patient's symptoms and diagnosed the patient as having a duodenal ulcer, we must next decide what general treatment direction to follow. Should it be surgery, diet, medication therapy, or a life-style change approach? At this point the physician does not decide on a specific treatment regimen. That step comes later. Brainstorming is helpful at this point, and the client system should be involved as much as possible in the process. Make a list of all the reasonable broad alternatives, and then analyze them thoroughly to determine the advantages, disadvantages, possible consequences, and risks involved in each. For the parents, we could consider general alternatives such as family counseling, a support group, or education in family life. Each of these alternatives has some advantages and disadvantages toward meeting the parents' need for confidence in their roles.

Next, we analyze each alternative. For example, the counseling solution could provide insight and awareness into family behavior. It would give family members opportunities to express feelings and gain understanding of how other members feel. However, it would not provide a frame of reference that they could use to compare their own parenting behaviors with other acceptable ones, nor would it provide adult peer support for the parents. The consequences of this alternative would most likely be to promote parents' self-understanding and better family communication. Risks would include the possibility that children, especially teenagers, might not be willing to participate and that parents might not gain self-confidence in their roles. We study each alternative to determine its usefulness and feasibility. We also go to the literature again and to other resources, such as consultants, to learn all we can about the best ways to meet the parents' need for change.

STEP 4. SELECT THE CHANGE

Having carefully analyzed all the alternatives, we now select the best solution. The parents agree with us that the best solution seems to be a parenting support group. We reexamine the risks involved in the change choice; sometimes a possible course of action may be too costly in time, money, or potential for failure. Also, there may be ways to reduce the risks.

It is important to know what the change is aiming to accomplish; we need a clearly stated goal. For the parenting group, our mutually agreed-upon goal is to provide a supportive, reinforcing climate while increasing members' parenting skills.

STEP 5. PLAN THE CHANGE

This step is at the heart of planned change because it is now that the change agent prepares the design, the blueprint that guides the change action. In steps 1 through 4, data are gathered, a diagnosis made, resources assessed, and a goal established, all preparatory actions for planning the change. The plan tells the change agent and client system how to meet that goal. Preferably they develop the plan together.

We talk with the parents about ways to meet their goal, considering such possibilities as weekly discussion groups on selected topics, monthly meetings with an informed speaker, or reading books and articles on parenting with regular sessions to discuss their application. After analysis and discussion, we decide to meet one evening a month, rotating the location between members' homes. Group sessions will include a variety of approaches: a speaker will be invited every three months; a book or article discussion will be held quarterly; and the remaining meetings will be spent on topics of the group's choice. All sessions will provide opportunities for parents to discuss their concerns or problems. We design this plan around a set of objectives.

The most important activity in planning is to have clear, specific objectives. They should be measurable and, preferably, stated as outcomes. For example, the objective, "By the end of the second session, each parent in the group will have participated in the discussion at least once," is measurable and describes an outcome. Make a list of activities to help you accomplish each objective and develop a time plan. It is also important to assess the potential costs in terms of time, money, number of people and materials needed and to determine the resources available. Design the evaluation plan, and start a list of ways to stabilize (refreeze) the change. During planning, it is useful to perform a force field analysis, a technique developed by Kurt Lewin (1947) for examining all the positive and negative forces in a change situation.

In any situation, there are both driving and restraining forces that influence change. Driving forces push for change. Examples might be clients' desire to be healthier, more productive, or have a safe environment. These are influencing forces in favor of change. Restraining forces, such as apathy, fear of something new, or hostility, work against change, decreasing its possibility. When the strength of the driving forces is equal to the strength of the restraining forces, equilibrium exists. To introduce a change and move the client system to a higher level, that balance must be altered. To do so, the change agent either increases the driving forces, decreases the restraining forces, or both. Force field analysis is a technique that the change agent utilizes to study both sets of forces and to develop strategies to influence them in favor of the change (see Fig. 20-5).

The procedure for conducting a force field analysis follows a few simple steps. As change agent, you may conduct it alone, but preferably, you will consult your clients, a change-planning resource group, such as your nursing team, or both. The steps for force field analysis are given below:

1. Brainstorm to produce a list of all driving and restraining forces. (For the parenting group, one driving force is the parents' desire to be better parents; a restraining force might be lack of group agreement on discussion topics.)
2. Estimate the strength of each force.

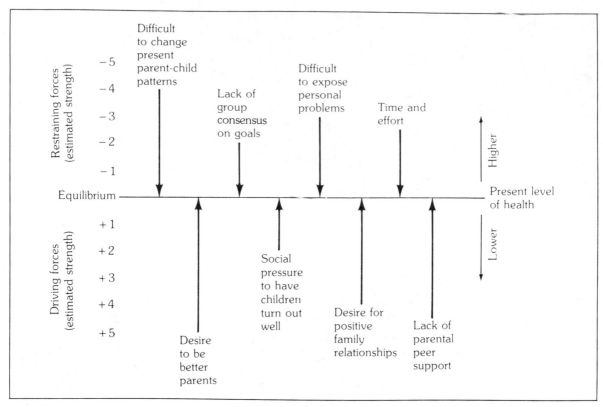

Figure 20-5
Analysis of restraining and driving forces.

3. Plot them on a chart such as the one shown in Figure 20-5.
4. Note the most important forces; then research and analyze them.
5. List and document possible responses or action steps that might strengthen each important driving force or weaken each important restraining force.

Finally, as a consideration in planning the change and in analyzing the driving and restraining forces, study the social network and interaction of the system involved in the change. The change agent needs to be aware of formal and informal leaders, cliques within larger groups, influential persons, the grapevine, and all the other possible social network influences on the change process. For instance, one nurse attempting to change the infant-feeding practices of a young mother failed to consider the strong influence of the grandmother living next door. Another nurse was making no headway with a group of teenage drug addicts until she discovered that their real leader was one of the boys who always sat in the back, not the "captain" appointed by the center director.

STEP 6. IMPLEMENT THE CHANGE

The implementation step involves enacting the change plan. Because their objectives and activities have been clearly defined, change agent and client system know exactly what needs to be done and now proceed to do it. The parenting group and their nurse–change agent, for instance, can start the discussion sessions because they know what they want to accomplish and how to go about it. The change plan tells them where they will meet, how often, what they will discuss, and who will be involved. As they move through implementation, they will also know when their objectives have been met and will have a ready-made plan for evaluation and stabilization of the change, once it has been completed.

At the start of implementation, it is important to make certain that all persons concerned are prepared for the change. When working with a family, for example, the nurse may do most of the planning with one or two key members. Do the other family members, who will also be affected by the proposed change, know what to expect? Do they understand the meaning of the change and what will be required of them in adapting to it? An unprepared client system, especially in a large group or organization, may often spell disaster; no matter how well a change effort is planned, people who are unprepared for it may resist it strongly and render it useless.

In some instances, such as introduction of a mass immunization program or a new clinic procedure, it is helpful to do a pilot study. The study is done to try out the change on a small scale, iron out the problems, and revise the change before implementing it into the whole system. One advantage of a pilot study is that it demonstrates to the client system how the change will work on a scale that is small enough not to require any major adaptation or pose any serious threats to present security. It gives people time to adjust their thinking and to discover that the change may not be so bad after all. It is another way of introducing evolutionary change.

STEP 7. EVALUATE THE CHANGE

The success of this step also depends on how well the change is planned. Well-written objectives with specific criteria for their measurement will make the evaluation step much simpler. However, evaluation does not end with saying whether or not the objectives were met. Each objective requires analysis: (1) Was it met? (2) What evidence (documentation) shows that it was met? and (3) Were the best means used to accomplish it, or would some other method have been better? The objective mentioned earlier for the parenting group could be evaluated by saying, yes, it was met. The fact that every person had entered into the discussion by the end of the second session, a point noted by the nurse–leader, would be evidence that the objective was met. However, the method used to encourage participation might have been to call on individuals who were not contributing, thus in a sense coercing them into participation. A better method would have been to suggest that some individuals seem more involved than others and that the more active ones might like to solicit ideas from those who had not had an opportunity to speak. Finally, considering the evaluation, the change agent makes needed modifications in the change before stabilization.

Figure 20-6
Positive health behaviors, such as these joggers' regular exercise, must be maintained and reinforced for change to be stabilized and health goals achieved.

STEP 8. STABILIZE THE CHANGE

The final step in the planned change process requires taking measures to reinforce and maintain the change (Figure 20-6). A well-developed change

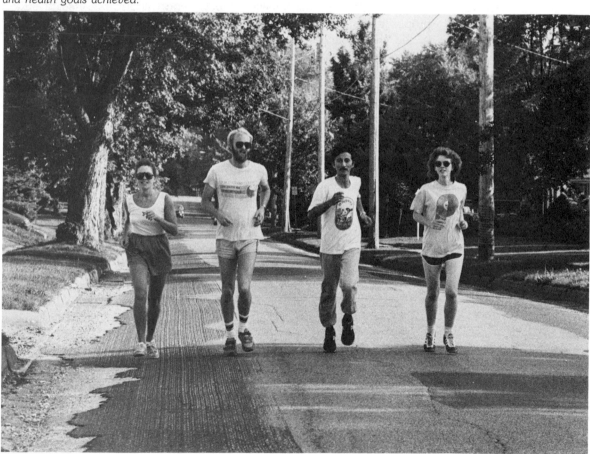

plan includes a design for stabilization. The change agent actively encourages continued use of the innovation by establishing two-way communication; thus any future resistance can be overcome, and the client's full commitment to the change can be maintained. Stabilization occurs through soliciting reactions from the client system. Do the clients perceive any potential problems? Do they have doubts? Reinforcing the desired behavior and following up on the change as long as necessary will help assure its permanence. Alcoholics Anonymous, for example, stabilizes the change to nondrinking by providing a regular support group that reinforces the nondrinking pattern. The group rewards compliance with praise and replaces drinking with other satisfying experiences, such as social acceptance, to keep the alcoholic from returning to the old behavior. We stabilize our parenting group's changed behavior by calling attention to their increased confidence in their parenting roles and by pointing out the greater number of successes they are having in coping with their children. The group itself decides to give a "Parent of the Month" plaque to the member who demonstrates the most growth in his or her parenting skills. The members also agree to nominate one member as "Parent of the Year" in the community newspaper contest. When stabilization occurs, the system achieves a new equilibrium (see Fig. 20-5), and the change agent–client system relationship, at least for this particular change effort, can be terminated.

We have viewed the planned change process primarily in the context of introducing change to smaller aggregates. Community health nurses also utilize these eight steps when managing change at the organization, population group, community, and larger aggregate levels. For example, a nurse may suspect that there is a widespread lack of confidence among young parents. This hypothesis could be tested through an epidemiologic survey to determine parenting needs among the entire community's population of young parents. If symptoms are present (step 1), the nurse, in collaboration with health department personnel or other appropriate professionals, could analyze the symptoms and reach a diagnosis (step 2), perhaps that a large percentage of young parents in the community are lacking in confidence and knowledge of parenting skills. Several approaches to meeting this need could be considered, such as instituting a parenting center in the community with satellite clinics; organizing churches, clubs, or both to sponsor parenting support groups; or working through the community college system to hold workshops and classes on parenting skills (step 3). The most feasible and useful alternative could be selected (step 4), and a parenting program for the community planned (step 5) and implemented (step 6). The nurse, with the other professionals involved, would then evaluate the outcomes (step 7) and make any necessary adjustments in the parenting program before finally stabilizing it (step 8), making certain that this change, undertaken to meet a population group need, remained an established and effectively functioning service.

Planned Change Strategies

The literature describes three general change strategies (Bennis, Benne, Chin, & Corey, 1976; Fischman, 1973; Zaltman & Duncan, 1977). In any given situation, the change agent may use one or a combination of these strategies to effect a change. They are (1) empirical-rational, (2) normative-reeducative, and (3) power-coercive.

EMPIRICAL-RATIONAL

This set of strategies assumes that men and women are rational. When presented with empirical data, people will adopt a new practice because it appears to be in their own best interest. To use this approach, which is common in community health, one simply offers or makes new information available to clients. For instance, most family planning programs use empirical-rational strategies (Fischman, 1973). Clients are given basic information on reproductive anatomy and physiology, and they are told about the benefits of contraception with an explanation of a variety of birth control methods. Health workers hope that once clients have this information, they will adopt some form of birth control. Some clients respond well to this approach, while others do not. The difference lies in client ability and interest in self-help. The nurse–change agent uses empirical-rational strategies with clients who can assume a relatively high degree of responsibility for their own health. In some respects, this set of strategies parallels the participative leadership style, described in Figure 20-2, that fosters maximum client autonomy.

NORMATIVE-REEDUCATIVE

A second set of change strategies goes beyond merely informing to actively influencing the client system. This approach assumes that attitudes and practices are determined by cultural norms; thus knowledge is necessary but not enough to change behavior (Chin & Benne, 1976). Nurse–change agents who use this set of strategies seek to modify the normative orientations of clients through reeducation. They directly influence clients' values, attitudes, skills, and relationships as well as offer new information. This approach attempts to strengthen client self-understanding, self-control, and commitment to new patterns through direct persuasion or manipulation. For example, a health-teaching program that aims to increase safety practices in an industrial setting will, if employing normative-reeducative strategies, not only provide safety information such as posters and warning signs but will also use persuasive tactics such as individual rewards for safe practices, division recognition for minimum number of accidents, or discipline for noncompliance. Nurses use normative-reeducative strategies with clients who have a measure of self-care skill but, at the same time, need external assistance to effect lasting behavior change. This type of client is found in teaching, counseling, and therapy situations.

POWER-COERCIVE

The third set of change strategies uses power to effect change. Change agents may derive power from the *law* (such as health regulations or administrative policies), from *position* (such as political, social, or managerial positions), from a *group* (such as a social, work, or professional group), or from *personal power* (such as personal magnetism, competence, or respect of followers). They use this power to coerce change; the result is more or less forced compliance by the client system. Some situations, particularly those that are life-threatening, may require power-coercive strategies. In community health practice, power-coercive strategies may be used with people who cannot help themselves or in situations that threaten the public's health. If officials find a restaurant in violation of health codes, for example, they will most likely require forced compliance or close down the restaurant. Occasionally clients cannot exercise responsibility, perhaps because they are experiencing temporary physical or psychological incapacitation caused, for example, by severe illness or family abuse. In such cases, the nurse may need to use power to effect changes that are in the clients' best interests. Although power-coercive strategies are appropriate in some situations, they should be used with caution because they can rob clients of opportunities to grow in autonomy and capacity for self-care.

Planned change strategies may be combined; for instance, a normative-reeducative approach might have a power backup. We see this combination in programs that, for example, educate and persuade groups of people to be immunized against an impending epidemic or to keep their garbage contained to avoid insect and rodent infestation. Behind this normative-reeducative strategy is an implied power threat of official disapproval, or worse, for noncompliance.

The effectiveness of a change strategy, then, varies with each situation and particularly with the degree of client capacity for self-care. As in the approach to leadership styles discussed earlier in the chapter, the nurse–change agent adapts strategies to fit each change situation.

Principles for Managing Change

Community health nurses introduce change every day that they practice. Every effort to solve a problem, prevent another from occurring, meet a potential community need, or promote optimal client health requires changes.

To make these changes truly successful so that desired outcomes are reached, they must be managed well. We shall examine six principles that provide some guidelines for effective management of change.

INVOLVE PERSONS AFFECTED BY THE PROPOSED CHANGE

Persons affected by a proposed change should participate as much as possible in every step of the planned change process. This involvement is important for several reasons. Collaboration with those who have a vested interest in the change can produce a wealth of ideas and insights that can greatly improve the change plan. Furthermore, such participation can help remove obstacles and reduce resistance. Participation ensures a greater likelihood of the change's acceptance and maintenance. One nurse, for instance, when planning for a grandmother's care, involved all the family members, including the grandmother; as a result, she automatically secured their support and cooperation, gained many helpful suggestions that she herself had not considered, and discovered that the grandmother was happier and more responsive to care because the change plan was specifically tailored to her needs.

BE PREPARED FOR RESISTANCE TO CHANGE

Because all systems instinctively preserve the status quo, the change agent can expect people to resist change. The homeostatic mechanism operating in any system seeks to maintain equilibrium; change poses a threat to that stability and security. Furthermore, all systems experience inertia, that is, they resist beginning movement. People do not undertake a change until they are convinced of its worth. Resistance may also come from a conflict over goals and methods or from misunderstanding about what the change will mean and require. Involving clients in the planned change process, discussed in the last section, is one way to overcome resistance. Another way is establishing and maintaining open lines of communication in order to make ideas clearly understood and to resolve disagreements quickly. Prepare people thoroughly for the change, provide support and patience during the changing process, and encourage response and expression of feelings.

PROPER TIMING IS IMPORTANT IN PLANNING FOR CHANGE

The Bible says, that for everything there is a time and a season. Sometimes a change, even a well-designed and much needed one, must be postponed because the present is not the right time to introduce it. The client system may now be experiencing too many other changes to handle the stress of another change. Other projects or activities in which the client system is currently engaged may compete for energy and other resources, depleting

578

those needed to make the proposed change successful. For example, some young mothers, eager to start a book club that focused on discussion of child rearing, had to postpone the project because Christmas was approaching. Shopping, entertaining, and vacations made it impossible to give the kind of time and energy needed to make the book club effective.

Proper timing is as important to a planned change as proper seed planting is to a good harvest. The change idea must be appropriate, the change recipient prepared, the climate right, and the resources available before the change can be fostered to grow into full maturity and usefulness.

VIEW CHANGE IN TERMS OF POTENTIAL IMPACT ON SYSTEMS OR SUBSYSTEMS

Every system has many subsystems that are intricately related to and interdependent upon one another. A change in one part of a system affects its other parts, and a change in one system may affect other systems. A county community nursing agency made a change in its use of home health aides. Because many homebound clients needed more care than the agency staff could provide, the agency contracted with a private home-care service for extra home health aides. These paraprofessionals worked in the homes of agency clients, supplementing the care given by agency staff. The private company preferred to supervise its own aides, whereas the county agency had a policy of using community health nurses to supervise aides. The county agency was legally responsible and professionally accountable for the quality of care given to clients. The private company wanted to retain control of its workers. The matter was resolved by contracting with another private service. The change, however, had affected the roles of nurses and aides within the system as well as the relationships between the two systems.

This principle reminds the nurse that change does not take place in a vacuum. When workers learn new health and safety practices associated with their jobs, their relationships with each other and with their bosses and their overall productivity in the organization may easily be affected. One must anticipate and prepare for the impact of the proposed change on the clients involved, other persons, departments, organizations, or even geographic areas.

BE FLEXIBLE

Unexpected events can occur in every situation. This fifth principle emphasizes two points; first, you need to be able to adapt to unexpected events and make the most of them. Perseverance and flexibility are the marks of a good change manager. One community health nurse had tried unsuccessfully to contact a young mother who was reportedly abusing her two-year-old son. After several phone calls and visits to an empty house, she finally found the mother at home but accompanied by a neighbor who insisted on staying for the entire visit. At first the nurse was angry that the neighbor was interfering with her goal of getting to know the mother. Then she realized that this situation offered an opportunity to learn more about the mother through an acquaintance's eyes and possibly to influence another client as well. She included them both in the discussion, explained what she had to offer in terms of health teaching and support, and eventually won their combined respect and confidence.

The second point to remember about flexibility is that a good change planner anticipates possible blocks or problems by preparing strategies and alternate plans. During step 3 of the planned change process, it is helpful to rank the alternative solutions considered. Then, if the first choice does not work out for some reason, a second alternative is ready to be put into action. Flexibility involves a willingness to consider a variety of options and suggestions from many sources.

KNOW YOURSELF

Self-understanding is essential for an effective change agent. As a leader and change agent, how do you define your role? How do others see it? What are your values and motives in relation to each change that you might ask clients to make? What is your personality like and how will it affect the change process? What is your typical leadership style, the one that you most often revert to when not consciously adapting it to the situation? The answers to these questions about yourself will give you much insight into personal behaviors that you may wish to alter and must be considered when planning for change in community health.

Summary

Community health nurses, at every level of practice, are leaders and change agents. They influence individuals and families to adopt healthier behaviors. They lead groups of people to change their health practices. Formally or informally, they act as leaders to bring about organizational change. At the community level, they are involved in changing people's health beliefs and practices and in promoting organized responses to community health problems.

Leadership is an interpersonal process in which one person influences the activities of another person or group of persons toward accomplishment of a goal in a specific situation. It has three major characteristics. First, it is purposeful; it always has a goal. Second, it is interpersonal; it always involves a social transaction. Third, it means influencing; it always affects other people by altering their beliefs and practices in some manner. Community health nursing leadership aims to influence people toward optimal health as well as upgrade professional nursing practice.

580

Effective leadership incorporates five essential functions. Exercising the *creative function,* the leader generates ideas and develops innovative plans for action. With the *initiating function,* the leader introduces changes and sets their processes in motion. Good leaders take calculated risks, evidence of the *risk-taking function.* They use the *integrative function* to strengthen the ties among their followers and unite them through a strong sense of purpose. Finally, with the *instrumental function,* effective leaders facilitate the movement of followers in the right direction. Community health nurses utilize these leadership functions in the context of ever-widening spheres of potential influence. They influence consumers; other nurses; health service organizations; other professionals; resources and programs affecting health; and state, regional, national, and even international programs and organizations.

Leadership styles have been studied for many years. The original view that some individuals are born with leadership qualities has been refuted. More recent research supports the fact that leader behavior, rather than leader personality, determines effectiveness. From this research we have drawn three styles of leadership. *Autocratic* leadership is authoritative; orders are given that people are expected to follow. *Participative* leadership is democratic and involves followers in the decision-making process. This style tends to promote followers' self-esteem and to increase their productivity. *Laissez-faire* leadership gives followers complete freedom of choice; they are essentially independent of the leader. Some would argue that this style is not a form of leadership at all.

Leadership encompasses two important dimensions: a concern for accomplishing goals and a concern for relationships with people. The different leadership styles emphasize these dimensions to varying degrees. An autocratic style tends to be task oriented, while a democratic style tends to be relationship oriented. Situational leadership integrates both task and relationships by emphasizing one or the other depending upon the situation. This more recent leadership approach has evolved as the most effective because it tailors to each situation the style of leadership one should use.

Change is an outcome of leadership. Our job in community health nursing is to effect change by preventing illness and promoting health. Change, however, is disruptive. Evolutionary change is gradual and requires adjustment on an incremental basis. We introduce this kind of change in many situations. Revolutionary change tends to occur suddenly and is more drastic. It may be necessary to introduce revolutionary change under certain conditions, such as an emergency.

Change occurs in three major stages. First, there is *unfreezing.* It is during this stage that the need for change develops. People become receptive. *Moving,* the second stage, occurs when people accept and try out the innovation. The third stage, *refreezing,* involves maintaining the change as an accepted, established part of the system.

Planned change is a purposeful, designed effort to effect improvement in a system with the assistance of a change agent. It involves a process of eight steps that nurses can follow to manage change:

1. Recognize the symptoms that indicate a need for change.
2. Diagnose the need by analyzing the symptoms and reaching a conclusion about what needs changing.
3. Analyze alternative solutions by first identifying a variety of possible general directions to pursue and then analyzing each of these in relation to their advantages, disadvantages, and possible outcomes and risks.
4. Select the change alternative that is most feasible and most likely to meet the identified need. Decide on the goal for this change project.
5. Plan the change by developing specific objectives and a set of activities to meet the stated goal. Force field analysis is a useful tool to facilitate change planning.
6. Implement the change by enacting the change plan, making certain that the client system is properly prepared.
7. Evaluate the change, measuring its outcomes and making needed adjustments.
8. Stabilize the change, instituting measures to reinforce and maintain (refreeze) the change.

During planned change, we can use one or a combination of three major strategies. *Empirical-rational* strategies provide basic information and assume that people are rational and will act on this new knowledge because to do so serves their own best interest. *Normative-reeducative* strategies not only give information but also directly influence people to change. *Power-coercive* strategies use power to force change.

Six principles provide community health nurses with guidelines for managing change:

1. Involve the persons affected by the proposed change.
2. Be prepared for resistance to change.
3. Proper timing is important in planning for change.
4. View any change in terms of its potential impact on systems or subsystems.
5. Be flexible.
6. Know yourself.

Study Questions

You have been asked to chair an ad hoc committee in a community health nursing agency. The committee's task is to plan a health fair for the local community.

1. Discuss how you would exercise each of the five leadership functions as you chair the planning committee.
2. What would your leadership style be and how would you know whether it was appropriate for this situation?
3. What strategies would you use to ensure that the health fair was viewed by community members as an evolutionary change?
4. Six principles for managing change were presented in this chapter. Briefly discuss how you would use each one as you and your committee develop the health fair.

References

Argyris, C. (1976). *Increasing leadership effectiveness.* New York: John Wiley.

Bennis, W. G., Benne, K. D., Chin, R., & Corey, K. (1976). *The planning of change* (3rd ed.). New York: Holt, Rinehart and Winston.

Chin, R., & Benne, D. (1976). General strategies for effecting changes in human systems. In W. G. Bennis, K. D. Benne, R. Chin, & K. Corey (Eds.), *The planning of change* (3rd ed.). New York: Holt, Rinehart and Winston.

Fischman, S. (1973). Change strategies and their application to family planning programs. *American Journal of Nursing, 73,* 1771.

Gerlach, L., & Hine, V. (1973). *Lifeway leap: The dynamics of change in America.* Minneapolis: University of Minnesota Press.

Hennes, K., Sr. (1979). *Expansion of the aide's role in home care.* Unpublished manuscript, University of Minnesota, Minneapolis.

Hersey, P., & Blanchard, K. (1977). *Management of organizational behavior: Utilizing human resources* (3rd ed.). Englewood Cliffs, NJ: Prentice-Hall.

Lewin, K. (1947). Frontiers in group dynamics: Concept, method, and reality in social science; social equilibria and social change. *Human Relations, 1,* 5.

Lippitt, G. L. (1973). *Visualizing change: Model building and the change process.* La Jolla, CA: University Associates.

Lippitt, R., Watson, J., & Westley, B. (1958). *The dynamics of planned change.* New York: Harcourt, Brace & World.

Moloney, M. (1979). *Leadership in Nursing: Theory, Strategies, Action.* St. Louis: C. V. Mosby.

Spradley, B. (1980). Managing change creatively. *Journal of Nursing Administration, 10*(5), 32–37.

Spradley, J., & McCurdy, D. (1980). *Anthropology: The cultural perspective* (2nd ed.). New York: Wiley.

Uris, A. (1964). *Techniques of leadership.* New York: McGraw-Hill.

Zaltman, G., & Duncan, R. (1977). *Strategies for planned change.* New York: Wiley.

Selected Readings

Aeschleman, D. (1976). A strategy for change. *Nurse Practitioner, 1*(1), 121–124.

Argyris, C., & Schon, D. A. (1974). *Theory in practice: Increasing professional effectiveness.* San Francisco: Jossey-Bass.

Aspree, E. S. (1975). The process of change. *Supervisor Nurse, 6*(10), 5–24.

Bennis, W. G., Benne, K. D., Chin, R., & Corey, K. (Eds.). (1976). *The planning of change* (3rd ed.). New York: Holt, Rienhart and Winston.

Brooten, D., Hayman, L., & Naylor, M. (1978). Leadership for change: A guide for the frustrated nurse. *American Journal of Nursing, 78,* 1526–1529.

Brooten, D., Hayman, L., & Naylor, M. (1978). *Leadership for change: A guide for the frustrated nurse.* Philadelphia: Lippincott.

Burns, J. M. (1978). *Leadership.* New York: Harper & Row.

Chin, R., & Benne, D. (1976). General strategies for effecting changes in human systems. In W. G. Bennis, K. D. Benne, R. Chin, & K. Corey (Eds.), *The planning of change* (3rd ed.). New York: Holt, Rinehart and Winston.

Conway, M. E. (1978). Clinical research: Instrument for change. *Journal of Nursing Administration, 8*(12), 27–32.

Deal, J. (1977). The timing of change. *Supervising Nurse, 8*(9), 73–79.

Dyer, W. G. (1973). Planning change in the family. In A. Reinhardt & M. Quinn (Eds.), *Family-centered community nursing: A sociocultural framework.* St. Louis: C. V. Mosby.

Fischman, S. (1973). Change strategies and their application to family planning programs. *American Journal of Nursing, 73,* 1771.

Gerlach, L., & Hine, V. (1973). *Lifeway leap: The dynamics of change in America.* Minneapolis, MN: University of Minnesota Press.

Green, L. W. (1976). Change process models in health education. *Public Health Reviews, 5*(1), 5–33.

Grissum, M. (1976). How you can become a risk taker and a role breaker. *Nursing '76 6*(11), 89–98.

Guest, R., Hersey, P., & Blanchard, K. (1977). *Organizational change through effective leadership.* Englewood Cliffs, NJ: Prentice-Hall.

Havelock, R. G., & Havelock, M. C. (1973). *Training for change agents: A guide to the design of training programs in education and other fields.* Ann Arbor, MI: University of Michigan, Institute for Social Research.

Hein, E. & Nicholson, M. J., (1982). *Contemporary leadership behavior: Selected readings.* Boston: Little, Brown.

Hersey, P., & Blanchard, K. (1977). *Management of organizational behavior: Utilizing human resources* (3rd ed.). Englewood Cliffs, NJ: Prentice-Hall.

Lancaster, J. (1980). An ecological orientation toward change: Considerations for leadership in nursing. *Image, 3*(4), 12–15.

Leary, P. A. (1972). The change agent. *Journal of Rehabilitation, 1,* 30–33.

584

Lippitt, G. L. (1973). *Visualizing change: Model building and the change process.* La Jolla, CA: University Associates.

Lippitt, R., Watson, J., & Westley, B. (1958). *The dynamics of planned change.* New York: Harcourt, Brace & World.

Longest, B. (1976). Managing change: The management imperative. In B. Longest (Ed.), *Management practices for the health professional* (pp. 223–238). Reston, VA: Reston Publishing.

Mirvis, P. H., & Berg, D. N. (1977). *Failures in organization development and change: Cases and essays for learning.* New York: Wiley.

Moloney, M. (1979). *Leadership in nursing: Theories, strategies, action.* St. Louis, C. V. Mosby.

Rodgers, J. (1973). Theoretical considerations involved in the process of change. *Nursing Forum, 12,* 161–174.

Rothman, J., Erlich, J., & Teresa, J. (1981). *Changing Organizations and Community Programs.* Beverly Hills, CA: Sage Publications.

Rothman, J. (1974). *Planning and organizing for social change: Action principles from social science research.* New York: Columbia University Press.

Rubin, I., Plovnich, M., & Fry, F. (1974). Initiating planned change in health care systems. *Journal of Applied Behavioral Science, 10,* 107–124.

Sanders, I. T. (1975). Professional roles in planned change. In R. M. Kramer & H. Specht (Eds.), *Readings in community organization practice* (2nd ed.). Englewood Cliffs, NJ: Prentice-Hall.

Schaller, L. E. (1972). *The change agent: The strategy of innovative leadership.* Nashville, TN: Abingdon.

Sims, L. S. (1979). The community nutritionist as change agent. *Family and Community Health, 1*(4), 83–92.

Spradley, B. (1980). Managing change creatively. *Journal of Nursing Administration, 10*(5), 32–37.

Stevens, B. J. (1975). Effecting change. *Journal of Nursing Administration, 5*(2), 23–28.

Watzlawick, P., Weaklund, J., & Fisch, R. (1974). *Change: Principles of problem formation and problem resolution.* New York: Norton.

Wheelis, A. (1973). *How people change.* New York: Harper & Row.

Williams, C. (1981). Nursing leadership in community health: A neglected issue. In J. McCloskey & H. Grace (Eds.), *Current Issues in Nursing* (pp. 289–297). Oxford, England: Blackwell Scientific Publications.

Zaltman, G., & Duncan, R. (1977). *Strategies for planned change.* New York: Wiley.

Zaltman, G., Duncan, R., & Holbek, J. (1973). *Innovations and organizations.* New York: Wiley.

Zimmerman, B. M. (1979). Changes of the second order. *Nursing Outlook, 27,* 199–201.

Political Involvement and Community Health Advocacy

Terry W. Miller

Community health has undergone many changes since its inception in the late 1880s and so has health policy. Historically and dangerously, nurses have placed blind trust in other health care providers, such as physicians, insurance companies, and politicians, to develop, regulate, and finance the U.S. health care system. Underneath all legislation and health care regulation are power struggles. The outcome determines the types and quality of all social services. To a great extent, health policy and nursing practice rest upon legislative action at the state and federal levels. Having only an institutional or local perspective is not enough to ensure the future of community health, much less nursing. Many people, even a health care bill's originator, are unaware of a bill's total impact on health care. In other words, the intent of a policy is not always its actual outcome. Consultation with nurses and other important implementers of the policy may not be considered. Clearly, nurses develop an operational knowledge of health policy and political process to protect individuals, families, communities, and nursing practice.

This chapter focuses on health policy and the political process as they relate to community health nursing. The aim is not to isolate or differentiate community health nursing from other health professions or even other nursing specialties. The purpose is to emphasize the need for community health nurses to understand their role and power in providing an essential determinant and unique perspective in health care.

586

What Is Policy?

Many definitions of social or public policy have been proposed in recent years as the study of policy has become a more formalized and highly funded academic field. Many of the most respected universities in the country support a school of public affairs. Nursing's representation in such schools has been minimal. These schools arose out of need and demonstrate the relevancy, as well as the complexity, of understanding policy and political process today.

Basically, policy is what an institution, organization, agency, or government chooses to do or not to do. Policy can be formally written, as it should be, but many policies are unwritten, unclear, or "hidden" to prevent public or legal review. Either way, policy includes all actions of an institution, organization, agency, or government. Government policy, whether the government is local, state, or federal, is public policy (Dye, 1978).

More specifically, health policy pertains to the deliberative allocations of resources to health care. Resources include people, facilities, time, and money. To see health policy only from the economic perspective is a mistake. Not to consider the costs of health care is a greater mistake, as the outcry of the public, followed by politicians, demonstrates. Policy usually begins as health laws but may be secondary to other types of legislation. For instance, military policy on nuclear defense affects health policy, whether intentionally or not. Since resources are limited, distribution in one area affects or determines the availability of resources in another area.

Most policies are created to express the collective interests and beliefs of the social system or institution that generates them. Unfortunately, many people within a social system or institution allow others to determine policy for them instead of with them. The community health nurse's primary mission is to promote and preserve the health of aggregates or populations. In order to fulfill this mission, nurses should be policymakers, as well as policy followers. Even within the profession, some nurses lack the vision to promote community health. They define the client as a hospitalized patient and nothing more.

Various health policies can be categorized by their social impact or outcomes. *Distributive* health policies promote nongovernmental activities thought to be beneficial to society as a whole. Title VIII, the Nurse Training Act, of the Public Health Service Act is such a distributive policy. This establishes a federal subsidy for nursing education. *Redistributive* health policy changes the allocation of resources from one group to usually a broader or different group. Medicare illustrates this type of redistributive policy. *Competitive* regulation through health policy limits or structures the provision of health services by designating who can deliver them. Nurse licensure is a form of such regulation at a state level. Protective regulation sets conditions under which various private activities can be undertaken. Although professional licensure is most commonly identified by professions as first and foremost protecting the public, such policy is competitive regulation in terms of social impact. Professional standards review organizations or certificates of need are more clearly defined as protective regulation.

Health policy comes from many sources. On the surface it appears that it emanates from the government. But, in reality, policymakers take their cues from many sources. Community health nurses should be one of the major sources, even though many strong and well-organized forces resist nursing's direct involvement in the politics and policy-making of health care.

Policy Systems and Policy Analysis

All people are political creatures in the sense that they live within the context of many political systems. The more obvious political systems are the state and federal governments. The political system within a community may be less formalized or apparent but also has a profound influence on the collective health and well-being of its people.

Political systems, such as city and county governments, are interrelated, complex, and generate policies. Therefore, they are also policy systems. A community health nurse needs a simple policy analysis framework for determining the intentions and possible capacity of political and policy systems. This framework allows the nurse to protect herself and, most important, protect the client, whether it be a community or individual.

Policy analysis is the systematic identification of causes or consequences of policy and the factors that influence it. Often nurses confuse policy advocacy with policy analysis. This mistake can be detrimental in community health nursing. Policy advocacy is subjective; policy analysis should be objective. What is most important is that policy analysis should come before policy advocacy.

When the nurse looks at a policy, for example, mandatory preschool immunizations, affecting the health of a community or target population, several approaches may be taken. Focusing on the policy's consequences makes the policy an independent variable and the social, economic, or political conditions in the community dependent variables. This impact approach to policy analysis requires two general questions to be answered: (1) Who benefits from this policy? and (2) Who loses from this policy? Whether or not the policy should be advocated by the community as a whole depends upon the degree to which the policy benefits the community without being detrimental to individuals or the country.

Figure 21-1 provides a simple model for studying health policy. If nurses know something about the forces shaping health policy and the policy process, then they are in a better position to influence policy outcomes. The model identifies four major stages in the policy process: formulation, adoption, implementation, and evaluation. Policy formulation has to do with identifying goals, problems, and potential solutions. Policy adoption refers to the authorized selection and specification of means to achieve goals, resolve problems, or

588

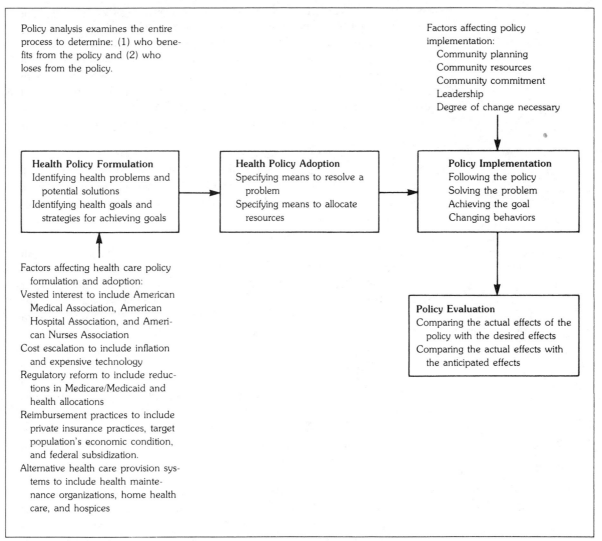

Figure 21-1
Policy analysis model.

both. Implementation follows adoption and occurs when the policy is put to use. Policy evaluation means comparing policy outcomes or effects with the intended or desired effects.

POLICY FORMULATION AND ADOPTION

Health policy formulation is the stage at which a policy is conceptualized and ultimately defined. It is approached in at least two ways. Most commonly, a health problem is identified, such as the increased infant mortality rate associated with a teenage pregnancy. Health policy is developed to correct the particular health problem. Another approach to policy formulation emphasizes health planning more than corrective actions, at least initially. Health goals and strategies for achieving the goals are identified. In this more proactive approach, resources may be created as well as allocated for health services. Whereas both approaches to policy formulation may lead to the solution of a health problem, the goal-oriented approach is less reactive in that it does not require problem identification before the making of health policy.

The social and political conditions that affect policy formulation are limitless, but public need and public demand should be the strongest. Health care providers can stimulate a community to identify its health needs and demand health policies to alleviate or fulfill its needs. During this process the community health nurse recognizes that each community is unique with its mix of health services and public expectations.

There are increasing demands for (a) better quality health services, (b) better access to health services, (c) better cost control of health services, and (d) more health services. Expensive technologies, consumer naïveté, and reimbursement procedures that reward inefficiency while disassociating care from actual costs, hinder the fulfillment of these demands. Americans have grown to believe that health care is a basic human right, and nursing has supported this belief. But Americans are no longer capable nor willing to pay for the present system with its rapidly escalating costs. Indeed, health care is undergoing a metamorphosis.

What should be the role of community health nurses in policy formulation? All professions face the continuing problem of making their knowledge useful to society (Dye, 1978, p. 13). Community health nursing, as does all of nursing, faces the challenge of determining its appropriate relationship with the government. In this determination there are certain requirements to be met.

Community health nurses are community advocates. Their role is to increase the community's health awareness and to support the community's decisions regarding health policies. This recognition of a community's rights in determining its health policies inherently involves conflict. Nurses as decision makers are often under pressure to define specific goals, delegate or implement actions to achieve these goals, and even to establish controls to see that a community moves toward these goals. Sometimes, specific health goals prove elusive or they have no validity save that they are agreed upon. One thing is certain, the goals, constraints, and consequences of actions are seldom known precisely at a community level.

POLICY IMPLEMENTATION

Implementation of health policy occurs when an individual, group, or community puts the policy into use. It involves overt behavior changes as the

590

policy is put into nursing practice. The degree and extent of compliance to a policy is the most direct measure of the policy's implementation. Non-compliance refers to the conscious or unconscious refusal to follow the policy directives. Community health nurses have always been health policy implementers and, recently, evaluators, regardless of whether or not these roles were consciously chosen.

Implementation of health policy is an essential part of effective, comprehensive client care for many documentable reasons. It should now be apparent that policies come in many forms and may have statutory or nonstatutory origins. Nurses are most cognizant of the latter in the form of procedure manuals and institutional guidelines. Communities are most aware of policies that limit or restructure their activities and growth, for example, curfews and zoning regulations.

Once a health policy is written and adopted, its successful implementation depends heavily upon the manipulation of many variables. For example, the implementation of day care standards depends, in part, on how they are interpreted and what resources are available to enforce them. The community health nurse as an implementer assesses the capacity of the community to formulate and define strategies that will enhance the community's compliance to the policy. This phase of policy analysis does not focus on the merits or shortcomings of the policy as is done in policy formulation, adoption, and evaluation.

POLICY EVALUATION

Comparing what a health policy does with what it is supposed to do is evaluation. Evaluation of a policy should result in continuance of the policy in its original form, revision or modification of the policy, or termination of the policy. Laws and policies are created to express the collective and powerful interests of the political system that generated them. The need for a particular health policy may be temporary, but a policy is difficult to change once adopted and implemented. Once a policy system is in operation, vested interests evolve as a result and become political influences. These vested interests under the guise of jobs, positions, titles, and wealth are perceptibly jeopardized by any change in the health policy that helped create them. Hence, tradition or old policies tend to prevail.

Regardless of the factors that affect policy evaluation, continual comparison of what a community believes about and wants in health care with what it is getting is necessary. As community advocates, nurses have a responsibility to increase the community's awareness of health issues. They help the community recognize and demand that its health needs are met through productive, desirable health policies.

Perhaps the major premise that should underlie the evaluation is that the goal of health policy is to design a system whereby health services are equitably distributed and appropriate care is given to the right people at a reasonable cost (Donley, 1982, p. 844). This premise leads to the basic criteria for evaluation:

1. Are the health services appropriate?
2. Are the health services accessible?
3. Are the health services comprehensive?
4. Is there continuity of care?
5. Is the quality of the services adequate?
6. Is the efficiency of the services adequate?
7. Is there an ongoing evaluation of the services?
8. Is appropriate action taken based on the findings of the evaluation?

Determining a Community's Health Policy Needs

It is essential that the community health nurse take an active role in community organization. The nurse serves as a facilitator in assessing the community's unique health care needs in relation to its existing health care policies. Legislation and policy must be reviewed from the community's viewpoint as opposed to an individual's viewpoint. Both public health efforts and community health systems are confronted with conflicting interests when individual rights interfere with aggregate rights. However, the community health nurse's primary mission is to promote and preserve the health of populations or aggregates for the benefit of the entire community.

To identify the health policy needs of a community requires an ongoing comprehensive assessment of the community or what some policy analysts call a "community diagnosis." Chapter 13 identifies the dimensions or variables of a community that are important in making a community assessment. Performing a community assessment is one important major component of community organization.

Steps in Community Organization for Political Action

Organizing a particular community is a multistep process in which several major steps have been identified. They follow:

1. *As the community health nurse, identify yourself as a potential community organizer.* In this beginning step, nurses must perform a self-assessment in terms of what they have to offer the community.
2. *Identify problems, concerns, and issues.* This information should come from the community's perspective, not merely that of individuals. Such information may be obtained directly by conducting a survey in the community and indirectly by looking at vital statistics, voting practices, and the life-style of the community.

3. *Assess the physical community.* The physical environment can have a significant influence on the community. Characteristics of the setting in which a population lives sets the stage for particular health problems and practices. Information about the physical environment can be obtained from a variety of resources, described in chapter 13.

4. *Assess community strengths, resources, and interests.* This information is an important indicator of the community's health potential. A wealth of untapped information may be lying dormant until it is identified and valued by the community. In this step, the nurse identifies community skills and assesses community strengths and limitations.

5. *Assess political influences in the community.* Each community has its own power base and political structure. The community health nurse must understand that power is an essential and primary concept inherent to all political and policy systems (Kalisch & Kalisch, 1982). Power is perceived as a limited entity and therefore is not given freely, even when "deserved" or "earned." Historically, the four most powerful health interest groups have been physicians, hospitals, insurance companies, and the drug industry (Lee, Estes, & Ramsey, 1984, p. 332). Gaining knowledge of community political systems enables the nurse to identify key people and operations that are essential to the successful implementation of health goals. The community health perspective has a political advantage in terms of votes if the community is clearly defined and can be unified on a particular health issue.

6. *Evaluate alternative courses of action.* Community decision making is facilitated when the community is well informed. The nurse can play an important role in the decision-making process by helping to identify possible outcomes and alternative courses of action to meet health goals. Each community, as well as each individual, is different in its perspective of a situation. Decision making will be influenced by the impact the decision can have on the social systems of the community.

7. *Redefine objectives, priorities, and the community health nurse's goals.* After a careful assessment of the community's needs, the community health nurse must compare the relationship between existing programs and policies as they relate to the defined needs and goals. If an incongruent relationship does exist, plans must be made to redefine and reshape existing and future policy directions.

8. *Develop a plan of action.* Planning for an entire community requires the nurse to collaborate with other professionals and representatives of the community's social systems. Each member of the planning team is considered an equal resource, and each member's input is vital to the successful implementation of the plan.

9. *Implement the plan.* Implementation of a plan requires several important considerations: involvement by representatives of the population to be affected, proper timing, and preparedness.

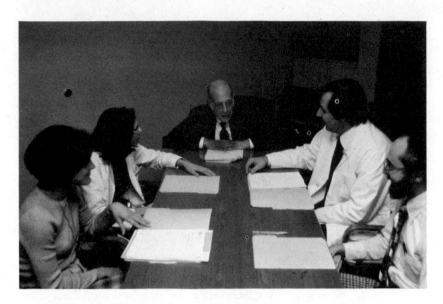

Figure 21-2
This group of professionals is meeting to accomplish a health planning task.

10. *Evaluate the outcome of the planned action.* Evaluation of a plan or program requires an analysis between the outcomes observed and the specific goals, objectives, and criteria that were adopted. Evaluation is a continuous consideration of community organization, and change is inherent before stabilization can occur.

The Legislative Process and Influencing Legislation

Theoretically, at the local level health policies are guidelines for the implementation of health laws. A community's policy system exerts its control in distributing its health resources through its health policies. Sometimes nurses and clients come to think of policies as statutes and therefore as difficult to change as law. In reality, community health policies are often an interpretation of health laws and at best serve as a strategy for implementing health laws, whether they be state or federal.

The nurse's role as an indirect care provider includes active involvement in the community's political arena. Nurses particularly have a responsibility in generating new ways of providing health care and in modifying or improving existing health care. In order to influence and initiate changes in the health care system, the nurse needs to know about the legislative process. The nurse also needs to know how to influence the passage of legislation or modify existing legislation. These skills are essential for all professional nurses

594

because they are major ways that nurses can provide leadership in the improvement of health care.

How a Bill Becomes Law

In the United States, all nurses have opportunities to provide input on the initiation, formulation, and revision of legislation at the local, state, and federal levels. Proposed drafts of bills originate from many places because the sources of legislative ideas are relatively unlimited. An idea may be forwarded to a legislator by individuals, groups, government agencies, or other interested parties. The process can be initiated simply by a concerned citizen or group writing or talking to a legislator.

The legislative process is well defined and governed by rules at all levels of government. The process is similar at the state and federal levels with the exception of some minor peculiarities. Public libraries have copies of a state's legislative process, or the nurse may write to the state's printing office for information.

There is a requirement that certain types of bills be started in the U.S. House of Representatives, as opposed to the U.S. Senate. This may not be true at the state level, depending upon the particular state's Constitution. Once a senator or representative is found who is willing to author a bill, discussion takes place about what current law needs changing or what needs to be added to existing laws. When authoring a bill, a senator or representative consults with a Legislative Council. This council consists of legal specialists who assist legislators with the drafting of bills. The drafted bill is returned to its originator in the form of an "author copy." Content is carefully reviewed to ascertain that the bill does in fact state what it was intended to state.

A bill can be introduced at any time while the House is in session as long as the sponsoring representative has endorsed the bill and placed the proposal in the House's hopper. The procedure is more formal for the Senate, and any Senator can postpone a bill by raising objections to it. All sponsored bills are assigned a legislative number and referred to committee. Presently there are 16 standing committees of the U.S. Senate and 22 standing committees of the U.S. House of Representatives. Most standing committees have two or more subcommittees.

Formal statements and details pertaining to the bill are published in the *Congressional Record*. Also the bill will be printed for distribution. At the federal level, a bill may be considered at any time during the two-year life of that Congress.

The chairperson of the committee to which a bill has been referred must submit the bill to the appropriate subcommittee within a specified time period, usually two weeks. The exception is when the majority of the committee members of the majority party vote to have the bill considered by full committee. Traditionally, many committees and subcommittees have held to a policy that any member who insists on a committee hearing on a particular bill should have it. Standing committees must have regular meetings at least once per month, and the chairperson may call additional meetings.

The legislators appointed to a committee conduct the hearing on a bill. At the federal level a bill may have no hearings or several hearings at one time in different committees. At the federal level, the author of a bill is seldom a member of the committee hearing the bill, while at the state level, the bill's author may have privileges not available to other legislators or the audience.

The committee chairperson selects individuals to present testimony first at hearings. Individuals or representatives of groups who have requested to speak about the bill may or may not be called for testimony. It is frustrating political reality that one may go to committee hearings planning to speak or expecting to hear witnesses, only to find that the voting action was determined before the meeting. Astute individuals and groups not only monitor legislation, but they tactfully lobby legislators before committee and subcommittee hearings.

After studying a bill and possibly hearing testimony, a committee may approve a bill in its original form and forward it. More commonly, the bill is revised and then forwarded or set aside. If a committee votes to pass a bill, a committee report is written that includes the bill's purpose, scope, and the reasons for the committee's approval. Containing a section-by-section analysis of the bill, the report is one of the most valuable sources of information regarding policy formulation and adoption.

Amendments to state bills and federal bills are handled differently. At the state level, the original bill retains its assigned number throughout the legislative process regardless of amendments. At the federal level, amending occurs in "mark-up" sessions. A new bill is printed and reintroduced with a new number following each mark-up session. Obviously, it is more difficult to follow a bill through the federal process. Also, it should be noted that over 25,000 bills and joint resolutions are introduced in the average two-year U.S. Congress. Less than 10 percent of these are enacted as laws (U.S. House of Representatives, 1981, p. 46).

In summary, there are three types of recommendations the committee can make. First, *due pass* means the committee approves the bill and is ready to forward it. Second, *due pass with amendments* means the committee has revised the bill. Third, the committee may refer the bill to another committee. If the bill is set aside by any committee it will eventually die; therefore, committees constitute veto points for bills.

Following committee action, the bill goes on the calendar and awaits being read before the originating house. The house considers the bill and at this point its author states reasons why the bill is needed and responds to questions. Only legislators of the house may speak at the floor vote. The house may pass the bill or defeat the bill at the third reading. If the author knows in advance there are not enough votes for the bill's passage, he or she will take action to delay the vote. At this point considerable compromise, negotiating, trade-offs and other strategies come into play. Success greatly depends upon the author's power base and political maneuvering.

If a bill passes the first house, it is forwarded to the second house. For example, if a bill passes the Senate, it then goes to the House of Representatives. It enters as a new bill with an introduction and first reading. In the second house the bill will again be assigned to committee. The committee will recommend due pass, due pass as amended, or amend and rerefer. Following this committee's actions, the bill has a second reading on the floor of the second house. The third reading results in a floor vote. If there are any changes in the bill by the second house, it is returned to the originating house for concurrence. When significant differences prevent concurrence, the bill is referred to a conference committee, consisting of members from both houses.

The conference committee action is a very important step to which the public has no access. This committee determines which version of the bill, or a compromise of the bill, will go forward in the conference report. After adoption by both houses, the bill is enrolled and goes to the president.

The president has three options; he may sign, hold, or veto the bill. Signing the bill causes it to become law. Holding the bill without signing it causes the bill to become law after a delay of ten days if Congress is still in session. Vetoing the bill sends it back to Congress with the president's objections attached. Congress can override this veto by a two-thirds majority vote in both houses, but if the veto is overridden, the bill becomes law despite the president's objections.

Figure 21-3 outlines the process by which a bill becomes law. The fact remains that statutory law is only the beginning. The legislature enacts statutory law that enables a government agency to administer that law by means of regulation. Law is only measured in court. There are few laws other than criminal law by which one may be cited for noncompliance without going through a report mechanism. The government agency administers the law through regulation. In the case of registered nurses, it is the Board of Registered Nursing that administers those laws relating to nursing education, licensure, and practice, most often called the Nurse Practice Act. That is the group accountable for disciplining registered nurses who do not meet the law.

A Political Strategy

Community health nursing must be clearly defined as having a necessary and integral role with clear-cut responsibilities in the health care system. The role must be understood and appreciated by the public and legislators. The "selling" or marketing of the role can begin at the community or grass-roots level but must also occur at the state and national levels. Ideas of opposition

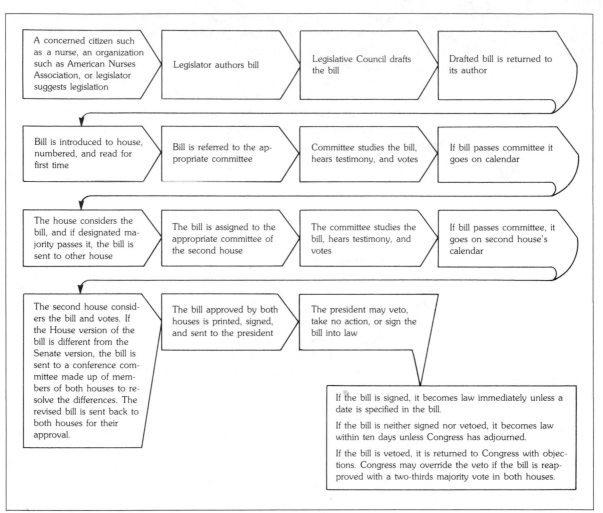

Figure 21-3
This flow chart diagrams the legislative process through which a bill becomes a federal law.

groups or interest groups with conflicting goals must be met with constructive criticism and compromise. During this process of defining and marketing nursing, nurses should present a positive and unified image to the public, the legislators, and opposition groups. Nursing, like all other professions, has internal struggles and disagreements, but politically successful professions avoid public disclosure of internal discontent. Nursing holds a great deal of power, but it remains unexerted. A change in image is coming. Nurses outnumber all other health care providers and are as well educated as most. They have enhanced the health care system throughout all its struggles. Nurses need to improve their individual and collective self-concept. They must assist each other in achieving the highest level of maturity, education, public service, and professionalism possible. Again, the focus should be on construction and growth.

Nurses must give each other credit for their accomplishments. Community health as a movement was created by nurses, yet others are ready to take the credit. Many leaders in nursing have received little recognition by nurses themselves. People in other fields who have done less and even borrowed heavily from nursing's ideas and practices have received tremendous recognition because they sell their accomplishments and have their colleagues' respect. Nurses must learn to support and assist one another.

Policy research has shown that economic resources continue to be the major determinant of public policy although the attitudes of political leaders appear to be increasingly important (Dye, 1978, p. 31). The fact that the bulk of federal law presently originates in the executive branch of the government supports this conclusion. A great deal of emphasis has been placed on pluralistic political variables such as voter participation, party competition, and majority party control.

A greater financial base for promoting nursing will have to be established. Remarkably, while nurses willingly give their services and energy, they hesitate to share their money. As with any investment, nurses must first put money into the investment before expecting any returns. Also, it must be recognized there is an inherent risk to be taken before any short-term or, more realistically, long-term gains can be expected. That is, gains for clients and for the profession as a whole because of nursing's present stage of political development. Once the profession assumes the authority, autonomy, and recognition it deserves, individual nurses will have the economic freedom to achieve their personal goals.

Individual Guidelines for Political Involvement

Three major goals should be accomplished by the nurse as an individual in the political arena. They are generating support, creating legitimacy, and resolving conflicts (Monsama, 1979; Archer & Goehner, 1982). These goals are fulfilled when you, as the community health nurse, follow certain guidelines.

GENERATING SUPPORT

1. Present yourself well by promoting a positive and professional image. Dress and act accordingly.
2. Communicate your ideas effectively. Be knowledgeable, prepared, and state your position well. Use clear, concise, and understandable terms.
3. Learn the importance of socialization skills. Being a legislator is a 24-hour a day position. Invite a legislator to a social event at which a subject can be discussed in a relaxed manner.

599

4. Get yourself known. Network both within and outside the profession.
5. Recognize your skills to initiate, organize, and participate as well as use nursing process skills. Apply these skills to the political process.
6. Know your representatives at the local, state, and federal levels. Know allies in legislation. Keep in touch with them and keep them informed of health issues and their potential impact.
7. Make a concerted effort to influence a legislator to take a particular position on prospective legislation. Become involved in lobbying, writing, and presenting testimony when legislators hold hearings on prospective legislation.
8. Support a candidate's campaign by donating money or by volunteering time and energy. Campaign for candidates who support nursing and community health provided the rest of their political platform is agreeable.
9. Join a political action committee (PAC). PACs are formed to permit a group to endorse candidates who will support the group's position on issues and to make monetary contributions to these candidates' campaigns.

CREATING LEGITIMACY

1. Keep abreast of current issues in health care and nursing. Share your information with your colleagues.
2. Register to vote. Encourage others to do so. Hold a voters' registration drive. Be sure to vote and communicate with legislators when a health issue surfaces.
3. Belong and become involved in nursing's professional organizations, such as the American Nurses Association and the National League for Nursing, and outside professional organizations, such as the American Public Health Association and the American Hospital Association.
4. Become involved on committees and boards within your agency and community, such as boards of directors, state boards of registered nursing, health planning boards and committees, city planning boards, and the League of Women Voters.
5. Run for office. Start by running for an office at the local level, or, if you are known in your community, consider state or national office. Nurses need representation from nurses in the governmental system at all levels.
6. Become knowledgeable of the political process. Become familiar with committees handling health care legislation.

RESOLVING CONFLICT

1. Plan your strategies well. Be able and willing to negotiate and compromise, or you may lose the entire battle. However, do not sell out your profession to meet the goals of other professions.
2. Be proactive rather than reactive on health issues whenever possible. It

gives you time to anticipate, accumulate resources, and more freedom to negotiate — all for better control.

3. Communicate with tact and respect. Each person has a right to his own beliefs. Avoid insults and overly aggressive behavior. Balance cooperation, collaboration, strength, and assertiveness.

4. Put politics into perspective. Every political position has pros and cons. Weigh each carefully and avoid tunnel vision.

Communicating with Public Officials

One form of political participation is communicating with legislators. The purpose of this contact is to sway the public official's views toward or against a specific bill or political position. The nurse can influence a legislator's opinion by means of oral and written communication through telephone calls, personal visit, telegrams, mailgrams, and letters. To be effective as a private citizen or as a member of a group, the nurse needs to know the process and appropriateness of each type of communication.

Legislators are more likely to be influenced by letters that express personal opinion and provide useful data than by form letters or mass telegrams. Form communications are tallied by a secretary or administrative assistant, but personal communication often reaches legislators directly. A considerable amount of data convincingly presented is necessary to change a legislator's opinion.

Effective communication persuades with facts, logic, and brevity. It requires the nurse to be well prepared. In writing a public official, the following points should be considered:

1. A neat, clear handwritten letter is acceptable, although a typewritten letter is preferable. Always address the letter appropriately with name and address on the letter and envelope.

President | The President
The White House
Washington, D.C. 20500

My dear Mr. President:
Most respectfully yours,

U.S. Senator | The Honorable Terry Miller
Senate Office Building
Washington, D.C. 20510

My dear Senator Miller:
Yours very truly,

U.S. Congressperson | The Honorable Terry Miller
House Office Building
Washington, D.C. 20515

	My dear Mr. or Ms. Miller: Yours very truly,
Governor	The Governor State Capitol City, State Zip
	Dear Governor: Respectfully yours,
Mayor or City Councilperson	Mayor Terry Miller (or) Councilperson Terry Miller City Hall City, State Zip
	Dear Mayor Miller: (or) Dear Mr. or Ms. Miller: Yours very truly,

2. When a bill is in committee, correspond with all members of the committee. The content of the letter may be the same but each letter should be individually typed or handwritten.
3. There are no extra points for length, so plan the wording to make points concisely. The following is a content outline of what is appropriate to include in the correspondence:
   a) One sentence that clearly states the issue
   b) One sentence that clearly states your individual or group position
   c) A statement that delineates the status of the proposed legislation (for example, where it is in the legislative process and what appears to be its disposition)
   d) A list of the reasons to support or oppose the pending legislation
      (1) Financial
      (2) Groups adversely affected
      (3) Weaknesses of opposing view
      (4) Specific benefits that override weaknesses of your view, benefits of the opposing view, or both
   e) Specific data that support these reasons
      (1) Dollar amounts
      (2) Number of groups affected and their names
      (3) Numbers within those groups
      (4) Delineation of processes, systems, equipment, and loopholes that have adverse or positive effects
   f) A clear concise statement of the action that you want the legislator to take on the piece of legislation; meet with you or your organization; ask for additional information; convey contents of letter to interested, influential persons; provide you with those persons' names and titles so that you can contact them, or other similar action.

Personal Visits

An amazing number of bills are enacted with no input from constituents. Lobbyists exert great influence as do other legislative colleagues and persons who use the physical proximity of sitting close to a legislator or the persuasive tactic of trading favors to sway legislator's decisions.

Personal visits by nurses to their legislators can have a profound impact. Many legislators welcome additional expert information and respect the professional commitment involved in making the visit. Because legislators are very busy, with as little as three to five minutes for an interview, the nurse will make the visit more profitable by sending a briefing sheet or letter prior to the meeting. Discussion with a legislator's staff members can also be worthwhile. These individuals do the legislator's background research and help to develop the positions and language contained in the bills. Staff members are often more knowledgeable about the issues and have more time to discuss them.

Community health nurses, as advocates for a health issue, must know the opposition's arguments and be prepared to counter them. The prepared nurse will communicate far more effectively with the legislator and his or her staff.

Attending Hearings

Community health nurses attending a legislative hearing can have considerable impact on a pending bill or proposed regulation. Singly or as an organized group, the nurses' physical presence communicates to legislators that they are concerned, informed, and ready to take action. Again, nurses need to be prepared in advance of the hearing. Resources, such as a government relations committee or the state nurses' association, can provide useful information on the issues surrounding the bill. Other existing communication networks, such as nurses involved in political action committees, can provide additional information.

Providing Testimony

Once a community health nurse is versed in the particular topic of a bill, he or she may want to provide testimony (Figure 21-4). Testimony may be verbal at the time of a hearing or it may be written in advance. What should be included in it differs little from what should be included in a letter, with the exception of supportive materials, such as actual research or survey data.

Party has significant impact on the conduct of legislative business. Legislators have a party or partisan affiliation, and the numbers of any given party in one of the houses make a considerable difference in the conducting of business. At times votes follow party lines and platforms rather than respond

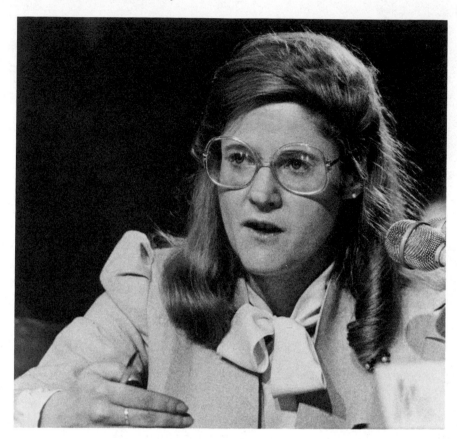

Figure 21-4
Advanced preparation enables the nurse to communicate clearly and convincingly as this nurse does while testifying before a legislative committee.

to the information provided at the hearing or through letters. For this reason an organized lobbying group can be one helpful means to facilitate change.

All the standing committees of the legislature use the hearing process to discuss bills. During a hearing, amendments are introduced and discussed, and it is the hearing process that government agencies use to discuss proposed regulations. Legislative protocol favors the bill's author and the committee chairperson. They have more rights and privileges for the conduct of business.

If you as a community health nurse are in support of a bill and wish to testify, contact the author. If you are opposed to a bill and wish to testify, notify the author and the chairperson. Organized groups with registered lobbyists are most familiar with the process and may provide the best entrée to providing testimony. Remember, votes are counted by the author before a committee meets, and if the number is not sufficient for a due pass, there are many ways to keep from taking an official vote.

604

Resources

The following is a brief compilation of resources covering some major facets of the policy studies area. There is no pretense that it is comprehensive. The chief objective is to provide directions in which political contacts and knowledge can be developed by the community health nurse.

A full-time clearinghouse with an extensive full-time staff would be required to review all the government publications in circulation. The nurse has to focus her reading and depend upon professional and political organizations and current nursing literature for guidance. The office of the *Federal Register* is responsible for the publication of laws, presidential documents, and the *United States Government Organization Manual*. Each act of Congress and public laws are accumulated for each congressional session in the *United States Statutes at Large*. Five times each week the *Federal Register* lists the regulations of government agencies, notices, executive orders, and presidential proclamations having general applicability and legal effect at the time. The annually updated *Code of Federal Regulations* lists all government regulations currently in effect. Presidential materials such as speeches and messages are available in the *Weekly Compilation of Presidential Documents*. Both the U.S. Senate and the U.S. House of Representatives keep a journal of their proceedings, but neither includes debates. The *Congressional Record* contains a complete record of everything said on the floor of both houses. It is printed bimonthly by the U.S. Government Printing Office and available by writing the Superintendent of Documents, U.S. Government Printing Office, Washington, D.C. 20402. Health statistics may be obtained from the National Center for Health Statistics, Hyattsville, Maryland 20872.

Just as there is an overwhelming number of federal publications, there is an overwhelming number of national, state, and local organizations. The *Encyclopedia of Associations*, published annually, is a comprehensive source of detailed information concerning nonprofit American organizations. The inclusion of for-profit groups in the list suggests that they are voluntary or not primarily for the purpose of profit generation. Citizen action groups, projects, and programs are also included. It is available in libraries and through the Gale Research Company in Detroit, Michigan.

Organizations politically significant to community health nurses are numerous. A listing of some of them at the national level is included at the end of this chapter.

The very diversity of policy articles requires a variety of journals. There are currently several publications that include articles and research directly related to health and health care from a policy analysis perspective. In the United States, the oldest of these journals is probably *Public Policy*. It offers detailed, theory-based case studies. Some other journals are *Policy Sciences, Policy Studies Journal,* and *Policy Analysis*.

An excellent resource specifically for nursing is the American Nurses Association Government Relations Division, that publishes *From the Washington Office*. This bulletin overviews federal policy and laws, the voting records of legislators, and the action needed for nursing at the national level. The address of the division is 1030 15th Street, NW, Washington, D.C. 20005.

Conclusion

It is logical to anticipate that the remainder of the 1980s will be characterized by increasing regulations regarding the costs, quantity, and quality of health care (American Nurses Association, 1980). Hence, the community health nurse must set forth an analysis framework that realistically assesses the capacity of a policy system to formulate, define, and implement health laws. The economic structure of a policy system or a community is integral to understanding its limits. More essential, the economic structure reveals what motivates the policy system. Although the nurse knows a well-planned community program based on disease prevention and health promotion is more cost-effective than a disease treatment program, many policymakers do not.

A community's health is strongly affected by many forces outside it. Funding limitations and reimbursement policies from third-party payers often dictate how nurses spend their time. Now diagnosis-related groupings are undergoing rapid growth as a significant financial base of health care agencies. The home health care boom has forced public health agencies to compete with private institutions. Social security benefits have been cut off to many recipients. A nurse's evaluation of a law or policy in relation to a community should identify these external forces and their impact on the population.

The role of government in the organization, provision, and subsidization of health care has evolved from that of a protector of public health and provider of limited services to the role of being the policy setter and major underwriter of the entire health care system. The nurse must be political because, as Litman and Robins (1984, p. 16) point out, he who pays the piper calls the tune.

Both nurses and communities have a common goal, and that is the best possible health care for all. Nurses and communities can formulate, implement, and evaluate health policies to achieve this goal. Nurses cannot solve problems by blaming others nor wait passively for others to solve a community's health problems. Communities are learning what they want at the same time that they are learning how to get it.

Understanding the policy process requires an integration of the findings and insights of many disparate studies into a reasonably comprehensive and verifiable framework. This framework should serve as a guide for future research and lead to a theory of policy process for nursing practice. The research information will make health policy formulation and implementation more cost-effective and community oriented.

Summary

Community health nurses need to understand and become involved in the development of health policy and in the political process to protect the public's health. Furthermore, nurses need to exercise decision-making power in the political arena to enhance their own professional image and practice.

Social policy is what an institution, organization, agency, or government chooses to do or not to do. It may be written or unwritten. Health policy refers to the choices made regarding distribution of resources — people, facilities, time, and money — to health care. Policies ideally reflect the collective interests and beliefs of the group affected by them. However, in many instances a few individuals determine policy for the rest of the group. If community health nurses are to fulfill their mission of promoting, protecting, and preserving the health of aggregates, they must become policy makers as well as policy implementers.

Political systems, such as city government, generate policies and thus are policy systems. To determine the intentions of political systems, the nurse needs a framework for objective policy analysis, in contrast to the subjective activity of policy advocacy. One such framework for studying health policy involves analyzing the four stages of the policy process. Policy formulation includes identifying goals, problems, and potential solutions. Policy adoption refers to authorizing the selection and specification of the means to achieve the goals, resolving the problems, or both. Policy implementation is putting the policy to use. Policy evaluation means comparing policy outcomes with intended effects.

Legislation and policy related to community health must be analyzed from an aggregate perspective. Therefore, the community health nurse benefits from being able to diagnose the community and from assuming an active role in community organization. Steps in community organization for political action include: (1) identify self as a community organizer, (2) identify problems, (3) assess the physical community, (4) assess community resources and interests, (5) assess community politics, (6) evaluate alternative actions, (7) redefine objectives and priorities, (8) develop a plan, (9) implement the plan, and (10) evaluate the outcomes.

Community health policies are guidelines for implementing health laws. As such, they are subject to interpretation and change. Community health nurses can influence the development of policies as well as laws by learning about the legislative process and becoming appropriately involved.

A bill becomes law by going through various stages at any of which nurses can have input. These stages are governed by rules at all levels of government. Each bill undergoes a prescribed series of reviews before passage or rejection. Information about the process and the content of bills is available to the nurse from several sources.

A political strategy available to community health nurses is to define and market nursing to the public and to legislators. Prerequisite to this is nursing's need to be internally supportive and reinforcing (in every way, including financially) in order to present a strong, unified front and have an impact on the health care system.

The politically involved nurse aims to accomplish the three goals of generating support, creating legitimacy, and resolving conflicts. The nurse can influence legislation by oral or written communication with public officials, by personally visiting legislators, by attending hearings, and by providing testimony.

Many resources exist to assist the nurse with political contacts and information. Community health nurses must recognize societal changes and their potential impact on community health, and become active in the political process.

Study Questions

Select one bill related to health currently (or recently) under consideration by your state legislature.

1. Describe it and the issues involved in it.
2. Who is sponsoring it and why?
3. Who is opposing it and why?
4. Who will it affect, if passed, and in what ways will it affect them?
5. Discuss what you, as a community health nurse, could do to be involved in this bill.
6. Write a letter to your legislator regarding this bill (or some other health issue of concern to you).

References

American Nurses Association. (1980). *Nursing: A social policy statement* (ANA Pub. NP-63 35M). Kansas City, MO: Author.

Archer, S. E., & Goehner, P. A. (1982). *Nurses: A political force.* Monterey, CA: Wadsworth Health Sciences Division.

Donley, R. (1982). Nursing and the politics of health. In N. L. Chaska (Ed.), *The nursing profession: A time to speak* (pp.884–857). New York: McGraw-Hill.

Dye, T. R. (1978). *Policy analysis: What governments do, why they do it, and what difference it makes.* Tuscaloosa, AL: University of Alabama.

Kalisch, B. J., & Kalisch, P. A. (1982). *Politics of nursing.* Philadelphia: J. B. Lippincott.

Lee, P. R., Estes, C. L., & Ramsey, N. (1984). *The nation's health* (2nd ed.). San Francisco: Boyd & Fraser.

Litman, T. J., & Robins, L. S. (1984). *Health politics and policy.* New York; Wiley.

Monsama, S. V. (1979). *American politics: A systems approach.* New York: Holt, Rinehart and Winston.

U.S. House of Representatives. (1981). *Our American government: What is it? How does it function? 150 questions and answers* (House Document No. 96-351). Washington, DC: U.S. Government Printing Office.

Selected Readings

Aiken, L. H. (Ed.). (1982). *Nursing in the 1980's: Crises, opportunities, challenges.* Philadelphia: J. B. Lippincott.

American Nurses Association. (1980). *Nursing: A social policy statement.* (ANA Pub. NP-63 35M). Kansas City, MO: Author.

Archer, S. E., & Goehner, P. A. (1982). *Nurses: A political force.* Monterey, CA: Wadsworth Health Sciences Division.

Bagwell, M. (1980). Motivating nurses to be politically aware. *Nursing Leadership, 3*(4), 4–6.

Baker, N. and Hart, C. (1981). Nurses in action. *Nursing and Health Care, 2*(3), 130–132.

Berg, M., Taylor, B., Edwards, L., & Hakanson, E. Y. (1979). Prenatal care for pregnant adolescents in a public high school. *Journal of School Health, 49*(1), 32–35.

Binder, J. (1983). Toward a policy perspective for nursing. *Nursing Economics, 1*(1), 47–50.

Braden, C. J., & Hervan, N. L. (1976). *Community health: A systems approach.* New York: Appleton-Century-Crofts.

Davis, A. J., & Aroskar, M. A. (1978). *Ethical dilemmas and nursing practice.* New York: Appleton-Century-Crofts.

de Kieffer, D. (1981). *How to lobby Congress.* New York: Dodd, Mead.

Donley, R. (1982). Nursing and the politics of health. In N. L. Chaska (Ed.), *The nursing profession: A time to speak* (pp. 844–857). New York: McGraw-Hill.

Dye, T. R. (1978). *Policy analysis: What governments do, why they do it, and what difference it makes.* Tuscaloosa, AL: University of Alabama.

Ellis, J. R., & Hartley, C. L. 1984. *Nursing in today's world: Challenges, issues, and trends.* Philadelphia: J. B. Lippincott.

Fisher, F. (Ed.). (1980). *Politics, values, and public policy: The problem of methodology.* Boulder, CO: Westview Press.

Goodwin, R. (1982). *Political theory and public policy.* Chicago: The University of Chicago Press.

Hambrick, R., Jr. (1980). A guide for the analysis of policy arguments. In F. Fisher (Ed.), *Politics, values, and public policy: The problem of methodology.* Boulder, CO: Westview Press.

Hein, E. C., & Nicholson, M. J. (1982). *Contemporary leadership behavior: Selected readings.* Boston: Little, Brown.

Jenkins, W. I. (1978). *Policy analysis: A political and organizational perspective.* New York: St. Martin's Press.

Kalish, B. J., & Kalisch, P. A. (1982). *Politics of nursing.* Philadelphia: J. B. Lippincott.

Lee, P. R., Estes, C. L., & Ramsey, N. B. (1984). *The nation's health.* San Francisco: Boyd & Fraser.

Levine, M. (1981). Conditions contributing to effective implementation and their limits. In J. Crecine (Ed.), *Research in public policy analysis and management.* Greenwich, CT: Jai Press.

Litman, T. J., & Robins, L. S. (1984). *Health politics and policy.* New York: Wiley.

McLaughlin, M. (1976). Implementation as mutual adaptation. In W. Williams & R. Elmore (Eds.), *Social program implementation* (pp. 167–180). New York: Academic Press.

Moore, E., & Oakley, D. (1983). Nurses, political participation, and attitudes toward reforms in the health care system. *Nursing and Health Care, 4*(9), 504–506.

Monsama, S. V. (1979). *American politics: A systems approach.* New York: Holt, Rinehart & Winston.

Nakamura, R., & Smallwood, F. (1980). *The politics of policy implementation.* New York: St. Martin's Press.

National League for Nursing. (1979). *The emergence of nursing as a political force* (NLN Pub. No. 41-1760). New York: Author.

National League for Nursing. (1982). Political action committees (PAC's). *Public Policy Bulletin, 1*(4).

National League for Nursing. (1982). Reimbursement for nurses in the primary care arena: A cost savings for health care. *Public Policy Bulletin, 1*(5).

Raven, B. H., & Haley, R. W. (1980). Social influence in a medical context. *Policy Studies Review Annual, 4,* pp. 626–648.

Sabatier, P., & Mazmanian, D. (1980). The implementation of public policy: A framework for analysis. *Policy Studies Review Annual, 4,* 181–203.

Sabatier, P., & Mazmanian, D. (1981). *Effective policy implementation.* Lexington, MA: Lexington Books.

Somers, A. R. (1983). Competition or regulation — or both. *CHA Insight, 7*(19).

Somers, A. R. (1983). New marching order for health care. *CHA Insight, 7*(18).

Stevens, K. R. (Ed.). (1983). *Power & influence: A source book for nurses.* New York: Wiley.

Thompson, T. (1980). An ordinal evaluation of the consumer participation process in community health programs. *Nursing Research, 29,* 50–54.

U.S. House of Representatives. (1978). *Adolescent Health, Service, and Pregnancy Prevention Act of 1978* (House of Representatives Report 12146). Washington, DC: U.S. Government Printing Office.

U.S. House of Representatives. (1981). *How our laws are made* (House Document No. 97-120). Washington, DC: U.S. Government Printing Office, 1981.

U.S. House of Representatives. (1981). *Our American government: What is it? How does it function? 150 questions and answers* (House Document No. 96-351). Washington, DC: U.S. Government Printing Office.

Van Meter, D., & Van Horn, C. 1975. The policy implementation process: A conceptual framework. *Administration and Society, 6*(4), 85–89.

Williams, F. C. & Williams, C. A. (1972). Ethical issues in health care policy. In Miller & Flynn (Eds.), *Current perspectives in nursing,* pp. 121–132. St. Louis: C. V. Mosby.

Williams, C. A. (1983). Making things happen: Community health nursing and the policy arena. *Nursing Outlook, 31,* pp. 225–228.

Zaretsky, H. W. (1983). Planning for competition. *CHA Insight, 7*(10), Special issue.

American Academy of Nurses
c/o American Nurses Association
2420 Pershing Road
Kansas City, MO 64108

American Association of Nursing Service Administrators
840 North Lake Shore Drive
Chicago, IL 60611

American Association of Occupational Health Nurses
3500 Piedmont
Suite 400
Atlanta, GA 30305
Publications include *AAOH Newsletter* and *Occupational Health Nursing*

American Civil Liberties Union
132 W. 43rd Street
New York, NY 10036
Publications include the newsletter *Civil Liberties Alert*

American College of Nurse Midwives
1522 K Street, NW
Suite 1120
Washington, DC 20005
Publications include *Journal of Nurse Wifery* and the newsletter *Quickening*

American Indian Nurses Association
P.O. Box 1588
Norman, OK 73071
Publications include the *Newsletter of the AINA*

American Nurses Association
2420 Pershing Road
Kansas City, MO 64108
Publications include the *American Journal of Nursing* and *The American Nurse*

American Public Health Association
1015 15th Street, NW
Washington, DC 20005
Publications include the *American Journal of Public Health*, *The Nation's Health*, and *Washington Newsletter*

Association of Rehabilitation Nurses
2506 Gross Point Road
Evanston, IL 60201
Publications include *Rehabilitation Nurses*

Association of State Democratic Chairs
1625 Massachusetts Avenue, NW
Washington, DC 20036

Chamber of Commerce of the United States
Public Affairs Department
1615 H Street, NW
Washington, DC 20006
Publications include *Elections Guide* and *They Grade the Congress*

International Council of Nurses
Box 42
1211 Geneva, Switzerland

League of Women Voters
1730 M Street, NW
Washington, DC 20005

National Association of Hispanic Nurses
12400 7th Avenue, NW
Seattle, WA 98177

National Association of School Nurses
7395 South Kramer Street
Englewood, CO 80112
Publications include *School Nurse*

National Black Nurses Association, Inc.
P.O. Box 1835B
Boston, MA 02118

National League for Nursing
10 Columbus Circle
New York, NY 10019
More significant policy publications include *Public Policy Bulletin* and *Nursing Health Care*

National Organization for Women
425 13th Street, NW
Suite 1048
Washington, DC 20004

National Student Nurse Association
10 Columbus Circle
New York, NY 10019
Publications include *Imprint*

National Women's Political Caucus
1411 15th Street, NW
Suite 1110
Washington, DC 20005
Publications include *Women's Political Times*

Nurses' Coalition for Action in Politics
1030 15th Street, NW
Suite 408
Washington, DC 20005

Public Citizen
P.O. Box 19404
Washington, DC 20036

Republican National Committee
310 First Street, SE
Washington, DC 20003

Some organizations politically significant to community health nurses.

(*continued from p. iv*)

Table 15–3: Adapted from E. Duval, *Family Development,* 5th edition, 1977. Reprinted by permission of Lippincott Publishing Company.

Tables 15–4 and 15–5: From *The Family Life Cycle,* edited by Elizabeth A. Carter and Monica McGoldrick. Copyright © 1980 by Gardner Press, Inc., New York. Reprinted by permission of the publisher.

Figures 16–5 and 16–6: Adapted from Holman, *Family Assessment* (1983), pp. 64–65 and p. 71. Reprinted by permission of Sage Publications, Inc.

Figure 20–3: Adapted from P. Hersey and K. Blanchard, *Management of Organizational Behavior: Utilizing Human Resources,* 3rd Edition (1977). Reprinted by permission of Prentice-Hall Publishing Company.

PHOTO CREDITS

Figure 1–4: Photograph by Dirck Halstead for *Time* © 1978, Time, Inc. *Figure 1–7*: From M. Blackwell, *Care of the Mentally Retarded.* Boston: Little, Brown, 1979. *Figure 2–1*: Paul Conklin. *Figure 2–6*: WHO Photo. *Figure 2–7*: Courtesy of the Harvard Community Health Plan, Boston. *Figure 3–1*: Courtesy of the Visiting Nurses' Association, Boston Collection. *Figure 3–2*: Courtesy of the Visiting Nurses' Association, Boston Collection. *Figure 3–4*: Courtesy of the American Red Cross. *Figure 4–1*: From M. Blackwell, *Care of the Mentally Retarded.* Boston: Little, Brown, 1979. *Figure 4–2*: From M. Blackwell, *Care of the Mentally Retarded.* Boston: Little, Brown, 1979. *Figure 4–3*: Courtesy of the Harvard Community Health Plan, Boston. *Figure 5–1*: David Conklin. *Figure 5–3*: Edward Slaman. *Figure 6–2*: The Picture Cube/Carol Palmer. *Figure 6–3*: Courtesy of the *Mt. Vernon News.* *Figure 6–4*: Photograph by Burk Uzzle, Magnum. *Figure 6–5*: Photograph by Michael O'Brien. © 1976 Time, Inc. *Figure 6–6*: Photograph by John Dominis for *Life* © 1961, Time, Inc. *Figure 6–7*: Mimi Forsyth/ Monkmeyer Press Photo Service. *Figure 7–2*: Courtesy of the *Mt. Vernon News.* *Figure 7–5*: Courtesy of Beth Israel Hospital, Boston. *Figure 8–1*: Edward Slaman. *Figure 8–4*: Jamie Cope. *Figure 9–1*: Paul Conklin. *Figure 9–2*: Courtesy of Beth Israel Hospital, Boston. Photograph by Michael Lutch. *Figure 9–4*: Courtesy of Beth Israel Hospital, Boston. *Figure 9–5*: Courtesy of the *Mt. Vernon News. Figures 10–1 and 10–2*: Courtesy of the Harvard Community Health Plan, Boston. *Figure 11–1*: From C. Schuster and S. Ashburn, *The Process of Human Development: A Holistic Approach.* Boston: Little, Brown, 1980. Photograph by Glenn Jackson. *Figure 11–2*: Courtesy of Lake Charles Louisiana Press. *Figure 11–3*: Courtesy of Beth Israel Hospital, Boston. Photograph by Michael Lutch. *Figure 12–1*: Courtesy of the *Mt. Vernon News. Figure 12–2*: Ted Carland/American Red Cross. *Figure 12–3*: Paul Conklin. *Figure 12–5*: Courtesy of the *Mt. Vernon News. Figure 13–2*: Photograph by Robert Isaacs for *Time.* © 1969 Time, Inc. *Figure 13–3*: Photograph by Kevin Byron for *Time.* © 1979 Time, Inc. *Figure 13–6*: Courtesy of the *Mt. Vernon News. Figure 14–1*: Andrew Brilliant/Carol Palmer. *Figure 14–2*: Paul Conklin. *Figure 14–3*: Paul Conklin. *Figure 14–4*: Andrew Brilliant/Carol Palmer. *Figure 14–5*: Edward Slaman. *Figure 14–6*: Courtesy of La Esperanza Developmental Center, San Mateo, CA. *Figure 15–1*: From C. Schuster and S. Ashburn, *The Process of Human Development: A Holistic Approach.* Boston: Little, Brown, 1980. Photograph by Glenn Jackson. *Figure 15–2*: Michael O'Brien/Archive. *Figure 15–3*: Photograph by Jeffrey Manditch-Prottas. *Figures 15–4 and 15–5*: Edward Slaman. *Figure 15–6*: From C. Schuster and S. Ashburn, *The Process of Human Development: A Holistic Approach.* Boston: Little, Brown, 1980. Photograph by Glenn Jackson. *Figure 16–1*: Courtesy of the *Mt. Vernon News. Figure 16–2*: Paul Conklin. *Figure 16–3*: Photograph by John Neubauer for *People.* © 1979 Time, Inc. *Figure 16–4*: Courtesy of the Harvard Community Health Plan, Boston. *Figure 17–1*: Photograph by Marilee Caliendo. *Figure 17–2*: Michael O'Brien/Archive. *Figure 17–3*: Photograph by Denny Lorentzen from *Newsletter,* National Swedish Board of Occupational Safety and Health, January, 1981. *Figure 17–4*: Courtesy of the Harvard Community Health Plan, Boston. *Figure 18–1*: Paul Conklin. *Figure 18–2*: Photograph by David Franklin. © 1979 Time, Inc. *Figures 18–3 and 18–4*: Paul Conklin. *Figure 18–5*: Jean Liftin/Archive. *Figure 19–1*: Dave Schaefer. *Figures 19–2, 19–3, and 19–5*: Paul Conklin. *Figure 20–2*: Courtesy of Beth Israel Hospital, Boston. *Figure 20–6*: David Conklin. *Figure 21–2*: Courtesy of the Harvard Community Health Plan, Boston. *Figure 21–4*: Copyright 1983 *The American Nurse.*

Index